Studies in Computational Intelligence

Volume 1016

The series "Studies in Computational Intelligence" (SCI) publishes new developments and advances in the various areas of computational intelligence—quickly and with a high quality. The intent is to cover the theory, applications, and design methods of computational intelligence, as embedded in the fields of engineering, computer science, physics and life sciences, as well as the methodologies behind them. The series contains monographs, lecture notes and edited volumes in computational intelligence spanning the areas of neural networks, connectionist systems, genetic algorithms, evolutionary computation, artificial intelligence, cellular automata, self-organizing systems, soft computing, fuzzy systems, and hybrid intelligent systems. Of particular value to both the contributors and the readership are the short publication timeframe and the world-wide distribution, which enable both wide and rapid dissemination of research output.

Indexed by SCOPUS, DBLP, WTI Frankfurt eG, zbMATH, SCImago.

All books published in the series are submitted for consideration in Web of Science.

More information about this series at https://link.springer.com/bookseries/7092

Khalid Raza
Editor

Computational Intelligence in Oncology

Applications in Diagnosis, Prognosis and Therapeutics of Cancers

Springer

Editor
Khalid Raza
Department of Computer Science
Jamia Millia Islamia
New Delhi, India

ISSN 1860-949X ISSN 1860-9503 (electronic)
Studies in Computational Intelligence
ISBN 978-981-16-9220-8 ISBN 978-981-16-9221-5 (eBook)
https://doi.org/10.1007/978-981-16-9221-5

This Springer imprint is published by the registered company Springer Nature Singapore Pte Ltd.
The registered company address is: 152 Beach Road, #21-01/04 Gateway East, Singapore 189721, Singapore

This volume is dedicated to my parents (Late Abdul Jabbar Qauis and Late Zulekha Khatoon), my beloved wife (Farhat), and my son (Arham).

Preface

Cancer has been known as a heterogeneous disease categorized into several different subtypes. According to WHO's recent report, cancer is a leading cause of death worldwide, accounting for over 10 million deaths in the year 2020. Therefore, its early diagnosis, prognosis, and classification to a subtype have become necessary as it facilitates the subsequent clinical management and therapeutics plan. Computational intelligence methods, including artificial neural networks (ANNs), fuzzy logic, evolutionary computations, various machine learning and deep learning, and nature-inspired algorithms, have been widely utilized in various aspects of oncology research, viz. diagnosis, prognosis, therapeutics, and optimized clinical management.

Appreciable progress has been made toward understanding the hallmarks of cancer development, progression, and its effective therapeutics. However, notwithstanding the extrinsic and intrinsic factors which lead to drastic increment in incidence cases, the detection, diagnosis, prognosis, and therapeutics remain an apex challenge for the medical fraternity. With the advent of computational intelligence-based approaches, including nature-inspired techniques, and the availability of clinical data from various high-throughput experiments, medical consultants, researchers, and oncologists have seen a hope to devise and employ computational intelligence methods in various aspects of oncology. The main aim of the book is to occupy state-of-the-art applications of computational intelligence methods that have been derived from core computer sciences to back medical oncology.

New Delhi, India — Kalid Raza

Acknowledgments The editor and contributors are thankful to all the anonymous reviewers for their valuable expert comments and suggestions on the chapters. Thanks go to the series editor, editors, publication and production manager, and other editorial staff of Springer Nature for their overwhelming support during the production of this book. Special thanks go to Ms. Sahar Qazi (DST-Inspire Fellow, Department of Computer Science, Jamia Millia Islamia) for her consistent and overwhelming support.

About This Book

This volume of the book encapsulates the recent applications of computational intelligence methods in the field of computational oncology, especially cancer diagnosis, prognosis, and its optimized therapeutics. It covers artificial neural networks, fuzzy logic and fuzzy inference systems, various nature-inspired algorithms, and hybrid intelligent systems which are widely appreciated for the diagnosis, prognosis, and optimization of therapeutics of various cancers. Besides, this volume also covers multi-omics exploration, gene expression analysis, gene signature identification of cancers, genomic characterization of tumors, anticancer drug design and discovery, drug response prediction through computational intelligence, and applications of blockchain technology in cancer research. This edited volume has 25 chapters which are divided into four parts.

The first part contains four introductory chapters that cover the present, past, and future of oncology, computational oncology; state-of-the-art computational intelligence methods that are used for the diagnosis, prognosis, and therapeutics of different cancers; computational intelligent toward translational healthcare; and comprehensive analysis of various computational resources available for oncology research.

The second part comprises eight chapters that cover applications of computational intelligence in cancer diagnosis, detection, survival prediction, breast cancer survival prediction, brain tumor classification, cancer recurrence prediction, detection of malignant or premalignant oral lesions, and fuzzy logic-based hybrid models for clinical decision support systems in cancers.

The third part is a collection of nine chapters that demonstrate the application of computational intelligence methods in biomarkers and therapeutics targets prediction in cancer; cancer biomarker discoveries; chemoinformatics-based models for cancer therapeutics; gene expression signature prediction and drug discovery in ovarian cancer; early diagnosis of breast cancer using biomarkers and gene expression profiles; exosomes as supramolecular biomarker conduit in cancer; therapeutic role of medicinal phytochemicals in the treatment of cancer; drug response prediction; and incipient role of computational intelligence in anticancer drug design, discovery, and development.

The fourth part has four chapters that attempt to present the role of computational intelligence in gene expression analysis of colorectal cancer; multi-omics approach for cancer diagnosis, prognosis, and therapeutics; cancer susceptibility prediction using SNP data; and application of blockchain technology in cancer research.

The contributing authors of this volume are experts in their fields, and they are from various reputed universities and institutions across the globe. This volume is a valuable and comprehensive resource for computational and medical oncologists, computational biologists, researchers from computer science, computational biology, medical sciences, bioinformatics, medical informatics, health informatics, and data science, along with graduate and research students of bioinformatics, computational biology, and computational & medical oncology.

Contents

Editor and Contributors

About the Editor

Dr. Khalid Raza is Assistant Professor at the Department of Computer Science, Jamia Millia Islamia (Central University), New Delhi. Dr. Raza has also served as "ICCR Chair Professor" at Faculty of Computer and Information Sciences, Ain Shams University, Cairo, Egypt. He has over 10 years of teaching & research experience in the field of computational intelligence and its various applications. He has contributed over 80 research articles in reputed journals and edited books, one single-authored book. Dr. Raza has reviewed over 100 research articles for reputed journals/conferences in the last 5 years. He has also edited three books with different publishers including Springer, Elsevier, and CRC Press. He is Academic Editor of *PeerJ Computer Science*. Dr. Raza has delivered several keynote addresses, invited talks, public lectures, and seminars in national and international conferences and workshops and chaired technical sessions in various national and international conferences. He has also executed two Indian governments funded research projects. Dr. Raza is Member of MIR Lab (USA), CSI (India), and SCRS (India). His research interest lies in computational intelligence and its applications in bioinformatics, viro-informatics, and health informatics.

Contributors

Naeem Ahmad Department of Computer Applications, National Institute of Technology, Raipur, India

Shaban Ahmad Department of Computer Science, Jamia Millia Islamia, New Delhi, India

Sarra Akermi Annotation Analytics Pvt. Ltd., Gurgaon, Haryana, India

Wasim Akram Accenture India, Gurgaon, India

Afroz Alam Department of Computer Application, Integral University, Lucknow, India

Muhammad Mohsin Ali Faisal Institute of Health Sciences Faisalabad, Affiliated with Government College University Faisalabad, Faisalabad, Pakistan

Vivek Anumala Department of Vegetable Science, College of Horticulture and Forestry, Central Agricultural University, Pasighat, Arunachal Pradesh, India

Punuri Jayasekhar Babu Biomaterials and Bioengineering Research Laboratory, Department of Biotechnology, Pachhunga University College, Mizoram University (A Central University), Aizawl, Mizoram, India

Ibrahim Badi Libyan Academy, Misrata, Libya

Rejaul Karim Barbhuiya National Council of Educational Research and Training, New Delhi, India

Anam Beg Department of Computer Science, Jamia Millia Islamia, New Delhi, India

Jean Bernard Insight Biosolutions, Rennes, France

Piyush Bhardwaj Centre for Advanced Computational Solutions (C-fACS), Lincoln University, Lincoln, New Zealand

Ritushree Biswas Annotation Analytics Pvt. Ltd., Biswa, Amarpura, Gurgaon, Haryana, India

Naorem BidyaLeima Chanu Department of Vegetable Science, College of Horticulture and Forestry, Central Agricultural University, Pasighat, Arunachal Pradesh, India

O. S. Dada Computer Science Department, Federal University of Kashere, Gombe, Nigeria

Abira Dey Indian Science and Technology Foundation (ISTF), New Delhi, India

Nancy Emmanuel Division of Research, Hospital das Clinicas, Faculty of Medicine of the University of Sao Paulo, Sao Paulo, Brazil

Muhammad Mazhar Fareed Faculty of Life Sciences, Department of Bioinformatics and Biotechnology, Government College University, Faisalabad, Pakistan

Ahmed Abba Haruna College of Computer Science & Engineering, University of Hafr Al Batin, Al Jamiah, Hafar Al Batin, Saudi Arabia

Yasha Hasija Department of Biotechnology, Delhi Technological University, New Delhi, Delhi, India

Punabati Heisnam Department of Natural Resource Management, College of Horticulture and Forestry, Central Agricultural University, Pasighat, Arunachal Pradesh, India

Naiyar Iqbal Department of Computer Science and IT, Maulana Azad National Urdu University, Hyderabad, India

Abdullahi Isa Department of Mathematical Sciences, Faculty of Science, University of Maiduguri, Maiduguri, Nigeria

Chandramohan Jana Department of Chemistry, Michael Madhusudan Memorial College, Durgapur, West Bengal, India

Sunil Jayant Indian Science and Technology Foundation (ISTF), New Delhi, India; Annotation Analytics Pvt. Ltd., Gurgaon, Haryana, India

Surabhi Johari Institute of Management, Studies University Courses Campus Ghaziabad, Ghaziabad, Uttar Pradesh, India

Ritu Karwasra ICMR-National Institute of Pathology, Safdarjung Hospital Campus, New Delhi, India

Manmeet Kaur Department of Microbiology, Punjab Agricultural University, Ludhiana, India

Arvind Keprate Department of Mechanical, Electronics and Chemical Engineering, Oslo Metropolitan University, Oslo, Norway

Fatima Nazish Khan Department of Education in Science and Mathematics, NCERT, New Delhi, India

Kushagra Khanna Department of Pharmacy, Lloyd Institute of Management and Technology (Pharm), Greater Noida, India

Mritunjay Kr. Ranjan Department of Computer Science, Magadh University, Bodh Gaya, India

Arif Md.Sattar Department of Computer Science, Anugrah Memorial College, Gaya, India

Ainura Mitalipova International Medical Faculty, Osh State University, Osh City, Kyrgyzstan

I. A. Mohammed Department of Computer Science, Yobe State University, Damaturu, Yobe, Nigeria

Azaroual Mouna Tambov State Medical University, Tambov City, Russia

L. J. Muhammad Computer Science Department, Federal University of Kashere, Gombe, Nigeria

Gregory Nicolas Department of Plastic and Reconstructive Surgery, Hospital das Clinicas, Faculty of Medicine of the University of Sao Paulo, Sao Paulo, Brazil

Anshul Nigam Amity University Mumbai, Bhatan Post-Somathne, Panvel, Mumbai, Maharashtra, India

Rina Ningthoujam Department of Vegetable Science, College of Horticulture and Forestry, Central Agricultural University, Pasighat, Arunachal Pradesh, India

Obiadul Ola Maulana Mazharul Haque Arabic and Persian University, Patna, India

Manasa Kumar Panda CSIR—Institute of Minerals and Materials Technology, Bhubaneswar, India

Rishabh Panesar Annotation Analytics Pvt. Ltd., Biswa, Amarpura, Gurgaon, Haryana, India;
Amity University Mumbai, Bhatan Post-Somathne, Panvel, Mumbai, Maharashtra, India

Rafat Parveen Department of Computer Science, Jamia Millia Islamia, New Delhi, India

Srimay Pradhan Department of Botany, School of Applied Sciences, Centurion University of Technology and Management, Bhubaneswar, Odisha, India

Ria Puri Institute of Management, Studies University Courses Campus Ghaziabad, Ghaziabad, Uttar Pradesh, India

Sahar Qazi Department of Computer Science, Jamia Millia Islamia, New Delhi, India

Waaris Qazi Department of Biotechnology, Jamia Millia Islamia, New Delhi, India

Syed Ali Abbas Rahat International Medical Faculty, Osh State University, Osh City, Kyrgyzstan

Sarah I. Rahman School of Biotechnology, Jawaharlal Nehru University, New Delhi, India

Sandhya Rai Department of Biotechnology, Motilal Nehru National Institute of Technology, Allahabad, India

Ayyagari Ramlal Division of Genetics, Indian Agricultural Research Institute (ICAR-IARI), New Delhi, India

Khalid Raza Department of Computer Science, Jamia Millia Islamia, New Delhi, India

Sagarika Sahoo Annotation Analytics Pvt. Ltd., Biswa, Amarpura, Gurgaon, Haryana, India;
Amity University Mumbai, Bhatan Post-Somathne, Panvel, Mumbai, Maharashtra, India

Ankita Sahu Tumor Biology, ICMR-National Institute of Pathology, New Delhi, India

Manjeet Kaur Sangha Department of Biochemistry, Punjab Agricultural University, Ludhiana, India

Shazmeen Shamsi School of Computational and Integrative Sciences, Jawaharlal Nehru University, New Delhi, India

Ashok Sharma Department of Biochemistry, All India Institute of Medical Sciences, New Delhi, India

Kayenat Sheikh Department of Computer Science, Jamia Millia Islamia, New Delhi, India

Mohd Faizan Siddiqui International Medical Faculty, Osh State University, Osh City, Kyrgyzstan

Astha Singh Tumor Biology, ICMR-National Institute of Pathology, New Delhi, India

Manish Pratap Singh Department of Biotechnology, Motilal Nehru National Institute of Technology, Allahabad, India

Surender Singh Department of Pharmacology, All India Institute of Medical Sciences, New Delhi, India

Yengkhom Disco Singh Biomaterials and Bioprocessing Research Laboratory, Department of Post-Harvest Technology, College of Horticulture and Forestry, Central Agricultural University, Pasighat, Arunachal Pradesh, India

Diksha Singla Department of Biochemistry, Punjab Agricultural University, Ludhiana, India

Subrata Sinha Centre for Biotechnology and Bioinformatics, Dibrugarh University, Dibrugarh, Assam, India

H. S. Sodhi Department of Microbiology, Punjab Agricultural University, Ludhiana, India

Mohamed Soudy Bioinformatics Program, Faculty of Computer Science and Information Technology, Ain Shams University, Cairo, Egypt

Ankit Srivastava Department of Biotechnology, Motilal Nehru National Institute of Technology, Allahabad, India

Sameer Srivastava Department of Biotechnology, Motilal Nehru National Institute of Technology, Allahabad, India

Mitali Tarika Institute of Management, Studies University Courses Campus Ghaziabad, Ghaziabad, Uttar Pradesh, India

Nazgul Tashmatova International Medical Faculty, Osh State University, Osh City, Kyrgyzstan

Parul Tiwari Centre for Advanced Computational Solutions (C-fACS), Lincoln University, Lincoln, New Zealand

Ashish Tyagi Department of Forensic Medicine and Toxicology, SHKM Govt. Medical College, Nalhar, Haryana, India

Saurabh Verma Tumor Biology, ICMR-National Institute of Pathology, New Delhi, India

Saanya Yadav Department of Biotechnology, Delhi Technological University, New Delhi, Delhi, India

Malik Yousef Department of Information System, Zefat Academic College, Jerusalem, Israel

Preliminaries

Computational Intelligence in Oncology: Past, Present, and Future

Khalid Raza, Sahar Qazi, Ankita Sahu, and Saurabh Verma

Abstract Computational Intelligence (CI) methods are being widely used in different fields of studies including medical sciences and oncology research. CI methods are applied in different facets of oncology including tumor classification, early prediction and diagnosis, survival prediction, modeling and simulation of cell growth, therapy optimization, and overall cancer management. This chapter aims to present introductory background about the field of Oncology, computational Oncology, roles of CI in various aspects of oncology research including classification, Prediction, risk analysis, therapy, optimized cancer treatment, management, etc. It also describes the current trends and future of CI in oncology research.

Keywords Oncology · Cancer research · Computational oncology · Data science in cancer · Cancer data analysis

1 Introduction

The concept of computational intelligence (CI) revolves around the concept of developing human-like capabilities, rationality, and reasoning in computers that can help humans in making better decisions in complex situations and problems. The term CI is synonymously used with the term soft computing, however, there is still no perfect definition of the same. The term "*computational intelligence*" was coined by the IEEE [4]. To better understand CI, researchers take help from domains such as—biological and linguistic approaches and then deploy them as motivation for problem-solving and optimization. Initially, there were three main subfields of CI,

K. Raza (✉) · S. Qazi
Department of Computer Science, Jamia Millia Islamia, New Delhi, India
e-mail: kraza@jmi.ac.in

S. Qazi
e-mail: rs.sahar1900560@jmi.ac.in

A. Sahu · S. Verma
Tumor Biology, ICMR-National Institute of Pathology, New Delhi, India

K. Raza (ed.), *Computational Intelligence in Oncology*, Studies in Computational Intelligence 1016, https://doi.org/10.1007/978-981-16-9221-5_1

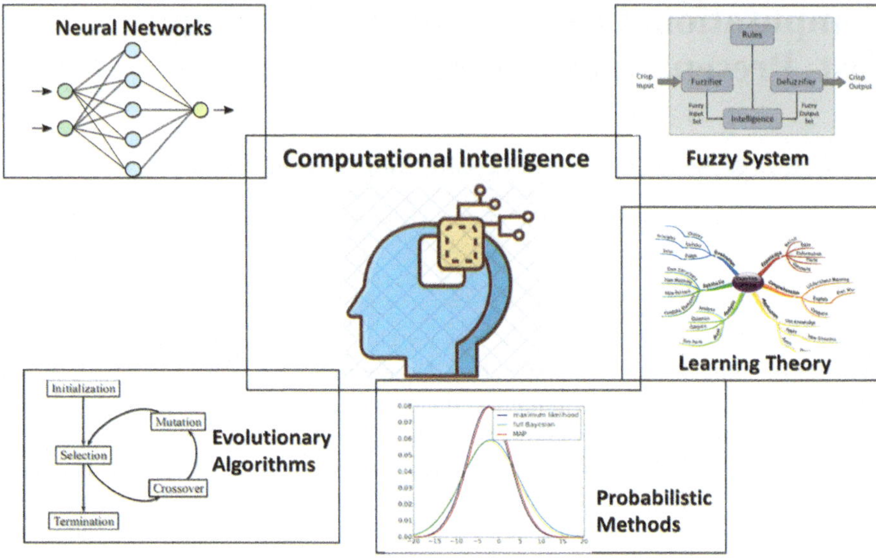

Fig. 1 The five subfields of computational intelligence

namely *fuzzy logic* (FL), *artificial neural networks* (ANNs), and *evolutionary algorithms* (EAs), however, with the advent of CI in almost all fields of science and technology, two new fields have been added, namely—*learning theory* and *probabilistic approaches*, thus, making a total of five important subfields [48]. Figure 1 showcases the five subfields of CI.

1.1 From AI to Computational Intelligence: The Transition

Generally, artificial intelligence (AI) and computational intelligence (CI) seem to go hand in hand, although they intend to achieve the same goal viz., human-like intelligence or *rationality with reasonability*, they are completely different in their approach. Many researchers believe that CI is simply a subset of AI [4].

It is important to cite here that this intelligence is of two kinds—artificial intelligence refers to hard computing, while natural intelligence refers to soft computing based on adaptation to complexities. Hard computation follows the binary logic based on Boolean values [0, 1], while soft computation follows the fuzzy logic where the values are not descriptively finite but fuzzy (that don't necessarily fall into one class of values) in nature. Therefore, AI is where the machines have a restricted learning capacity, whereas, CI allows the machines to "*think-like*" humans and to make their own decisions based on the severity of a situation.

1.2 Motivation: CI in Oncology

CI has significantly contributed to various biomedical problems, including the field of oncology. Over the past decade, CI techniques, such as ANN, fuzzy logic, evolutionary algorithms, deep learning, and nature-inspired techniques, have been substantially used in various aspects of cancer research including *diagnosis*, *prognosis*, and *treatment*. The ability to automatically learn the patterns, handle imprecision, noise, and the optimization capability to concise the solution space make the CI suitable for both basic and clinical cancer research. In other words, CI helps oncologists in developing intelligent systems to aid cancer diagnosis, prognosis, and optimized treatments [38].

This chapter aims to introduce the readers to the basic background of oncology and computational oncology research, and how CI methods are strengthening better diagnosis, prognosis, treatment, and management of cancers.

2 Oncology: Origin, Evolution, Current Status, and Future

2.1 Origin

In the second century AD, the Roman physician of Greek origin Galen (130–200) used the word "Oncology"; which is made up of a combination of two root words [12]. The prefix ὄγκος (*onkos*) means tumor, burden, volume, bulk or mass while suffix λόγος (logos) means "study of". The term oncology literally means a specialized branch of medicine that deals with the prevention, diagnosis, analysis, treatment, and research of tumors or cancer. The oncologic disease is a chronicle of ancient disease and one of the known increased risk health behaviors in a large number of diseases in mankind. The disease was first called cancer by the Greek physician Hippocrates (460–370 BC) who is traditionally known as the father of medicine, describes the several types of cancer including breast, skin, uterus, rectum, and stomach perceived the distinction between benign and malignant tumors. The connection between the lymphatic system and cancer was discovered by the Gaspare Aselli (1581–1625 AD). The French physician Claude Gendron (1663–1750 AD) discovered after eight years of research that cancer arises from severe irritation in the tissues. The founder of the cellular pathogen, Rudolf Virchow (1858 AD) proposed many hypotheses to explain how do cancer cells originally form, how do cancer develops, and progresses in various levels such as morphology, metastatic capacity, and invasion of tissue behavior [19]. In the 19th century, human cancer appeared in ancient Egyptian manuscripts, especially two distinct papyri the Edwin Smith and George Ebers papyri that define the surgical technique [15]. The manuscripts were written between the period 1500 and 1600 BC. Several theories have been formulated, but the most protuberant and accepted mutation theory models are confronted by an increasing amount of experimental data and arguments that could either not be explained by the model, or that contradicted this model. Cancer came in diverse forms including lung, skin, breast, stomach, prostate, colorectal, kidney (renal), bladder, leukaemia, Non-Hodgkin, lymphoma, cervical cancer, and so on. James Watson and Francis Crick (1916–2004 AD) indicated that DNA plays a key role in carcinogens which are strongly linked at the cellular level and understanding the cancer mechanisms.

A book written by Siddhartha Mukherjee's "**The Emperor of All Maladies: A Biography of Cancer**" published on 16th November 2010 defines the various factors that have contributed to the perception of cancer. There are more than 100 types of cancer that can affect nearly every system of the body. It could be indolent, causing little or no pain. The most common global cancers are listed in Table 1. The morbidity and mortality of this disease are notable due to inadequate clinical expertise, lack of appropriate services, and low awareness of the growing population.

Table 1 Origin of the most common types of cancer

Cancer type	Origin	Discovered cancer
Ovarian cancer	A single layer of epithelial cells comprises the ovarian surface epithelium	In 1809 by Jane Todd Crawford
Breast cancer	Epithelial cells of the breast	In 1600 BC by Edwin Smith Papyrus
Lung adenocarcinoma (LUAD)	Fusions of macrophages and neoplastic lung epithelial cells	In 1929 by the German physician, Fritz Lickint first recognized the potential connection between smoking and lung cancer
Skin cancer	The outermost layer (epidermis) of the skin	In early 1800 by French physician Rene Theophile Hyacinthe Laënnec
Bladder cancer	Transitional cells of the bladder mucosal epithelium	In 1895 by Maximilian Nitze, a German urologist
Cervical cancer	Cells lining the cervix which is the lower part of the uterus (womb)	In the 1970s by Harald Zur Hausen detected the human papillomavirus in warts and cervical cancer
Pancreatic cancer	The tissue of the pancreas	In 1761 by Giovanni Battista Morgagni
Prostate cancer	Basal and luminal cells constitute most of the prostate epithelium	In 1853 by J. Adams
Colorectal cancer	Epithelial cells lining the colon or rectum of the gastrointestinal tract	Egyptian and Peruvian mummies dating back to ~1500 BC
Stomach cancer	Mucus membrane lining the stomach (mucus-producing cells)	Ancient Egypt in 1500 BC recorded on papyrus

2.2 Evolution

Cancer is a complex and dynamic system where the cancer-causing cells invade into the nearby area (body's cells grow uncontrollably) and travel to other body parts. The individual factors that influence cancer development also come under the evolutionary process. The continuous evolution of life is prompted by two mechanisms: on the one hand by cellular alterations in biopsies of tumors or genetic changes, likely to be passed to the next generation, and on the other hand by the biological properties of the organisms in a skirmish with their characteristic environment. A precise effective guide for understanding the conceptual model of cancer has been evolutionary theory, which has a throughout history in the treatment and research.

The secret of battling cancer is to find means to uncontrolled mutated cells growth outpaces the growth of single cell in the normal tissue. Malignant growth and normal growth are so genetically intertwined that unbraiding the two might be one of the most significant scientific challenges faced by the species. The genes that unmoor normal cell division contribute to the development of cancer that expands to form a tumor mass from the normal host cells [10].

The key concept of the evolution of cancer is the idea that the environment shapes (phenotypes and the fitness values of phenotypes), leading to a fitness landscape [51]. The cancer evolution theory can be directly understood by sampling precursor lesions or by exploiting the computational methods to deduce the timing of driver events. The somatic/clonal evaluation process suggests that the genetic and epigenetic alteration occur expansion of the cancer cells population in an individual single cell under a changing environment [33, 49]. Tumor initiation and progression are heavily influenced by the drift. The bottleneck effect amplifies the effect of genetic drift which explains the reduces the gene variants with spatial population size represented in Fig. 2 [33].

2.3 Current Status and Future

In 2020, the novel coronavirus disease 2019 (COVID-19) outbreak hampered the global pandemic for the diagnosis and treatment of cancer. The major areas of oncology for diagnosis, treatment, and research are *therapeutic oncology,* which treats cancers using chemotherapy, hormone, and targeted and immunotherapy; *radiation oncology* which is a unique branch in the field of medicinal biology for the use of radiation therapy by damaging their DNA to treat cancer; and *surgical oncology* focuses on surgical methods to diagnose the stage of cancerous or tumor to treat different types of cancer. All things for identifying, diagnosis, and treatment of cancer from the beginning to twentieth centuries considered that the advances in technology and information-based medical research that plays a remarkable contribution to work on oncology, occurred as a result of effective solutions for physicians, surgeons, scientists, and basic researchers.

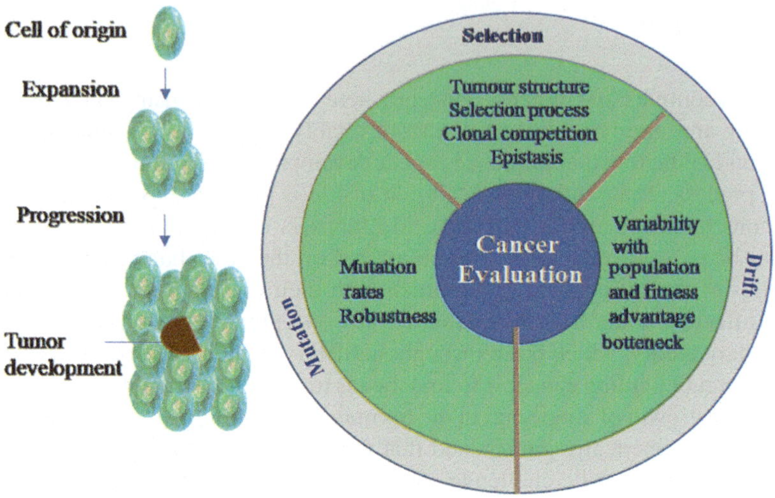

Fig. 2 Cancer origin and evolution

The accumulation of knowledge over time has changed numerous types of cancer from an incurable condition to specific biological aberrations, computational intelligence systems, clinical behaviors, and patterns of response to current systemic treatment. These improvements are a significant achievement for quality of life. Refining our understanding of oncology, several strategies have focused on cancer screening, cell therapy development, anti-tumor vaccines, biological drug development, and patient-specific computational model, therefore, for the foreseeable future, many landmark discoveries will undeniably support an innovative revolution in the field of oncology. To continue this legacy, and take it to a new level of excellence, efforts in further understanding and refining the oncology are being conducted.

3 Computational Oncology

3.1 Background and History

Tumor and cancer biology are going through a transformational change whereby biological and clinical quantitative big data, and modern computing are powering the research and discoveries. The remarkable advances in computing methods, such as computational intelligence (fuzzy logic, neural networks, evolutionary algorithms, nature-inspired algorithms), machine learning, deep learning, data mining, cloud computing, data engineering, and rich cancer data are combining to answer major questions in oncology and cancer biology, called Computational Oncology.

Computational Oncology is defined as a field of study encompassing the application of computer-based modeling to tumor and cancer biology [6]. This field is still emerging and that is why it has been loosely defined in the literature. Alan T. Lefor defines as "*Computational oncology is the application of techniques from the physical sciences (e.g., physics, mathematics, and engineering) to problems in tumor biology*" [29]. Computational oncology can be seen as an interdisciplinary field of studies focussing on the molecular aspects of cancer. Mathematics, statistics, computational models, tumor growth pathways, tumor biology, computational biology, bioinformatics, tumor marker profiles, large-scale genomics, transcriptomic, and proteomics data are used to develop predictive models for the diagnosis, prognosis, and treatments of cancers.

As far as the history of computational oncology is concerned, [29] traces it to 1943 when Erwin Schrodinger (Novel Prize in Physics, 1933) delivered talks at Trinity College (Dublin) addressing how the laws of physics, and thermodynamics can be utilized for a better understanding of the human organism, and how the concept of entropy relates to biological systems. Schrodinger further concluded that the laws of physics are inefficient to explain biological systems due to the fact that biological systems are not closed systems by their nature, and they utilize an external source of energy to avoid the law of thermodynamics [29]. As per our finding in PubMed, the term "computational oncology" first appeared in the year 2008 in the paper by Rosenfeld and Kapetanovic [43], however, computational oncology has grown for a long time. Some of the instances of earlier attempts in computational oncology are (i) two-stage mathematical model of carcinogenesis by Armitage and Doll in 1954 [5], (ii) Gomertzain model of tumor growth kinetics in 1964 [28], (iii) modeling and simulation of the regenerative processes in liver cancer [46], (iv) mathematical model of growth and spread of breast cancer [7], (v) astochastic model for the growth of cells in cancer [24], and so on.

3.2 Data Analysis and Applications

Computational oncology is an integrative approach where multidisciplinary teams such as oncologists, biologists, bioinformaticians, physicists, mathematicians, and engineers work jointly to enhance our understanding of cancers. Mathematical modeling helps to describe, simplify, and analyze complex systems, while computational simulation aids in the analysis and observations to steer hypotheses [37]. However, biological experiments are important for the validation and refinement of hypotheses [14]. With the increased processing power of modern computers, the availability of cheaper computing infrastructure through the computer cloud, the computational sciences, and mathematical sciences are advancing their applications in the field of oncology. It was reported that computational oncology has been implemented mostly in systems biology studies [6].

Some of the prominent data analysis in computational oncology and its applications are as follows [6, 11, 25]:

- To refine drug dosing and scheduling by modeling the pharmacokinetics (PK) and pharmacodynamics (PD) relationship.
- To predict tumor responses, efficacy, and toxicity during treatment planning.
- To improve stipulation of personalized and precision medicine for treatment using systems biology approaches by using multiscale modeling and PK/PD modeling to ascertain a better efficacy-toxicity balance.
- To integrate various layers of biological descriptors (e.g., multi-omics, medical imaging, single-cell sequencing, etc.) into a consistent framework using pure mathematical models, machine learning network approaches, and various computational intelligence methods.
- To model spatial architecture of three-dimensional tumors, tumor development, progression, and treatment response.
- To develop tools for the prediction of susceptibility, recurrence, and survival of cancers.
- To discover biomarkers, develop classification and association models for the interpretation of molecular studies in cancer.
- To develop and progress towards virtual clinical trials by integrating (i) standard-of-care patient data, (ii) evaluation of data for the purpose of diagnosis, (iii) quantitative data profiling, screening, and analysis, (iv) design, calibration, and simulation of mathematical models, (v) testing and validation with an organ-on-chip platform, (vi) tool for clinical decision making based on mathematical and organ-on-chip predictions, (vii) collection of longitudinal data for treatment monitoring as reported in [25].

One of the recent global projects on computational oncology is PRIMAGE (https://www.primageproject.eu/), "*PRedictive In-silico Multiscale Analytics to support cancer personalized diaGnosis and prognosis, Empowered by imaging biomarkers*". It is one of the largest and more ambitious projects funded by the European Union (EU) and launched as Horizon 2020 in late 2018. It has 16 European partners who are internationally recognized in in-silico technologies and clinical experts in paediatric cancer. PRIMAGE proposes an open cloud-based platform to support decision making in the clinical management of most frequent paediatric cancers, offering predictive tools to assist diagnosis, prognosis, therapies options, and treatment follow up, based on the usage of novel imaging biomarkers, a computational model of tumor growth simulation, advanced visualizations, and machine learning-based predictors of the most relevant, disease-specific clinical endpoints.

4 How CI is Strengthening Oncology Research?

Computational intelligence (CI) has proved to epitomize the field diagnosis and prognosis for various diseases including various cancers. It has allowed the development of effective and reliable clinical decision support systems (CDSS) that aid medical practitioners and staff to diagnose the disease and also to classify its subtype. Furthermore, these CI expert systems have also played a pivotal role in selecting the best drugs for the treatment of diseases. The five subfields of CI (refer to Sect. 1, Fig. 1) have become quintessential in various oncology research domains such as classification of the disease into subtypes, prediction of the disease in its initial stages, risk assessment, drug discovery, therapeutics, providing an optimized treatment approach, etc.

4.1 Classification

Researchers have deployed a multi-layered Mamdani fuzzy inference system (Ml-MFIS) for diagnosing and classifying the subtypes of hepatitis B as normal, severe, and chronic [3]. Furthermore, a fuzzy control model (FCM) has been discerned to be effective in diagnosing liver-based diseases in humans [20].

4.2 Imaging Identification and Analysis

CI has been doing significantly well in imaging and radiodiagnosis [58]. The drastic improvement in image analysis has been possible because of the deep learning architecture, called the Convolutional Neural Network (CNN). The deep learning architecture has the potential to analyze pixel-level information from medical images [42]. Moreover, they can judge the picture orientation of the pixels allowing the CNN model to check for lines, curves, and patterns within images. Their performance has been discerned to be greatly equivalent to human assessment and judgment of identifying tumors [45]. They have been successful in segmenting tumor volumes that now have been employed as a new strategy for radiotherapy treatment planning in lung cancer [56]. In addition, computational methods, including generative adversarial network (GAN), helps in the ad-hoc generation of biomedical images [50].

4.3 Risk Assessment

Myriad commercial applications employ computational intelligent systems in achieving better clinical decisions in cancers [47]. In order to identify cancers at an early stage, it becomes mandatory to predict the risk of the disease in individuals first! With the crucial task of forecasting the risk of developing cancers in individuals, CI systems have been improved to prevent the poor performance of prediction on new patient populations. In 2019, MIT's Computer Science and Artificial Intelligence

Laboratory (CSAIL) and Jameel Clinic deployed a deep learning model to prophesize cancer risk using mammograms. Their CI system showcased robust results as it accurately predicted the risk of breast cancer in both white and black women [17].

4.4 Cancer Therapy

Since the past decade, CI systems have been used to identify specific anticancer medications or have been dexterously deployed in anticancer drug design and development. Various cancers may use the same drugs, but their mode of action differs in the different cancers it is being used for [31]. A random forest model was developed by Lind and Anderson [32] by combining screening data and machine learning to predict anticancer drug activity according to cancer cell alterations in the human genome. A machine learning-based model was developed by [57] to predict drug sensitivity which was called Elastic Net Regression (ENR). For ovarian cancer too, many CI learning systems have been used to predict drug activity [21, 40], for gastric cancers [35, 53], endometroid cancer [18, 52]. The CI models deployed for ovarian cancer drug prediction suggested that the patients must be treated with tamoxifen, while in the case of gastric cancer, patients must be treated with 5-FU. For endometroid cancer CI drug prediction suggested the treatment with paclitaxel.

4.5 Cancer Treatment Optimization

As far as treatment of cancer is concerned, chemotherapy is the main choice to control metastatic cancer [8]. Optimization of cancer therapies is one of the important tasks that would be carried out by the oncologist. Computational intelligence-based methods, namely genetic algorithms, and nature-inspired optimization methods can be utilized to optimize the treatment plan, strategies, and management. For instance, beam orientation optimization using genetic algorithm and simulated dynamics hybrid [22], beam-angle optimization in radiotherapy planning using genetic algorithm [30] and neuro-genetic hybrid [13], optimizing beam intensities in intensity-modulated radiotherapy [2], multiple-drug chemotherapy schedule optimization using genetic algorithm and iterative genetic programming, called named as memetic algorithm [54], optimization of temperature field and magnetic nanoparticles optimal approximation for cancer therapy [23], radiotherapy pre-treatment scheduling using genetic algorithm [41], corrector magnets layout optimization for a proton therapy beamline using genetic algorithm [34], optimization of adaptive cancer therapy using dynamic programming and evolutionary game theory [16], optimizing therapies with multiple types of nanoparticles using genetic algorithms [55], and so on.

4.6 Diagnosis and Screening in Radiology

Convolutional neural networks (CNNs) have been used and approved by radiologists in providing a better screening and diagnostic endoscopy. Yamada et al. (2019) developed a CNN model that outperformed radiologists by rectifying cancerous and early cancerous abrasions with a sensitivity of 97% and a specificity of 99% in real-time. There are several other CI-based models that have been successful in identifying lesions at an early stage, howbeit, further work and validation are required in the same to prove CNN as the best and reliable early diagnosis and screening model for endoscopy [38].

5 Promises and Challenges of CI in Oncology

Computational intelligence (CI) has myriad applications in oncology and its related domains as already described in detail in the previous sections. However, with such rapid development and fulfilling promises, there still are a few limitations of CI systems in cancer research. The deployment of computational intelligence (CI) in myriad aspects of research domains is growing various digital revolutions too! From the perception change in healthcare management, personalized medicines (PM), and wearable biosensors to creating awareness in the general public has have been huge! The education and research sectors have also shown a magnanimous growth in computational intelligence (CI). When a drastic and ongoing paradigm shift occurs, there are obvious and easily visible consequences that are not uniformly adopted. Therefore, we chalk out four crucial challenges of CI in oncology: (a) The impact of CI in oncology must not be restricted in simple diagnosis and prognosis, but must extend to person-centric treatment strategies too!, (b) it must include the potential to explain the clinical decision that has been taken by the CI model, must provide dataset bias transparency to ensure the reliability of the system, (c) individuals must be given proper training of CI systems and there is a need to provide better infrastructure to learn and gain expertise in the field [27]. Table 2 highlights the fulfilled promises and existing challenges of CI systems in oncology.

6 Discussion and Conclusion

Computational intelligence (CI) is a group of computational methods that mimic human-like capabilities, rationality, and reasoning in computers. These methods help us develop intelligent systems that can help humans in making better decisions in complex situations and problems. CI has been significantly utilized for solving complex problems in various fields of study, including biomedical sciences and oncology. Past decades witnessed significant applications of CI techniques, such

Table 2 Promises and challenges of CI systems in oncology

S. No.	Promise	Limitation/challenge	Source
1	*Generalizability*	Currently, only a few CI-based models have been successfully used in cancer research. The main limitation of providing generalizability of CI systems in oncology is its poor translation into real-world complex problems	[60]
2	*Easy free access of data*	Medical data is siloed, i.e., it is not easily accessible to other medical institutions or medical staff. Thus, this is another limitation and a challenge for CI systems to consider the complete, heterogeneous medical data for better functionality. In fact, *findable, accessible, interoperable, reusable* (FAIR) data must be used by CI systems	[36, 44], ORIEN; Academics and hospitals. Flatiron health; [9, 59]
3	*Interpretability*	Currently, our CI models function as a black box, viz., we cannot interpret the accurate reasoning behind its prediction	[26]
4	*A good expertise*	Presently, medical consultants and staff receive little to no knowledge about CI systems and how they function. There is a need to create education and require skills to handle CI systems in oncology-based research	https://www.sciencedaily.com/releases/2018/09/180927083327.htm

as ANN, fuzzy logic, evolutionary algorithms, deep learning, and nature-inspired techniques, in various aspects of oncology research. CI facilitates oncologists in developing intelligent systems for better cancer management.

The term "oncology" is generally defined as a specialized branch of medicine that deals with the prevention, diagnosis, analysis, treatment, and research of tumors or cancers. There is a slight paradigm shift in tumor and cancer biology as biological and clinical quantitative big data, and modern computing is powering and accelerating scientific research and discoveries. The advances in computing methods, such as computational intelligence (fuzzy logic, neural networks, evolutionary algorithms, nature-inspired algorithms), machine learning, deep learning, data mining, cloud computing, data engineering, and rich cancer data are combining to answer major questions in oncology and cancer biology, called Computational Oncology. With the increased processing power of modern computers, availability of cheaper computing infrastructure through the computer cloud, the computational sciences, and mathematical sciences are advancing their applications in the field of oncology. Apart from the basic background of oncology, computational intelligence, and computational oncology, this chapter also reported some of the prominent data analysis and its applications in the field of oncology. Further, this chapter also addresses the question "*how computational intelligence is strengthening oncology research*"? Despite myriad applications of CI in the field of oncology and its related subfields, there are still a few limitations of CI systems in cancer research that includes lack of generalizability and interpretability of the CI models, inaccessibility, or unavailability of free access to cancer-related data, and need for the appropriate methods to integrate heterogeneous cancer data.

Acknowledgements SQ is supported by the DST-INSPIRE fellowship provided by the Department of Science & Technology, Govt. of India.

References

1. Academics & Hospitals. (2021). Flatiron Health. https://flatiron.com/academics/ (Accessed on 11th August, 2021).
2. Ahmad, S. U., & Bergen, S. W. (2010, July 1). A genetic algorithm approach to the inverse problem of treatment planning for intensity-modulated radiotherapy. *Biomedical Signal Processing and Control*, *5*(3), 189–195.
3. Ahmad, G., Khan, M. A., Abbas, S., Athar, A., Khan, B. S., & Aslam, M. S. (2019). Automated diagnosis of hepatitis B using multilayer mamdani fuzzy inference system. *Journal of Healthcare Engineering*, 1–11. https://doi.org/10.1155/2019/6361318
4. ANDATA. (2016). *Artificial intelligence, computational intelligence, soft computing, natural computing—What's the difference?* (Accessed 4th August, 2021). https://www.andata.at/en/answer/artificial-intelligence-computational-intelligence-softcomputing-natural-computation-whats-the-difference.html
5. Armitage, P., & Doll, R. (1954). The age distribution of cancer and a multi-stage theory of carcinogenesis. *British Journal of Cancer*, *8*(1), 1–12.
6. Barbolosi, D., Ciccolini, J., Lacarelle, B., Barlési, F., & André, N. (2016, April). Computational oncology—Mathematical modelling of drug regimens for precision medicine. *Nature Reviews Clinical Oncology, 13*(4), 242–254.
7. Blumenson, L. E., & Bross, I. D. (1969 March). A mathematical analysis of the growth and spread of breast cancer. *Biometrics, 1*, 95–109.
8. Chamseddine, I. M., Frieboes, H. B., & Kokkolaras, M. (2020, May 19) Multi-objective optimization of tumor response to drug release from vasculature-bound nanoparticles. *Scientific Reports, 10*(1), 1–1.
9. Chavan, V., & Penev, L. (2011). The data paper: A mechanism to incentivize data publishing in biodiversity science. *BMC Bioinformatics, 12*(15), S2.ed. 15:e1002683.
10. Davis, A., Gao, R., & Navin, N. (2017). Tumor evolution: Linear, branching, neutral or punctuated? *Biochimica et Biophysica Acta, 1867*(2), 151–161. https://doi.org/10.1016/j.bbcan.2017.01.003
11. de Anda-Jáuregui, G., & Hernández-Lemus, E. (2020, April 7) Computational oncology in the multi-omics era: State of the art. *Frontiers in Oncology, 10*, 423.

12. Di Lonardo, A., Nasi, S., & Pulciani, S. (2015). Cancer: We should not forget the past. *Journal of Cancer, 6*(1), 29–39. https://doi.org/10.7150/jca.10336
13. Dias, J., Rocha, H., Ferreira, B., & do Carmo Lopes, M. (2014 September) A genetic algorithm with neural network fitness function evaluation for IMRT beam angle optimization. *Central European Journal of Operations Research, 22*(3), 431–55.
14. Enderling, H., & Rejniak, K. A. (2013 September 13) Simulating cancer: Computational models in oncology. *Frontiers in Oncology, 3*, 233.
15. Faguet, G. B. (2015). A brief history of cancer: Age-old milestones underlying our current knowledge database. *International Journal of Cancer, 136*(9), 2022–2036. https://doi.org/10.1002/ijc.29134
16. Gluzman, M., Scott, J. G., & Vladimirsky, A. (2020 April 29). Optimizing adaptive cancer therapy: dynamic programming and evolutionary game theory. *Proceedings of the Royal Society B, 287*(1925), e20192454.
17. Gordon, R. (2021). *Robust artificial intelligence tools to predict future cancer*. Retrieved August 11, 2021, from MIT News | Massachusetts Institute of Technology website: https://news.mit.edu/2021/robust-artificial-intelligence-tools-predict-future-cancer-0128
18. Günakan, E., Atan, S., Haberal, A. N., Küçükyıldız, İ. A., Gökçe, E., & Ayhan, A. (2018). A novel prediction method for lymph node involvement in endometrial cancer: Machine learning. *International Journal of Gynecologic Cancer, 29*(2), 320–324. https://doi.org/10.1136/ijgc-2018-000033
19. Hanselmann, R. G., & Welter, C. (2016). Origin of cancer: An information, energy, and matter disease. *Frontiers in Cell and Developmental Biology, 4*, 121. https://doi.org/10.3389/fcell.2016.00121
20. Hashmia, A., & Khan, M. S. (2015). Diagnosis blood test for liver disease using fuzzy logic. *International Journal of Sciences: Basic and Applied Research, 20*, 151–183.
21. Hossain, M. A., Saiful Islam, S. M., Quinn, J. M. W., Huq, F., & Moni, M. A. (2019). Machine learning and bioinformatics models to identify gene expression patterns of ovarian cancer associated with disease progression and mortality. *Journal of Biomedical Informatics, 100*, 103313. https://doi.org/10.1016/j.jbi.2019.103313
22. Hou, Q., Wang, J., Chen, Y., & Galvin, J. M. (2003, September) Beam orientation optimization for IMRT by a hybrid method of the genetic algorithm and the simulated dynamics. *Medical Physics, 30*(9), 2360–2367.
23. Hu, G., Li, Y., Yang, S., Bai, Y., & Huang, J. (2015, April 23) Temperature field optimization and magnetic nanoparticles optimal approximation of MFH for cancer therapy. *IEEE Transactions on Magnetics, 51*(3), 1–4.
24. Iyer, K. S., & Saksena, V. N. (1970, September) A stochastic model for the growth of cells in cancer. *Biometrics, 1*, 401–410.
25. Karolak, A., Markov, D. A., McCawley, L. J., Rejniak, K. A. (2018, January 31) Towards personalized computational oncology: from spatial models of tumour spheroids, to organoids, to tissues. *Journal of The Royal Society Interface, 15*(138), 20170703.
26. Kuang, C. (2017). *Can A.I. be taught to explain itself? The New York Times*. November 21, 2017. https://www.nytimes.com/2017/11/21/magazine/can-ai-be-taught-to-explain-itself.html (Accessed 11th August, 2021).
27. Kusters, R., Misevic, D., Berry, H., Cully, A., Le Cunff, Y., Dandoy, L., & Wehbi, F. (2020) Interdisciplinary research in artificial intelligence: Challenges and opportunities. *Frontiers in Big Data, 3*. https://doi.org/10.3389/fdata.2020.577974
28. Laird, A. K. (1964) Dynamics of tumor growth. *British Journal of Cancer, 18*, 490–502.
29. Lefor, A. T. (2011, August 1) Computational oncology. *Japanese Journal of Clinical Oncology, 41*(8), 937–947.
30. Li, Y., & Lei, J. (2009, October 9) A feasible solution to the beam-angle-optimization problem in radiotherapy planning with a DNA-based genetic algorithm. *IEEE Transactions on Biomedical Engineering, 57*(3), 499–508.
31. Liang, G., Fan, W., Luo, H., & Zhu, X. (2020). The emerging roles of artificial intelligence in cancer drug development and precision therapy. *Biomedicine & Pharmacotherapy, 128*, 110255. https://doi.org/10.1016/j.biopha.2020.110255

32. Lind, A. P., & Anderson, P. C. (2019). Predicting drug activity against cancer cells by random forest models based on minimal gsssenomic information and chemical properties. *Plos One, 14*(7), e0219774. https://doi.org/10.1371/journal.pone.0219774
33. Lipinski, K. A., Barber, L. J., Davies, M. N., Ashenden, M., Sottoriva, A., & Gerlinger, M. (2016). Cancer evolution and the limits of predictability in precision cancer medicine. *Trends in Cancer, 2*(1), 49–63. https://doi.org/10.1016/j.trecan.2015.11.003
34. Liu, X., Chen, Q., Liao, Y., Wang, W., Chen, A., & Qin, B. (2020, December 1) Layout optimization of corrector magnets for a proton therapy beamline via genetic algorithm. Nuclear instruments and methods in physics research section A: Accelerators, spectrometers. *Detectors and Associated Equipment, 982*, 164560.
35. Liu, C., Qi, L., Feng, Q.-X., Sun, S.-W., Zhang, Y.-D., & Liu, X.-S. (2019). Performance of a machine learning-based decision model to help clinicians decide the extent of lymphadenectomy (D1 vs. D2) in gastric cancer before surgical resection. *Abdominal Radiology, 44*(9), 3019–3029. https://doi.org/10.1007/s00261-019-02098-w
36. London, J. W. (2018). Cancer research data-sharing networks. *JCO Clinical Cancer Informatics. 2*, 1–3.
37. Mumenthaler, S., D'Antonio, G., Preziosi, L., & Macklin, P. (2013, July 26) The need for integrative computational oncology: An illustrated example through MMP—Mediated tissue degradation. *Frontiers in Oncology, 3*, 194.
38. Nagy, M., Radakovich, N., & Nazha, A. (2020). Machine learning in oncology: What should clinicians know? *JCO Clinical Cancer Informatics, 4*, 799–810. https://doi.org/10.1200/cci.20.00049
39. ORIEN. (2021). *Oncology research information exchange network*. http://oriencancer.org/ (Accessed 11th August, 2021).
40. Paik, E. S., Lee, J.-W., Park, J.-Y., Kim, J.-H., Kim, M., Kim, T.-J., & Seo, S. W. (2019). Prediction of survival outcomes in patients with epithelial ovarian cancer using machine learning methods. *Journal of Gynecologic Oncology, 30*(4). https://doi.org/10.3802/jgo.2019.30.e65
41. Petrovic, S., & Castro, E. (Eds.). (2011, April 27). A genetic algorithm for radiotherapy pre-treatment scheduling. In: *European conference on the applications of evolutionary computation* (pp. 454–463). Springer.
42. Raza, K., & Singh, N. K. (2021, January 27) A tour of unsupervised deep learning for medical image analysis. *Current Medical Imaging. 17*(9), 1059–1077.
43. Rosenfeld, S., & Kapetanovic, I. (2008, January). Systems biology and cancer prevention: All options on the table. *Gene Regulation and Systems Biology, 2*, GRSB-S1114.
44. Ross, J.S., & Waldstreicher, J., et al. (2018). Overview and experience of the YODA project with clinical trial data sharing after 5 years. *Science Data, 5*, 180268.
45. Russakovsky, O., Deng, J., et al. (2015). ImageNet large scale visual recognition challenge. *International Journal of Computer Vision, 115*, 211–252.
46. Sendov, B., & Tsanev, R. (1968). Computer simulation of the regenerative processes in the liver. *Journal of Theoretical Biology, 18*(1), 90–104.
47. Sennaar, K. (2019). AI and machine learning for clinical trials: Examining 3 current applications. *Emerj—Artificial Intelligence Research and Insight*. https://emerj.com/ai-sector-overviews/ai-machine-learning-clinical-trials-examining-x-current-applications/ (Accessed 5th August, 2021).
48. Sharma, M., Agrawal, S., & Deswal, S. (2020). Application of hybrid computational intelligence in health care. *Hybrid Computational Intelligence*, 123–148. https://doi.org/10.1016/b978-0-12-818699-2.00007-x
49. Shlush, L. I., & Hershkovitz, D. (2015). Clonal evolution models of tumor heterogeneity. In *American society of clinical oncology educational book. American society of clinical oncology. Annual meeting* (pp. e662–665). https://doi.org/10.14694/EdBook_AM.2015.35.e662
50. Singh, N. K., & Raza, K. (2021). Medical image generation using generative adversarial networks: A review. *Health Informatics: A Computational Perspective in Healthcare*, 77–96.
51. Somarelli, J. A., Gardner, H., Cannataro, V. L., Gunady, E. F., Boddy, A. M., Johnson, N. A., Fisk, J. N., Gaffney, S. G., Chuang, J. H., Li, S., Ciccarelli, F. D., Panchenko, A. R., Megquier,

K., Kumar, S., Dornburg, A., DeGregori, J., & Townsend, J. P. (2020). Molecular biology and evolution of cancer: From discovery to action. *Molecular Biology and Evolution, 37*(2), 320–326. https://doi.org/10.1093/molbev/msz242

52. Stanzione, A., Cuocolo, R., Del Grosso, R., Nardiello, A., Romeo, V., Travaglino, A., Raffone, A., Bifulco, G., Zullo, F., Insabato, L., & Mainenti, P. P. (2021). Deep myometrial infiltration of endometrial cancer on MRI: A radiomics-powered machine learning pilot study. *Academic Radiology, 28*(5), 737–744. https://doi.org/10.1016/j.acra.2020.02.028
53. Taninaga, J., Nishiyama, Y., Fujibayashi, K., Gunji, T., Sasabe, N., Iijima, K., & Naito, T. (2019). Prediction of future gastric cancer risk using a machine learning algorithm and comprehensive medical check-up data: A case-control study. *Scientific Reports, 9*(1). https://doi.org/10.1038/s41598-019-48769-y
54. Tse, S. M., Liang, Y., Leung, K. S., Lee, K. H., & Mok, T. S. A memetic algorithm for multiple-drug cancer chemotherapy schedule optimization. *IEEE Transactions on Systems, Man, and Cybernetics, Part B (Cybernetics), 37*(1), 84–91.
55. Tsompanas, M. A., Bull, L., Adamatzky, A., & Balaz, I. (2021). In silico optimization of cancer therapies with multiple types of nanoparticles applied at different times. *Computer Methods and Programs in Biomedicine, 1*(200), 105886.
56. Wang, S., Zhou, M., Gevaert, O., Tang, Z., Dong, D., Liu, Z., & Jie, T. (2017). A multi-view deep convolutional neural networks for lung nodule segmentation. In *Conference proceedings of the IEEE engineering medicine biology society* (pp. 1752–1755).
57. Wang, Y., Wang, Z., Xu, J., Li, J., Li, S., Zhang, M., & Yang, D. (2018). Systematic identification of non-coding pharmacogenomic landscape in cancer. *Nature Communications, 9*(1). https://doi.org/10.1038/s41467-018-05495-9
58. Wani, N., & Raza, K. (2018, January 1). Multiple kernel-learning approach for medical image analysis. In *Soft computing based medical image analysis* (pp. 31–47). Academic Press.
59. Wilkinson, M. D., Dumontier, M., Aalbersberg, I. J., Appleton, G., Axton, M., Baak, A., & Mons, B. (2016). The FAIR Guiding Principles for scientific data management and stewardship. *Scientific Data, 3*, 160018.
60. Zech, J.R., Badgeley, M.A., Liu, M., Costa, A. B., Titano, J. J., & Oermann, E. K. (2018). Variable generalization performance of a deep learning model to detect pneumonia in chest radiographs: A cross-sectional study. *PLOS*. MLambin, P., Roelofs, E., & Reymen, B., et al. (2013) 'Rapid learning health care in oncology': An approach towards decision support systems enabling customised radiotherapy. *Radiother Oncology, 109*, 159–64.

Machine Learning-Based Models in the Diagnosis, Prognosis and Effective Cancer Therapeutics: Current State-of-the-Art

Fatima Nazish Khan, Malik Yousef, and Khalid Raza

Abstract Currently, the advancement of computational intelligence (CI) and machine learning (ML) leading to the integration of methods. Cancer, one of the major challenges in organisms, is considered a heterogeneous disease that has been classified into various subtypes. Therefore, the classification of cancer subtypes led the researchers from the bioinformatics and biomedical field, to focus on the major applications of ML methods. From the last decades, various research has been done for the prediction, treatment, and prognosis of cancer, yet there is a challenge of morbidity and mortality of cancer patients. In order to limit these challenges, effective prediction and diagnosis methods are essential. Many researchers in this field have implemented ML-based models with high-performance such as Support Vector Machines, Decision Trees, Artificial Neural Networks, and Bayesian Networks, and their ensembling for the prediction and early diagnosis, prognosis, and effective cancer therapeutics. This chapter presents recent advancements in ML-based models in the prediction, prognosis, and effective cancer therapeutic research. We also focus on ML-based models in various types of cancers like lung, breast, head, brain, liver, neck, gynecological, esophagus, and prostate cancers.

Keywords Cancer diagnosis · Machine learning in cancer · AI in cancer · Cancer prognosis

F. N. Khan
Department of Education in Science and Mathematics, NCERT, New Delhi 110016, India

M. Yousef
Department of Information System, Zefat Academic College, Jerusalem, Israel

K. Raza (✉)
Department of Computer Science, Jamia Millia Islamia, New Delhi 110025, India
e-mail: kraza@jmi.ac.in

K. Raza (ed.), *Computational Intelligence in Oncology*, Studies in Computational Intelligence 1016, https://doi.org/10.1007/978-981-16-9221-5_2

1 Introduction

A common branch and subdivision of Artificial Intelligence (AI) known as Machine Learning (ML) was originated in the year 1950 by Arthur Lee Samuel, one of the pioneers in AI, for playing strategic games such as chess. In this, the machines learn automatically without being programmed and are in many fields like retail, finance, social data as well as in health care [108]. It correlates the learning problem from samples of the dataset and provides outcomes for each problem, and is utilized for various classification problems, estimation, and prediction. This field is generally used in various biomedical research applications, with different biological samples and algorithms. Majorly, supervised and unsupervised learning methods of ML have been utilized. Yet, some more additional types of ML have also been found such as reinforcement learning, semi-supervised learning; evolutionary learning, and deep learning (Fig. 1). Supervised learning deals with the training dataset that is labeled and is utilized for estimation or mapping of input data onto desirable output, for example, decision tree (DT), k-nearest neighbor (kNN), artificial neural network (ANN), Naïve Bayes (NB), random forest (RF), support vector machine (SVM) and ensemble learning. But, with unsupervised learning, the training dataset has not been labeled and there is no desired output in the learning process like the k-means clustering algorithm. Semi-supervised learning, one of the widely applied methods of ML is a linkage of both commonly used methods (supervised and unsupervised learning), that generally links both labeled and unlabelled datasets for the construction of accurate and desirable learning models. This type of learning method is widely used when an unlabelled dataset is huge, compared to the labeled dataset. The performance of

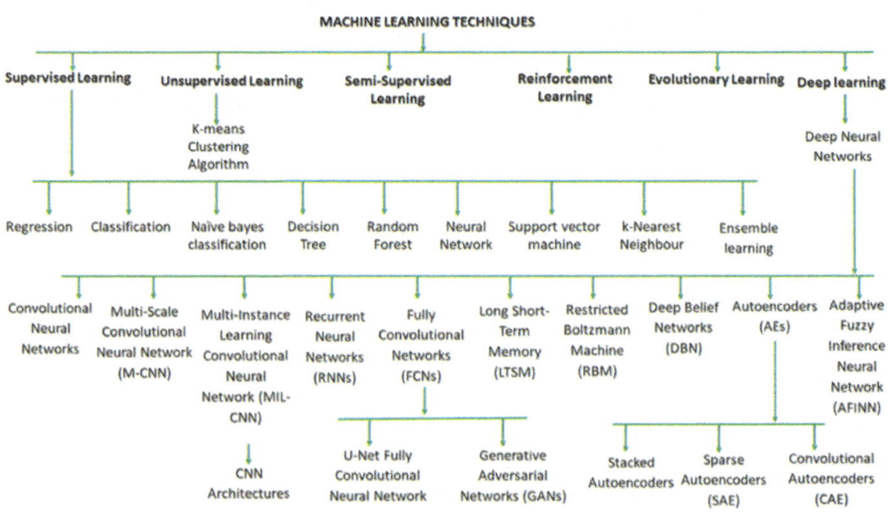

Fig. 1 Taxonomy of machine learning (ML) techniques

each model can be calculated and analyzed on the basis of performance such as sensitivity, specificity, area under the curve (AUC), and accuracy [51, 88, 102].

Deep Learning (DL), a branch of ML is based on a number of ML algorithms, that build high-level abstraction models like deep neural networks (DNN) which include convolutional neural networks, multi-instance learning convolutional neural networks (MIL-CNN), multi-scale convolutional neural network (M-CNN), recurrent neural networks (RNNs), fully convolutional networks (FCNs), long short-term memory (LTSM), restricted Boltzmann machine (RBM), autoencoders (AEs), adaptive fuzzy inference neural network (AFINN), and deep belief networks (DBN). It generally utilizes the deep graph having a number of processing layers, consisting of linear and nonlinear transformation [111]. According to input and output training data, DL performs the prediction of new output whenever there is induction of new input, for example, Model Regression Network [114]. In healthcare, the DL algorithms like Deep Belief Networks (DBNs), Convolutional Neural Network (CNN), and Fully Connected Convolutional Networks (FCNs) are used to study and examining of X-Ray, MRI, and computed tomography (CT) images [5, 87].

From the last three decades, various ML methods, as well as algorithms for feature selection, have been widely used for the prediction and prognosis of the disease like cancer (cells rapidly multiply and grow inside the body) [73, 79]. Most of the previous work utilized ML methods to model the cancer progression and help in the identification of various factors used for classification problems. ML techniques such as ANNs, SVMs, BNs, and DTs are majorly used to detect and prognosis of different types of cancer using the clinical, histological, and population-based datasets [5, 52, 79]. Additionally, the features such as age, weight, history, diet, family, habits of high-risk, and exposure to environmental carcinogens helped in identifying and prognosis of cancer development.

With the accessibility of a huge number of online pharmacogenomics as well as oncological datasets, research in this field has been continuously increasing. Instead of traditional computational and statistical methods, bioinformaticians are utilizing ML technologies for improving the treatment of genetic disorders. With the advancement of computational biology and ML, one can easily find biomarkers that cause diseases and help in accurately diagnosis and prognosis of genetic profiles of patients [73]. To produce functional therapies for oncological research, one can better understand the complexities that are present in the cancer microenvironment. Although there are lots of methods described in the literature, yet the mortality due to cancer still persists. In this regard, AI or ML is providing a fast, efficient, and reliable method for the prognosis and diagnosis of cancer [68].

Here, the chapter presents an overview of the current state of the ML-based models in prediction, diagnosis, prognosis, and effective cancer therapeutics. We also focus on ML-based models and techniques and their applications in various types of cancers such as lung, breast, head, prostate, esophagus, liver, neck, gynaecological, and brain cancers. Along with their applications, we finally focus on possible challenges and future cancer research based on ML models.

2 Machine Learning in Prediction and Prognosis of Cancer

During the previous two decades, a number of feature selection algorithms as well as ML techniques were used for disease prediction and prognosis [79]. Successful detection and prognosis of disease generally depend on medical diagnosis quality, however, instead of only the decision of diagnosis, one should also deal with prognostic prediction methods. If cancer prediction/prognosis is taken into account one can deal with three tasks of prediction: susceptibility of cancer prediction (risk assessment), recurrence of cancer prediction, and cancer survival prediction (Table 1).

Most feature selection algorithms that are applied to gene expression data are based on statistics and ML. However, most of them do not use biological knowledge, related to the analyzed data, which could contribute to better feature selection. Combining traditional gene selection with external biological knowledge is an emerging field in bioinformatics. Traditional approaches are still predominantly used in current practice and external knowledge is manually incorporated and applied in specific cases. We suggest that the information about biological processes/functions/pathways should be taken into consideration upfront during the biomarkers selection process. Since the integrative approach attracted attention in the gene expression domain, lately the gene selection process shifted from being purely data-centric to being more incorporative in terms of additional biological knowledge [122–124]. See for a recent review of such approaches [126].

2.1 Cancer Susceptibility Prediction

With the help of a literature survey, we collected publications that used ML approaches for different types of cancer susceptibility prediction [107]. Among the recently published work on the prediction of cancer risk assessment, very interesting research has been found that estimates the risk of breast cancer by using ANNs [7]. It is a study that used demographic and mammographic datasets and predicted the characteristics of the model proposed. Most of the authors developed tools that make decisions and distinguish malignant and benign findings in breast cancer. On the basis of their knowledge, these studies along with computer models utilized ML approaches like ANNs for risk assessment of patients suffering from breast cancer. Radiologists then reviewed each record of mammographic findings for obtaining reading information, which was further used to enter as input in the ANN model, and then performance has been interpreted using ten-fold cross-validation. Also, for prevention of overfitting, they utilized the method of ES, which generally prevents the network error at the time of training and pauses it when overfitting is seen. With training, testing, and also ten-fold cross-validation, they finally calculated the AUC value of the model (i.e., 0.965) and drew the ROC curve, and showed that the model can predict the breast cancer risk of patients accurately using a huge amount of datasets. Apart from these outcomes, there are limitations of the mix of diagnostic

Table 1 List of ML methods used for cancer susceptibility, cancer recurrence, and cancer survival prediction

ML approaches	Type of cancer	Number of patients	Type of data	Accuracy	Salient features	References
Cancer susceptibility prediction						
ANN	Breast	62,219	Demographic, mammographic	AUC = 0.96	Mammography findings, age	[7]
SVM	Multiple myeloma	80	Single nucleotide polymorphisms	71%	snp994532, snp521522, snp739514 (SNPs in myeloma)	[113]
SVM	Breast	174	Single nucleotide polymorphisms	69%	(+)4536 T/C site of the aldosterone synthase gene CYP11B2 at amino acid residue 386 Val/Ala (T/C) (rs4541); (+)4328C/G site of the aryl hydrocarbon hydroxylase CYP1B1 at amino acid residue 293 Leu/Val (C/G) (rs5292)	[62]
BN	Colon carcinomatosis	53	Pathological, clinical	AUC = 0.71	Histology of primary tumor, stage of node formation, peritoneal cancer	[99]
Cancer recurrence prediction						
BN	Oral	86	Blood genomic, clinical, imaging tissue genomic	100%	p53 stain, smoker, extra-tumor spreading, SOD2, TCAM	[31]
SVM	Breast	679	Clinical, epidemiological, pathological	89%	Tumor local invasion	[54]

(continued)

Table 1 (continued)

ML approaches	Type of cancer	Number of patients	Type of data	Accuracy	Salient features	References
Graph-based SSL algorithm	Colon	437	Protein–protein interactions, Gene expression	76.70%	CCNB1, BRCA1, STAT1,CCND1	[78]
	Breast	374		80.70%		
SVM	Cervical	168	Pathological, clinical	68%	Pathologic_T, pathologic_S, target summary of RT cell type	[106]
SVM	Breast	547	Population, clinical	95%	Age at diagnosis and menarche	[3]
Cancer Survival Prediction						
ANN	Lung	440	Gene expression, clinical	83.50%	Age,sex, N_stage, T_stage, ERBB2 and LCK genes	[15]
Graph-based SSL algorithm	Breast	1,62,500	SEER	71%	Size of tumor, nodes count, age at diagnosis	[79]
SVM	Oral	31	Genomic, clinical	75%	p63 gene, drink, invasion	[13]
SVM	Breast	295	Genomic	97%	50-gene signature	[119]
BN	Breast	97	Microarray, clinical	AUC = 0.85	NA	[35]
SVM	Oral	69	Molecular, clinical	98%	TNM_stage, recurrences count	[91]
DT	Breast	2,00,000	SEER	93%	Size of tumor, histology, age at diagnosis, nodes count	[24]
SSL Co-training algorithm	Breast	1,62,500	SEER	76%	Size of tumor, age at diagnosis, nodes count, tumor extension	[53]

data and screening which cannot accurately separate with input to the ANN, and hence applied pre-processing steps for converting raw dataset into a suitable format for further analysis.

2.2 Cancer Recurrence Prediction

On the basis of a literature search, we present the recently published literature that utilizes the techniques of ML that predict the recurrence of cancer. In one study, prediction of oral squamous cell carcinoma (OSCC) recurrence has been proposed [79]. The authors of this study analyzed the evolution of OSCC of cancer patients by using a multiparametric Decision Support System. They used different types of datasets such as clinical, genomic, and imaging for predicting OSCC relapse and further recurrence of cancer. Eighty-six patients were taken in this study, out of which 13 were considered as relapses and the remaining were normal. By integrating algorithms of feature selection such as wrapper algorithm and correlation-based feature selection (CFS), a particular procedure of feature selection has been applied, and also biasing has been avoided when feature selection algorithms are used on the heterogeneous dataset. Initially, there were a total number of 65, 40, and 17 feature selection methods for clinical, genomic, and imaging datasets. Further, integration of CFS algorithm, total 8, 7, and 6 datasets were used in each classifier, respectively. This study followed the basic idea of patient's discrimination with disease relapse and normal individuals using 5 classification approaches such as ANNs, BNs, SVMs, RF, and DTs classifiers. These algorithms then employed the technique of ten-fold cross-validation to evaluate the model, and further accuracy, specificity, and sensitivity were also calculated to compare these classifiers. In terms of outputs of these classifiers, authors predicted that the BN classifier scheme has better performance for clinical and imaging datasets with an accuracy of 78.6% and 82.8%, respectively, but the classification of BN along with the CFS algorithm gave the best performance having an accuracy of 91.7% in terms of cancer recurrence.

2.3 Cancer Survival Prediction

In one of the studies, there was a development of a predictive model that generally evaluates and predicts survival of cancer in females with breast cancer [79]. The authors did a comparison of three classification models such as ANN, self-supervised learning (SSL), and SVM according to the cancer database [42]. For the analysis, the dataset consists of key features (16) and records (162,500). A variable class like survivability is taken for patients presenting as survived and not survived. Among all the features, the age, size of the tumor, and nodes count were considered, and then classifiers were applied. After comparison of these three models, it has been found that accuracy for SVM, ANN, and SSL was calculated as 51%, 65%, and 71%, respectively. For the evaluation of the predictive model's performance, five-fold cross-validation was utilized. For survival analysis, the authors claimed that the SSL model is considered the best model for clinical experts. Similarly, another study was also published on non-small cell lung cancer (NSCLC) for assessing the prediction of a patient's survival by using ANNs [15]. The raw dataset consisted of clinical as well as NSCLC patients' gene expression from the NCI Array database. The authors initially pre-process the raw datasets and choose important genes associated with survival like ERBB2 and LCK genes that are further utilized for the training of ANN classifiers. Four clinical variables such as age, sex, N_stage, and T_stage were also taken for input into the ANN model. The number of ANN architectures have also been performed for predicting cancer survival, and overall, 83% of accuracy has been predicted.

3 Chronological Review

According to a PubMed search result with the MeSH term "cancer" AND "machine learning", approximately 7,650 articles have been published by 2021. These publications mainly deal with ML algorithms and linked datasets from different sources for tumor detection and also prognosis and prediction of different types of cancer. We have done a literature review and collected a set of literature using the keywords cancer prognosis, diagnosis, and ML techniques of more than 50 years, which is

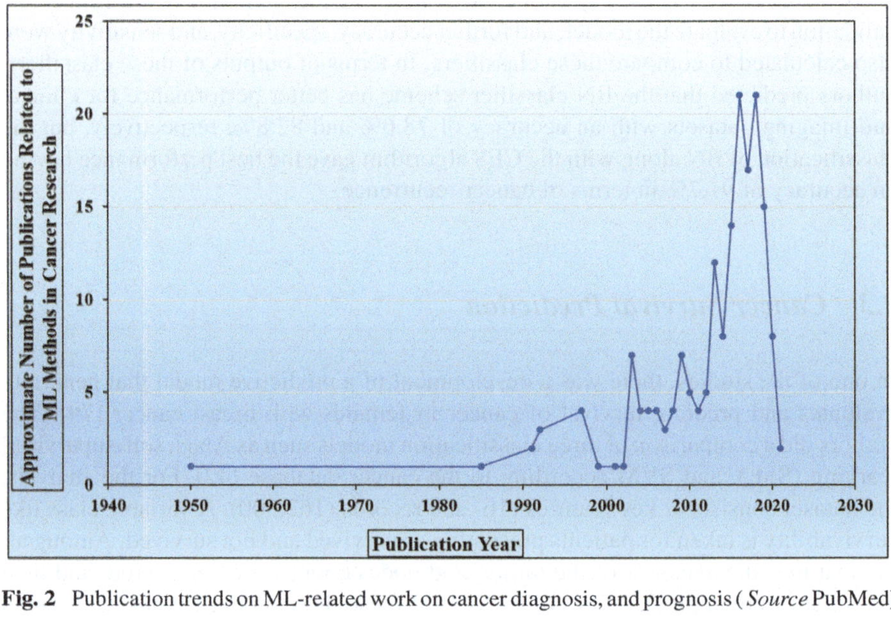

Fig. 2 Publication trends on ML-related work on cancer diagnosis, and prognosis (*Source* PubMed)

further manually checked. The year-wise publication trend is depicted in Fig. 2, showing an exponential increase after 2010.

4 Machine Learning-Based Cancer Diagnosis System: A General Pipeline

Cancer has been described as a complex disorder with a wide range of subgroups with thousands of genetic and epigenetic variations. The need of classifying cancer patients into a level of risk as low or high-risk classes has given rise to numerous bioinformatics as well as biomedical researchers who identify utilization of ML algorithms for physicians and pathologists could be a major help for disease prediction, treatment, diagnosis, and prognosis. Clinical utilization of AI and ML in the treatment and diagnosis of cancer serves as medical guidance in future faster identification of new treatment at the individual level [47]. There are 3 main steps in cancer diagnosis-based image, Pre-Processing, Image Segmentation, and Post-Processing. First, pre-processing step helps to eliminate noise from the image while keeping this noise will harm the classification task by the machine learning algorithm. Beeravolu et al., in their study, implemented techniques of image pre-processing and by using training data, Deep Convolutional Neural Networks improved classification performances [9]. This approach was implemented on breast cancer images by applying various methods for image enhancements, removal of background, and pectoral muscle. Additionally, Hoshyar et al., have surveyed different pre-processing methods for images of skin cancer, where those approaches are based on Image Enhancement, Image Restoration, and Removing Thick Hairs [41]. For more information, we refer to the review of Breast Cancer pathological image processing [129]. Image Segmentation is the second step, which is the process of segmenting images into segments or regions. This method is very important for mining, extracting, and interpreting knowledge from digital images. Vu et al., have developed an algorithm for segmentation that has multiscale aggregation of deep residual networks that accurately segment nuclear material which was further separated as individual nuclei from clumped nuclei [112]. Xu et al., offer one automatic method that segments skin cancer and pigmented lesions images [118]. In this method, initially, a color image converts to an intensity image, then uses intensity thresholding to roughly partition the image. The segmentation is then fine-tuned using picture edges. The third step is post-processing, in which features are generally extracted. There are many techniques for feature extraction such as wavelet Packet Transform (WPT), principal component analysis (PCA), Fourier power spectrum (FPS) [40], grey level co-occurrence matrix (GLCM), decision boundary features, and Gaussian derivative kernels. For example, the GLCM technique is helpful to extract texture features like contrast, extracted-autocorrelation, correlation, cluster prominence, dissimilarity, cluster shade, homogeneity, energy, maximum probability, entropy, variance, and the sum of squares from any target image [6].

5 Models for Detection of Various Cancers Types

5.1 Breast Cancer

A few years back, lots of studies have been done on the detection of breast cancer. Based on deep learning, [4] in their study designed and developed a model for feature extraction on breast histopathological images, particularly, focused on mitosis detection. By this proposed model, the features were extracted from CNN that was further given to SVM for its training, and hence, the breast mitosis has been detected [4, 72]. To construct the CNN, AlexNet was utilized to classify benign and malignant mitosis using histopathological images [98]. Similarly, for the detection of breast mitosis from histology slides, a deep cascade network has developed [16]. Further, with the help of a trained FCN model, the mitosis candidates from histology slides were extracted, which was then finely tuned by the CaffeNet model [85]. And for classification of mitosis, images were pre-trained from the model ImageNet. Then, fully connected layers of three networks were trained with different configurations and thereafter generated output as multiple probabilities/scores. Final results are then generated by averaging probabilities. In one of the studies, an algorithm of stacked sparse autoencoder (SSAE) was used for nuclei classification from histopathological images of the breast [117]. The greedy approach was utilized for SSAE optimization, where only a single hidden layer is trained at a time, and the output of the previous layer serves as the input to the next hidden layer.

Along with histopathological images which detect breast cancer, the dataset of mammographic images is also utilized to identify breast cancer. Authors in one of the studies introduced a hybrid model (a combination of CNN and SVM) on digital mammograms for mass detection [72]. During CNN model training, mammogram patches have been utilized, and also from results of a fully connected layer at the end, representation of high-level features has been produced [115]. Similarly, Ertosun et al. proposed a model that initially identifies the availability of mass of mammogram, which further locates this mass from mammographic images [29]. For features learning from mammograms, Kallenberg et al. used stacked convolutional sparse autoencoders (SCAE) to train the model, sparsity regularizer, then was utilized for enhancing model's robustness [50]. Dhungel et al. used SVM, random forest classifiers, and DL to detect mass using mammographic pictures [26].

5.2 Lung Cancer

Along with breast cancer, various ML methods like deep learning were used to predict lung cancer [86]. Paul et al. adopted pre-trained CNN (i.e., trained on large-scale datasets) for detecting lung cancer using features extraction from CT images [80]. In [38], authors applied CNN and DBN algorithms on raw images of lung cancer, and for the classification of pulmonary nodes, they utilized 2D images of CT, whereas, in another study with the same approach [45], authors utilized 3D images of CT for model training. From 3D images, they take out patches in 2D format and further utilize them for extracting features on CNN, which are then fused and given as input to the classifier. In [96], the authors constructed a multi-variant convolutional neural network (Mc-CNN), that helps in overcoming the problem of nodule size of variables. Convolutional operation is given by the equation:

$$y^l = \mathrm{RReLU}\left(\sum\nolimits_K c^{kl} * h^k + b^l\right)$$

where, y^1, the lth output map, h^k, the kth input map, c^{kl}, the link between input map and output map of convolutional kernels, b^1, bias of the lth output map. RReLU is defined as:

$$\mathrm{RReLU} = \begin{cases} x & \text{if } x \geq 0 \\ x/a & \text{if } x < 0, a \sim U(b_l, b_u) \end{cases}$$

where, U (b_l, b_u), is uniform distribution, b_l and b_u are lower and upper bound of distribution.

5.3 *Brain Cancer*

Brain cancer, one of the major types of cancer, is an uncontrolled growth of cell mass in any region of the brain, which is more challenging to detect. However, the most challenging task is brain segmentation of the healthy and cancerous parts of the brain. ML techniques such as DL have been successfully used to combat these challenges in brain images. Gao et al. proposed two algorithms on the basis of 2D and 3D CNN with the help of 2D and 3D images, respectively. These two models were then finally combined to form a hybrid model which outperformed 2D and 3D scale-invariant features swift (SIFT) with good outcomes. In [82], authors discussed a CNN-based method called the automatic magnetic resonant image segmentation, which detected the augmentation and normalization intensity in brain cancer. Also, found global and local features from the CNN model, and utilized a fully connected layer in the CNN model for enhancement of the system's speed that easily detected cancer within the brain. Conditional random fields (CRFs) and fully connected convolutional neural networks (FCNs) were also utilized to segment brain cancer.

5.4 Skin Cancer

"Melanoma", a skin cancer, is treated easily when it is detected much earlier but is much hard to differentiate between benign and malignant melanoma as they seem similar at earlier stages. There are lots of methods like the seven-point checklist method, ABCD rule, pattern analysis, and Menzies method that can easily differentiate malignant and benign melanoma. Pomponiu et al. classified benign melanoma by using 399 images that were taken from standard cameras [83]. For the classification of lesions, the method of K-nearest neighbor was utilized, which achieved 93.62% of accuracy, 95.18% of specificity, and 92.1% of sensitivity. Esteva et al., in their study, used a total of 129,450 images for CNN pretraining, out of which only 2032 were taken from skin lesions and the rest were from dermatoscopic devices [30, 72]. The classifications such as benign nevi and benign seborrheic keratosis classification from malignant melanoma and keratinocytes carcinomas respectively were there and utilized transfer learning their classifications. For both carcinomas and melanomas, the AUC value was 0.96. In the same way, Han et al. by utilizing 19,398 images that trained the ResNet model, proposed a classifier that helps in the classification of 12 types of skin cancer [38]. Masood et al. proposed a self-advised semi-supervised learning model for the detection of melanoma. This system was made up of two self-advised support vector machines (SA-SVM) and a deep belief network that was trained by three types of datasets [66]. The utilization of deep neural networks along with images mapping has been used by Sabbaghi et al. for increasing the accuracy of classification into bag-of-feature (BoF) space [93]. To train CNN model, Demyanov et al. utilized stochastic gradient descent, which is further helpful in detecting regular globules patterns and typical network in another study [25]. Sumithra et al. in their work analyzed lesions with the use of kNNSVM [101]. He et al., utilized a method of backward-propagation in the CNN model of eight layers, nine hundred images were utilized for testing of this classification, with accuracy of 89.5 and 91.92% on test and training sets, respectively [40].

5.5 Prostate Cancer

The third highest type of cancer that leads to death in males is prostate cancer [37]. The method of deep learning along with sparse patch matching proposed by authors in [37] for segmentation of prostate. And for the extraction of feature representation from a dataset of MR images, they utilized the technique of SSAE. In [121], the authors gave a method that identifies prostate cancer by using an SAE classifier, then features that are collected were improved by the SSAE model. Similarly, Tian et al. with the help of a fully convolutional network segmented the prostate [104]. Yu et al., in their study, made prostate segmentation with the help of volumetric convolutional networks using 3D MR images [127]. Ma et al. detected prostate cancer with the help of patch-based CNN [65], which was further used in other studies [56].

6 Models for Predicting Toxicity in Various Cancerous Types

A number of variables lead to toxicity in cancerous cells, and therefore ML techniques are used to build models that relate these variables to side effects induced by treatment (Fig. 3). The models that are successfully built, enhance the probability of positive outcomes and minimize side effects in clinical practices. From previous studies, it has been found that large numbers of studies are present that are based on ML models to predict the toxicity and side effects in cancer types. Till the year 2020, most of these studies focused on prostate, lung, and neck and head cancers. Minor studies are breast, gynecology, esophagus, brain, and liver cancers [48] (Table 2).

6.1 Brain

In brain cancer, a single study has been found on ML-based models for toxicity prediction [23]. The authors compared the performance of various classifiers of machine learning on multiple datasets of patients with lung and neck and head cancers with that of brain cancers. Total 12 different types of datasets were tested from 3496 patients using neural networks, decision trees, SVM, RF, LogitBoost, and elastic net LR classifiers. Both blood marker and dosimetry datasets from neck and head cancer

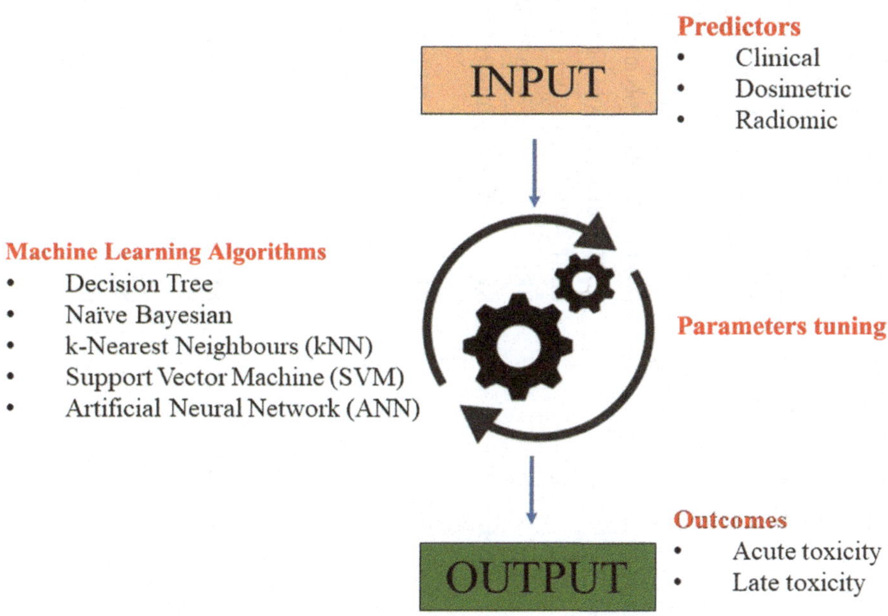

Fig. 3 General workflow of ML-based models for prediction of clinical toxicity

Table 2 ML-based models that predict toxicity in various cancerous types

Cancer type	No. of patients	Type of RT	Type of predicted toxicity	Features type	Classifier	Results[a]	References
Breast	90	RT	Dermatitis	R	RF	Acc = 0.87%	[95]
	2277	N/A	Moist desquamation, dermatitis, chest pain, fatigue	D, C	LR, RF, GB	0.56–0.85	[90]
Esophagus	101	IMRT or 3D-CRT	Pneumonitis	D, C	LR	Acc = 0.63	[39]
Gyneco	42	EBRT + BRT	Rectal toxicity	D	SVM	0.82–0.91	[17]
	42	EBRT + BRT	Rectal toxicity	D	CNN	1.29	[130]
	35	BRT	Fistula formation	D, C	SVM	1.3	[103]
Head and Neck	437	RT (397) PT (40)	Toxicity (grade $\geq$ 3)	C	LR, RF, XGBoost	0.63–0.65	[116]
	2121	RT	Unplanned hospitalizations, feeding tube placement, weight loss	D, C	LR, DB, RF	0.64–0.76	[89]
	153	RT	Xerostomia	D, R, C	6 ML algorithms	SVM and extra-trees 0.74–0.89	[34]
	86	RT	Trismus	D	IBDM	Identification of a cluster of voxels related to toxicity	[8]
	427	RT	Xerostomia	D, C	LR, LASSO, RF	Best LR (0.70)	[49]
	173	RT	Acute dysphagia	D, C	SVM, RF	0.82	[22]

(continued)

Table 2 (continued)

Cancer type	No. of patients	Type of RT	Type of predicted toxicity	Features type	Classifier	Results[a]	References
	297	IMRT	Xerostomia (grade ≥ 2)	D, C	LR	Model updating is beneficial	[74]
	134	IMRT and PT	Esophagitis	R, D	LASSO	0.75	[75]
	47	3D-CRT	Sensorineural hearing loss	R, C	DS; Hoeffding	Acc = 76.08%, Pr = 75.9%	[1]
	37	IMRT	Parotid shrinkge, xerostomia	D, C	FL, NB	Acc = 0.79–0.86	[84]
	249	IMRT	Xerostomia, sticky saliva	R, D	Multivariate LR	0.77	[110]
	351	IMRT	Mucositis	D, C	LR, SVM, RF	0.71 (RF)	[21]
	1 (H&N); 1 (Prostate)	IMRT	Xerostomia (H&N); rectal bleeding (prostate)	D	DT, SVM	0.42% MAE (H&N); Acc = 97% (Prostate)	[128]
Liver	125	SBRT	Hepatobiliary toxicity	D, C	CNN	1.25	[46]
Lung	203	IMRT or PT	Pneumonitis	C	RF	1.06	[64]
	192	IMRT and 3D-CRT	Radiation pneumonitis	R, D, C	LASSO	0.68	[55]
	197	SBRT	Chest wall syndrome	D, C	DT, RF	n/a	[14]
	3496 (lung + brain + H&N)	RT	Classifiers comparison	D, C	DT, RF, ANN, SVM, elastic net, logit-boost	Best: elastic net, LR, and RF	[23]

(continued)

Table 2 (continued)

Cancer type	No. of patients	Type of RT	Type of predicted toxicity	Features type	Classifier	Results[a]	References
	14	SBRT	Lung injuries	R, D	LR	0.64–0.78	[69]
	115	RT	Esophagitis	D, C	LASSO	0.78	[44]
	54	3D-CRT	Pneumonitis	D, C	BN, LR, Single variable	0.66–0.83	[59]
	748	RT	Esophagitis	D, C	LR	0.83	[43]
	219	3D-CRT	Pneumonitis	D, C	SVM	1.16	[18]
	55 (H&N) 219 + 166 (Lung)	3D-CRT	Xerostomia, pneumonitis (166), esophagitis (216)	D, C	LR, SVM, ANN	Best: modified SVM	[27]
	219	RT	Radiation pneumonitis	D, C	DT, ANN, SVM, SOM	0.79	[19]
	234	RT	Radiation pneumonitis	D, C	DT	0.72	[20]
	142	3D-CRT	Pneumonitis	D	ANN	0.61–0.85	[100]
Prostate	64	IMRT (52 pts); 3D-CRT (12 pts)	Urinary toxicity; gastro-intestinal toxicity	R, D, C	LR	0.65–0.77	[70]
	33	IMRT	Cystitis	R	LR	0.62–0.75	[2]
	33	IMRT	Rectal wall changes	R	LR	0.46–0.81	[1]

(continued)

Table 2 (continued)

Cancer type	No. of patients	Type of RT	Type of predicted toxicity	Features type	Classifier	Results[a]	References
	351	RT	Rectal bleeding, fecal incontinence, urinary incontinence, nocturia	R, D, C	LR	0.58–0.73	[92]
	598	RT	Late fecal incontinence	D, C	ANN	0.78	[12]
	593	RT	Rectal bleeding	D, C	ICA	0.83, 0.80, 0.78	[32]
	324	BRT + -EBRT	GU toxicity symptoms	D, C, G	RF	0.7	[59]
	118	EBRT, BRT	GI toxicities	D	LR	Identification of spatial constraint for toxicity reduction	[71]
	368	RT	Rectal bleeding; erectile dysfunction	C, G	RF, LR	0.71 (rectal bleeding); 0.68 (erectile dysfunction)	[76]
	79	IMRT	Rectal toxicity (grade ≥ 2)	D, C	LR	1.28	[63]
	754	EBRT	Dysuria, hematuria, incontinence, frequency	D, C	LR, Elastic-net, SVM, RF, ANN, MARS	Best: LR, MARS AUC = 0.65	[120]

(continued)

Table 2 (continued)

Cancer type	No. of patients	Type of RT	Type of predicted toxicity	Features type	Classifier	Results[a]	References
	99	EBRT	Rectal bleeding	D	LDA, SVM, k-means, kNN, PCA, CP-DMA	Best: CP-DMA	[33]
	261	3D-CRT	Rectal toxicity, rectal bleeding	D, C	RF NTCP, NTCP	0.76, 0.66	[77]
	718	RT	Rectal bleeding	N/A	LR, ANN	0.655, 0.704	[105]
	321	RT	Acute bladder and rectal toxicity	D, C	ANN, SVM	0.70	[81]
	119	RT	Rectal bleeding; Nocturia	D	ANN	Sn & Sp > 55%	[36]

3D-CRT 3D conformal RT; *Acc* accuracy; *ANN* artificial neural network; *AUC* area under the curve; *BRT* brachytherapy; *CNN* convolutional neural network; *CP-DMA* canonical polyadic decomposition–deterministic multi-way analysis; *DS* decision stump; *DFS* disease free-survival; *DT* decision tree; *EBRT* external beam RT; *FL* fuzzy logic; *GB* gradient boosting; *GI* gastrointestinal; *GU* genitourinary; *H&N* head and neck; *IBDM* image-based data mining; *ICA* indipendent component analysis; *IMRT* intensity-modulated RT; *kNN* *k*-nearest neighbors; *LASSO* least absolute selection; *LC* local normal tissue complication probability; *OS* overall survival; *PCA* principal component analysis; *Pr* precision; *PT* proton therapy; *RF* random forest; *RT* radiotherapy; control; *LDA* linear discriminant analysis; *LR* logistic regression; *MAE* mean absolute error; *MARS* multivariate adaptive regression splines; *ML* machine learning; *n/a* not available; *NB* naïve bayes; *NTCP* shrinkage operator; *RUSBoost* random under-sampling boost; *SBRT* stereotactic body RT; *Sn* sensitivity; *Sp* specificity; *SOM* self-organizing maps; *SVM* support vector machine. Features were classified as clinical (C), dosimetric (D), genomic (G), or radiomic (R).

[a] If not specified, AUC values are reported

patients and (non)-small-cell lung cancer (NSCLC), as well as meningioma were taken for further study. Not any particular classifiers used were found to provide better results for all the datasets used, but net LR and RF performed comparatively better than others. On the basis of outcomes, authors used approaches to preselect classifier and inferred classifier's empirical selection provides better results with an increase in the mean AUC as 0.02.

6.2 *Breast*

Three studies have been found that used ML-based models to predict toxicity [67, 90, 95]. Saednia et al. proposed a novel method that detects the increasing temperature of the body surface by radiation dermatitis. With this irradiation, thermal images of breasts have been taken from ninety patients at four different points (i.e., before RT as well as after 5, 10, and 15 RT fractions). Common Terminology Criteria for Adverse Events (CTCAE) guidelines have been used to assess the toxicity of skin after RT [95]. In their study, Reddy et al., gave training to classifiers of three different types such as gradient boosted DT, LR, and RF using 2277 patients for identification of radiation toxicities like radiation dermatitis, fatigue, the pain of breast/chest wall, and moist desquamation occurrence. After validation, the performance of AUC reached up to 0.82, 0.56, 0.77, and 0.85, respectively, which proves that model predicts RT toxicities very precisely [90]. In their study, Mbah et al. highlighted the major causes of failure of models for prediction of toxicity. They used a dataset from two different studies in Germany that had 827 breast cancer patients treated with RT. The model is known as Least Absolute Selection and Shrinkage Operator (LASSO) LR has been utilized for the prediction of telangiectasia for all the available datasets separately. Then they tested these models on another dataset and surprisingly found that one variable tested for example hypertension with a negative coefficient on one available dataset, whereas a positive coefficient on the other [67].

6.3 *Esophagus*

Hart et al. published an ML-based model that predicted patients' toxicity suffering from esophagus cancer [39]. They identified how radiation pneumonitis clinical symptoms are related to metabolic activity of pulmonary after the treatment of [18F]-fluorodeoxyglucose positron emission tomography (FDG PET). They took up 101 patients having oesophageal cancer who initially completed thoracic RT, followed by computed tomography (CT) imaging/FDG PET in 3–12 weeks. A number of LR models were built pertaining to various treatment combinations and measuring variables, observing accuracy as 0.63 having $p \leq 0.032$, which usually demonstrated the significant relation of radiation pneumonitis and the response of pulmonary metabolic radiation.

6.4 Gynecological Cancers

There are three studies that majorly describe the prediction of toxicity outcomes in gynecological cancers following with only brachytherapy or along with external beam RT (EBRT). A limited number of datasets, for example only 35–42 patients having gynecological cancers, were utilized for training all the models with the help of SVM or CNN classifiers. In their study, Tian et al. proposed a model that predicts the formation of fistula with the help of an SVM classifier [103]. They used thirty-one varieties of features as predictor variables from samples of 35 patients having interstitial brachytherapy. With the limited number of datasets used they found that their model has 0.901 of accuracy. Similarly, in another study done by Chen et al., they observed a relationship between toxicity of rectal (CTCAE grade $\geq$ 2) and dosimetric features. They performed feature calculations on both the 2D accumulated rectal surface that is deformed and the 3D rectum surface on 42 patients. The models on which they utilized SVM classifiers showed 0.91 and 0.82 AUC values on a variety of features selection procedures [17]. In their cohort, Zhen et al., by using the transfer learning method, tested the feasibility of CNN to predict the toxicity of rectum on the ImageNet datasets [130].

6.5 Head and Neck

All published ML-based models that predict toxicity in head and neck cancers worked only on 37-2121 patients as training datasets. The toxicity outcomes that were predicted were acute mucositis, weight loss, late xerostomia, unplanned hospitalization, and parotid shrinkage by using RF, LR, fuzzy logic-based, and gradient boosting classifiers. Additionally, one study majorly focused on comparing the performance of a number of classifiers on a variety of datasets used [23]. The two major studies used three types of classifiers such as LR, RF, and gradient boosting models for identifying the placement of feeding tubes, weight loss, unplanned hospitalizations, and $\geq$3 toxicity [89, 116]. Reddy et al., took up huge datasets (2,121 patients) and compared about 700 clinical and treatment-related variables. After comparison, they achieved AUC values like 0.751, 0.755, and 0.640 for LR, gradient boosting, and RF, respectively [89]. Similarly, Wojcieszynski et al., in their cohort predicted grade $\geq$3 toxicity in datasets of 437 patients prior to 90 days and 180 days having c-statistic values of 0.65 and 0.63, respectively. It has also been observed that age, body mass index (BMI), an integral dose of the planning target volume (PTV), and integral dose to outside regions have shown the best statistical outcomes [116]. In another study, Nakatsugawa et al., through comparison of updating strategies demonstrated the implementation and role of continuous model revising [74]. Beasley et al. aimed to identify trismus that is induced by radiation by searching the specific image regions of CT with dose and toxicity association in patients suffering from head and neck cancers treated with RT. For achieving this goal, the image-based data mining

(IBDM) framework has been used on 86 patients in the study. The IBDM method helped in identifying voxel clusters linked with trismus, which was further internally validated by a method of DVH (86 patients) as well as externally on 35 patients [8]. By using a dataset of 427 head and neck cancer patients (RT treated), Jiang et al. identified xerostomia. Non-dosimetric features and classifiers such as LASSO LR, RF, and ridge LR were trained by using a dataset of planned dose that identified the effect of patterns of dose on xerostomia. Among the three classifiers used, ridge LR was the best of AUC as 0.70. This study reported combination of radio-morphology and ML approaches that shows the dose patterns effective on xerostomia and improved the planning of radiation treatment [49].

Dean et al. developed a new model that helps in predicting severe acute dysphagia among patients having head and neck cancer after treatment with RT. SVM, RF, and penalized LR (PLR) models were trained with clinical and dosimetric datasets and further validated internally on 173 and externally on 90 patients. It has been found from their outcomes that PLR model performance was better with an AUC value of 0.82 [22]. Gabry et al. identified whether a risk assessment of xerostomia can be treated with ML-based models consisting of demographic, radiomic, and dosimetric features instead of utilizing only the NTCP model. In this, the authors compared the outcomes of 10 techniques of data cleaning/class balancing, seven algorithms of classification, and six methods of feature selection using analysis of Nemenyi post-hoc and Friedman test. This study of 153 patients having head and neck cancer helps in the prediction of xerostomia at various stages of time that achieve AUC in the range of 0.74–0.88, where the SVM model performs better [34]. Abdollahi et al. aimed for predicting hearing loss in patients with head and neck cancer after treatment with radio-chemotherapy. From a study of 47 patients, CT images produce 490 image features of 94 cochleae and for performing each feature selection, prediction, and classification, 10 approaches of machine learning have been tested. In each case, the precision, accuracy, and AUC of ML algorithms were more than 0.70, where Hoeffding modeling and Decision Stump obtained the best precision and accuracy of 75.9% and 76.08%, respectively [1]. Pota et al., by using a very small dataset (37 patients) treated with IMRT, used a classifier based on fuzzy logic for predicting the occurrence of12-month xerostomia and parotid shrinkage. They used dosimetric parameters, clinical features, predictor variables combinations, and CT-based radiomic features and observed accuracies of up to 0.79 for xerostomia and 0.86 for parotid shrinkage and having performance comparable with naïve Bayes classifier [84].

Van Dijk et al., build a model using CT image biomarkers (IBMs) for predicting sticky saliva and xerostomia having cancer of the head and neck. For extracting IBMs, they collected planning CT scans (249 head and neck cancer patients) then utilized them for the creation of multivariable LR models and internally validated them with bootstrapping methods. They selected 24 features correlated with sticky saliva and 26 with xerostomia. The outcomes were identified as IBM "maximum CT intensity" was useful for predicting sticky saliva and "short-run emphasis" for xerostomia prediction [110]. Authors in research of Dean et al. worked on 351 patients having head and neck cancer and compared three classifiers like RF, SVM, and LR for predicting severe acute mucositis using variables such as dose-volume (DV) parameters, spatial dose metrics, and clinical datasets. Among all the classifiers used RF classifier performs best having an AUC of 0.71 [21]. On single head and neck cancer patients, Zhang et al. discovered SVM and DT models to predict the flow rate of saliva with tailored plan properties and DV constraints as input variables. They found that the mean absolute error (MAE) of the flow rate of saliva was very low (0.42%), and outcomes suggested, ML methods have been utilized for guiding planners for choosing DV constraint settings in a predictable manner [128]. In one of the studies, the authors identified different types of linear and non-linear kernels for generating interactions and finding the appropriate function of treatment responses. These parameters helped in capturing the accurate and potential interactions of heterogeneous variables. They used the dataset of 55 patients having head and neck cancer and also 2 patients with prostate cancer (PCa) datasets for the investigation of xerostomia. By analyzing the distributions of patients with principal component analysis (PCA), authors found SVM classifier performs best [27].

6.6 Liver

In their study, Ibragimov et al. utilized a CNN model (pre-trained) on 3D dose maps for predicting liver toxicity prior to SBRT. They also used variables of non-dosimetric patients as an additional number of inputs to put up into the network. With the help of the network's saliency maps, they predicted anatomical regions that were difficult to identify during SBRT. Using a dataset of 125 liver cancer patients, they managed the model that further helped in predicting hepatobiliary toxicity having an AUC of 0.85. Additionally, the authors found their deep learning model gave the prominent outcomes with two times lesser number of false-positive cases of toxicity compared with DVH-based predictions. Finally, they also predicted that the proximal portal vein's irradiation was majorly linked with two times larger number of toxicity cases [46].

6.7 Lung

The size of the datasets utilized for predicting lung cancers toxicity was ranging from 54 to 235 patients. A large number of studies focused on radiation-induced pneumonitis, whereas few were based on xerostomia, esophagitis, chest pain, and sticky saliva datasets. Chest pain may be caused by lung cancer RT due to fracture in ribs, radiation-induced neuropathy, chest wall edema, nerve branches, or chest wall fibrosis [14]. By using 197 patients, the authors used RF and decision tree methods with univariate and multivariate analyses, for investigating robust predictive features of chest wall pain. With the help of 219 patients having lung cancer given treatment with the RT dataset, Das et al. worked in two studies for predicting pneumonitis [19,

20]. Their first study in 2007, initiated with 234 RT-treated patients having lung cancer and then they trained model for pneumonitis (grade 2+) induced with radiation. The model combined the Lyman NTCP model (parametric) with weighted DTs (non-parametric) having an AUC value of 0.72 [20]. In their other study (2008), the authors developed a consensus model by linking four types of non-linear multivariate models like self-organizing maps, neural networks, decision trees, and SVMs that have an average AUC of 0.79 [19]. One common side effect in RT of lung cancer is esophagitis, but only two studies have been published yet [27, 28]. Their first study dealt with searching of variable selection methods as well as model building for assessing multivariate dose-response using 166 NSCLC patient's datasets. The authors used the LR classifier and suggested, performance will further improve with the fusion of DV factors having clinical variables considering input parameters [28]. In the second study, they used 219 lung cancer patients and identified different kernels (linear and non-linear) for finding functions of treatment-response. These parameters helped in capturing the accurate and potential interactions of heterogeneous variables. By analyzing the distributions of patients with principal component analysis (PCA), they observed SVM classifier performs best [27].

Niedzielski et al. proposed a new approach for utilizing CT imaging biomarkers for quantification of radiosensitivity of patients as well as predicting risk factors associated with esophagitis. They used a total of 134 NSCLC patient datasets treated with IMRT in 85 patients and passive-scatter PT in 49 patients. Instead of lower doses of radiation, patients who highly responded to radiation have been labeled as radiosensitive, by using K-means clustering having three nodes. And hence, the authors found that the addition of radiosensitive variables helped in improving the performance of the LASSO LR model with a mean AUC value of 0.75, in comparison to models not having radiosensitivity (average AUC value as 0.69) [75]. For predicting radiation-induced pneumonitis NSCLC patients of stage I who received SBRT, Valdes et al. developed "big data" clinical decision tools specific for these patients. They used 201 patients with lung cancer and their performance was evaluated by three different algorithms namely, random under-sampling (RUS) Boost, RF, and Decision Trees. In their feature selection studies, the most relevant feature for predicting pneumonitis was the ability of carbon monoxide that is diffused to and from the lungs and also the doses to bronchus, trachea, and heart [109]. For predicting esophagitis, Huang et al. worked in two studies. In their former study, they developed a model that assesses esophagitis in RT-treated NSCLC patients. They utilized a total of 748 patients that were tested with 3 various datasets from Washington University for testing LR models with clinical as well as dosimetric variables as well for correlation analysis. They found AUC as 0.83 on the best bivariate model they developed using variables such as concurrent chemotherapy and mean esophagus dose [43]. Their second research utilized new data of 115 NSCLC patients for testing the previously published model for predicting risk factors associated with severe acute esophagitis. By using the same logistic function having previously used predictor variables such as concurrent chemotherapy and mean esophagus dose, the authors found that this model had the AUC of 0.78 [44]. By using the dataset of NSCLC patients (54) after treatment with 3D conformal RT (3D-CRT), Lee et al. proposed a Bayesian network method with the addition of clinical, blood biomarker, and DV datasets. With this, they compared their Bayesian network method for managing AUC of 0.83 along with univariate predictors (AUC $\leq$ 0.69) as well as LR classifier (AUC = 0.77) [59]. For similar types of studies, for comparing testing and training errors in the discovery process, Valdes et al., utilized a stage I dataset for 201 NSCLC patients for developing various ML-based models along with decision trees, RF, and RUSBoost classifiers. They found, among these classifiers, RUSBoost performs best [109].

Su et al. identified a method for building an ANN, to compare three different methods of validation. They took DV data (from a 142 patients' dataset) with 3D-CRT treatment, and the ANN gave AUC as 0.85 [100]. Similarly, Chen et al. used a dataset of 219 patients to test an SVM model and also did a comparison of two models having dose variables only and having dose and non-dose variables, at an AUC of 0.71 and 0.76, respectively [18]. Using 203 NSCLC (stage II–III) treated people and RF approach Luna et al., evaluated 32 clinical features to predict the role of volume of lung receiving 20% of the dose, pack-year, and lung mean as identifiers of radiation pneumonitis. They analyzed both univariate and multivariate datasets and identified one new indicator [64]. Instead of using clinical- and dosimetric-based predictors, the models of image-based variables were also used to predict RT-related toxicity outcomes in patients with lung cancer. In this regard, Bousabarah et al. utilized radiomic features based on CT for predicting lung injuries up to fibrosis induced by radiation, with 110 stage I/IIa NSCLC patients that were given treatment with stereotactic body RT. Outcomes were known to work like image biomarkers, help in supporting the process of clinical decision, benefitted oncologists as well as patients [11]. In the same way, Moran et al. identified the role of radiomic features based on CT for the characterization of post-SBRT injuries of the lung. They assess the lung injury with the help of a classifier known as logistic regression, and AUC values ranging between 0.64 and 0.75 [69]. For radiation pneumonitis, Krafft et al. constructed a predictive model with the help of radiomic features extracted from CT. In their study, they used a combination of dosimetric and clinical features from a dataset of NSCLC patients (192), among them 152 (80%) patients given the treatment of IMRT and remaining by 3D-CRT. They built a classifier named LASSO logistic regression and found an average AUC of 0.68 [55].

6.8 Prostate

The toxicity outcomes from RT of prostate cancer (PCa) are gastrointestinal (GI) disorders, genitourinary (GU) side effects, erectile dysfunction (ED), and rectal toxicity. For predicting these outcomes, a number of ML classifiers such as ANN, SVM, multivariate adaptive regression splines (MARS), and RF as well as datasets in the range of 79–754 were used to train models. Lee et al., adopt gene ontology analysis and predicted the symptoms of GU toxicity using the dataset of 324 PCa patients with only models that were clinically valid and found to have an AUC of 0.7 [58]. With the use of ANN classification approaches, Carrara et al., in their study predicted late fecal incontinence in patients with PCa treated with RT. A total of 598 PCa patients were tested and their information was recorded as previous abdominal surgeries, dose distribution, drug treatments, and comorbidities, for identification of best-performing ANNs. They selected the best performing ANN model that showed a specificity of 63.7% and sensitivity of 80.8% as well as an AUC value of 0.78 [12]. To predict RB in 593 RT-treated PCa patients, Fargeas et al. used a model named independent component analysis (ICA), with clinical and dosimetric parameters. Their model was tested for three years of RB prediction, like 3 (AUC 0.68), 5 (AUC 0.66), and 8 (AUC 0.64) years. Interestingly, with the addition of ICA parameters, AUC values were enhanced for 3, 5, and 8 years, respectively [32]. A new classification algorithm is known as pre-conditioned random forest regression (PRFR) developed by Oh et al. used in single-nucleotide polymorphisms (SNPs) and genome-wide association studies (GWAS). They used a dataset of 368 RT-treated PCa patients and developed a predictive model of ED and rectal bleeding, with the inclusion of useful SNPs. And hence, by this method, they found AUC of 0.68 for ED as well as 0.71 for bleeding of the rectum [76]. Applying the Wilcoxon rank test and logistic regression model on 118 treated patients by combining EBRT/high-dose-rate brachytherapy, Moulton et al. identified how GI toxicities related to spatial dose distribution including stool frequency, tenesmus, diarrhea, and rectal bleeding [71]. Using patient clinical and dosimetry characteristics by treatment of 3D-CRT and IMRT, respectively, both Pella et al. [81] and Liu et al. [63] modeled rectal toxicity for people having prostate cancer. The model developed by Liu and Li using a combination of dosimetric and clinical variables achieved a better AUC value (0.88) [63]. Using the dataset of 321 conformal RT-treated patients, Pella et al. did a comparison of the ANN and SVM model after training them by clinical as well as dosimetric dataset and showed comparative performance of AUC of up to 0.7 [81].

Yahya et al. used a dataset of 754 PCa patients and compared classifiers like elastic-net, RF, SVM, MARS LR, and neural network for various urinary symptoms. Using comorbidities, medication intake, and dose-surface data as input parameters, their study analyzed hematuria, frequency, clinical endpoints dysuria, and incontinence, and found that MARS and LR perform best with 0.65 of AUC [120]. A novel method was developed by Fargeas et al., that predicts patients having bleeding of the rectum known as CP-DMA (canonical polyadic decomposition). Their outcomes were compared to various models and algorithms such as SVM, kNN, linear discriminant analysis, NTCP model, K-means, unsupervised multidimensional classification, and PCA-based unsupervised algorithm and have AUC of 0.85 [33]. On 261 3D-CRT treated PCa patients, Ospina et al. did a comparison of performances of classical and RF NTCP models for prediction of late rectal toxicity. They used both dosimetric and clinical features for the training of three RF models for predicting rectal toxicity endpoints. Their model predicted the performance ranging between 0.66 and 0.76, depending on toxicity [77]. By using only a single PCa patient, Zhang et al. proposed SVM and DT models for the prediction of rectal bleeding (RB) with tailored plan properties and DV constraints as input variables. This prediction has achieved an average of 97.04% of accuracy [128]. Tomatis et al. used a total of 718 PCa patients and compared the performances of ANN and LR models for the prediction of late

RB using DVH-based and clinical parameters. The authors concluded that the ANN model performs best with an AUC of 0.704 [105].

Gulliford et al. used ANN for predicting biological outcomes such as nocturia and rectal bleeding in 119 PCa patients followed by RT. Their analysis suggested that specificities and sensitivities of approximately 0.55 [36]. Mostafaei et al. investigated the importance of CT radiomics that help in predicting toxicities related to prostate RT, rectal acute, and bladder injuries in 64 PCa patients. The results showed that combining features of CT radiomic with dosimetric and clinical data helps in the enhancement of the predictive model's performance [70]. For investigation of urinary toxicity in PCa patients, Abdollahi et al. predicted magnetic resonance imaging (MRI) images of 33 PCa patients with different radiomics features. Overall, changes with features resulted in a better correlation having toxicity of radiation-induced and radiation of urinary dose [2]. Similarly, with an analysis of radiomics, Abdollahi et al. predict imaging biomarkers for the prediction of rectal toxicity on pre/post images of IMRT MRI [1]. Finally, using predictors like non-treatment related (NTR), texture features 3D dose distributions of patients, and DVH parameters, Rossi et al., developed predictive models like multivariate LR models for GU and GI toxicities. They considered fecal incontinence, RB, urinary incontinence, and nocturia for their study. For urinary incontinence, fecal incontinence, and RB, the values of AUC are enhanced with the addition of texture features and DVH to NTR features (from 0.68, 0.63, and 0.58 to 0.73 for each). While in the case of nocturia, the addition of parameters related to DVH leads to a little improvement (from 0.64 to 0.66) [92].

7 Challenges and Future of Machine Learning in Cancer Research

In the previous decades, techniques of ML have been evolved as one of the methods to screen disease, including cancers, and predict it at an early stage before they cause symptoms. Further, the availability of the large volume of cancer-related data made machine learning a suitable choice for cancer screening, diagnosis, classification, prognosis, and developing a treatment plan. Despite several promises, there are various obstacles and challenges associated with the machine learning applications in cancer research, some of them are being discussed in the following section.

(a) *Need for large-scale structured data*: The accuracy and success of machine learning models, including deep learning, depending on the availability of large-scale structure data. Further, the variability in the datasets pose challenges to creating a cohesive dataset for training and analysis [10, 57].

(b) *Imbalance class problem in high-dimensional data*: A dataset having the unequally distributed majority as well as minority classes is known as a class imbalance problem which may lead to poor accuracy in the minority class prediction as most of the standard classification algorithms favor the majority class. However, several approaches were reported in the literature that handles the class imbalance problem [60, 61].

(c) *Model and data biasedness*: A model bias is a phenomenon that arises due to prejudiced and erroneous assumptions adopted in the machine learning process. For example, giving more importance to some of the features in order to achieve better generalization. Data bias is also an important and prevalent problem that must be addressed. Some of the common data biases are *exclusion bias, sample bias, recall bias, measurement bias, racial bias, association bias,* and *observer bias.* Some of the methods to remove data bias in ML are: (i) Take care of general use-cases and potential outliers, (ii) Be sure that annotators and data labelers are consistent, diverse, create a gold standard, and get it reviewed by domain experts, (iii) Ensure data diversity by combining inputs from multiple sources, and (iv) Include bias testing an essential step in the data analysis process.

(d) *Efficient feature selection technique*: Feature selection is necessary for the reduction of dimension in high dimensional data. It helps in the selection of relevant features by filtering out redundant and irrelevant features, leading to a reduction of computational and storage costs without affecting the learning performance. The availability of big data poses challenges for the traditional feature selection algorithms, including scalability and stability issues.

(e) *Model scalability*: A machine learning algorithm is considered "scalable" if it is capable to deal with any amount of data without consuming growing amounts of resources. During this era, where the dataset is present in large numbers, scalable ML approaches are needed.

(f) *Heterogeneity in drug responses*: It is defined as the differential response of different patients to similar treatment. A drug that is effective for one person may induce adverse effects on another. Hence, heterogeneity in drug responses poses a serious challenge to machine learning applications in drug response modeling [94].

(g) *Drug synergy prediction issue*: Combinations of drugs are widely used for the treatment of cancer that provides several benefits such as lower toxicity, higher efficacy, and delay in onset of acquired drug resistance [97]. Unfortunately, synergistic combinations prediction with the use of experimental methods is a challenging task. Machine learning-based approaches help in predicting the possible combinations of large compound libraries among all synergistic.

(h) *Gain the trust of stakeholders*: Trust is an important parameter to gain popularity and reliability. Machine learning must again the significant trust of various stakeholders such as clinicians, researchers, and medical experts through interpretability, and prospective validation in clinical settings [10].

8 Conclusion

The availability of large-scale cancer genomics, proteomics, pharmacogenomics, and oncological datasets brought lots of hope for fighting against cancers. Apart from disease diagnosis, and identification of biomarkers, researchers are continuously working on the development of ML algorithms for personalized therapies for cancer patients, that generally identify drug synergy and responses of the drug to specific disease and drug-target interactions [68, 73]. This chapter presents an overall idea of the current state of the ML-based models in prediction, diagnosis, prognosis, and effective cancer therapeutics. It also focuses on ML-based models and techniques and their applications in various types of cancers. Finally, it presents possible challenges and the future aspects of oncological research based on ML models.

References

1. Abdollahi, H., Mostafaei, S., Cheraghi, S., Shiri, I., Mahdavi, S. R., & Kazemnejad, A. (2018). Cochlea CT radiomics predicts chemoradiotherapy induced sensorineural hearing loss in head and neck cancer patients: A machine learning and multi-variable modelling study. *Physica Medica, 45*, 192–197.
2. Abdollahi, H., Tanha, K., Mofid, B., Razzaghdoust, A., Saadipoor, A., Khalafi, L., Bakhshandeh, M., & Mahdavi, S. R. (2019). MRI radiomic analysis of IMRT-induced bladder wall changes in prostate cancer patients: a relationship with radiation dose and toxicity. *Journal of Medical Imaging and Radiation Sciences, 50*(2), 252-260.
3. Ahmad, L. G., Eshlaghy, A. T., Poorebrahimi, A., Ebrahimi, M., & Razavi, A. R. (2013). Using three machine learning techniques for predicting breast cancer recurrence. *Journal of Health and Medical Informatics, 4*(124), 3.
4. Albayrak, A., & Bilgin, G. (2016, November). Mitosis detection using convolutional neural network-based features. In *2016 IEEE 17th International symposium on computational intelligence and informatics (CINTI)* (pp. 000335–000340). IEEE.
5. Alkadi, R., Taher, F., El-Baz, A., & Werghi, N. (2019).A deep learning-based approach for the detection and localization of prostate cancer in T2 magnetic resonance images. *Journal of Digital Imaging, 32*(5), 793–807.
6. Ankita, R., Kumari, C. U., Mehdi, M. J., Tejashwini, N., & Pavani, T. (2019). Lung cancer image-feature extraction and classification using GLCM and SVM classifier. *International Journal of Innovative Technology Exploring Engineering, 8*(11), 2211–2215.
7. Ayer, T., Alagoz, O., Chhatwal, J., Shavlik, J. W., Kahn, C. E., Jr., & Burnside, E. S. (2010). Breast cancer risk estimation with artificial neural networks revisited: Discrimination and calibration. *Cancer, 116*(14), 3310–3321.
8. Beasley, W., Thor, M., McWilliam, A., Green, A., Mackay, R., Slevin, N., Olsson, C., Pettersson, N., Finizia, C., Estilo, C., Riaz, N., & van Herk, M. (2018). Image-based data mining to probe dosimetric correlates of radiation-induced trismus. *International Journal of Radiation Oncology* Biology* Physics, 102*(4), 1330–1338.
9. Beeravolu, A. R., Azam, S., Jonkman, M., Shanmugam, B., Kannoorpatti, K., & Anwar, A. (2021). Preprocessing of breast cancer images to create datasets for deep-CNN. *IEEE Access, 9*, 33438–33463.
10. Bertsimas, D., & Wiberg, H. (2020). Machine learning in oncology: Methods, applications, and challenges. *JCO Clinical Cancer Informatics, 4*, 885–894.

11. Bousabarah, K., Temming, S., Hoevels, M., Borggrefe, J., Baus, W. W., Ruess, D., Visser-Vandewalle, V., Ruge, M., Kocher, M., & Treuer, H. (2019). Radiomic analysis of planning computed tomograms for predicting radiation-induced lung injury and outcome in lung cancer patients treated with robotic stereotactic body radiation therapy. *Strahlentherapie und Onkologie, 195*(9), 830–842.
12. Carrara, M., Massari, E., Cicchetti, A., Giandini, T., Avuzzi, B., Palorini, F., Stucchi, C., & Valdagni, R. (2018). Development of a ready-to-use graphical tool based on artificial neural network classification: application for the prediction of late fecal incontinence after prostate cancer radiation therapy. *International Journal of Radiation Oncology* Biology* Physics, 102*(5), 1533–1542.
13. Chang, S. W., Abdul-Kareem, S., Merican, A. F., & Zain, R. B. (2013). Oral cancer prognosis based on clinicopathologic and genomic markers using a hybrid of feature selection and machine learning methods. *BMC Bioinformatics, 14*(1), 1–15.
14. Chao, H. H., Valdes, G., Luna, J. M., Heskel, M., Berman, A. T., Solberg, T. D., & Simone, C. B. (2018). Exploratory analysis using machine learning to predict for chest wall pain in patients with stage I non-small-cell lung cancer treated with stereotactic body radiation therapy. *Journal of Applied Clinical Medical Physics, 19*(5), 539–546.
15. Chen, Y. C., Ke, W. C., & Chiu, H. W. (2014). Risk classification of cancer survival using ANN with gene expression data from multiple laboratories. *Computers in Biology and Medicine, 48*, 1–7.
16. Chen, H., Qi, X., Yu, L., & Heng, P. A. (2016). DCAN: Deep contour-aware networks for accurate gland segmentation. In *Proceedings of the IEEE conference on computer vision and pattern recognition* (pp. 2487–2496).
17. Chen, J., Chen, H., Zhong, Z., Wang, Z., Hrycushko, B., Zhou, L., Jiang, S., Albuquerque, K., Gu, X., & Zhen, X. (2018). Investigating rectal toxicity associated dosimetric features with deformable accumulated rectal surface dose maps for cervical cancer radiotherapy. *Radiation Oncology, 13*(1), 1–10.
18. Chen, S., Zhou, S., Yin, F. F., Marks, L. B., & Das, S. K. (2007). Investigation of the support vector machine algorithm to predict lung radiation-induced pneumonitis. *Medical Physics, 34*(10), 3808–3814.
19. Das, S. K., Chen, S., Deasy, J. O., Zhou, S., Yin, F. F., & Marks, L. B. (2008). Combining multiple models to generate consensus: Application to radiation-induced pneumonitis prediction. *Medical Physics, 35*(11), 5098–5109.
20. Das, S. K., Zhou, S., Zhang, J., Yin, F. F., Dewhirst, M. W., & Marks, L. B. (2007). Predicting lung radiotherapy-induced pneumonitis using a model combining parametric Lyman probit with nonparametric decision trees. *International Journal of Radiation Oncology Biology Physics, 68*(4), 1212–1221.
21. Dean, J. A., Wong, K. H., Welsh, L. C., Jones, A. B., Schick, U., Newbold, K. L., Bhide, S. A., Harrington, K. J., Nutting, C. M., & Gulliford, S. L. (2016). Normal tissue complication probability (NTCP) modelling using spatial dose metrics and machine learning methods for severe acute oral mucositis resulting from head and neck radiotherapy. *Radiotherapy and Oncology, 120*(1), 21-27.
22. Dean, J., Wong, K., Gay, H., Welsh, L., Jones, A. B., Schick, U., & Gulliford, S. (2018). Incorporating spatial dose metrics in machine learning-based normal tissue complication probability (NTCP) models of severe acute dysphagia resulting from head and neck radiotherapy. Clinical and translational radiation oncology, 8, 27–39.
23. Deist, T. M., Dankers, F. J., Valdes, G., Wijsman, R., Hsu, I. C., Oberije, C., & Lambin, P. (2019). Erratum: Machine learning algorithms for outcome prediction in (chemo) radiotherapy: An empirical comparison of classifiers, *Medical physics, 45*(7), 3449–3459.
24. Delen, D., Walker, G., & Kadam, A. (2005). Predicting breast cancer survivability: A comparison of three data mining methods. *Artificial Intelligence in Medicine, 34*(2), 113–127.
25. Demyanov, S., Chakravorty, R., Abedini, M., Halpern, A., & Garnavi, R. (2016, April). Classification of dermoscopy patterns using deep convolutional neural networks. In *2016 IEEE 13th International symposium on biomedical imaging (ISBI)* (pp. 364–368). IEEE.

26. Dhungel, N., Carneiro, G., & Bradley, A. P. (2015, November). Automated mass detection in mammograms using cascaded deep learning and random forests. In *2015 International conference on digital image computing: techniques and applications (DICTA)* (pp. 1–8). IEEE.
27. El Naqa, I., Bradley, J. D., Lindsay, P. E., Hope, A. J., & Deasy, J. O. (2009). Predicting radiotherapy outcomes using statistical learning techniques. *Physics in Medicine & Biology, 54*(18), S9.
28. El Naqa, I., Bradley, J., Blanco, A. I., Lindsay, P. E., Vicic, M., Hope, A., & Deasy, J. O. (2006). Multivariable modeling of radiotherapy outcomes, including dose–volume and clinical factors. *International Journal of Radiation Oncology* Biology* Physics, 64*(4), 1275–1286.
29. Ertosun, M. G., & Rubin, D. L. (2015, November). Probabilistic visual search for masses within mammography images using deep learning. In *2015 IEEE International conference on bioinformatics and biomedicine (BIBM)* (pp. 1310–1315).IEEE.
30. Esteva, A., Kuprel, B., Novoa, R. A., Ko, J., Swetter, S. M., Blau, H. M., & Thrun, S. (2017). Dermatologist-level classification of skin cancer with deep neural networks. *Nature, 542*(7639), 115–118.
31. Exarchos, K. P., Goletsis, Y., & Fotiadis, D. I. (2011). Multiparametric decision support system for the prediction of oral cancer reoccurrence. *IEEE Transactions on Information Technology in Biomedicine, 16*(6), 1127–1134.
32. Fargeas, A., Acosta, O., Arrango, J. D. O., Ferhat, A., Costet, N., Albera, L., Azria, D., Fenoglietto, P., Créhange, G., Beckendorf, V., Hatt, M., & de Crevoisier, R. (2018). Independent component analysis for rectal bleeding prediction following prostate cancer radiotherapy. *Radiotherapy and Oncology, 126*(2), 263–269.
33. Fargeas, A., Albera, L., Kachenoura, A., Dréan, G., Ospina, J. D., Coloigner, J., Lafond, C., Delobel, J. B., De Crevoisier, R., & Acosta, O. (2015). On feature extraction and classification in prostate cancer radiotherapy using tensor decompositions. *Medical Engineering & Physics, 37*(1), 126–131.
34. Gabryś, H. S., Buettner, F., Sterzing, F., Hauswald, H., & Bangert, M. (2018).Design and selection of machine learning methods using radiomics and dosiomics for normal tissue complication probability modeling of xerostomia. *Frontiers in Oncology, 8*, 35.
35. Gevaert, O., Smet, F. D., Timmerman, D., Moreau, Y., & Moor, B. D. (2006). Predicting the prognosis of breast cancer by integrating clinical and microarray data with Bayesian networks. *Bioinformatics, 22*(14), e184–e190.
36. Gulliford, S. L., Webb, S., Rowbottom, C. G., Corne, D. W., & Dearnaley, D. P. (2004). Use of artificial neural networks to predict biological outcomes for patients receiving radical radiotherapy of the prostate. *Radiotherapy and Oncology, 71*(1), 3–12.
37. Guo, Y., Gao, Y., & Shen, D. (2015). Deformable MR prostate segmentation via deep feature learning and sparse patch matching. *IEEE Transactions on Medical Imaging, 35*(4), 1077–1089.
38. Han, F., Wang, H., Zhang, G., Han, H., Song, B., Li, L., Moore, W., Lu, H., Zhao, H., & Liang, Z. (2015). Texture feature analysis for computer-aided diagnosis on pulmonary nodules. *Journal of Digital Imaging, 28*(1), 99–115.
39. Hart, J. P., McCurdy, M. R., Ezhil, M., Wei, W., Khan, M., Luo, D., Munden, R. F., Johnson, V. E., & Guerrero, T. M. (2008). Radiation pneumonitis: correlation of toxicity with pulmonary metabolic radiation response. *International Journal of Radiation Oncology* Biology* Physics, 71*(4), 967–971.
40. He, J., Dong, Q., & Yi, S. (2018, May). Prediction of skin cancer based on convolutional neural network. In *International conference on mechatronics and intelligent robotics* (pp. 1223–1229). Springer.
41. Hoshyar, A. N., Al-Jumaily, A., & Hoshyar, A. N. (2014). The beneficial techniques in preprocessing step of skin cancer detection system comparing. *Procedia Computer Science, 42*, 25–31.
42. Howlader, N. N. A. K. M., Noone, A. M., Krapcho, M., Garshell, J., Neyman, N., Altekruse, S. F., Kosary, C. L., Yu, M., Ruhl, J., Tatalovich, Z., Cho, H., & Cronin, K. (2013). *SEER cancer statistics review*, 1975–2010. Bethesda, MD: National Cancer Institute, 21, 12.

43. Huang, E. X., Bradley, J. D., El Naqa, I., Hope, A. J., Lindsay, P. E., Bosch, W. R., Matthews, J. W., Sause, W. T., Graham, M. V., & Deasy, J. O. (2012). Modeling the risk of radiation-induced acute esophagitis for combined Washington University and RTOG trial 93–11 lung cancer patients. *International Journal of Radiation Oncology* Biology* Physics, 82*(5), 1674–1679.
44. Huang, E. X., Robinson, C. G., Molotievschi, A., Bradley, J. D., Deasy, J. O., & Oh, J. H. (2017). Independent test of a model to predict severe acute esophagitis. *Advances in Radiation Oncology, 2*(1), 37–43.
45. Hussein, S., Gillies, R., Cao, K., Song, Q., & Bagci, U. (2017, April). Tumornet: Lung nodule characterization using multi-view convolutional neural network with gaussian process. In *2017 IEEE 14th International Symposium on Biomedical Imaging (ISBI 2017)* (pp. 1007–1010). IEEE.
46. Ibragimov, B., Toesca, D., Chang, D., Yuan, Y., Koong, A., & Xing, L. (2018). Development of deep neural network for individualized hepatobiliary toxicity prediction after liver SBRT. *Medical Physics, 45*(10), 4763–4774.
47. Iqbal, M. J., Javed, Z., Sadia, H., Qureshi, I. A., Irshad, A., Ahmed, R., Malik, K., Raza, S., Abbas, A., Pezzani, R., & Sharifi-Rad, J. (2021). Clinical applications of artificial intelligence and machine learning in cancer diagnosis: looking into the future. *Cancer Cell International, 21*(1), 1–11.
48. Isaksson, L. J., Pepa, M., Zaffaroni, M., Marvaso, G., Alterio, D., Volpe, S., Corrao, G., Augugliaro, M., Starzyńska, A., Leonardi, M. C., Orecchia, R., & Jereczek-Fossa, B. A. (2020). Machine learning-based models for prediction of toxicity outcomes in radiotherapy. *Frontiers in Oncology, 10*, 790.
49. Jiang, W., Lakshminarayanan, P., Hui, X., Han, P., Cheng, Z., Bowers, M., Shpitser, I., Siddiqui, S., Taylor, R.H., Quon, H., & McNutt, T. (2019). Machine learning methods uncover radiomorphologic dose patterns in salivary glands that predict xerostomia in patients with head and neck cancer. *Advances in Radiation Oncology, 4*(2), 401–412.
50. Kallenberg, M., Petersen, K., Nielsen, M., Ng, A. Y., Diao, P., Igel, C., Vachon, C. M., Holland, K., Winkel, R. R., Karssemeijer, N., & Lillholm, M. (2016). Unsupervised deep learning applied to breast density segmentation and mammographic risk scoring. *IEEE Transactions on Medical Imaging, 35*(5), 1322–1331.
51. Khan, F. N., Ahmad, S., & Raza, K. (2021). Clinical Applications of Next-Generation Sequence Analysis in Acute Myelogenous Leukemia. In *Translational bioinformatics applications in healthcare* (pp. 41–66). CRC Press.
52. Khan, F. N., Khanam, A. A., Ramlal, A., & Ahmad, S. (2021). A review on predictive systems and data models for covid-19. In *Computational intelligence methods in COVID-19: Surveillance, prevention, prediction and diagnosis* (pp. 123–164). Springer.
53. Kim, J., & Shin, H. (2013). Breast cancer survivability prediction using labeled, unlabeled, and pseudo-labeled patient data. *Journal of the American Medical Informatics Association, 20*(4), 613–618.
54. Kim, W., Kim, K. S., Lee, J. E., Noh, D. Y., Kim, S. W., Jung, Y. S., Park, M.Y., & Park, R. W. (2012). Development of novel breast cancer recurrence prediction model using support vector machine. *Journal of Breast Cancer, 15*(2), 230–238.
55. Krafft, S. P., Rao, A., Stingo, F., Briere, T. M., Court, L. E., Liao, Z., & Martel, M. K. (2018). The utility of quantitative CT radiomics features for improved prediction of radiation pneumonitis. *Medical Physics, 45*(11), 5317–5324.
56. Källén, H., Molin, J., Heyden, A., Lundström, C., &Åström, K. (2016, April). Towards grading gleason score using generically trained deep convolutional neural networks. In *2016 IEEE 13th International symposium on biomedical imaging (ISBI)* (pp. 1163–1167). IEEE.
57. Landhuis, E. (2020). Deep learning takes on tumours. *Nature, 580*(7804), 551–554.
58. Lee, S., Kerns, S., Ostrer, H., Rosenstein, B., Deasy, J. O., & Oh, J. H. (2018). Machine learning on a genome-wide association study to predict late genitourinary toxicity after prostate radiation therapy. *International Journal of Radiation Oncology* Biology* Physics, 101*(1), 128–135.

59. Lee, S., Ybarra, N., Jeyaseelan, K., Faria, S., Kopek, N., Brisebois, P., Bradley, J. D., Robinson, C., Seuntjens, J., & El Naqa, I. (2015). Bayesian network ensemble as a multivariate strategy to predict radiation pneumonitis risk. *Medical Physics, 42*(5), 2421–2430.
60. Leevy, J. L., Khoshgoftaar, T. M., Bauder, R. A., & Seliya, N. (2018). A survey on addressing high-class imbalance in big data. *Journal of Big Data, 5*(1), 1–30.
61. Lin, W. J., & Chen, J. J. (2013). Class-imbalanced classifiers for high-dimensional data. *Briefings in Bioinformatics, 14*(1), 13–26.
62. Listgarten, J., Damaraju, S., Poulin, B., Cook, L., Dufour, J., Driga, A., Mackey, J., Wishart, D., Greiner, R., & Zanke, B. (2004). Predictive models for breast cancer susceptibility from multiple single nucleotide polymorphisms. *Clinical Cancer Research, 10*(8), 2725–2737.
63. Liu, X., Li, J., Wu, T., Schild, S. E., Schild, M. H., Wong, W., Vora, S., & Fatyga, M. (2016). Patient specific characteristics are an important factor that determines the risk of acute grade $\geq$2 rectal toxicity in patients treated for prostate cancer with IMRT and daily image guidance based on implanted gold markers. *OMICS Journal of Radiology, 5*(3).
64. Luna, J. M., Chao, H. H., Diffenderfer, E. S., Valdes, G., Chinniah, C., Ma, G., Cengel, K. A., Solberg, T. D., Berman, A.T., & Simone II, C. B. (2019). Predicting radiation pneumonitis in locally advanced stage II–III non-small cell lung cancer using machine learning. *Radiotherapy and Oncology, 133*, 106–112.
65. Ma, L., Guo, R., Zhang, G., Tade, F., Schuster, D. M., Nieh, P., Master, V., & Fei, B. (2017, February). Automatic segmentation of the prostate on CT images using deep learning and multi-atlas fusion. In *Medical imaging 2017: Image processing* (Vol. 10133, p. 101332O). International Society for Optics and Photonics.
66. Masood, A., Al-Jumaily, A., & Anam, K. (2015, April). Self-supervised learning model for skin cancer diagnosis. In *2015 7th International IEEE/EMBS conference on neural engineering (NER)* (pp. 1012–1015). IEEE.
67. Mbah, C., Thierens, H., Thas, O., De Neve, J., Chang-Claude, J., Seibold, P., Botma, A., West, C., & De Ruyck, K. (2016). Pitfalls in prediction modeling for normal tissue toxicity in radiation therapy: An illustration with the individual radiation sensitivity and mammary carcinoma risk factor investigation cohorts. *International Journal of Radiation Oncology* Biology* Physics, 95*(5), 1466–1476.
68. Mihaylov, I., Nisheva, M., & Vassilev, D. (2019). Application of machine learning models for survival prognosis in breast cancer studies. *Information, 10*(3), 93.
69. Moran, A., Daly, M. E., Yip, S. S., & Yamamoto, T. (2017). Radiomics-based assessment of radiation-induced lung injury after stereotactic body radiotherapy. *Clinical Lung Cancer, 18*(6), e425–e431.
70. Mostafaei, S., Abdollahi, H., Dehkordi, S. K., Shiri, I., Razzaghdoust, A., Moghaddam, S. H. Z., Saadipoor, A., Koosha, F., Cheraghi, S., & Mahdavi, S. R. (2020). CT imaging markers to improve radiation toxicity prediction in prostate cancer radiotherapy by stacking regression algorithm. *La Radiologia Medica, 125*(1), 87–97.
71. Moulton, C. R., House, M. J., Lye, V., Tang, C. I., Krawiec, M., Joseph, D. J., Denham, J.W., & Ebert, M. A. (2017). Spatial features of dose–surface maps from deformably-registered plans correlate with late gastrointestinal complications. *Physics in Medicine & Biology, 62*(10), 4118.
72. Munir, K., Elahi, H., Ayub, A., Frezza, F., & Rizzi, A. (2019). Cancer diagnosis using deep learning: A bibliographic review. *Cancers, 11*(9), 1235.
73. Murthy, N. S., & Bethala, C. (2021). Review paper on research direction towards cancer prediction and prognosis using machine learning and deep learning models. *Journal of Ambient Intelligence and Humanized Computing*, 1–19.
74. Nakatsugawa, M., Cheng, Z., Kiess, A., Choflet, A., Bowers, M., Utsunomiya, K., Sugiyama, S., Wong, J., Quon, H., & McNutt, T. (2019). The needs and benefits of continuous model updates on the accuracy of RT-induced toxicity prediction models within a learning health system. *International Journal of Radiation Oncology* Biology* Physics, 103*(2), 460–467.
75. Niedzielski, J. S., Yang, J., Stingo, F., Liao, Z., Gomez, D., Mohan, R., Martel, M., Briere, T., & Court, L. (2017). A novel methodology using CT imaging biomarkers to quantify radiation sensitivity in the esophagus with application to clinical trials. *Scientific Reports, 7*(1), 1–9.

76. Oh, J. H., Kerns, S., Ostrer, H., Powell, S. N., Rosenstein, B., & Deasy, J. O. (2017). Computational methods using genome-wide association studies to predict radiotherapy complications and to identify correlative molecular processes. *Scientific Reports, 7*(1), 1–10.
77. Ospina, J. D., Zhu, J., Chira, C., Bossi, A., Delobel, J. B., Beckendorf, V., Dubray, B., Lagrange, J. L., Correa, J. C., Simon, A., & de Crevoisier, R. (2014). Random forests to predict rectal toxicity following prostate cancer radiation therapy. *International Journal of Radiation Oncology* Biology* Physics, 89*(5), 1024–1031.
78. Park, C., Ahn, J., Kim, H., & Park, S. (2014). Integrative gene network construction to analyze cancer recurrence using semi-supervised learning. *PloS One, 9*(1), e86309.
79. Park, K., Ali, A., Kim, D., An, Y., Kim, M., & Shin, H. (2013). Robust predictive model for evaluating breast cancer survivability. *Engineering Applications of Artificial Intelligence, 26*(9), 2194–2205.
80. Paul, R., Hawkins, S. H., Hall, L. O., Goldgof, D. B., & Gillies, R. J. (2016, October). Combining deep neural network and traditional image features to improve survival prediction accuracy for lung cancer patients from diagnostic CT. In *2016 IEEE international conference on systems, man, and cybernetics (SMC)* (pp. 002570–002575). IEEE.
81. Pella, A., Cambria, R., Riboldi, M., Jereczek-Fossa, B. A., Fodor, C., Zerini, D., Torshabi, A.E., Cattani, F., Garibaldi, C., Pedroli, G., Baroni, G., & Orecchia, R. (2011). Use of machine learning methods for prediction of acute toxicity in organs at risk following prostate radiotherapy. *Medical Physics, 38*(6Part1), 2859–2867.
82. Pereira, S., Pinto, A., Alves, V., & Silva, C. A. (2016). Braintumor segmentation using convolutional neural networks in MRI images. *IEEE Transactions on Medical Imaging, 35*(5), 1240–1251.
83. Pomponiu, V., Nejati, H., & Cheung, N. M. (2016, September). Deepmole: Deep neural networks for skin mole lesion classification. In *2016 IEEE international conference on image processing (ICIP)* (pp. 2623–2627). IEEE.
84. Pota, M., Scalco, E., Sanguineti, G., Farneti, A., Cattaneo, G. M., Rizzo, G., & Esposito, M. (2017). Early prediction of radiotherapy-induced parotid shrinkage and toxicity based on CT radiomics and fuzzy classification. *Artificial Intelligence in Medicine, 81*, 41–53.
85. Quan, T. M., Nguyen-Duc, T., & Jeong, W. K. (2017). *Compressed sensing MRI reconstruction with cyclic loss in generative adversarial networks.* arXiv preprint arXiv:1709.00753.
86. Raoof, S. S., Jabbar, M. A., & Fathima, S. A. (2020, March). Lung Cancer prediction using machine learning: A comprehensive approach. In *2020 2nd International conference on innovative mechanisms for industry applications (ICIMIA)* (pp. 108–115). IEEE.
87. Raza, K., & Singh, N. K. (2021). A tour of unsupervised deep learning for medical image analysis current medical imaging. *Bentham Science, 17*(9), 1059–1077. https://doi.org/10.2174/1573405617666210127154257
88. Raza, K.. (2019). Improving the prediction accuracy of heart disease with ensemble learning and majority voting rule. In *In Advances in ubiquitous sensing applications for healthcare, U-healthcare monitoring systems: Design and applications.* Academic Press, Elsevier, pp. 179–196. https://doi.org/10.1016/B978-0-12-815370-3.00008-6.
89. Reddy, J. P., Lindsay, W. D., Berlind, C. G., Ahern, C. A., Holmes, A., Smith, B. D., Phan, J., Frank, S. J., Gunn, G. B., Rosenthal, D. I., Morrison, W. H., & Fuller, C. D. (2019). Applying a machine learning approach to predict acute radiation toxicities for head and neck cancer patients. *International Journal of Radiation Oncology, Biology, Physics, 105*(1), S69.
90. Reddy, J., Lindsay, W. D., Berlind, C. G., Ahern, C. A., & Smith, B. D. (2018). Applying a machine learning approach to predict acute toxicities during radiation for breast cancer patients. *International Journal of Radiation Oncology, Biology, Physics, 102*(3), S59.
91. Rosado, P., Lequerica-Fernández, P., Villallaín, L., Peña, I., Sanchez-Lasheras, F., & De Vicente, J. C. (2013). Survival model in oral squamous cell carcinoma based on clinicopathological parameters, molecular markers and support vector machines. *Expert Systems With Applications, 40*(12), 4770–4776.
92. Rossi, L., Bijman, R., Schillemans, W., Aluwini, S., Cavedon, C., Witte, M., Incrocci, L., & Heijmen, B. (2018). Texture analysis of 3D dose distributions for predictive modelling of toxicity rates in radiotherapy. *Radiotherapy and Oncology, 129*(3), 548–553.

93. Sabbaghi, S., Aldeen, M., & Garnavi, R. (2016, August).A deep bag-of-features model for the classification of melanomas in dermoscopyimages. In *2016 38th Annual international conference of the IEEE engineering in medicine and biology society (EMBC)* (pp. 1369–1372). IEEE.
94. Sacristán, J. A., & Avendaño-Solá, C. (2015). On heterogeneity of treatment effects and clinical freedom. *International Journal of Clinical Practice, 69*(1), 6–8.
95. Saednia, K., Tabbarah, S., Lagree, A., Wu, T., Klein, J., Garcia, E., Hall, M., Chow, E., Rakovitch, E., Childs, C., Sadeghi-Naini, A., & Tran, W. T. (2020). Quantitative thermal imaging biomarkers to detect acute skin toxicity from breast radiation therapy using supervised machine learning. *International Journal of Radiation Oncology* Biology* Physics, 106*(5), 1071–1083.
96. Shen, W., Zhou, M., Yang, F., Yu, D., Dong, D., Yang, C., Zang, Y., & Tian, J. (2017). Multi-crop convolutional neural networks for lung nodule malignancy suspiciousness classification. *Pattern Recognition, 61*, 663–673.
97. Sidorov, P., Naulaerts, S., Ariey-Bonnet, J., Pasquier, E., & Ballester, P. J. (2019). Predicting synergism of cancer drug combinations using NCI-ALMANAC data. *Frontiers in Chemistry, 7*, 509.
98. Spanhol, F. A., Oliveira, L. S., Petitjean, C., &Heutte, L. (2016, July). Breast cancer histopathological image classification using convolutional neural networks. In *2016 International joint conference on neural networks (IJCNN)* (pp. 2560–2567). IEEE.
99. Stojadinovic, A., Nissan, A., Eberhardt, J., Chua, T. C., Pelz, J. O., & Esquivel, J. (2011). Development of a bayesian belief network model for personalized prognostic risk assessment in colon carcinomatosis. *The American Surgeon, 77*(2), 221–230.
100. Su, M., Miften, M., Whiddon, C., Sun, X., Light, K., & Marks, L. (2005). An artificial neural network for predicting the incidence of radiation pneumonitis. *Medical Physics, 32*(2), 318–325.
101. Sumithra, R., Suhil, M., & Guru, D. S. (2015). Segmentation and classification of skin lesions for disease diagnosis. *Procedia Computer Science, 45*, 76–85.
102. Suzuki, S., Zhang, X., Homma, N., Ichiji, K., Sugita, N., Kawasumi, Y., Ishibashi, T., & Yoshizawa, M. (2016, September). Mass detection using deep convolutional neural network for mammographic computer-aided diagnosis. In *2016 55th Annual conference of the society of instrument and control engineers of Japan (SICE)* (pp. 1382–1386). IEEE
103. Tian, Z., Yen, A., Zhou, Z., Shen, C., Albuquerque, K., & Hrycushko, B. (2019). A machine-learning–based prediction model of fistula formation after interstitial brachytherapy for locally advanced gynecological malignancies. *Brachytherapy, 18*(4), 530–538.
104. Tian, Z., Liu, L., Zhang, Z., & Fei, B. (2018). PSNet: Prostate segmentation on MRI based on a convolutional neural network. *Journal of Medical Imaging, 5*(2), 021208.
105. Tomatis, S., Rancati, T., Fiorino, C., Vavassori, V., Fellin, G., Cagna, E., Mauro, F. A., Girelli, G., Monti, A., Baccolini, M., Naldi, G., & Valdagni, R. (2012). Late rectal bleeding after 3D-CRT for prostate cancer: development of a neural-network-based predictive model. *Physics in Medicine & Biology, 57*(5), 1399.
106. Tseng, C. J., Lu, C. J., Chang, C. C., & Chen, G. D. (2014). Application of machine learning to predict the recurrence-proneness for cervical cancer. *Neural Computing and Applications, 24*(6), 1311–1316.
107. Urbanowicz, R. J., Andrew, A. S., Karagas, M. R., & Moore, J. H. (2013). Role of genetic heterogeneity and epistasis in bladder cancer susceptibility and outcome: A learning classifier system approach. *Journal of the American Medical Informatics Association, 20*(4), 603–612.
108. Urgiriye, A., & Bhartiya, R. (2020).Review of s. *International Journal of Scientific Research & Engineering Trends, 6*(6).
109. Valdes, G., Solberg, T. D., Heskel, M., Ungar, L., & Simone, C. B., II. (2016). Using machine learning to predict radiation pneumonitis in patients with stage I non-small cell lung cancer treated with stereotactic body radiation therapy. *Physics in Medicine & Biology, 61*(16), 6105.
110. van Dijk, L. V., Brouwer, C. L., van der Schaaf, A., Burgerhof, J. G., Beukinga, R. J., Langendijk, J. A., Sijtsema, N. M., & Steenbakkers, R. J. (2017). CT image biomarkers

to improve patient-specific prediction of radiation-induced xerostomia and sticky saliva. *Radiotherapy and Oncology, 122*(2), 185–191.

111. Vial, A., Stirling, D., Field, M., Ros, M., Ritz, C., Carolan, M., Holloway, L., & Miller, A. A. (2018). The role of deep learning and radiomic feature extraction in cancer-specific predictive modelling: a review. *Translation Cancer Research, 7*(3), 803–816.
112. Vu, Q. D., Graham, S., Kurc, T., To, M. N. N., Shaban, M., Qaiser, T., Koohbanani, N. A., Khurram, S. A., Kalpathy-Cramer, J., Zhao, T., Gupta, R., & Farahani, K. (2019). Methods for segmentation and classification of digital microscopy tissue images. *Frontiers in Bioengineering and Biotechnology, 7*, 53.
113. Waddell, M., Page, D., & Shaughnessy Jr., J. (2005, August). Predicting cancer susceptibility from single-nucleotide polymorphism data: a case study in multiple myeloma. In *Proceedings of the 5th international workshop on bioinformatics* (pp. 21–28).
114. Wang, Y. X., & Hebert, M. (2016, October). Learning to learn: Model regression networks for easy small sample learning. In *European conference on computer vision* (pp. 616–634). Springer
115. Wichakam, I., &Vateekul, P. (2016, February). Combining deep convolutional networks and SVMs for mass detection on digital mammograms. In *2016 8th International conference on knowledge and smart technology (KST)* (pp. 239–244).IEEE.
116. Wojcieszynski, A. P., La Cava, W., Baumann, B. C., Lukens, J. N., Ghiam, A. F., Urbanowicz, R. J., Swisher-McClure, S. D., Doucette, A., Gabriel, P. E., Lin, A., Xiao, Y., & Metz, J. M. (2019). Machine learning to predict toxicity in head and neck cancer patients treated with definitive chemoradiation. *International Journal of Radiation Oncology, Biology, Physics, 105*(1), E139–E140.
117. Xu, B., Wang, N., Chen, T., & Li, M. (2015). *Empirical evaluation of rectified activations in convolutional network.* arXiv preprint arXiv:1505.00853.
118. Xu, L., Jackowski, M., Goshtasby, A., Roseman, D., Bines, S., Yu, C., Dhawan, A., & Huntley, A. (1999). Segmentation of skin cancer images. *Image and Vision Computing, 17*(1), 65–74.
119. Xu, X., Zhang, Y., Zou, L., Wang, M., & Li, A. (2012, October). A gene signature for breast cancer prognosis using support vector machine. In *2012 5th International conference on biomedical engineering and informatics* (pp. 928–931). IEEE.
120. Yahya, N., Ebert, M. A., Bulsara, M., House, M. J., Kennedy, A., Joseph, D. J., & Denham, J. W. (2016). Statistical-learning strategies generate only modestly performing predictive models for urinary symptoms following external beam radiotherapy of the prostate: A comparison of conventional and machine-learning methods. *Medical Physics, 43*(5), 2040–2052.
121. Yan, K., Li, C., Wang, X., Li, A., Yuan, Y., Feng, D., Khadra, M., & Kim, J. (2016, August). Automatic prostate segmentation on MR images with deep network and graph model. In *2016 38th Annual international conference of the IEEE engineering in medicine and biology society (EMBC)* (pp. 635–638). IEEE.
122. Yousef, M., Jung, S., Showe, L. C., & Showe, M. K. (2007). Recursive cluster elimination (RCE) for classification and feature selection from gene expression data. *BMC Bioinformatics, 8*(1), 1–12.
123. Yousef, M., Ketany, M., Manevitz, L., Showe, L. C., & Showe, M. K. (2009). Classification and biomarker identification using gene network modules and support vector machines. *BMC Bioinformatics, 10*(1), 1–7.
124. Yousef, M., Kumar, A., & Bakir-Gungor, B. (2021). Application of biological domain knowledge based feature selection on gene expression data. *Entropy, 23*(1), 2.
125. Yousef, M., Goy, G., Mitra, R., Eischen, C. M., Jabeer, A., & Bakir-Gungor, B. (2021). miRcorrNet: machine learning-based integration of miRNA and mRNA expression profiles, combined with feature grouping and ranking. *PeerJ, 9*, e11458.
126. Yousef, M., Ülgen, E., & Sezerman, O. U. (2021). CogNet: Classification of gene expression data based on ranked active-subnetwork-oriented KEGG pathway enrichment analysis. *PeerJ Computer Science, 7*, e336.
127. Yu, L., Chen, H., Dou, Q., Qin, J., & Heng, P. A. (2016). Automated melanoma recognition in dermoscopy images via very deep residual networks. *IEEE Transactions on Medical Imaging, 36*(4), 994–1004.

128. Zhang, H. H., D'Souza, W. D., Shi, L., & Meyer, R. R. (2009). Modeling plan-related clinical complications using machine learning tools in a multiplan IMRT framework. *International Journal of Radiation Oncology* Biology* Physics, 74*(5), 1617–1626.
129. Zhang, Y. N., Xia, K. R., Li, C. Y., Wei, B. L., & Zhang, B. (2021). Review of breast cancer pathologigcal image processing. *BioMed Research International*, 2021.
130. Zhen, X., Chen, J., Zhong, Z., Hrycushko, B., Zhou, L., Jiang, S., Albuquerque, K., & Gu, X. (2017). Deep convolutional neural network with transfer learning for rectum toxicity prediction in cervical cancer radiotherapy: a feasibility study. *Physics in Medicine & Biology, 62*(21), 8246.

Computational Intelligent Systems in Oncology: A Way Toward Translational Healthcare

Waaris Qazi, Ashok Sharma, and Sahar Qazi

Abstract *Cancer is a word and not a sentence!* However, cancer is one such malady in humankind with a low median survival rate, a complex examination process, and an expensive treatment. As per the GLOBOCAN 2020 report, the global cancer pattern map showcases incidence cases of eight different types of cancers in men, while for women is of seven different types. The most common cancer in men is prostate cancer, followed by lung cancer, whereas, in the case of females, breast cancer followed by cervical and ovarian cancers are more lethal. With the completion of the Human Genome Project in 2003, there has been a rise in the deployment of *Artificial Intelligence in Medicine (AIM),* aiding the rapid growth of *translational healthcare.* Advents in computer science, statistics, mathematics, computer engineering, and biological sciences have allowed researchers to deploy computational methods such as multivariate statistical analysis to understand the prognosis of the disease. The accuracy score of such analyses is better when compared to empirical approaches. Moreover, the rise of *Computational Intelligent Systems* (CIS) that encapsulates the power of both—machine learning and deep learning—has allowed some successful applications in clinical cancer research with a quick and robust cancer prediction performance in patients at a pocket-friendly cost. This chapter highlights the CIS used to diagnose, prognosis, and provide better treatment approaches for translational healthcare in oncology.

Keywords Artificial Intelligence in Medicine (AIM) · Computational Intelligent Systems (CIS) · Deep learning · Oncology · Translational healthcare

W. Qazi
Department of Biotechnology, Jamia Millia Islamia, New Delhi 110025, India

A. Sharma
Department of Biochemistry, All India Institute of Medical Sciences, New Delhi 110029, India

S. Qazi (✉)
Department of Computer Science, Jamia Millia Islamia, New Delhi 110025, India
e-mail: rs.sahar1900560@jmi.ac.in

K. Raza (ed.), *Computational Intelligence in Oncology*, Studies in Computational Intelligence 1016, https://doi.org/10.1007/978-981-16-9221-5_3

1 Introduction

When cells multiply abnormally and uncontrollably and ultimately spread in the entire body, this process is called cancer. Cancer can begin in any cell of the human body. Multiplication of cells is a normal phenomenon that takes place in any multi-cellular organism. Like humans, cells have a life cycle; they grow old, get weak and damaged, and die when new cells form eventually. Although this process may sound easy howbeit, it may not always be the case. Sometimes, forming new cells may get abnormally rapid, leading to the growth and multiplication of these damaged cells. These cells are then called—tumors, viz. they have agglomerated groups of tissues. These tumors can either be normal *(benign)* or cancerous (*malignant*) in nature. Cancerous tumors keep on dividing and eventually spread into the entire body in a matter of a short period. This movement of cancerous tumors from their original position to other parts is called—metastasis. Benign tumors do not show metastasis, and when surgically removed, they do not regrow. However, the same is not with malignant tumors. Cancer is a genetic disorder that develops because of the abnormal multiplication of cells in the human body. These genetic changes in cells occur because (What is cancer, 2021)—(a) *Erroneous division of cells*, (b) *Environmental stress and changes cause DNA damage*, and (c) *Family inheritance of the disease.* Figure 1 showcases stages of cancer development from normal cells.

The Global Cancer Observatory (GCO) is an interactive online platform that reports global cancer statistics to apprise cancer types and their current status based on gender and age group. As per the GLOBOCAN 2020 report, the estimated number of new incidence cases of all the cancers recorded in 2020 for both genders and all age groups was computed to be 19,292,789, respectively. Also, the cancer tomorrow approach helps us to understand that the prevalence of all the cancers in both sexes would grow manifolds by the year 2040 (https://gco.iarc.fr/today/online-analysis-pie). As per the GLOBOCAN 2020 report, the global cancer pattern map showcases incidence cases of eight different types of cancers in men, while for women is of seven different types. The most common cancer in men is prostate cancer, followed by lung cancer, whereas, in females, breast cancer, followed by the cervix and ovarian cancers, is more lethal. Figure 2 represents the number of incidence cases estimated in 2020, along with the growth of cancers worldwide in the form of a human chart. In 2020, there were 19.3 million incidence cases of all cancer types in both sexes, and this number would grow to be approximately 30.2 million by 2040 (https://gco.iarc.fr/tomorrow/en/dataviz/tables).

This reveals that the disease's prominence is such that even with hi-tech and fast technology, science, and research, we still cannot understand or control cancers. Though the medicine and pharmaceutical industries have tried to identify the best possible drug candidates that can aid consultants in treatment, there is still a long way to go!

With the rise of intelligent expert systems, there has been a drastic change in the approach to dealing with oncology. Advents in computer science, statistics, mathematics, computer engineering, and biological sciences have allowed researchers to

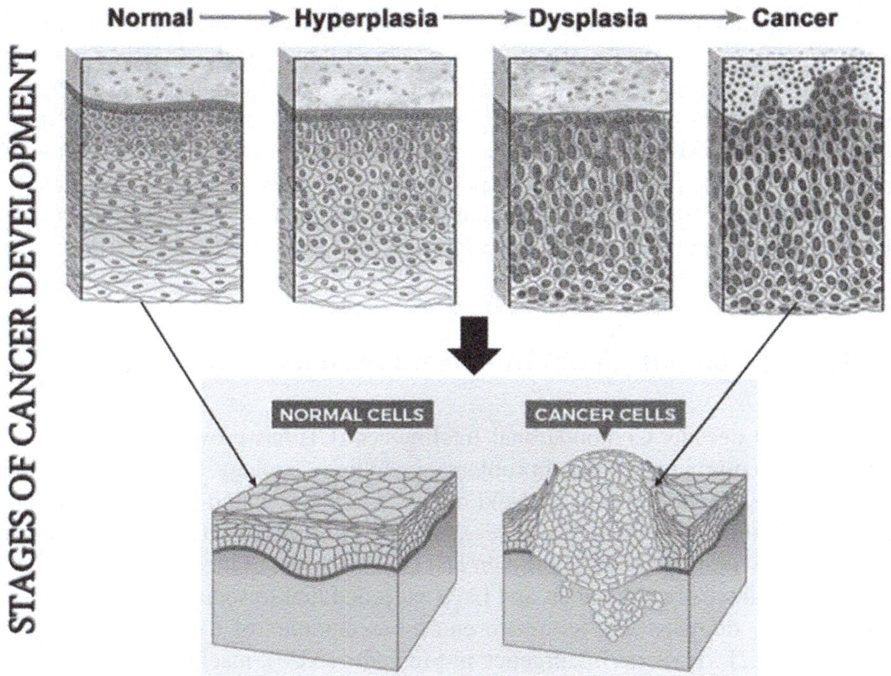

Fig. 1 Cancer developmental stages

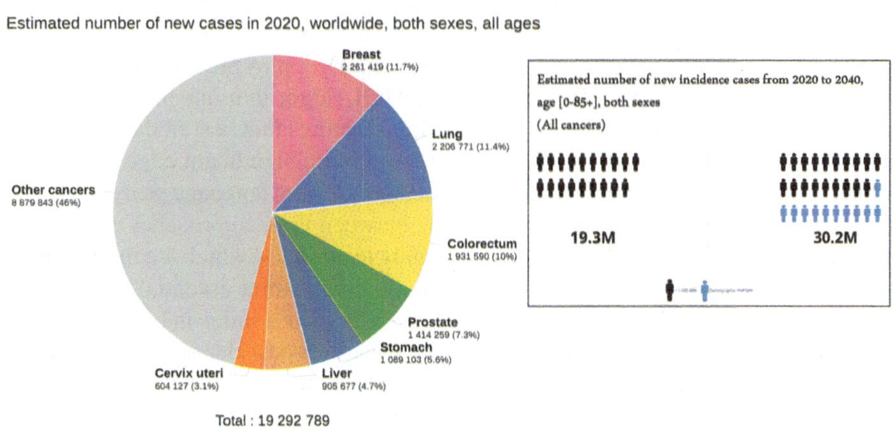

Fig. 2 GLOBOCAN 2020 estimates the incidence of cancers in both sexes and the prediction of the number of cases in cancers by 2040

deploy computational methods such as multivariate statistical analysis to understand the prognosis of the disease. The accuracy score of such analyses is better when compared to empirical approaches. Moreover, the rise of Computational Intelligent Systems (CIS) that encapsulates the power of both—machine learning and deep learning—has allowed some successful applications in clinical cancer research with a quick and robust cancer prediction performance in patients at a pocket-friendly cost. This chapter describes the CIS that is used to diagnose diseases and provide better treatment options for translational healthcare in oncology.

2 Rise of Computational Intelligent Systems in Oncology

Over the past decade, Computational Intelligence (CI) has proven to be a pivotal contributor to myriad biomedical problems, including oncology. Its extension, deep learning, viz. a highly flexible subfield of AI, aids in automatic feature extraction, helping in enormous clinical cancer research [17]. Biological sciences and medical sciences have become more data-driven and data-intensive as the applications of AI to genomics alone are equivalent and have exceeded that to social media and other data-intensive domains that automate enormous amounts of data generation and its analysis [22]. Artificial Intelligence in Medicine (AIM), machine learning algorithms, and deep learning techniques have been clubbed together and are now termed *Computational Intelligent Systems* (CIS). These intelligent systems extract essential data that allow understanding biological complex processes and aid in better and effective diagnosis and treatments, further paving the way for a holistic, personalized platform [21]. Traditional machine learning algorithms deploy pre-formatted features to give the best predictions, while deep learning (DL) algorithms are more innovative and quickly adapt and select the suitable optimal features that best fit the data by the training process. This is why deep learning has a more significant edge to real-life problem-solving approaches—image classification, natural language processing, and sequence prediction [11]. There is a fine line between these approaches of artificial intelligence, machine learning, and deep learning techniques, which are mainly interrelated. Figure 3 displays the flower representation of the three essential components of the Computational Intelligent Systems along with their utilities in biomedical and biological science research that have grown since the past decade. From disease identification using gene/protein markers to disease subtype classification, to find out the best drug candidate for disease treatment to developing a network-based disease diagnosis and prognosis approach; CIS is capable of and has proven to be an essential aid in disease detection, diagnosis, prognosis and in developing treatment approaches by using its extraordinary techniques [16].

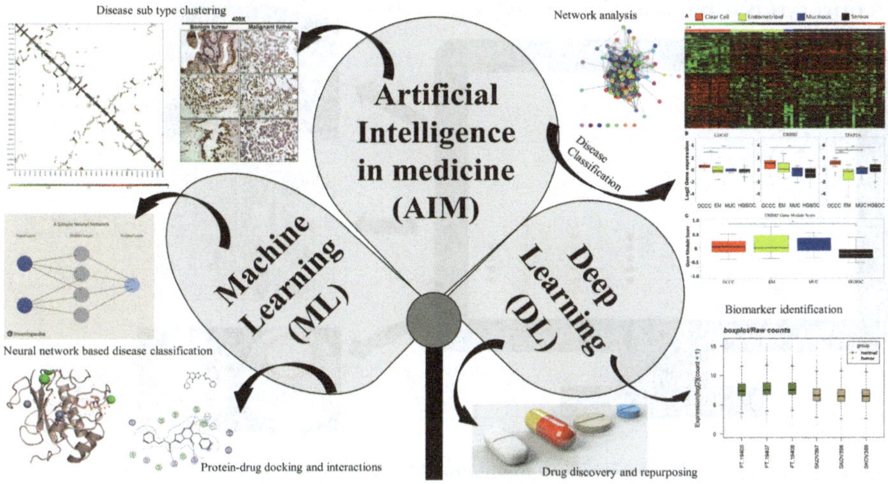

Fig. 3 A flower representation of the three essential components of Computational Intelligent Systems (CIS) and their multitudinous applications in biomedical and biological sciences research

3 Transition from Traditional Approaches to CIS

Medical communities have always preferred their manual, non-computational approach as they rely on human knowledge, expertise, and experience more when it comes to clinical decision making, diagnosis, prognosis, and suggesting treatments. This is known as the—"*traditional approach.*" However, scientific communities have always tried to innovate and improve the existing technologies and techniques that can aid physicians, consultants, and medical bodies in boosting clinical care. When it comes to adopting the practice of CIS in healthcare services, the transition has been smooth and rapid [23]. With the ever-growing pace of generating medical data from various streams, the channeling, optimization, and normalizing of the data become highly critical. This is where the CIS come in handy as they outperform in identifying complex and significant patterns in medical data such as X-rays, USG, MRI, or CT/PET scans, therein provides opportunities to transform a qualitative task into a quantifiable one.

Further, these systems can draw information that humans cannot easily understand or detect, thus aiding clinical decision making [4]. In addition, AI may quantify information from images that humans do not detect, thereby complementing clinical decision making. CIS has proved its efficiency in mainly three tasks—(a) *initial screening of the disease*, (b) *classification of the disease into subtypes,* and (c) *tumor identification and tracking* [16, 23]. Figure 4 displays the three clinical tasks of CIS.

Characterization encapsulates the segmentation (gives details about the tumor abnormality), diagnosis, and classification of tumors extending its prospects to prognosis for a given disease. Computational Intelligent Systems gather all such vital information and aid consultants in better clinical decisions regarding diagnosis

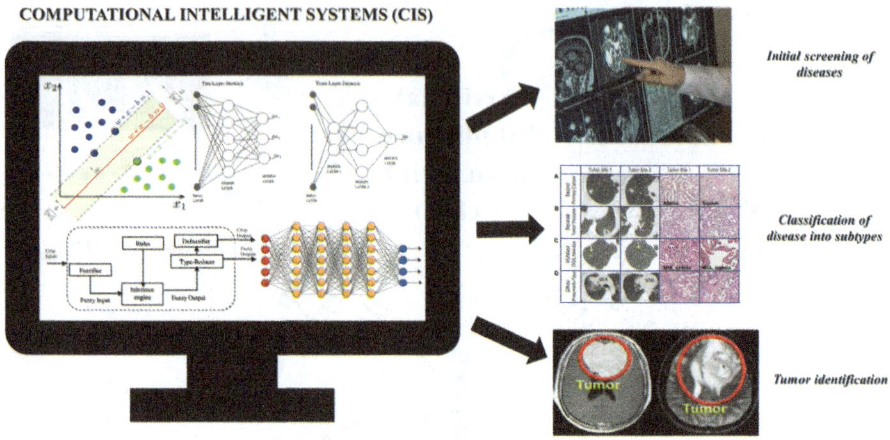

Fig. 4 Three major clinical tasks of Computational Intelligent Systems

and prognostications. Currently, cancers are manually identified using common biomarkers such as CA-125, human epididymis—4 (HE-4), PSA, EGFR, etc., while tumors are rectified using traditional techniques with various disadvantages, including interrater bias and difficult reproducibility and consumption of time and labor. Even though segmentation has been appreciated and is now used in a variety of clinical settings, however, it is still thought of as inferior compared to human analysis. CIS uses the segmentation techniques that let consultants diagnose the disease in its initial stages without any bias allowing reproducible and accurate tumor measurements with tumor stage classification too! Very similarly, fuzzy logic-based systems have been dexterously deployed in clinical decision support systems (CDSS) [1, 18, 19], while a random forest model was used to screen for anticancer drug compounds [12]. Table 1 summarizes all the CIS-based methods used in different domains of oncology research, mainly in—classification, diagnosis, and prescribing drug candidates or checking for drug specificity of a said drug compound that can be used to treat cancers.

4 CIS in Translational Healthcare

The primary purpose of science and development focuses on improving healthcare and providing better facilities to diagnose and treat diseases, especially cancer. Computational Intelligent Systems have magnanimously improved oncology research by providing an array of methods and techniques that help medical staff and consultants. CIS systems, namely neural networks, machine learning, fuzzy logic systems, hybrid systems, evolutionary algorithms along with big data analytics, and the Internet of Things (IoT), have been combined for real-time screening, diagnosis, prediction, and decision making [15, 18].

Table 1 Computational Intelligent Systems in various clinical oncology-based applications

S. No.	Computational Intelligent System	Applications	References
1	Artificial Neural Networks (ANN)	Cancer classification, cancer imaging, disease prediction, risk assessment of cancers	[9, 10]
2	Convolutional Neural Networks (CNN)	Digital pathology, clinical photography, radiographic imaging,	[5, 6, 24, 25]
3	Deep learning	Drug–target interaction analysis, anticancer drug synergy prediction, cell cycle reconstruction and disease prediction, drug repurposing	[3, 7, 14]
4	Decision trees	Drug sensitivity prediction	[13]
5	Fuzzy logic	Disease classification, diagnosis, clinical decision support systems	[1, 8]

CI systems have also helped people living in remote areas in monitoring and managing their healthcare needs. Tele-based healthcare is another essential service that has been easily achieved by Computational Intelligent Systems, including teleconsultation, telediagnosis, tele-based nursing, telepsychiatry consultations and therapies, tele-based treatment, tele-based rehabilitation, tele-education, and awareness programs [17].

Many smart and intelligent biosensors have been developed that deploy the Internet of Living Things (IoLT) technology that has shown a perception shift in the healthcare sector. It has connected all in one cycle at a single platform—the doctors, patients, nurses, pharmacists, medic staff via an intelligent sensor device that is readily available and pocket-friendly with high bandwidth networks [2].

5 Challenges and Future Prospects of CIS in Oncology

We have discussed the pros of CIS in oncology and how it has paved a way for translational healthcare management. However, there are a few challenges and limitations of CIS too that currently exist and there is a need to resolve these in order to enhance their potential in medical oncology. Following are the major limitations of CIS in oncology that needs to be addressed on an urgent basis [20].

(a) *Improved Equipment*: With CIS being added to the medical fraternity, a lot of pressure gets piled up on medical systems and equipment. In fact, there is a need of developing a computational-aided medical infrastructure that can hold easily manage the processing, storage of medical data, management.

(b) *Veracious medical data*: With each day passing by a humongous amount of medical big data is being generated. There is a need to boost up the capacity of such data's processing and storage.

(c) *Perfect clinical decision making*: With the existing hybrid systems in hand, for instance, fuzzy logic-based clinical decision support systems, there is a need to upgrade and expand this potential of CDSS in various other cancers too.
(d) *Expanding CIS systems*: Assisting CIS with expanded *virtual intelligence* (VI) for medical consultants.
(e) *Ethical, Legal, Social Issues (ELSI)*: There is a need to address the common concerns of the general public and consultants with rest to the ethical way of diagnosis and prognosis using CIS along with creating awareness about its boons to the public.
(f) *Training*: As CIS is growing, a lot of new sub-extensions have also grown which are new in the medical fraternity and there is an urgent need to train and make individuals aware of it. Individuals (consultants/medical staff) must be trained with each CIS system that can be deployed for different purposes in oncology. Growth in expertise and skill is a must!

6 Conclusions

Cancer is a word and not a sentence! It is a genetic disorder as it develops because of the abnormal multiplication of cells. However, cancer is one such malady in humankind with a low median survival rate, a difficult examination process, and an expensive treatment. As per the GLOBOCAN 2020 report, the estimated number of new incidence cases of all the cancers recorded in 2020 for both genders and all age groups were computed to be 19,292,789. This reveals that the disease's prominence is such that even with hi-tech and fast technology, science and research, we still cannot understand or control cancers. Artificial Intelligence in Medicine (AIM), machine learning algorithms, and deep learning techniques have been clubbed together and are now termed—*Computational Intelligent Systems* (CIS). These intelligent systems extract essential data that allow understanding biological complex processes and aid in better and effective diagnosis and treatments, further paving the way for a holistic, personalized platform.

There are three components of intelligent computational systems, namely machine learning, Artificial Intelligence in Medicine (AIM), and deep learning. From disease identification to disease subtype classification, to find out the best drug candidate to develop a diagnosis and prognosis approach, CIS is capable of and has proven to be an essential aid in disease detection, diagnosis, prognosis, and developing treatment approaches using its extraordinary techniques. The future seems bright for CI systems in oncology and other medical fields of study.

Acknowledgements SQ is supported by the DST-INSPIRE, Department of Science and Technology (DST), Government. of India.

Conflict of Interest None reported.

References

1. Ahmad, G., Khan, M. A., Abbas, S., Athar, A., Khan, B. S., & Aslam, M. S. (2019). Automated diagnosis of hepatitis b using multilayer mamdani fuzzy inference system. *Journal of Healthcare Engineering*, 1–11, https://doi.org/10.1155/2019/6361318
2. Alam, A., Qazi, S., Iqbal, N., & Raza, K. (2020). Fog, edge and pervasive computing in intelligent internet of things driven applications in healthcare: Challenges, limitations and future use. *Fog, Edge, and Pervasive Computing in Intelligent IoT Driven Applications*, 1–26, https://doi.org/10.1002/9781119670087.ch1
3. Aliper, A., Plis, S., et al. (2016). Deep learning applications for predicting pharmacological properties of drugs and drug repurposing using transcriptomic data. *Molecular Pharmaceutics, 13*, 2524–2530.
4. Bi, W. L., Hosny, A., Schabath, M. B., Giger, M. L., Birkbak, N. J., Mehrtash, A., & Aerts, H. J. W. L. (2019). Artificial intelligence in cassncer imaging: Clinical challenges and applications. *CA: A Cancer Journal for Clinicians*, https://doi.org/10.3322/caac.21552
5. Data Science Bowl. (2017). https://www.kaggle.com/c/data-science-bowl-2017 (Accessed 11th August, 2021).
6. Esteva, A., Kuprel, B., Novoa, R. A., et al. (2017). Dermatologist-level classification of skin cancer with deep neural networks. *Nature, 542*, 115–118.
7. Feng, Q., & Dueva, E., et al. (2018). *PADME: A deep learning-based framework for drug-target interaction prediction.* http://arxiv.org/abs/1807.09741
8. Hashmia, A., & Khan, M. S. (2015). Diagnosis blood test for liver disease using fuzzy logic. *International Journal of Sciences: Basic and Applied Research., 20*, 151–183.
9. Hirschberg, J., & Manning, C. D. (2015). Advances in natural language processing. *Science, 349*, 261–266.
10. Hopfield, J. J. (1988). Artificial neural networks. *IEEE Circuits and Devices Magazine, 4*, 3–10.
11. Kann, B. H., & Thompson, R., et al. (2019). Artificial Intelligence in Oncology: Current Applications and Future Directions. *Cancer Network. Oncology, 33*(2), 46–53, https://www.cancernetwork.com/view/artificial-intelligence-oncology-current-applications-and-future-dir
12. Lind, A. P., & Anderson, P. C. (2019). Predicting drug activity against cancer cells by random forest models based on minimal genomic information and chemical properties. *Plos One, 14*(7), e0219774. https://doi.org/10.1371/journal.pone.0219774
13. Menden, M. P., & Iorio, F., et al. (2013). Machine learning prediction of cancer cell sensitivity to drugs based on genomic and chemical properties. *Plos One, 8*, e61318.
14. Preuer, K., & Lewis, R. P. I., et al. (2018). DeepSynergy: Predicting anti-cancer drug synergy with Deep Learning. *Bioinformatics, 34*, 1538–1546.
15. Qazi, S., & Raza, K. (2020). Smart biosensors for an efficient point of care (PoC) health management. *Smart Biosensors in Medical Care*, 65–85, https://doi.org/10.1016/b978-0-12-820781-9.00004-8
16. Qazi, S., Raza, K., & Iqbal, N. (2021). Artificial intelligence in medicine (AIM): machine learning in cancer diagnosis, prognosis and therapy. *Artificial Intelligence for Data-Driven Medical Diagnosis. De Gruyter*, 103–126.
17. Qazi, S., Tanveer, K., ElBahnasy, K., & Raza, K. (2019). From Telediagnosis to Teletreatment. *Telemedicine Technologies*, 153–169. https://doi.org/10.1016/b978-0-12-816948-3.00010-6
18. Qazi, S. & Raza, K. (2021). Fuzzy logic-based hybrid knowledge systems for the detection and diagnosis of childhood autism. *Handbook of Decision Support Systems for Neurological Disorders*, 55–69. https://doi.org/10.1016/B978-0-12-822271-3.00016-5
19. Raza, K. (2019). Fuzzy logic based approaches for gene regulatory network inference. *Artificial Intelligence in Medicine, 97*, 189-203. https://doi.org/10.1016/j.artmed.2018.12.004
20. Shanthi, S. (2021, May 26). *Challenges and future of AI in healthcare.* Retrieved October 13, 2021, from Analytics India Magazine website: https://analyticsindiamag.com/challenges-and-future-of-ai-in-healthcare/
21. Shimizu, H., & Nakayama, K. I. (2020). Artificial intelligence in oncology. *Cancer Science, 111*(5), 1452–1460, https://doi.org/10.1111/cas.14377

22. Stephens, Z. D., Lee, S. Y., Faghri, F., Campbell, R. H., Zhai, C., Efron, M. J., Robinson, G. E. (2015). Big data: Astronomical or genomical? *Plos Biology, 13*(7), e1002195. https://doi.org/10.1371/journal.pbio.1002195
23. Svoboda, E. (2020). Artificial intelligence is improving the detection of lung cancer. *Nature, 587*(7834), S20–S22. https://doi.org/10.1038/d41586-020-03157-9
24. Wang, P., Xiao, X., et al. (2018). Development and validation of a deep-learning algorithm for the detection of polyps during colonoscopy. *Nat Biomed Engineering, 2*, 741.
25. Webster, D. E., Suver, C., & Doerr, M., et al. (2017). The Mole Mapper Study, mobile phone skin imaging and melanoma risk data collected using ResearchKit. *Scientific Data, 4*, 170005.
26. What Is Cancer? (2021, May 5). Retrieved August 11, 2021, from National Cancer Institute website: https://www.cancer.gov/about-cancer/understanding/what-is-cancer

Computational Resources for Oncology Research: A Comprehensive Analysis

Kayenat Sheikh, Ayyagari Ramlal, and Fatima Nazish Khan

Abstract Despite the efforts and clinical trials in the past for the production of novel and promising therapeutics against cancer, it remains a major challenge leading to mass morbidity and mortality. Cancer is an emerging field of research that requires early identification, diagnosis, prognosis, and therapeutics. The resources and web servers play pivotal roles in cancer genomics & medical image analyses and much more. The outburst of computational methods such as artificial intelligence and high-performance computing including computational intelligence (CI) have enabled thorough analysis of similar data at remarkable scales. CI is a set of computational methodologies involving design, application, and development used to solve complex real-world problems. CI has immense potential in the field of medicine from predictive modeling of cancers and medicines through computational approaches to image and microarray analyses. Hence, various computational resources such as tools, software, databases, packages, and web servers, accessible publicly have led to scientific advancement. The period of big data and bioinformatics has increased the demand for partnership, sharing data, and resources that help in the effective utilization of novel information and knowledge. These resources not only help in studying the diseases but also in the analysis, and diagnosis and development of personalized medicine. This chapter covers important computational resources including tools, software, databases, packages, and web servers in cancer research with a major focus on their nature and functioning strategies in oncology. It will enhance awareness and implement appropriate resources in future cancer research, safer development of therapeutics and critical questions can be answered.

K. Sheikh
Department of Computer Science, Jamia Millia Islamia, New Delhi 110025, India
e-mail: kayenat1903945@st.jmi.ac.in

A. Ramlal
Division of Genetics, Indian Agricultural Research Institute (ICAR-IARI), Pusa Campus, New Delhi 110025, India

F. N. Khan (✉)
Department of Education in Science and Mathematics, NCERT, New Delhi 110025, India

K. Raza (ed.), *Computational Intelligence in Oncology*, Studies in Computational Intelligence 1016, https://doi.org/10.1007/978-981-16-9221-5_4

Keywords Computational intelligence · Bioinformatics · Cancer · Tools · Software · Databases

1 Introduction

With the evolution of medical oncology, the major focus is continuously moving towards therapeutic strategies instead of methods that involve nonspecific cytotoxic treatment. Precision medicine aims to understand the treatment and diagnose a patient's biological profile and reduce the exposure to ineffective therapies. The goal has been fulfilled by using various bioinformatics software, tools, databases, and web servers, that help in the treatment and diagnosis of tumors. Bioinformatics is an interdisciplinary field that uses computers and biology and has grown rapidly from the 1980s and expanded the scope for storing genomic sequencing datasets and other information. The integration of wet lab experiments with computational or bioinformatics analysis greatly helps researchers to solve the majority of disease-related issues including human diseases, as it provided a means for both storing information and analysis of the data generated. Computational techniques such as artificial intelligence (AI), machine and deep learning have immense potential in different areas of healthcare, data analysis, drug repurposing, and discovery. The software and tools can explore genetic data and identify methods for precise medicine administration. Bioinformatics is a term utilized in computer-based algorithms as well as various resources for the extraction of a biological dataset [56]. The National Institutes of Health (NIH) defined bioinformatics as "research, development or application of computational tools and approaches for expanding the use of biological, medical, behavioral or health data, including those acquire, store, organize, analyze, visualize such data" [56]. Previously, several species have been utilized for looking into many events such as morphological, anatomical, molecular, biochemical, evolutionary, and inheritance-based studies. These processes generate a gigantic amount of biological information. There have been numerous pieces of evidence since the last three decades that generally support that cancer is a genome disease [41].

Cancer is one of the most complex diseases is being faced by human beings throughout the world. About 200 different subtypes of cancer have been recognized and characterized by various molecular profiles having particular therapeutic methods. Cancer in the genome of an organism is related to dynamic changes [73]. Each type of cancer is majorly linked with genetic aberrations like somatic mutations, epigenetic alterations, changes in gene expression profiles, and copy number variations. There is a need for better prediction and diagnosis of cancer, which is related to a better comprehension of genetic alterations in cancer. Many bioinformatics resources have been developed to analyze the dataset that is linked with cancer-related issues, and hence these resources allow prediction, diagnosis, treatment, and prevention of cancer. Nowadays, greater attention has been paid to precision medicine for the treatment of cancer. The resources of computational and artificial intelligence use the genetic profile of individual patients for the identification of suitable drugs for patients. These resources also provide significant proof and ideas for scientists and researchers working on cancer development and treatment. Despite several complexities, cancer continues an interesting field for human geneticists. However, instead of numerous diagnoses involved in cancer prevention, researchers still didn't know the causes for many cancers and their treatment. Therefore, for recovering meaningful biological results, the analysis has been done with particular tools. Storing, organization, and retrieval of data need particular databases such as the National Centre for Biotechnology Information (NCBI), European Molecular Biology Laboratory (EMBL), DNA Database of Japan (DDBJ), structural databases such as Protein Data Bank (PDB), nucleic acid database (NDB); metabolic pathways databases such as KEGG and MetaCyc; literature databases such as PubMed, Scopus; disease databases such as Online Mendelian Inheritance in Man (OMIM), Online Mendelian Inheritance in Animals (OMIA), Genecard, Pathcard; and many more.

The progress in the development of computational intelligence (CI), bioinformatics, and sequencing technologies has shed light on cancer [36, 62, 68]. The Cancer Genome Atlas (TCGA) as well as the International Cancer Genome Consortium (ICGC) two major projects launched in 2005 and 2008, respectively, accelerate the understanding of cancer genetics with the utilization of innovative genome analysis technologies that are majorly helpful in developing novel therapeutics of cancer, preventive and diagnostic methods [13, 73]. For the creation of "atlas" of profiles of cancer genomic, the TCGA Pilot Project has been launched through the National Institute of Health (NIH). This project has a goal to discover and catalog the majorly identified genomic alterations that cause cancer in a study of about 30 human tumors with the application of multi-dimensional and sequencing approach analyses. The openly accessible datasets of cancer genomics will aid in the enhancement of diagnostic and treatment methods and methodologies for further prevention of the disease [73].

The chapter deals with important computational resources including tools, software, databases, packages, and web servers in cancer research with a major focus on their nature and functioning strategies in oncology (Fig. 1). Firstly, it will provide some glimpses about cancer, followed by computational resources in oncological research such as software tools and databases for the study of cancer genomics; bioinformatics software for cancer metabolomics; web servers and software for analyzing prognosis of the disease (cancer); similarly tools involved and dedicated to cancer biomarker development; software tools for cancer hazard identification; online and offline tools for analyzing the dataset of TCGA; and other databases/tools/webservers in oncological research with more focus on the function of genes and tools for structure prediction. Secondly, it provides a brief overview of AI and computational biology technologies in the precision drug discovery of cancer. Finally, it deals with the limitations and prospective of cancer-related resources. These resources will enhance awareness and might help in implementing appropriate resources in future cancer research for the safer development of therapeutics.

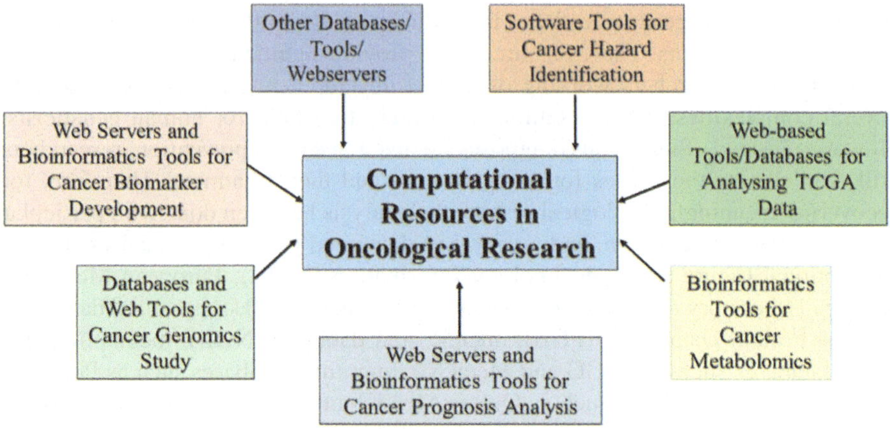

Fig. 1 Various computational resources in oncological research

2 Computational Resources in Oncological Research

Computational techniques such as machine learning, deep learning, and fuzzy logic have immense potential in the domains of healthcare, data analysis, drug repurposing, and discovery. The present software and tools can explore genetic data and identify methods for precise medicine administration. The advancements in sequencing techniques have led to greater accessibility to extensive data sets and genetic variations data accumulation. Several computational tools and resources are available to analyze datasets associated with genomic sequences. Such tools help in the prediction of the functions when genes are deleted. Some tools are designed with combinatorial properties such as protein sequence and structure information, evolutionary sequence analysis, functional properties of sequence with genetic variations, and much more. The AI technique uses the genetic profile of an individual patient and identifies the appropriate drug for his needs. The advantage of computational tools is the ability to refine important information in a very short period. The reason for employing computational resources for oncological studies is to accelerate the process of identification of precision drugs and enhance pharmaceutical research [51]. In this section, the recent computational resources, web tools, software, methods that are used in oncological research will be discussed.

2.1 Resources for Cancer Genomics Study

The primary cause for cancer disease arises from the genome. With the enormous flow of genomic data through high-throughput sequencing techniques, cancer genomic studies have become more feasible [81]. The following sections describe various tools and databases used in analyzing the cancer genomic data (Figs. 2 and 3).

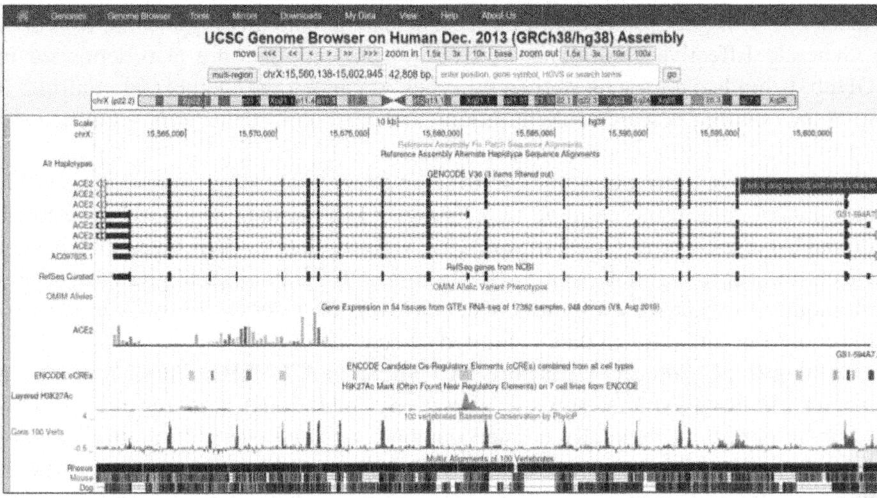

Fig. 2 Interface of UCSC cancer genomics browser

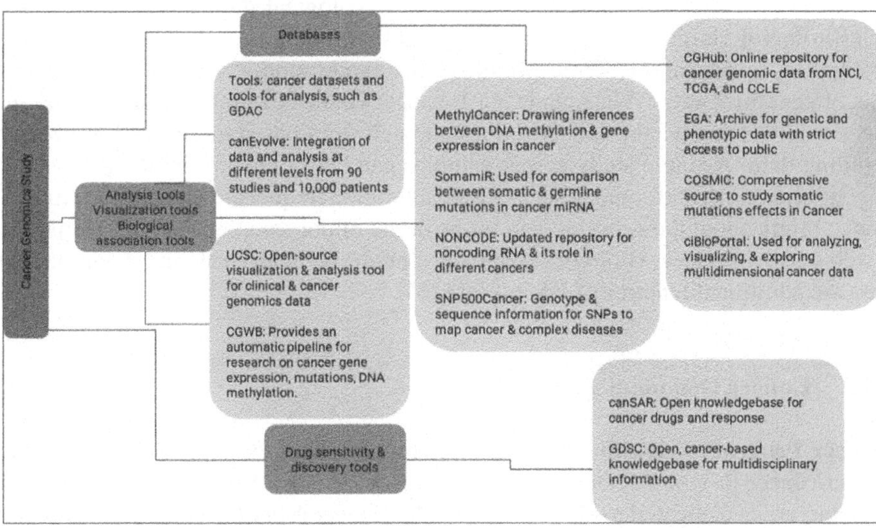

Fig. 3 Resources for cancer genomics study

2.1.1 Cancer Genomics Study Databases

Cancer Genomics Hub or CGHub (https://gdc.cancer.gov) is a cancer genomic information archive. It is handled by the University of California (UCSC), which allows very limited access and maintains data privacy. It stores the data generated by The Cancer Genome Atlas (TCGA), National Cancer Institute (NCI), and the

Cancer Cell Line Encyclopedia (CCLE). The Therapeutically Applicable Research to Generate Effective Treatments (TARGET) projects data are also deposited in CGHub. It holds data for more than 42 types of cancer and the normal controls. It allows data sharing, research collaborations, and personalized medicine identification [76].

European Genome-phenome Archive or EGA (https://ega-archive.org/) holds experimental data from genotype sequencing. It has the data generated from International Cancer Genome Consortium (ICGC). Holds data from more than 50 cancer projects and approximately from 12,000 samples. ICGC data portal gives full access to the somatic variant data which is open. However, the access to germline mutations, raw sequences, and clinical data is limited or controlled [35].

Catalogue of Somatic Mutations in Cancer or COSMIC (https://cancer.sanger.ac.uk) holds maximum somatic alterations (mutations) data and their effects on human cancer. A manually curated database updated every 2 months includes personal details of patients and diseases. Relevant works of literature on whole-genome shotgun sequencing are available for reference. It has data on rearrangements in the genome, whole-genome, mutations, fusions, CNVs, and abnormal expression variants. The query can be conducted using keywords. Output is available for download by the user. A valuable resource for oncological studies [72].

cBioPortal (http://www.cbioportal.org/public-portal/) is a dynamic portal for researchers on Cancer Genomics. It allows the exploration, visualization, and analysis of genomics data. TCGA and CCLE cancer studies datasets are integrated into this portal. It contains the cancer tissues and cell lines based on original molecular profiling data. A single study across samples can help in exploring the patterns of genetic alterations and comparisons of gene alteration frequencies in multiple studies. It also briefs about the genomic variations in the tumor sample of an individual via a web query interface. Biological pathways, analysis of survival, and downloading data are additional features of this portal [18].

2.1.2 Cancer Genomics Analysis Tools

Cancer Program Scientific Tool and Resources (https://www.broadinstitute.org/cancer/cancer-program-scientific-tools-and-resources) by Broad Institute of MIT and Harvard is dedicated to cancer studies. The cancer program is primarily focused on cancer mechanisms investigation and clinical uses. It provides many tools for cancer research hosted by the Broad Cancer Program Gateway (CPRG). For instance, the Genome Data Analysis Center (GDAC) of Broad Institute is efficient in analyzing data by extending the TCGA pilot for other diseases too. The firehose system of GDAC can analyze around 40 TB of TCGA data (TCGA processed every 2 weeks) and run around 6000 pipelines every month. Firehose has multiple pipelines for cancer genomic analysis. The public has access to the computational setup for running their tools. Due to high computation speed and less time consumption, Broad Institute provides recent data and different layers of results (analyses reports, standard datasets, and user-friendly) [45].

canEvolve (www.canevolve.org/) tool is used for cancer genome profiling. It enables data integration and interpretation. More than 10,000 patients' data from 90 clinical studies are integrated into canEvolve. A public platform used for analyzing the functional genomics data. Visualization of data in tabular and graphical forms. Analysis of data is performed at different tiers. The primary analysis tier is for miRNA, mRNA, protein expression, variation in the genome, protein-protein interactions, and more. The second tier is the gene and miRNA expression, CNVs and gene set enrichment analyses. The third tier involves analysis of the network. The fourth-tier analysis is survival analysis [62].

2.1.3 Cancer Genomics Data Visualization Tools

UCSC Cancer Genomics Browser (https://genome-cancer.soe.ucsc.edu/) is a publicly available visualization and analyzing tool for cancer genomic-related data. It has information on single experiment measurements and related clinical data for multiple samples. Comparative study of CNV and Gene Expression across the different data types of cancer is possible at the same time. Heatmaps are generated for clinical data along with data download. Most data sources are TCGA and CCLE [19].

Cancer Genome WorkBench (CGWB) (https://cgwb.nci.nih.gov/) is a widely used tool for gene expression and mutation studies. Also provides CNV and mutation data. It is effective in producing automated research pipelines. It facilitates data visualization and genomic analysis and gives information on gene expression variation in each sample. Two types of CGWB viewers are present—Genome browser and Heatmap viewer. Both the browsers provide information on gene expression, somatic mutations, and pathways. Not an open tool, permission is required for accessing data [85].

2.1.4 Cancer Genomics Data and Biological Association Tool

MethyCancer (http://methycancer.psych.ac.cn) is a helpful tool in cancer studies and related cancer activities. It constitutes different data types—DNA methylation, CpG Island clones, CNV and cancer, and correlations between datasets. MethyCancer is used for the interpretation between biological processes and cancer. It identifies the inter-relationship between three biological aspects—Gene Expression, DNA methylation, and cancer. Useful in studies of gene silencing-tumor suppression and instability in chromosomes [23].

SomamiR (http://compbio.uthsc.edu/SomamiR/) is a huge database with mutation data from Gene Expression Omnibus (GEO). It also holds data from child cancer projects such as the Pediatric Cancer Genome Project (PCGP). The miRNA data is collected from the miRBase release 18. This resource is used for the investigation of miRNA and its role in cancer. The main purpose of SomamiR is to find the association between somatic and germline mutations with miRNA's role in cancer. Genome-Wide

Association Studies (GWAS), KEGG pathways, genes associated with cancer, and mutations are some methods to find the non-germline (somatic) mutations affecting target sites of miRNA. It assists in predicting the miRNA binding and functions after mutations [7].

NONCODE (http://www.noncode.org/) is an up-to-date database holding data for noncoding RNAs (ncRNAs). It plays an important role in many cancer types. There are more than 5 lakh ncRNA entries in NONCODE. Around 80% of data is obtained experimentally, thus indicating the reliability of data. It provides long ncRNA profiles for tissues and an online pipeline that is used to analyze RNA-seq data. This pipeline is called iLncRNA. Functions of ID conversion from RefSeq IDs or Ensembl IDs to NONCODE IDs are available too [78].

SNP500Cancer (http://snp500cancer.nci.nih.gov) is a part of the Cancer Genome Anatomy Project (CGAP). A database for verification of sequence and genotype for SNPs in diseases, specifically cancer. The purpose of SNP500 is to conduct epidemiology studies. It is used for resequencing the reference samples to identify novel SNPs for cancer research. For unknown DNA samples, this database can be used for retrieving sequence information. The query is made through the gene, GO pathways, SNP Database ID, chromosome, SNP500Cancer SNP ID. Due to high accuracy, the SNP500Cancer is used for meaningful insights and SNPs selection [52].

2.1.5 Cancer Genomics Tool for Drug Sensitivity and Discovery

Genomics of Drug Sensitivity in Cancer (GDSC) (http://www.cancerrxgene.org) database is an openly accessible knowledge base on drug sensitivity in cancer cells. It has more than 200 therapeutic responses for more than 1000 cancer cell lines. Helps in the identification of molecular markers for cancer drug response. Drug sensitivity queries are made by the cancer gene, cell line, and compound. Results can be downloaded in different graphical representations [80].

canSAR (https://cansar.icr.ac.uk/) is an open database used frequently by researchers to facilitate translational cancer research. It holds data from multidisciplinary fields. It holds huge proteome data for human proteins at present. Also contains cancer annotation data, non-transformed cell lines data, and 3D protein structure details [14].

2.2 Bioinformatics Tools for Cancer Metabolomics

Metabolomics is a new field of study. It is gaining momentum in cancer studies. Metabolomics techniques help in different data generation and analysis of such data takes place in three steps—targeted analysis, metabolite profiling, and metabolic fingerprinting [8]. In this section, the tools and databases used for cancer metabolomics studies are discussed (Fig. 4).

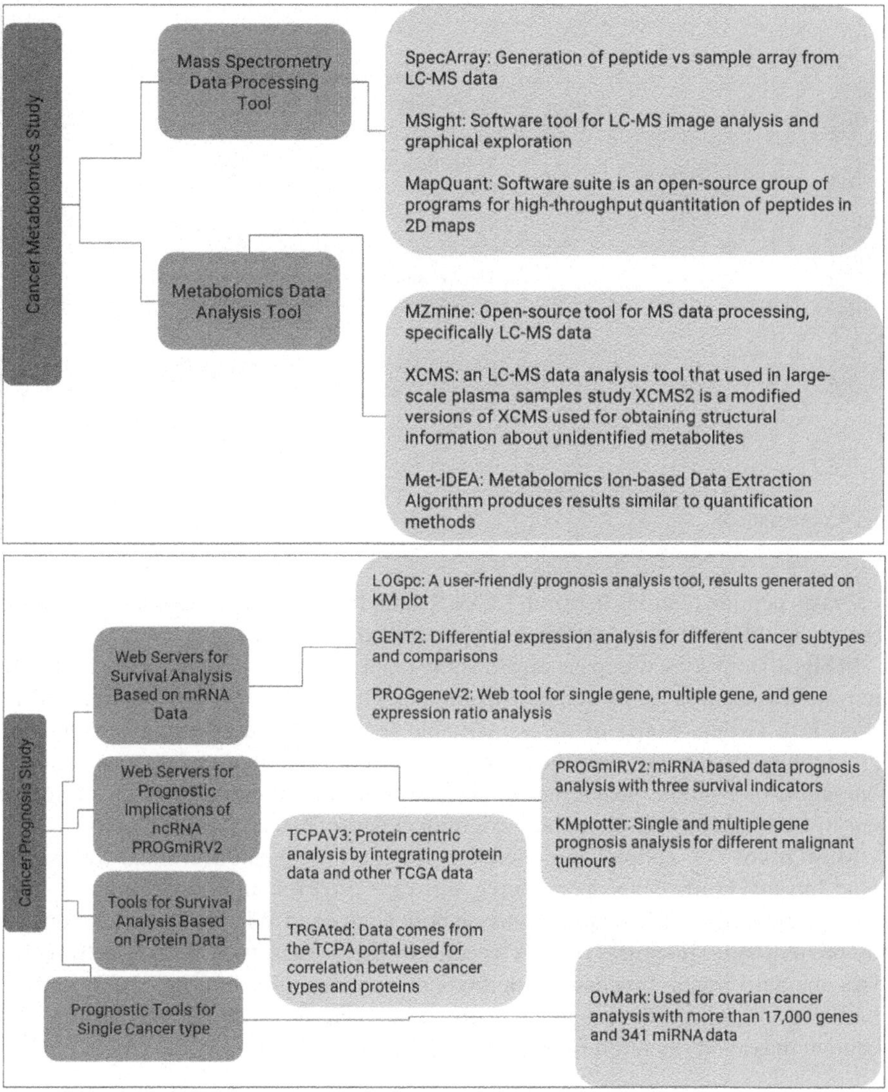

Fig. 4 Bioinformatics tools and web servers for cancer metabolomics, cancer prognosis analysis, and cancer biomarker development

2.2.1 Mass Spectrometry Data Processing Tool

SpecArray (https://sourceforge.net/projects/sashimi/files/SpecArray/)%20 software used for the generation of a peptide vs sample expression array from an LC-MS dataset by analyzing peptides through LC-MS settings. It contains programs such as Pep3D that generates 2D gel-type images from the LC-MS data, PepList which

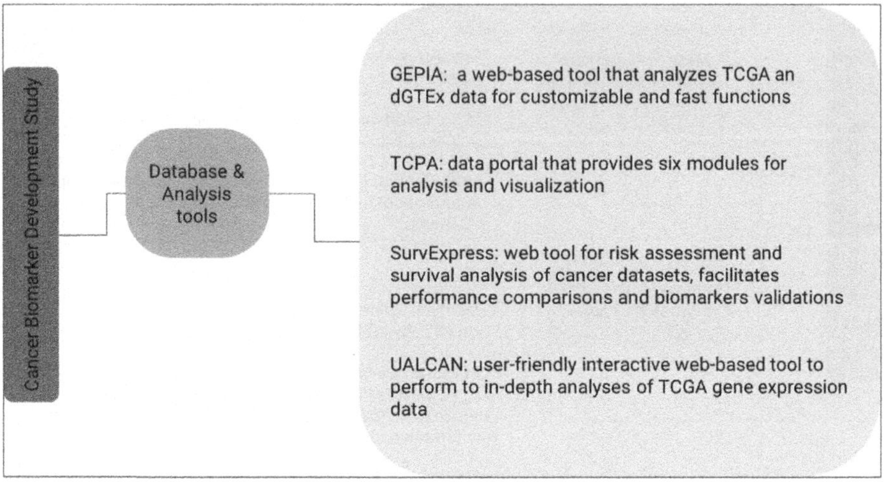

Fig. 4 (continued)

generates peptide features list from LC-MS data, PepMatch for alignment of peptide features of different samples, PepArray, and mzxml2dat [40].

MSight (http://www.expasy.org/MSight/) is a freely accessible tool for LC-MS analysis. Developed by Proteome Informatics Group in 2005, now maintained by Swiss-Prot Group. Some of the remarkable features are user-friendly navigation across a huge volume of data, fast and provides multi-resolution data visualization, generation of isotopic peaks, noise filtering, data sets comparisons for proteome analysis, data quality assessment, designing experiments, and much more [53].

MapQuant (https://arep.med.harvard.edu/MapQuant/download-forms/download-bin-msi.html) is an open-source software used for high-throughput identification of peptides in 2D maps. It runs on both Linux and Windows environments. It comprehensively quantifies organic species in large datasets of mass spectrometry. Uses standard image processing methods to execute noise filtering, peak finding, clustering, fitting, carbon content estimation, and more. Possesses features of accurate mass and retention time of isotopic clusters [37].

2.2.2 Metabolomics Data Analysis Tool

MZmine (http://mzmine.sourceforge.net/) is an open-source and user-friendly tool for the processing and visualizing of MS-based molecular profile data. It has the ability of parallel processing. It estimates the peak areas by employing an algorithm of post-alignment peak picking. Sammon's mapping is implemented for curvilinear distance analysis used for data observation and exploration. The tool supports mzXML file format and can perform batch processing for voluminous data files [28].

XCMS (http://metlin.scripps.edu/download/) is an open-access tool that includes nonlinear retention time alignment, peak matching, peak detection, matched filtration, and many more. It identifies lots of endogenous metabolites that are used as standards, calculating a non-linear retention time correction profile for every sample. This tool is freely available under the open license [67].

Met-IDEA (http://noble.org/) is an open-access tool for users that solves the problem of metabolomics high-throughput data conversion of raw chromatographically coupled MS datasets. MET-IDEA produces results similar to traditional methods of quantification, reduces time and effort in producing organized datasets. Rapid extraction of semiquantitative data from raw datasets, thus allowing quick biological insights [11].

2.3 Tools and Web Servers for Cancer Prognosis Analysis

The estimation of prognosis in cancer patients is highly significant to facilitate the clinical treatments and mechanism of tumorigenesis. There are several factors for determining the prognosis such as clinical performance, understanding of cancer, disease stage, and more [88]. This section will focus on the wide range of tools available for different data types used in cancer prognosis analysis (Fig. 4).

2.3.1 Web Servers for Survival (mRNA) Based Analysis

LOGpc (http://bioinfo.henu.edu.cn/DatabaseList.jsp) is a web server that holds huge datasets for survival analysis. The datasets from more than 28,000 cancer patients are stored here. Data of 26 types of malignant tumors and online prognostic tools are included here. TCGA and GEO are the main sources for patient sample collection. LOGpc is a user-friendly tool. The gene symbol input is accepted in this program. The results are displayed on the output web page when the user clicks on the Kaplan-Meier plot. The parameters are simple to adjust [69].

GENT2 (http://gent2.appex.kr) is a tool that provides analysis for Differential Expression (DE) and prognosis of different cancer types. Gene expression profiles are available for different issues and comparison between expression levels is feasible. It also provides the Kaplan-Meier plot with the log-rank test. It establishes Cox proportional risk model for meta-analysis. Presently, there are 27 cancer types of survival analysis data [54].

PROGgeneV2 (http://genomics.jefferson.edu/proggene/) is an online tool used in the prognosis analysis of different cancer types. Presently, there are 193 data sets from 27 cancer types. An analysis is performed for a single or multiple genes, and two gene expression ratios. Researchers can upload customized gene datasets for prognosis analysis of the gene of interest and compare the results with previous studies [22].

2.3.2 Web Servers for Prognostic Implications of ncRNA

PROGmiRV2 (http://xvm145.jefferson.edu/progmir/) is a database based on miRNA prognostics Collected from TCGA and GEO. The data sets from samples are huge and improved prognosis analysis is possible. This version is better than the previous one for the analysis of pan-cancer. There are three survival indicators called overall survival, metastasis-free, and recurrence-free. It allows users to upload data set for prognosis analysis [21].

KMplotter, also called a Kaplan–Meier plotter (http://kmplot.com/analysis/) is a tool for prognosis analysis for a single gene and multiple genes for different kinds of malignant tumors. It executes the pan-cancer analysis to study the effects of both mRNA and miRNA expressions on the survival rate of 21 cancers. The user can input gene names and choose the correct cut-off point for gene expression. The results of the comparison between the two groups are displayed with a confidence interval of 95% [74].

2.3.3 Tools for Survival (Protein) Based Analysis

TCPAV3 (http://tcpaportal.org/) is an updated tool used for the analysis and exploration of protein expression data extracted from TCGA RPPA data. It provides protein-centric analysis by integrating protein data and other TCGA data. A helpful tool in identifying protein markers and pathway events based on the survival of a patient. It uses Cox proportional risk model and log-rank test. Pan-cancer analysis facilitates the identification of proteins that enable the prognosis of different types of cancer [87].

TRGAted (https://nborcherding.shinyapps.io/TRGAted) is a tool for analyzing correlation. An integrative tool to identify a correlation between 31 cancer types and 200 proteins. The data in this tool comes from the TCPA portal. The users can apply the Cox proportional hazard model for the prognosis analysis of proteins for each cancer type. The patient information is comprehensive. It provides several survival indicators and functions for visualization as well. The users can download and modify the tool according to their needs [9].

2.3.4 Prognostic Tools for Single Cancer Type

OvMark (http://glados.ucd.ie/OvMark/index.html) is a prognostic tool for ovarian cancer analysis. More than 17,000 genes and 341 miRNAs are detected for potential prognostic analysis. A user-friendly tool that uses the OvMark algorithm for combining data from multiple microarray platforms and later correlates them with clinical parameters [43].

2.4 Servers and Tools for Cancer Biomarker Development

Molecular biomarkers in cancer play crucial roles in diagnosis, prognosis, and treatment. Lack of sufficient biomarkers poses difficulty in cancer prognosis. The high throughput MicroArray and sequencing technologies and databases such as TCGA and GEO have increased dramatically. These resources on full exploitation can be used in bioinformatics research to identify potential biomarkers for cancer [77] (Fig. 4).

GEPIA (http://gepia.cancer-pku.cn/) offers various interactive and customizable functions such as differential expression analysis, profiling plotting, patient survival analysis, correlation analysis, similar gene detection, and dimensionality reduction analysis. It allows data mining, scientific discussion, and therapeutic discovery processes. It is the binding tool between cancer genomics big data and information transfer at the customer end [71].

2.5 Software Tools for Cancer Hazard Identification

Several online tools focus on health assessment in a systematic method. One such tool is health assessment workplace collaborative HAWC for literature searches and another one called table builder for analysis of tabulated data [65] (Fig. 5).

HAWC is an online open-access software specifically designed to inspect the environment and perform human health assessments. It is developed using the python-based Django web framework and relational PostgreSQL database. Open-source code and available for reuse by the public (https://hawcproject.org). It consists of a series of modules used independently or together for achieving the steps of the work pipeline. It helps in the evaluation of data on hazards and the response to drugs and chemicals in humans, animals, and similar information. This application is a content management system in which the users perform assessments in public or private mode with a tiered permission system. The literature search and review components are the most widely used module by IARC and NTP [49].

Table builder is a web-based content management system that is specifically designed to extract tabular data from published literature and execute qualitative and quantitative analysis. Developed using the meteor JavaScript web framework. It uses a document-based MongoDB database. An open-source software with codes available for public reuse (https://table-builder.com/). These executions help in human health assessments for potential carcinogens. It also meets the needs of NTP and IARC. The customization of this software allows the standardization of key fields of extracted data from different studies. It is flexible and incorporates innovations that are not widely implemented yet. The vocabulary for data extraction and fields are fixed. It is done to promote consistency in reporting of data and terminology usage across assessments. There are four data types in the data extraction templates by

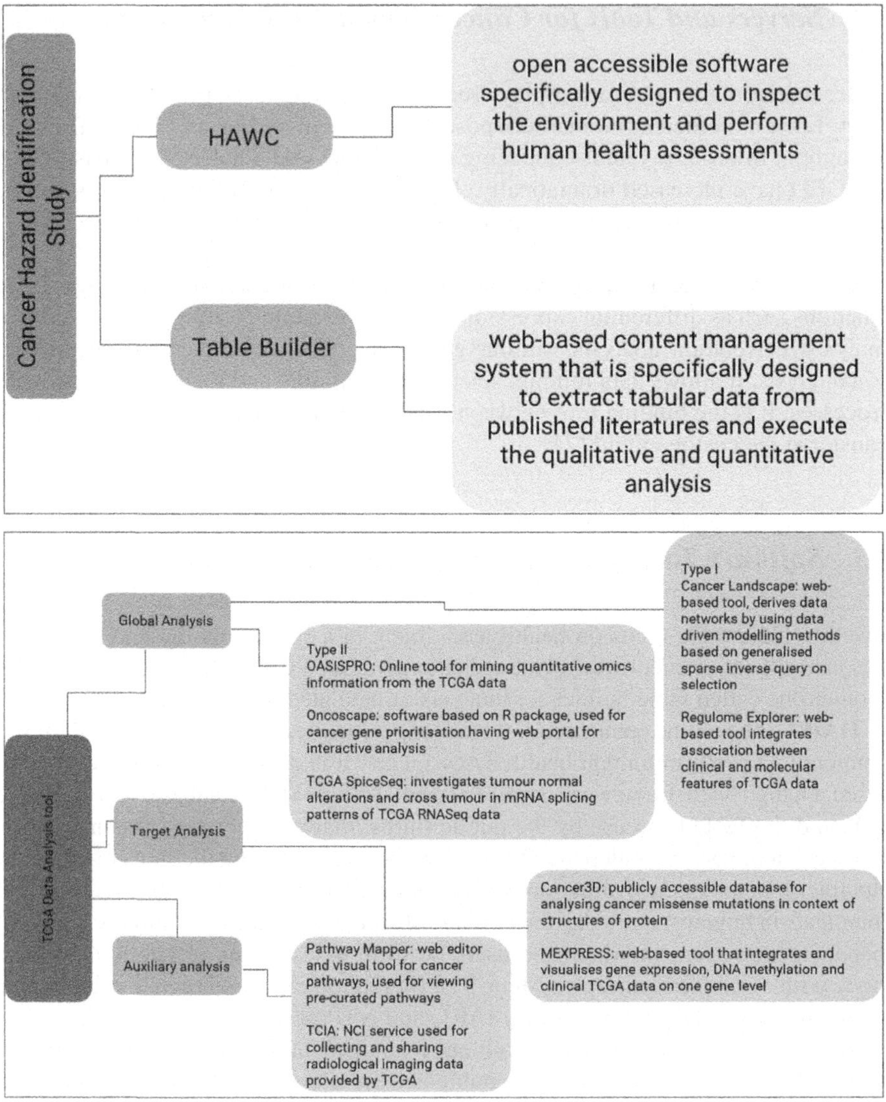

Fig. 5 Software tools and databases for cancer hazard identification and analysis of TCGA data

the name of—details relevant to human exposure to the substance, epidemiological evidence, animal bioassay evidence, and genotoxicity data [65].

2.6 *Web-Based Tools/Databases for Analyzing TCGA Data*

A huge amount of genomic data needs a specialized web store to help researchers in interpretation in a meaningful way [86] (Fig. 5).

2.6.1 Global Analysis

The global analysis tools let the researchers understand the complete features of the cancer genome. It is usually used to initiate cancer genomics studies. There are mainly two types of such tools—type one and type two. Type one provides global analysis while type two is used for target analysis [86].

Type I

Cancer landscapes (http://cancerlandscae.org/) is a tool for deriving networks of data by using data-driven modeling methods based on sparse inverse covariance selection. It includes data such as genetic data, epigenetic data, and transcriptional data from multiple cancers. It is an interactive web used for visualizing network models [33].

Regulome explorer (http://explorer.canceregulome.org/all_pair/) tool finds associations and allows the integration of clinical and molecular features of TCGA. It helps in searching and visualizing analytical data and filtering it according to user parameters. Several viewing options are available for the evaluation of associations such as graphs and tables [44].

Type II

Omics analysis system for precision oncology (OASISPRO) (http://tinyurl.com/oasispro) is a web-based tool built specifically for mining quantitative omics information from TCGA data. Extensively used for visualization of clinical profiles of patients. Evaluation of prediction performance is feasible. It uses different machine learning methods [82].

OncoScape (http://oncoscape.nki.nl/) is software-based on R language package. It is used for cancer gene prioritization also has an interactive analysis portal. It accesses five types of data across 11 different cancer types. It identifies cancer-causing genes and uses a fusion of genomic data to explore the cancer aberrations [46].

TCGA SpliceSeq is an investigative tool used for tumor-normal alterations and cross tumor in mRNA splicing patterns of TCGA RNASeq data. The PSE values are collected from 33 types of tumors. Investigation on splicing factors of interest gene in various cancer types. It also offers knowledge discovery through genome-wide PSI splicing event searches [84].

2.6.2 Target Analysis

The target analysis web-based tools are often used by researchers. These tools help in the investigation of a targeted interest via analysis of genes and miRNAs [86].

Cancer3D (http://www.cancer3d.org) is a publicly accessible database that analyses missense mutations in cancer in the context of the structures of protein. It helps in exploring different cancer-based problems simultaneously. It assists in biomarker identification, drug sensitivity, and prediction of cancer drivers as well [64].

MEXPRESS (http://mexpress.be/) is a very simple to use web-based tool that allows the integration and visualization of gene expression data, DNA methylation, and TCGA data on a single gene level. It enables finding correlations among data sets. It is easy to use tool that integrates visualization of different data types from hundreds of samples [29].

2.6.3 Auxiliary Analysis

These web-based tools help in translating TCGA data into online resources which are easily accessible and downloadable. It helps users in complementing their experimental results or as additional evidence to their experiments [86].

PathwayMapper (http://pathwaymapper.org) is an online Web editor tool for cancer pathways. It allows viewing of pre-curated Cancer pathways. It provides an intuitive editing choice for graphics to build and edit the pathways. Multiple users can cooperate curation in real-time. Users are allowed to import data from different portals and export images of the pathways [5].

TCIA (http://www.cancerimagingarchive.net) is a tool provided by the National Cancer Institute for the collection and sharing of radiological imaging data. TCGA data supports imaging phenotype-genotype research. The users have the feasibility to find relevant research-based clinical image data and download the image files [70].

2.7 Other's Databases/Tools/Webservers in Oncological Research to Identify Gene Function and Structure Prediction

In this section, we have listed software used in organizing microarray data and retrieving annotation information for genes from public databases. The microarray data repositories, function prediction of genes, protein structure prediction methods, and gaining useful insights are also described. Databases of protein-protein interaction describing the function of genes are mentioned [32]. The list of all the tools and web servers based on gene function and structure prediction for oncological studies has been provided below Table 1.

Table 1 Various other tools and web servers used in cancer studies

Type	Resources	Features	Websites	References
Cancer Metabolomics tools	XCMS2	XCMS2 is a modified version of XCMS used for obtaining structural information about unidentified metabolites. It is used for the development of automatic search tandem mass spectrometry MS/MS data against high-quality MS/MS data from the METLIN database	http://mathdamp.iab.keio.ac.jp/	[6]
	Ingenuity Pathway Analysis (IPA)	The web-based commercial tool allows users to upload results of data analysis from experiments (NGS, microarray) for functional analysis	http://www.ingenuity.com/products/ipa-metabolomics.html	[38]
Web servers of ncRNA	SurvMicro	miRNA data-based prognosis analysis using Cox multiple fitting for risk evaluation	http://bioinformatica.mty.itesm.mx/SurvMicro	[1]
Cancer biomarker development tools	TCPA	TCPA is a data portal that provides six modules for analysis and visualization	http://bioinformatics.mdanderson.org/main/TCPA:Overview	[39]
	SurvExpress	SurvExpress is a web tool for risk assessment and survival analysis of cancer datasets, facilitates performance comparisons and biomarkers validations	http://bioinformatica.mty.itesm.mx/SurvExpress	[2]

(continued)

Table 1 (continued)

Type	Resources	Features	Websites	References
	UALCAN	UALCAN is a user-friendly interactive web-based tool to perform in-depth analyses of TCGA gene expression data	http://ualcan.path.uab.edu	[12]
Survival analysis based on DNA tool	MethSurv	A web-based tool containing more than 7000 samples, based on the DNA methylation data for survival analysis	https://biit.cs.u.ee/methsurv/	[48]
Single cancer prognosis tool	BreastMark	A cancer prognostic tool used for the analysis of breast cancer, evaluation of miRNA and genes	http://glados.ucd.ie/BreastMark/miRNA_list.html	[42]
Cancer biomarker development tools/web servers	OncoLnc	OncoLnc tool is extensively used for interactive exploration of survival correlations. It allows downloading clinical data	http://www.oncolnc.org	[3]
TCGA data analysis tools/web servers	TCGA next-generation clustered heat maps	Classic heat map approach used for creating interactive large-scale visualization of data	http://bioinformaticsmdanderson.org/chm	[86]
	TCGA SpliceSeq	This tool investigates tumor-normal alterations and crosses tumors in mRNA splicing patterns of TCGA RNASeq data	http://bioinformatics.mdanderson.org/TCGASpliceSeq/	[84]

(continued)

2.7.1 Microarray Data Management and Analysis Software

GoMiner (http://discover.nci.nih.gov/gominer/) is a software that creates a list of genes of interest for biological interpretation in Gene Ontology. It produces statistical results and quantitative outputs. There are two visualization methods—the first is the

Table 1 (continued)

Type	Resources	Features	Websites	References
	TANRIC	An open resource that provides three modules for investigating functional and clinical relevance of long non-coding RNA in cancer	http://ibl.mdanderson.org/tanric/_design/basic/index.html	[31]
	Vanno	A tool for variant annotation used for visualization and analysis of genetic alteration profiles	http://cgts.cgu.edu.tw/vanno	[25]
Protein function prediction tools	BLAST	Basic Local Alignment Search Tool is used to find the best sequence matches to the query sequence; many versions are available	http://www.ncbi.nlm.nih.gov/BLAST	[27]

tree-like structure and the second is a compact and interactive directed acyclic graph [83].

caGEDA (http://bioinformatics.upmc.edu/GE2/GEDA.html) is a web-based application for the integrated analysis of global gene expression patterns in cancer. It uploads gene expression profiles from cDNA or microarrays and conducts linear normalization. It helps in the identification of differentially expressed genes using different tests. It produces tabular data with a list of literature references [55].

2.7.2 Microarray Data Repositories

CIBEX (http://cibex.nig.ac.jp) also called the Centre for Information Biology Gene Expression Database is a publicly accessible repository. It has a data retrieval system in compliance with MIAME. It has a wide range of high throughput experimental data based on gene expressions such as MicroArray based experiments and SAGE tags [26].

Standard Microarray Database (SMD) (http://smd.stanford.edu/) microArray research data for Stanford researchers and collaborators. It is a source of data for the entire scientific community. It is freely accessible and has open-source code. It offers various analysis tools for that data. It holds more than 3,500 microarrays from 85 publications [20].

2.7.3 Protein Function Prediction Tools

Pfam (http://pfam.wustl.edu) is a database of curated protein and its families. Each protein family is defined by two alignments and a profile Hidden Markov Model (HMM). The HMM is a probabilistic model for statistical inference of homology. The data is available in different formats such as flat files and relational table dumps. It provides both a graphical representation and interactive access to the data [17].

2.7.4 Protein Structure Prediction Tools

PSIPRED (http://bioinf.cs.ucl.ac.uk/psipred/) is a protein structure prediction web server that allows users to submit protein sequences. There are three methods of prediction available, PSIPRED for secondary structural prediction, MEMSAT2 for transmembrane topology prediction, and GenTHREADER For protein fold recognition [47].

SWISS-MODEL (http://swissmodel.expasy.org) is a web server used for automated comparative modeling of 3-D protein structures. A widely used tool that provides user interaction through a web interface. The entire process is automated such as template selection, alignment, and model building. The project mode allows complex modeling tasks using a Swiss PDB viewer. A highly reliable tool under constant developments [63].

2.7.5 Protein-Protein Interaction Databases

BIND (http://bind.ca/) also called the biomolecular interaction network database used popularly for identifying biomolecular interactions. It also provides complex pathway information. It is a graphical analysis tool that provides the domain composition of proteins and the ability to relate the protein interactions with functional domains. It is also our interaction network clustering tool focusing on regions of interest [4].

IntAct (http://www.ebi.ac.uk/intact/) is a freely accessible tool for studying molecular interaction, storing and representing those interactions. It has both graphical and textual representation of data and also allows interaction networks exploration for the GO annotations. Approximately 2200 binary and complex interactions are stored in it which is imported from the Swiss-Prot. [24]. Table 1 shows various other tools and webservers available and widely used from the identification to analysis in cancer.

3 Cancer Precision Drug Discovery: Computational Biology and AI

Cancer is a major global issue causing mass morbidity, mortality and characterized by some hallmarks of cancer including deregulated growth, angiogenesis, evading apoptosis, and others. It involves several modifications [15]. Computer-assisted tools are used for the identification of DNA/RNA or protein sequences, single nucleotides polymorphisms (SNPs), and microarrays can be carried out and analyzed. According to the report by the International Agency for Research on Cancer (IARC) 2018, around 18.1 million new cases and 9.6 million deaths have occurred due to cancer globally [10, 30]. Nowadays, newer alternative technologies are being used and identified for targeted cancer therapy. Artificial intelligence, machine learning, and computational technologies have proven to be better alternatives for precision cancer therapy [51]. The concept of artificial intelligence came as a boon to the fields of drug discovery and analysis of biomedical data (Fig. 6). AI has great importance in precision medicine and drug discovery. Precision medicine is an upcoming modern method wherein prevention and treatment of any disease will be much easier as compared to traditional methods as it evaluates the person's genetic variation, style, and other aspects. Furthermore, the availability of a huge amount of data that has been generated by the next-generation sequencing (NGS) methods and the incorporation of machine learning along with AI algorithms have tremendously increased the scope in the field [16, 51, 60]. Imaging-based analysis coupled with NGS has provided the easy identification, early diagnosis, and prognosis of cancer with the applications of AI. Some of the facets of NGS include whole-genome & whole-exome sequencing (WG/ES), target sequencing, methylome sequencing, RNA sequencing, and whole transcriptome sequencing which have paved the path for the identification of nucleotide aberrations which ultimately result in cancers [16, 34]. Some of the software which is available to identify functional and silent variations that occurred in the genome based on the computational approaches include PROVEAN, AlignGVGD, SIFT, MutationTaster & PolyPhen2, and NNSPLICE, GeneSplicer, Human Splicing

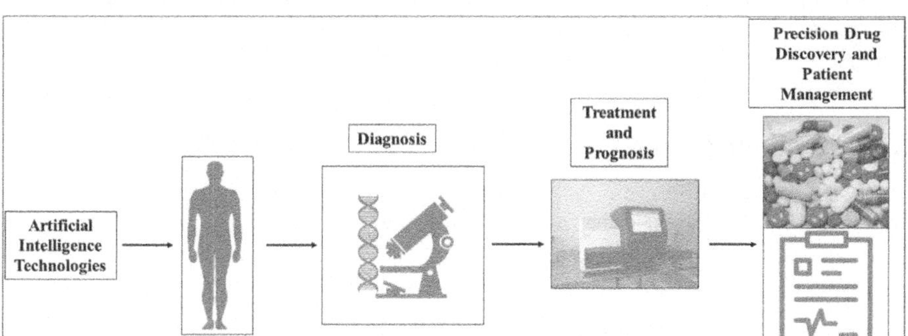

Fig. 6 Computational and artificial intelligence applications in precision drug discovery

Finder, MaxEntScan, SpliceSiteFinder [16, 50, 58, 79]. AI has many applications in cancer-related diagnostics through image-based identification and management which include digital pathology, ultrasounds, positron-emission tomography (PET), computed tomography (CT/CAT), X-rays, and magnetic resonance imaging (MRI) [16, 61, 66, 75].

4 Limitations and Prospects

There are various demerits associated with the usage and application of various webservers and tools available for cancer-related analyses and studies [15, 57, 59].

4.1 Terminology Inconsistency

Bioinformatics is a dynamic field and as a result, due to a lack of standard terminology (new terms are coming each day), it causes a barrier to free access of resources.

4.2 Lack of Interoperability

Every database communicates its resources, and this results in a lack of access to proper utilization of the websites properly.

4.3 Database Proprietary Issues

The databases are publicly available but, sometimes papers and resources are not. For instance, privately owned databases are not accessible easily and freely.

4.4 Payment Issues

Sometimes, some databases are not accessible and need payment for complete access to resources.

4.5 Inadequate Support

For the usage of these resources and tools, expertise is required wherein technical support is required for complete and proper utilization of the database/resource for obtaining desired results.

4.6 Misleading Results

Due to the occurrence of human or technical, sometimes, results can be falsely positive or deceiving.

4.7 Algorithms

The commands and algorithms are complex and require expertise in understanding and getting the correct results.

There are numerous databases for a single topic, the problem arises to choose the perfect and appropriate one, there should be an announcement or monthly release of issues mentioning the development and release of such databases publicly. The privately-owned databases issue can be resolved by making the databases available freely to the scientific community like with an annual subscription basis to the educational and research institutions. Training programs and workshops should be conducted either directly by the developer or from an expert learned in the educational/academic and research institutions to make the young researchers aware of those databases.

The physiochemical information and structural features of the ligands and their interactions with the target should be increased with the application of algorithms. Artificial intelligence and computational methods have gained momentum and will be required in all the sectors of healthcare which include a virtual screening of candidates, genetic variation analysis using deep machine learning, molecular docking, and simulations [51]. The above-mentioned plausible solutions can be treated as loopholes and missing gaps as future directions for bridging the gap between the source (database developer) and the sink (user).

5 Conclusions

The inclusion of bioinformatics and computational tools and resources play vital roles in delineating, observation (visualization), and analyzing the results obtained from the different sources of data generation methods (omics technologies). The multiple methods and approaches which are relevant have been discussed in the content which is being used for the cancer diagnosis, prognosis, and treatments using computational and artificial intelligence algorithms. These software, tools, and resources are robust and sensitive. Each of these databases, resources, and tools provide a vast scope for exploring and the ability to the research for submitting, sharing along analyzing their data. Cancer bioinformatics is a new field that involves the utilization of the tools and resources for identifying, preventing, and diagnosis of cancer.

References

1. Aguirre-Gamboa, R., & Trevino, V. (2014). SurvMicro: Assessment of miRNA-based prognostic signatures for cancer clinical outcomes by multivariate survival analysis. *Bioinformatics, 30*(11), 1630–1632.
2. Aguirre-Gamboa, R., Gomez-Rueda, H., Martínez-Ledesma, E., Martínez-Torteya, A., Chacolla-Huaringa, R., Rodriguez-Barrientos, A., Tamez-Pena, J. G., & Trevino, V. (2013). SurvExpress: An online biomarker validation tool and database for cancer gene expression data using survival analysis. *PloS One, 8*(9), e74250.
3. Anaya, J. (2016). OncoLnc: Linking TCGA survival data to mRNAs, miRNAs, and lncRNAs. *PeerJ Computer Science, 2*, e67.
4. Bader, G. D., Betel, D., & Hogue, C. W. (2003). BIND: The biomolecular interaction network database. *Nucleic Acids Research, 31*(1), 248–250.
5. Bahceci, I., Dogrusoz, U., La, K. C., Babur, Ö., Gao, J., & Schultz, N. (2017). PathwayMapper: A collaborative visual web editor for cancer pathways and genomic data. *Bioinformatics, 33*(14), 2238–2240.
6. Benton, H. P., Wong, D. M., Trauger, S. A., & Siuzdak, G. (2008). XCMS2: Processing tandem mass spectrometry data for metabolite identification and structural characterization. *Analytical chemistry, 80*(16), 6382–6389.
7. Bhattacharya, A., & Cui, Y. (2016). SomamiR 2.0: A database of cancer somatic mutations altering microRNA—ceRNA interactions. *Nucleic Acids Research, 44*(D1), D1005–D1010.
8. Blekherman, G., Laubenbacher, R., Cortes, D. F., Mendes, P., Torti, F. M., Akman, S., Torti, S.V., & Shulaev, V. (2011). Bioinformatics tools for cancer metabolomics. *Metabolomics, 7*(3), 329-343.
9. Borcherding, N., Bormann, N. L., Voigt, A. P., & Zhang, W. (2018). TRGAted: A web tool for survival analysis using protein data in the Cancer Genome Atlas. *F1000 Research, 7*.
10. Bray, F., Ferlay, J., Soerjomataram, I., Siegel, R. L., Torre, L. A., & Jemal, A. (2018). Global cancer statistics 2018: GLOBOCAN estimates of incidence and mortality worldwide for 36 cancers in 185 countries. *CA: A Cancer Journal for Clinicians, 68*(6), 394–424.
11. Broeckling, C. D., Reddy, I. R., Duran, A. L., Zhao, X., & Sumner, L. W. (2006). MET-IDEA: Data extraction tool for mass spectrometry-based metabolomics. *Analytical Chemistry, 78*(13), 4334–4341.
12. Chandrashekar, D. S., Bashel, B., Balasubramanya, S. A. H., Creighton, C. J., Ponce-Rodriguez, I., Chakravarthi, B. V., & Varambally, S. (2017). UALCAN: A portal for facilitating tumour subgroup gene expression and survival analyses. *Neoplasia, 19*(8), 649–658.
13. Chin, L., Andersen, J. N., & Futreal, P. A. (2011). Cancer genomics: From discovery science to personalized medicine. *Nature Medicine, 17*(3), 297–303.
14. Coker, E. A., Mitsopoulos, C., Tym, J. E., Komianou, A., Kannas, C., Di Micco, P., Villasclaras Fernandez, E., Ozer, B., Antolin, A. A., Workman, P., & Al-Lazikani, B. (2019). canSAR: update to the cancer translational research and drug discovery knowledgebase. *Nucleic Acids Research, 47*(D1), D917–D922.

15. de Anda-Jáuregui, G., & Hernández-Lemus, E. (2020). Computational oncology in the multi-omics era: State of the art. *Frontiers in Oncology, 10*, 423.
16. Dlamini, Z., Francies, F. Z., Hull, R., & Marima, R. (2020). Artificial intelligence (AI) and big data in cancer and precision oncology. *Computational and Structural Biotechnology Journal.*
17. Finn, R. D., Bateman, A., Clements, J., Coggill, P., Eberhardt, R. Y., Eddy, S. R., Heger, A., Hetherington, K., Holm, L., Mistry, J., Sonnhammer, E.L., & Punta, M. (2014). Pfam: The protein families database. *Nucleic Acids Research, 42*(D1), D222–D230.
18. Gao, J., Aksoy, B. A., Dogrusoz, U., Dresdner, G., Gross, B., Sumer, S. O., Sun, Y., Jacobsen, A., Sinha, R., Larsson, E., Cerami, E., & Schultz, N. (2013). Integrative analysis of complex cancer genomics and clinical profiles using the cBioPortal. *Science Signaling, 6*(269), pl1–pl1.
19. Goldman, M., Craft, B., Swatloski, T., Ellrott, K., Cline, M., Diekhans, M., Ma, S., Wilks, C., Stuart, J., Haussler, D., & Zhu, J. (2013). The UCSC cancer genomics browser: Update 2013. *Nucleic Acids Research, 41*(D1), D949–D954.
20. Gollub, J., Ball, C. A., Binkley, G., Demeter, J., Finkelstein, D. B., Hebert, J. M., Jin, H., Kaloper, M., Matese, J. C., Schroeder, M., & Sherlock, G. (2003). The Stanford Microarray Database: data access and quality assessment tools. *Nucleic Acids Research, 31*(1), 94–96.
21. Goswami, C. P., & Nakshatri, H. (2012). PROGmiR: A tool for identifying prognostic miRNA biomarkers in multiple cancers using publicly available data. *Journal of Clinical Bioinformatics, 2*(1), 1–8.
22. Goswami, C. P., & Nakshatri, H. (2014). PROGgeneV2: Enhancements on the existing database. *BMC Cancer, 14*(1), 1–6.
23. He, X., Chang, S., Zhang, J., Zhao, Q., Xiang, H., Kusonmano, K., Yang, L., Sun, Z.S., Yang, H., & Wang, J. (2007). MethyCancer: The database of human DNA methylation and cancer. *Nucleic Acids Research, 36*(suppl_1), D836–D841.
24. Hermjakob, H., Montecchi-Palazzi, L., Lewington, C., Mudali, S., Kerrien, S., Orchard, S., Vingron, M., Roechert, B., Roepstorff, P., Valencia, A., Margalit, H., & Apweiler, R. (2004). IntAct: an open source molecular interaction database. *Nucleic Acids Research, 32*(suppl_1), D452–D455.
25. Huang, P. J., Lee, C. C., Tan, B. C. M., Yeh, Y. M., Huang, K. Y., Gan, R. C., Chen, T. W., Lee, C. Y., Yang, S. T., Liao, C. S., Liu, H., & Tang, P. (2015). V anno: A visualization-aided variant annotation tool. *Human Mutation, 36*(2), 167–174.
26. Ikeo, K., Ishi-i, J., Tamura, T., Gojobori, T., & Tateno, Y. (2003). CIBEX: Center for information biology gene expression database. *Comptesrendusbiologies, 326*(10–11), 1079–1082.
27. Johnson, M., Zaretskaya, I., Raytselis, Y., Merezhuk, Y., McGinnis, S., & Madden, T. L. (2008). NCBI BLAST: A better web interface. *Nucleic Acids Research, 36*(suppl_2), W5–W9.
28. Katajamaa, M., Miettinen, J., & Orešič, M. (2006). MZmine: Toolbox for processing and visualization of mass spectrometry based molecular profile data. *Bioinformatics, 22*(5), 634–636.
29. Katopodis, P., Kerslake, R., Zikopoulos, A., Beri, N., & Anikin, V. (2021). p38β-MAPK11 and its role in female cancers. *Journal of Ovarian Research, 14*(1), 1–12.
30. Kaur, G., Gupta, S., Kaur, G., Verma, M., & Kaur, P. (2021). Bioinformatics: An important tool in oncology. *Biomedical Data Mining for Information Retrieval: Methodologies, Techniques and Applications*, 163–195.
31. Kaushik, A. C., Mehmood, A., Wang, X., Wei, D. Q., & Dai, X. (2020). Globally ncRNAs expression profiling of TNBC and screening of functional lncRNA. *Frontiers in Bioengineering and Biotechnology, 8.*
32. Kihara, D., Yang, Y. D., & Hawkins, T. (2006). Bioinformatics resources for cancer research with an emphasis on gene function and structure prediction tools. *Cancer Informatics, 2*, 117693510600200020.
33. Kling, T., Johansson, P., Sanchez, J., Marinescu, V. D., Jörnsten, R., & Nelander, S. (2015). Efficient exploration of pan-cancer networks by generalized covariance selection and interactive web content. *Nucleic Acids Research, 43*(15), e98–e98.
34. Kulski, J. (Ed.). (2016). Next generation sequencing: Advances, applications and challenges. *BoD–Books on Demand.*

35. Lappalainen, I., Almeida-King, J., Kumanduri, V., Senf, A., Spalding, J. D., Saunders, G., Kandasamy, J., Caccamo, M., Leinonen, R., Vaughan, B., Laurent, T., & Flicek, P. (2015). The European Genome-phenome Archive of human data consented for biomedical research. *Nature Genetics, 47*(7), 692–695.
36. Lengauer, C., Kinzler, K. W., & Vogelstein, B. (1998). Genetic instabilities in human cancers. *Nature, 396*(6712), 643–649.
37. Leptos, K. C., Sarracino, D. A., Jaffe, J. D., Krastins, B., & Church, G. M. (2006). MapQuant: Open-source software for large-scale protein quantification. *Proteomics, 6*(6), 1770–1782.
38. Li, G., Zhang, N., Geng, F., Liu, G., Liu, B., Lei, X., Li, G., & Chen, X. (2019). High-throughput metabolomics and ingenuity pathway approach reveals the pharmacological effect and targets of Ginsenoside Rg1 in Alzheimer's disease mice. *Scientific Reports, 9*(1), 1–11.
39. Li, J., Lu, Y., Akbani, R., Ju, Z., Roebuck, P. L., Liu, W., Broom, B. M., Verhaak, R. G., Kane, D. W., Wakefield, C., & Liang, H. (2013). TCPA: A resource for cancer functional proteomics data. *Nature Methods, 10*(11), 1046–1047.
40. Li, X. J., Eugene, C. Y., Kemp, C. J., Zhang, H., & Aebersold, R. (2005). A software suite for the generation and comparison of peptide arrays from sets of data collected by liquid chromatography-mass spectrometry* S. *Molecular and Cellular Proteomics, 4*(9), 1328–1340.
41. MacConaill, L. E., & Garraway, L. A. (2010). Clinical implications of the cancer genome. *Journal of Clinical Oncology, 28*(35), 5219.
42. Madden, S. F., Clarke, C., Gaule, P., Aherne, S. T., O'Donovan, N., Clynes, M., Crown, J., & Gallagher, W. M. (2013). BreastMark: an integrated approach to mining publicly available transcriptomic datasets relating to breast cancer outcome. *Breast Cancer Research, 15*(4), 1–14.
43. Madden, S. F., Clarke, C., Stordal, B., Carey, M. S., Broaddus, R., Gallagher, W. M., Crown, J., Mills, G.B., & Hennessy, B. T. (2014). OvMark: A user-friendly system for the identification of prognostic biomarkers in publically available ovarian cancer gene expression datasets. *Molecular Cancer, 13*(1), 1–11.
44. Madhavan, S., Gusev, Y., Natarajan, T. G., Song, L., Bhuvaneshwar, K., Gauba, R., Gauba, R., Pandey, A., Haddad, B. R., Goerlitz, D., Cheema, A. K., Juhl, H., & Weiner, L. M. (2013). Genome-wide multi-omics profiling of colorectal cancer identifies immune determinants strongly associated with relapse. *Frontiers in Genetics, 4*, 236.
45. Marx, V. (2013). Drilling into big cancer-genome data. *Nature Methods, 10*(4), 293–297.
46. McFerrin, L. G., Zager, M., Zhang, J., Krenn, G., McDermott, R., Horse-Grant, D., Silgard, E., Colevas, K., Shannon, P., Bolouri, H., & Holland, E. C. (2018). Analysis and visualization of linked molecular and clinical cancer data by using Oncoscape. Nature genetics, 50(9), 1203-1204.
47. McGuffin, L. J., Bryson, K., & Jones, D. T. (2000). The PSIPRED protein structure prediction server. *Bioinformatics, 16*(4), 404–405.
48. Modhukur, V., Iljasenko, T., Metsalu, T., Lokk, K., Laisk-Podar, T., & Vilo, J. (2018). MethSurv: A web tool to perform multivariable survival analysis using DNA methylation data. *Epigenomics, 10*(3), 277–288.
49. Molander, L., Hanberg, A., Rudén, C., Ågerstrand, M., & Beronius, A. (2017). Combining web-based tools for transparent evaluation of data for risk assessment: Developmental effects of bisphenol A on the mammary gland as a case study. *Journal of Applied Toxicology, 37*(3), 319–330.
50. Moles-Fernández, A., Duran-Lozano, L., Montalban, G., Bonache, S., López-Perolio, I., Menéndez, M., Santamariña, M., Behar, R., Blanco, A., Carrasco, E., López-Fernández, A., & Gutiérrez-Enríquez, S. (2018). Computational tools for splicing defect prediction in breast/ovarian cancer genes: how efficient are they at predicting RNA alterations?. Frontiers in genetics, 9, 366.
51. Nagarajan, N., Yapp, E. K., Le, N. Q. K., Kamaraj, B., Al-Subaie, A. M., & Yeh, H. Y. (2019). Application of computational biology and artificial intelligence technologies in cancer precision drug discovery. *BioMed Research International.*

52. Packer, B. R., Yeager, M., Staats, B., Welch, R., Crenshaw, A., Kiley, M., Eckert, A., Beerman, M., Miller, E., Bergen, A., Rothman, N., & Chanock, S. J. (2004). SNP500Cancer: a public resource for sequence validation and assay development for genetic variation in candidate genes. *Nucleic Acids Research, 32*(suppl_1), D528–D532.
53. Palagi, P. M., Walther, D., Quadroni, M., Catherinet, S., Burgess, J., Zimmermann-Ivol, C. G., Zimmermann-Ivol, C. G., Sanchez, J. C., Binz, P. A., Hochstrasser, D. F., & Appel, R. D. (2005). MSight: An image analysis software for liquid chromatography-mass spectrometry. *Proteomics, 5*(9), 2381–2384.
54. Park, S. J., Yoon, B. H., Kim, S. K., & Kim, S. Y. (2019). GENT2: An updated gene expression database for normal and tumour tissues. *BMC Medical Genomics, 12*(5), 1–8.
55. Patel, S., & Lyons-Weiler, J. (2004). caGEDA: a web application for the integrated analysis of global gene expression patterns in cancer. *Applied bioinformatics, 3*(1), 49–62
56. Pevsner, J. (2015). *Bioinformatics and functional genomics*. John Wiley & Sons.
57. Pool, R., & Esnayra, J. (2000). *Bioinformatics: Converting data to knowledge: A workshop summary*. National Academies Press.
58. Pshennikova, V. G., Barashkov, N. A., Romanov, G. P., Teryutin, F. M., Solov'ev, A. V., Gotovtsev, N. N., Nikanorova, A. A., Nakhodkin, S. S., Sazonov, N. N., Morozov, I. V., Bondar, A. A., & Fedorova, S. A. (2019). Comparison of predictive in silico tools on missense variants in GJB2, GJB6, and GJB3 genes associated with autosomal recessive deafness 1A (DFNB1A). *The Scientific World Journal*.
59. Ramlal, A., Ahmad, S., Kumar, L., Khan, F. N., & Chongtham, R. (2021). From molecules to patients: the clinical applications of biological databases and electronic health records. In *Translational bioinformatics in healthcare and medicine* (pp. 107–125). Academic Press.
60. Raza, K., & Ahmad, S. (2019). Recent advancement in next-generation sequencing techniques and its computational analysis. *International Journal of Bioinformatics Research and Applications, Inderscience, 15*(3), 191–220.
61. Raza, K., & Singh, N. K. (2021). A tour of unsupervised deep learning for medical image analysis current medical imaging. *Bentham Science, 17*(9), 1059–1077. https://doi.org/10.2174/1573405617666210127154257
62. Samur, M. K., Yan, Z., Wang, X., Cao, Q., Munshi, N. C., Li, C., & Shah, P. K. (2013). canEvolve: A web portal for integrative oncogenomics. *PLoS One, 8*(2), e56228.
63. Schwede, T., Kopp, J., Guex, N., & Peitsch, M. C. (2003). SWISS-MODEL: An automated protein homology-modeling server. *Nucleic acids research, 31*(13), 3381–3385.
64. Sedova, M., Iyer, M., Li, Z., Jaroszewski, L., Post, K. W., Hrabe, T., Porta-Pardo, E., & Godzik, A. (2019). Cancer3D 2.0: Interactive analysis of 3D patterns of cancer mutations in cancer subsets. *Nucleic Acids Research, 47*(D1), D895–D899.
65. Shapiro, A. J., Antoni, S., Guyton, K. Z., Lunn, R. M., Loomis, D., Rusyn, I., Jahnke, G. D., Schwingl, P. J., Mehta, S. S., Addington, J., & Guha, N. (2018). Software tools to facilitate systematic review used for cancer hazard identification. *Environmental Health Perspectives, 126*(10), 104501.
66. Singh, N. K., & Raza, K. (2021). Medical image generation using generative adversarial networks: A review. *Health Informatics: A Computational Perspective in Healthcare, Studies in Computational Intelligence, Springer, 932*, 77–96. https://doi.org/10.1007/978-981-15-9735-0_5
67. Smith, C. A., Want, E. J., O'Maille, G., Abagyan, R., & Siuzdak, G. (2006). XCMS: Processing mass spectrometry data for metabolite profiling using nonlinear peak alignment, matching, and identification. *Analytical Chemistry, 78*(3), 779–787.
68. Stratton, M. R., Campbell, P. J., & Futreal, P. A. (2009). The cancer genome. *Nature, 458*(7239), 719–724.
69. Sun, K., Zhang, X. D., Liu, X. Y., & Lu, P. (2021). YAP1 is a prognostic biomarker and correlated with immune cell infiltration in pancreatic cancer. *Frontiers in Molecular Biosciences, 8*, 504.
70. Taha, B., Li, T., Boley, D., Chen, C. C., & Sun, J. (2021). Detection of isocitrate dehydrogenase mutated glioblastomas through anomaly detection analytics. *Neurosurgery*.

71. Tang, Z., Li, C., Kang, B., Gao, G., Li, C., & Zhang, Z. (2017). GEPIA: A web server for cancer and normal gene expression profiling and interactive analyses. *Nucleic Acids Research, 45*(W1), W98–W102.
72. Tate, J. G., Bamford, S., Jubb, H. C., Sondka, Z., Beare, D. M., Bindal, N., Boutselakis, H., Cole, C. G., Creatore, C., Dawson, E., Fish, P., & Forbes, S. A. (2019). COSMIC: the catalogue of somatic mutations in cancer. Nucleic acids research, 47(D1), D941-D947.
73. Tomczak, K., Czerwińska, P., & Wiznerowicz, M. (2015). The cancer genome atlas (TCGA): An immeasurable source of knowledge. *Contemporary Oncology, 19*(1A), A68.
74. Turkistani, S., Sugita, B. M., Fadda, P., Marchi, R., Afsari, A., Naab, T., Apprey, V., Copeland, R. L., Campbell, M., Cavalli, L. R., & Kanaan, Y. (2021). *A panel of miRNAs as prognostic markers for African-American patients with triple negative breast cancer.*
75. Wani, N., & Raza, K. (2018). Multiple Kernel Learning Approach for Medical Image Analysis. In: N. Dey, A. Ashour, F. Shi, E. Balas (Eds.), *Soft computing based medical image analysis*, (pp. 31–47). Elsevier. https://doi.org/10.1016/B978-0-12-813087-2.00002-6
76. Wilks, C., Cline, M. S., Weiler, E., Diehkans, M., Craft, B., Martin, C., Murphy, D., Pierce, H., Black, J., Nelson, D., Litzinger, B., & Maltbie, D. (2014). The cancer genomics hub (CGHub): overcoming cancer through the power of torrential data. *Database.*
77. Xie, L., Wang, L., Zhu, W., Zhao, J., & Guo, X. (2020). Bioinformatics tools (and web server) for cancer biomarker development. *Frontiers in Oncology, 10.*
78. Xiyuan, L., Dechao, B., Liang, S., Yang, W., Shuangsang, F., Hui, L., Haitao, L., Chunlong, L., Wenzheng, F., Runsheng, C., & Yi, Z. (2017). Using the NONCODE database resource. *Current Protocols in Bioinformatics, 58*(1), 12–16.
79. Xu, J., Yang, P., Xue, S., Sharma, B., Sanchez-Martin, M., Wang, F., Beaty, K. A., Dehan, E., & Parikh, B. (2019). Translating cancer genomics into precision medicine with artificial intelligence: applications, challenges and future perspectives. *Human Genetics, 138*(2), 109–124
80. Yang, W., Soares, J., Greninger, P., Edelman, E. J., Lightfoot, H., Forbes, S., Bindal, N., Beare, D., Smith, J. A., Thompson, I. R., Ramaswamy, S., & Garnett, M. J. (2012). Genomics of drug sensitivity in cancer (GDSC): A resource for therapeutic biomarker discovery in cancer cells. *Nucleic Acids Research, 41*(D1), D955–D961.
81. Yang, Y., Dong, X., Xie, B., Ding, N., Chen, J., Li, Y., Zhang, Q., Qu, H., & Fang, X. (2015). Databases and web tools for cancer genomics study. *Genomics, Proteomics and Bioinformatics, 13*(1), 46–50.
82. Yu, K. H., Fitzpatrick, M. R., Pappas, L., Chan, W., Kung, J., & Snyder, M. (2018). Omics analysis system for PRecision oncology (OASISPRO): A web-based omics analysis tool for clinical phenotype prediction. *Bioinformatics, 34*(2), 319–320.
83. Zeeberg, B. R., Feng, W., Wang, G., Wang, M. D., Fojo, A. T., Sunshine, M., Narasimhan, S., Kane, D. W., Reinhold, W. C., Lababidi, S., Bussey, K. J., & Weinstein, J. N. (2003). GoMiner: a resource for biological interpretation of genomic and proteomic data. *Genome Biology, 4*(4), 1–8.
84. Zhang, B., Yang, L., Wang, X., & Fu, D. (2021). Identification of survival-related alternative splicing signatures in acute myeloid leukemia. *Bioscience Reports, 41*(7), BSR20204037.
85. Zhang, J., Finney, R. P., Rowe, W., Edmonson, M., Yang, S. H., Dracheva, T., Jen, J., Struewing, J. P., & Buetow, K. H. (2007). Systematic analysis of genetic alterations in tumours using Cancer Genome WorkBench (CGWB). *Genome Research, 17*(7), 1111–1117.
86. Zhang, Z., Li, H., Jiang, S., Li, R., Li, W., Chen, H., & Bo, X. (2019). A survey and evaluation of Web-based tools/databases for variant analysis of TCGA data. *Briefings in Bioinformatics, 20*(4), 1524–1541.
87. Zhao, X., Liu, X., & Cui, L. (2020). Development of a five-protein signature for predicting the prognosis of head and neck squamous cell carcinoma. *Aging (Albany NY), 12*(19), 19740.
88. Zheng, H., Zhang, G., Zhang, L., Wang, Q., Li, H., Han, Y., Xie, L., Yan, Z., Li, Y., An, Y., Dong, H., & Guo, X. (2020). Comprehensive review of web servers and bioinformatics tools for cancer prognosis analysis. *Frontiers in Oncology, 10*, 68.

Cancer Detection, Diagnosis, Survival, and Recurrence Prediction

Application of Convolutional Neural Networks in Cancer Diagnosis

Rejaul Karim Barbhuiya, Naeem Ahmad, and Wasim Akram

Abstract Early detection and treatment are crucial for recovery from cancer. Due to rapid advancement in medical imaging techniques, today doctors can scan various body parts from different perspectives to diagnose cancer or see the progress during a course of treatment. Such techniques are less painful and require less preparation and recovery. The recent evolution of AI, particularly deep learning algorithms have shown potential in computer-aided diagnosis of cancer. These include analysis of cancer images for detection of tumor region, prognosis, skin tissue inspection, etc. Convolutional Neural Network (CNN) based image processing techniques are showing promising results in the diagnosis of breast cancer, skin cancer, prostate cancer, lung cancer, etc. Literature shows many other CNN-based models such as feed-forward neural network, Deep CNN, Multi-Crop CNN, fully convolutional networks (FCNs), Deep Fully Convolutional Network (DFCNet), Recurrent neural networks, etc. The CNN focus solely on the image-specific features and hence require a lesser number of input parameters. A CNN model reduces the size of the input image vector without losing the features critical for making an accurate prediction. This makes it easier to process and reduces computational complexity. CNNs are also not sensitive to the object positioning in an image since the approximate position of image motifs relative to others is known. CNN deals with the variations in images through augmentation and other pre-processing techniques. This makes them robust to various straining conditions in images. This chapter presents an overview of a generic CNN architecture followed by a discussion on major advances in CNN models and their applications for cancer image analysis.

R. K. Barbhuiya (✉)
National Council of Educational Research and Training, New Delhi, India
e-mail: rejaul.ncert@nic.in

N. Ahmad
Department of Computer Applications, National Institute of Technology, Raipur, India
e-mail: nahmad.mca@nitrr.ac.in

W. Akram
Accenture India, Gurgaon, India

K. Raza (ed.), *Computational Intelligence in Oncology*, Studies in Computational Intelligence 1016, https://doi.org/10.1007/978-981-16-9221-5_5

Keywords Neural networks · Convolutional Neural Networks (CNNs) · Image classification · Image segmentation · Cancer detection · CNN architecture

1 Introduction

Cancer is a leading cause of death worldwide. According to the World Health Organization [1], cancer accounted for nearly 10 million deaths in 2020. The common types of cancers reported were breast, lung, colon and rectum, prostate, skin, and stomach. Early detection of cancer significantly increases the chance of successful treatment and thus recovery. Biomedical imaging techniques such as Computed tomography (CT) scan, Magnetic resonance imaging (MRI), bone scans, Positron Emission Tomography (PET) scans, Ultrasound, X-ray, Mammography, etc. are useful in all phases of cancer management starting with prediction, screening, staging, prognosis, as well as therapeutic guidance [2, 3].

The key steps involved in the diagnosis of cancer from images consist of image acquisition, segmentation (border detection), future classification/feature extraction. The key stages of cancer management are depicted in Fig. 1. The overall role of imaging in each of these stages is ever-increasing primarily due to its non-invasive nature.

There have been efforts in the application of neural network techniques in processing such images for accurate detection and diagnosis of cancer. Convolutional Neural Network (CNN) is found to be highly effective for processing such images. Before going to discuss in detail computer-aided cancer diagnosis, let us have a brief overview of neural networks.

1.1 Artificial Neural Network

Artificial neural networks (ANNs) are biologically inspired computer programs designed to simulate the processing of information by a human brain. ANNs gather their knowledge by detecting the patterns and relationships in the data and learn

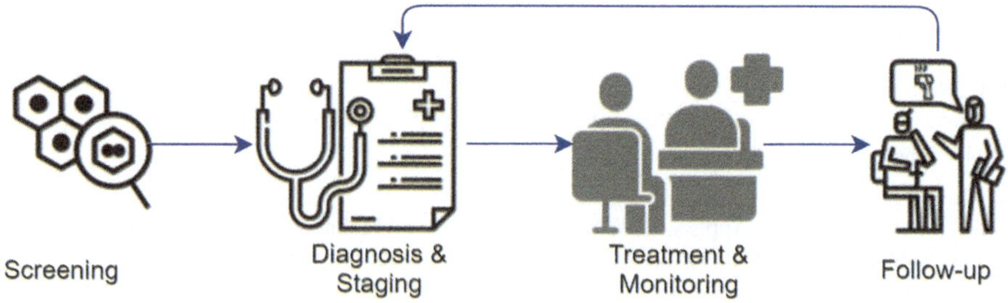

Fig. 1 Different stages of cancer management

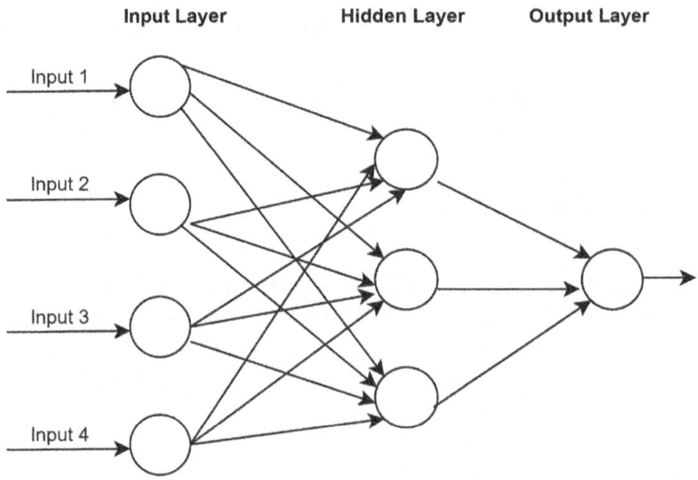

Fig. 2 A simple three-layered feedforward Artificial Neural Network (ANN)

through experience, and not from programming. It can be considered as a layered network of artificial neurons in our brain. The basic structure of an artificial neural network is shown in Fig. 2. The first layer of an ANN, called the input layer, is usually in the form of a multidimensional vector. The data gets distributed to the hidden layer(s) based on decisions made in the previous layer. This process is usually referred to as learning.

1.2 Convolutional Neural Network

Convolutional Neural Network (CNN) is a special type of ANN. Like ANN, a CNN also comprises neurons that self-optimize through learning. The neurons have three dimensions—height, weight, and depth. The input layer is usually a grayscale image while the output layer has binary or multi-class labels. The hidden layers consist of convolution layers, ReLU (rectified linear unit) layers, the pooling layers, and a fully connected Neural Network.

CNNs are useful in processing image contents and have been used in different tasks such as image detection, segmentation, classification, diagnosis, and retrieval [4]. Today, some of the best-known image processing and visual perception applications employ CNN models that are based on deep neural networks [5]. The advantage of CNN over an ANN is that it focuses only on image-specific features. Hence it requires a lesser number of input parameters, thereby reducing the computational complexity.

CNN and DCNN (Deep convolutional neural network) are widely used in cancer diagnosis and prognosis in the health care sector [15] leveraging medical images generated by medical imaging equipment. CNN has evolved over the period of time and with the advancement in the computing capacity of CPUs and GPUs, it is widely considered in other sectors too.

2 Architecture of a CNN

The generic architecture of a convolutional neural network is depicted in Fig. 3. A general model of CNN consists of a group of convolution, pooling, and fully connected layers. The arrangement of convolution and pooling layers is alternate, followed by fully connected layers at the end. These connected layers can be one or more depending on the need of architecture [6]. In this section, we will discuss the basic building blocks of CNN-based general architecture.

2.1 *Convolutional Layer*

Cancer images can be in different color spaces- RGB, grayscale, CMTK, etc. Multiple color channels result in huge volumes of data to work with. Any classification algorithm has to provide features of the images out of these data and classify them based on the obtained features into appropriate categories. A CNN model reduces the size of the image vector so that it becomes easier to process, but without losing the features critical for making an accurate prediction.

The Convolutional layer is the first layer of a CNN. This layer aims to learn feature representations of the input images. This layer is a set of convolutional kernels having different weights to extract features from the input. The input parameters consist of a set of learnable filters. Every filter is small in terms of width and height but extends through the full depth of the input volume. In the forward pass, each filter is convolved based on the height and width of the input values, and the dot product of the input values with filter values at a particular position is calculated. A two-dimensional activation map is generated that shows the result of that filter for every

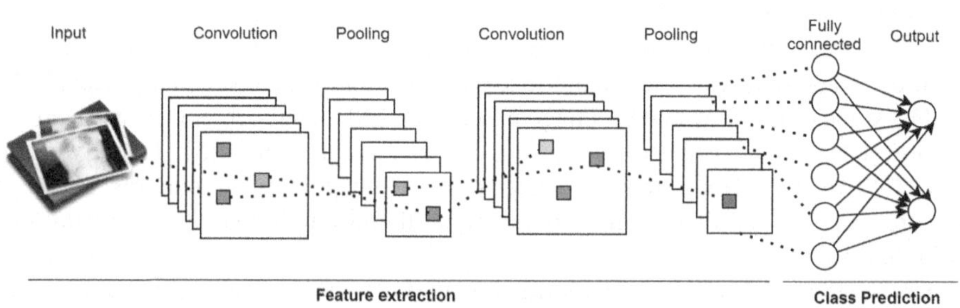

Fig. 3 Block diagram of a Convolutional Neural Network (CNN)

point. The network automatically learns filters that get activated on seeing some type of visual feature. A set of filters in each convolutional layer will produce a separate two-dimensional activation map. These activation maps are stacked along the depth dimension and the output volume is produced.

There can be more than one convolution layer depending on the complexity of the image. The first Convolution Layer captures the gradients whereas the second layer captures the edges.

2.2 Pooling Layer

Pooling, also called a down-sampling operation, is performed to sum up similar information in the neighborhood of the receptive field and output the dominant response within this local region. This reduces the computational complexity required to process the huge volume of image data. Pooling extracts a set of features that are invariant to any translational shifts or minor distortions. Once the features are extracted in a convolutional layer, we are not concerned about the exact location of the feature motifs since their approximate position relative to others is known. Reducing the size of the feature map to an invariant feature set helps regulate the complexity of the network while increasing the generalization and avoiding overfitting. It can be either *Max Pooling*, where the pooling kernel returns the maximum value from the portion of the image, or the *Average Pooling* where the pooling kernel returns that average value.

2.3 Activation Function

The output of each neuron or node is driven by an activation function [6]. The activation function thus acts as a decision function while learning complicated patterns. The selection of an appropriate activation function can expedite the overall learning process. There are various activation functions used in the literature such as *linear*, *sigmoid*, *maxout*, *tanh*, *ReLU* and its variants such as *leaky-ReLU*, *parametric ReLU*, *SWISH*, and *MISH*. These functions are used to inculcate non-linear combinations of features. Among these, ReLU and MISH have shown better results in most of the recently reported deep network models on benchmark datasets.

ReLU or rectified linear unit is the process of applying an activation function. This is done to increase the non-linearity of the network without affecting the receptive fields of convolution layers. ReLU is useful in faster training of the data, whereas Leaky ReLU is useful to handle the issue of vanishing gradient.

2.4 Fully Connected Layers

In this layer, neurons provide full connections to all activations in the previous layer. This layer creates a flattened representation of all the information obtained in the previous layer about the input image. Here, it is flattened, because neurons are unstructured and can be considered as a 1-D array of numbers. This flattened representation is produced by fewer neurons than the previous layers, which determines the specific target output of reaching the number of classes using pre-trained CNN. Eventually, the most probable class is obtained by choosing the highest score from the list of scores for each of the classes.

2.5 Weights and Biases

Neurons are the core of a neural network that processes the input they receive to compute an output value by applying a specific function. These neurons decide whether the next layer can use the obtained output as input or not. This decision is called bias and the function applied to the inputs is called the activation function. Here, each neuron has learnable weights and biases (typically real numbers) that are used as input to the activation function. This learning is an iterative process achieved by adjusting these biases and weights.

2.6 Dropouts

Overfitting and training are very common problems in such types of architecture. Generally, these problems occur if the model works well on training data but poorly works on test data. This means that the model exhibits low training error and high test error. In order to fix overfitting for CNN, a dropout approach is introduced, which means randomly dropping out nodes during training. Dropout applies regularization to minimize the risk of error within the network. It ultimately improves generalization by randomly dropping some nodes or connections with a certain probability. It is computationally cheap and a very effective regularization method for reducing the problem of overfitting and improving generalization error.

When multiple connections which learn in a non-linear relation are co-adapted, it can cause overfitting. This random dropping of some connections or nodes creates several thinned network architectures, of which, one representative network with small weights is selected. Dropout can be implemented on all layers in a network (hidden, visible or input layer) except the output layer.

2.7 Batch Normalization

Batch normalization addresses the issues related to the internal covariance shift within feature maps. Any such shift during the distribution of hidden units will change the learning rate to a small value, and thus slow down the convergence. It unifies the distribution of feature-map values by setting them to zero mean and unit variance. Batch normalization smoothens the flow of gradient. It also acts as a regulating factor thereby improving the generalization of the network.

3 Data Source, Preprocessing, and Model Performance

The effectiveness of the growing deep learning approach to analyze medical images depends on the amount of available heterogeneous raw data. We pass the input raw images or the pixel values in the form of a triplet (width, height, depth) in the input layer of the CNN for the further process. Different imaging techniques are used for each type of cancer, and thus the raw images also vary.

This section highlights various imaging techniques as well as the availability of standard datasets for the training and testing of models. It further talks about the pre-processing steps required to make the data ready to be input for a CNN model. Lastly, we talk about standard metrics to assess the performance and accuracy of a model.

3.1 Types of Medical Imaging for Cancer Diagnosis and Treatment

To successfully train deep CNN models, there is a need for adequate training data which should be labeled with the classes. Or else, there is a chance of overfitting the neural network and, consequently, an incompetent generalization of the network for unknown raw input data comes into existence. Images of body organs are used to diagnose cancer, its spread or to see the effect of a particular treatment. A few of the most common types of imaging tests are:

- CT-scan (Computed tomography)—a cross-section of the body or slice. The CT scan images highlight bones, organs, and soft tissues more clearly than standard x-rays imagining.
- MRI-scan (Magnetic resonance imaging)—creates images by taking cross-sectional slices (views) from many angles. Instead of radiation, MRI leverages enhanced magnets to make the images.
- X-rays—generate shadow-like images of certain organs, bones, and tissues. X-rays are generally fast, painless, and there's no special preparation needed.
- Mammography—low-dose x-rays that can help find breast cancer.

- Nuclear imaging (bone scans, PET scans)—generate images based on the different body's chemistry rather than on different physical shapes and forms. The particular type of nuclear scan depends on the organ under the examination.
- Ultrasound—creates sonograms pictures by transmitting high-frequency sound waves that go through the body. It is used to check for tumors in different areas of the body that don't show up on x-rays.

3.2 Open Cancer Datasets

A large-scale labeled dataset is needed to train and test CNN models. But, medical images are usually grayscale, and full-scale large image datasets are not readily available because of the intensive and time-consuming labeling work and expertise requirement. A few of the open-source datasets that can be used to train and test CNN models to diagnose cancer are listed below:

- MNIST (HAM10000)—It has a large collection of dermatoscopic images of pigment lesions. This dataset consists of 10,000 or more dermatoscopic images that could be used for skin cancer diagnosis [7].
- Breast Cancer Wisconsin Data Set—It has 570 instances with 33 attributes [8]. The features and characteristics are calculated from a scanned image of a fine needle aspirate (FNA) of a breast mass. It describes properties of the cell nuclei, such as radius, which is mean distances from the center to points on the perimeter, standard deviation of gray-scale values (texture), perimeter, area, local variation in radius lengths, compactness, concavity, concave points, fractal dimension, symmetry, etc.
- BACH 2018 dataset (The Breast Cancer Histology Challenge) [9]—It is a large public dataset having 400 microscopy and 30 whole-slide high-resolution H&E (Hematoxylin and eosin) stained histopathological images. These RGB images are of size 2048 × 1536 pixels.
- BreakHis dataset (The Breast Cancer Histopathological Image Classification)—Has 9,108 microscopic pictures of breast tumor tissue. These RGB images, each of 700 × 460 pixels, are in two classes—2,480 benign and 5,429 malignant[10].
- The cervical Cancer Risk Classification dataset—contains a general list of risk factors that causes cervical cancer leading to a biopsy examination.
- International Collaboration on Cancer Reporting dataset—It has cancer datasets of different body areas like reproductive organs, urinary and male genital, skin, head, neck, bone, central nervous system, breast, ophthalmic and endocrine organs, etc.

3.3 Pre-processing of Images

Medical images consist of noise, artifacts, and additional factors that may influence the interpretations. Therefore, we may require preprocessing data to enhance the image quality, contrast, and remove noise. Further, medical images are mostly imbalanced and have small sample sizes. It is difficult to know how best to prepare images data during the formation of a convolutional neural network for cancer diagnosis. Best practices to deal with the imbalanced data and small sample size involve both improving the pixel values by scaling and using data augmentation techniques at the training and evaluation stage of the model. Training and testing time augmentation achieve the highest performance on challenging cancer diagnosis datasets.

Image enhancement primarily focuses on suppressing noise and preserving important diagnostic characteristics. For example, in the case of breast cancer, we need to delineate the tumor if it is present in the background, extract the breast lines at the border, and abolish the pectoral muscle. To remove noise, we can use filters like wavelet transformation, adaptive median filter, mean & median filter, Gaussian filter, etc.

In recent times image augmentation is widely used to increase the size of the dataset to avoid overfitting. Some of the commonly used image augmentation techniques are image manipulations through rotation, flipping, feature space augmentation, transformation, kernel, mixing images, meta-learning, and random erasing.

Image segmentation involves the separation of region-of-interest like lesions, microcalcifications, and masses from the background of the pictures. Some of the CNN approaches have shown promising results on segmentation.

Before training the CNN model we should check the image datasets on the below points.

- The per-channel mean pixel values determined on the training dataset should probably be subtracted from the image data to centre it.
- Data augmentation should probably involve random rescaling, disruption of brightness, contrast and color, horizontal flips, and random cropping to increase the data size.
- Augmentation at test time should involve both a mixture of multiple rescaling of each image and predictions for multiple different systematic crops of each re-scaled version of the image.

3.4 Evaluating the Performance of a Model

This section talks about assessing the performance of a CNN model. Accuracy is the most commonly used metric to evaluate the model performance. Misclassification can be analyzed by the following Confusion Matrix, which helps in summarizing the performance of classification algorithms.

Confusion Matrix		
	Actual values	
Predicted values	**Positive (1)**	**Negative (0)**
	True Positive (TP)	False Positive (FP)
	False Negative (FN)	True Negative (TN)

In the above confusion matrix, rows of the matrix represent the occurrence of a predicted class while each column represents the occurrence in an actual class. True Positive (TP) class means those datasets which are actually malignant and the model has predicted as malignant. False Positive (FP) class means those datasets which are actually benign but the model has predicted as malignant. False Negative (FN) class means those datasets which are actually malignant but the model has predicted as benign. True Negative (TN) class means those datasets which are actually benign and the model has predicted as benign.

The diagonals part shows the classes that have been classified correctly. However, when the actual dataset has only a small percentage of true positive class, a very high misclassification score may not be sufficient to identify the accuracy of a mode. For example, in the case of a cancer dataset having 98% of benign class and 98% of malignant class, a model having 98% accuracy can still be a terrible one. For a better understanding of accuracy, we generally look for other scores such as Precision, Recall, F1-score.

- Precision—It is the proportion of correctly predicted true positive values out of total predicted true positives.

$$\text{Precision} = \text{TP}/(\text{TP} + \text{FP})$$

- Recall—It is defined as the number of true positives (TP) out of those that are correctly identified as positive samples.

$$\text{Recall} = \text{TP}/(\text{TP} + \text{FN})$$

- Accuracy—it indicates the global accuracy of a model and is calculated as,

$$\text{Accuracy} = (\text{TP} + \text{TN})/(\text{TP} + \text{TN} + \text{FP} + \text{FN})$$

- F1-Score—It is the weighted average of Precision and Recall.

$$F1 = \frac{2 * (\text{Precision} * \text{Recall})}{(\text{Precision} + \text{Recall})}$$

- ROC Curve is a graph-based method to analyze the performance of a model. We plot the TP (True Positive) in the y-axis against the FP (False Positive) in the x-axis as we vary the threshold. The AUC (area under the curve) summarizes the sensitivity and specificity for all possible threshold values. The ROC curve shows the diagnostic ability of the classifier system as its threshold values are varied.

4 Recent Advances in CNN Models for Cancer Diagnosis

In Sect. 2, we have discussed the architecture of a generic CNN model for computer-assisted cancer diagnosis. The image processing techniques vary since the imaging method and the nature of the input image vary for each type of cancer. Many researchers have developed different methods based on CNN, which improves the accuracy of the system. These methods are specific to different types of cancer. Given a suspicious region (I_x), the process of leveraging a pre-trained CNN-based model to predict the lesion malignancy can be formalized as:

$$y = F(I_x) = fn(f_{n-1}(\cdots(f(I_x))))$$

Here n is the number of hidden layers and f_i represents the activation function in the subsequent corresponding layer i [11].

In this section, we discuss different methodologies focusing on varieties of cancers such as breast cancer, myeloma cancer, lung cancer, etc. The main advantage of CNNs is that they replace manual features extraction with task-dependent automatic feature extraction. In CNN, transfer learning is used in which a convolutional neural network trained on one dataset is used on another dataset as per the requirement. This pre-trained network provides automatic feature extraction with or without a fine-tuned dataset. Sometimes fine-tuning shows better performance than direct feature extraction, the use of direct feature extraction is avoided. There are many popular CNN-based models including AlexNet, VGGNet, GoogLeNet, LeNet, VGG, Inception, DenseNet, Xception, and ResNet. In the latest literature, many other improvised approaches have also been proposed.

4.1 Breast Cancer Diagnosis

In 2020, the highest number of cancer cases were found in Breast cancer, which is the most deadly type of cancer among women. Some of the CNN models to diagnose breast cancer are integrated into mammographic mass segmentation information. In the CNN pipeline for automatic diagnosis, segmentation stages are included that specify the lesion boundaries differentiating it from background tissue. With this mammographic information, the objective is to locate the suspicious lesions in a mammogram. For this researchers use different methods based on CNN. In literature [11], features were extracted from mammographic masses by applying CNN, which is later classified using a linear SVM for classification. In another study [12], pre-trained CNN was used to draw out the ‘high-level’ and ‘middle-level’ features. These features are also combined with intensity information. Authors in [13] encourage the use of handcrafted features integrated with CNN features to improve performance. But this type of system requires human interaction. In other literature, the author added a detection stage with pre-trained CNN on regression to hand-crafted features for classification. This classification procedure processes both the gray-level image integrated with the segmentation map. Pre-training using hand-crafted features and assimilating segmentation is beneficial for the diagnosis performance. Some other methodologies are also proposed such as AlexNets, fully-integrated mass CAD system, CaffeNet, etc. As of now, this type of work was focused on differentiating CNN-based architectures from ML (machine learning) methods. The later proposed methodologies only consider the gray level characteristics of the input mammogram images, skipping any form of segmentation information.

4.2 Lung Cancer

Lung cancer is the second-highest reported category, which is also having a high mortality rate. CT scan is a very common approach to observe cancer in the lungs. However, in some cases the identification of cancer cells in the lungs may be delicate as the vessels or the walls of the chest may block the nodules.

The irregular shape of the cells due to noise makes it difficult to identify nodules in the early stages of cancer. Early detection of this cancer may save the life of the patient. In order to diagnose this type of cancer, many methodologies based on CNN are developed. Some of them are very popular like feed-forward neural network (FFNN), Deep CNN, Multi-Crop Convolutional Neural Network, feed-forward back-propagation neural network (FF-BNN), Deep Fully Convolutional Neural Network (DFCNet), Transfer learning based on CNN, attention-based fully CNN [14].

4.3 Skin Cancer

Skin cancer is another commonly reported type diagnosed primarily visually. The skin cells grow and further divide and create more cells. This way, a mass is formed called a tumor. The diagnostic process also involves dermoscopic analysis, biopsy, and histopathological examinations. Melanoma skin cancer is malignant in nature caused by an uncontrolled increase in pigment-producing cells. It starts from skin melanocytes that undergo a transformation that is malignant in nature.

Epiluminescence microscopy is a successful method that can do a scheming of light and filter out skin reflections to give better quality pictures of skin. In order to assist dermatologists in diagnosing outer cover disorders in the body, researchers are developing computer-based epiluminescence examination methods to study microscopic pictures.

The CNN-based approach for diagnosis of melanoma [15] has the following key steps:

(a) image acquisition of skin lesion image,
(b) segmentation, which involves separation of the skin lesion from nearby skin so that we can identify the region to be examined, extraction of parameters of the skin lesion, classification of image feature; and
(c) feature extraction for extracting those features that characterize a melanoma lesion accurately.

The CNN performs better in pattern recognition from medical images hence it is used for the diagnosis of skin melanoma from microscopic images of skin obtained through Epiluminescence technique. CNN models utilize the hyperparameters obtained from earlier tested structures in order to categorize skin patches for microscopic descriptions with more accuracy and sensitivity [13].

4.4 Multiple Myeloma

Another major category of cancer is Multiple Myeloma (MM). Like other cancers, this also requires prompt diagnosis to reduce the risk of mortality. Multiple Myeloma is also known as white blood cancer. In this type of cancer, unrestricted growth of plasma cells lead to their accumulation in the bone marrow. This generates abnormal proteins which block the normal generation of blood cells in bone marrow, resulting in a reduction of RBC, WBC counts. For this, microscopic blood cell imaging-based data is used to counter the challenges of visual similarity of healthy versus cancerous cells due to understaining or overstaining. CNN models based solutions learn the morphological features of images that are otherwise not visible to naked eyes.

The infected plasma cells can form different types of clusters, such as nuclei-nuclei, nuclei-cytoplasm, or cytoplasm-cytoplasm. Hence, detection and segmentation of images of plasma cells is difficult work as one has to apply segmentation on both nucleus and cytoplasm.

5 Limitations and Challenges

Although computer-assisted diagnosis systems provide positivity in analyzing the medical image and better performance, still there are many limitations and challenges in modeling and implementing such systems in a real-world environment. Due to these limitations, it is challenging to adopt these tools in a real-world environment.

High complexity and the large volume of data make the processing very challenging as computational power and huge memory storage are needed. This processing of huge data cannot be avoided because of the need to train models to produce a reliable and correct result. The reason behind it is that small datasets do not satisfy the requirement to train models having sufficient knowledge to be applicable in the real-world environment. Another limitation is bias and imbalanced class distribution. At the time of collecting data, errors may have been made. These errors come in the form of wrong class labels and bias sampling. This biased sampling leads to an imbalanced class distribution measured in percentages of the training dataset. It must be defined with respect to a particular dataset or distribution. For example, a dataset contains data about emails with labeling spam and not spam. Of 100 instances, 80 instances are with label spam and 20 with non-spam. This imbalance class distribution gives classification predictive modeling problems while building computer-assisted diagnosis systems upon such datasets. Thus it leads to the results being more likely to be biased and therefore produces the wrong diagnosis.

Several models have been proposed based on CNN and evaluated based on accuracy and other performance metrics. However, these models are not feasible to be applicable in a real-world hospital environment. Because general and large-scale diagnosis systems are required for effective and efficient cancer diagnosis. In the case of supervised learning, CNN models work on labeled input image data but it is always difficult to manually label cancer images as it needs specific medical expertise. These become very challenging when we have problems such as complex and high volume datasets, bias sampling, and imbalanced class distribution. For this reason, further extensive investigation in unpredictable real-world environments is needed to achieve reliable and effective computer-assisted systems for cancer diagnosis. These challenges and limitations are motivating the research community to continue to develop a diagnosis system to be able to gain credibility for clinical adoption in the future.

6 Conclusion

CNN has made significant progress, especially in image processing and vision-related tasks. CNNs have over the years significantly improved their learning and analyzing capacity by utilizing image depth and other types of structural changes. This has led to a renewed interest among neural network researchers. CNN gives the best performance in pattern recognition or image identification problems and even outperforms humans in some cases. Compared with other learning methods, deep learning models have certain advantages while processing pathology images. For example, in reduction of feature sets, auto-learning of features from raw images, ability to faster recognize complex objects, efficiency and less time taken due to parallel processing, and suitability for propagation or transfer learning. There is a rise in the application of deep learning methods to process pathological images of lung cancer. The performances of CNNs in relatively simpler tasks like tumor detection and histology classification are generally considered to be acceptable. However, the performance of CNN in more complex tasks like mutation and prediction of transcription status are less satisfactory.

Although the success of CNN-based models in cancer image analysis is still limited, however, with the advances in parallel computing systems and imaging techniques, it is expected that deep convolutional networks will have a major contribution to the development of cancer image diagnosis systems in the future. Therefore, cancer image processing using deep CNN models could have a potential impact on future cancer treatment.

References

1. Ferlay, J., Ervik, M., Lam, F., Colombet, M., Mery, L., & Piñeros, M., et al. (2020). *Global cancer observatory: Cancer today*. International Agency for Research on Cancer.
2. Fass, L. (2008). Imaging and cancer: A review. *Molecular Oncology, 2*(2), 115–152.
3. Hussain, T., & Nguyen, Q. T. (2014). Molecular imaging for cancer diagnosis and surgery. *Advanced Drug Delivery Reviews, 66*, 90–100.
4. Liu, X., Deng, Z., & Yang, Y. (2019). Recent progress in semantic image segmentation. *Artificial Intelligence Review, 52*, 1089–1106. https://doi.org/10.1007/s10462-018-9641-3
5. Khan, A., Sohail, A., Zahoora, U., et al. (2020). A survey of the recent architectures of deep convolutional neural networks. *Artificial Intelligence Review, 53*, 5455–5516. https://doi.org/10.1007/s10462-020-09825-6
6. Anwar, S. M., Majid, M., Qayyum, A., et al. (2018). Medical image analysis using convolutional neural networks: A review. *Journal of Medical Systems, 42*, 226. https://doi.org/10.1007/s10916-018-1088-1
7. Tschandl, P., Rosendahl, C., Kittler, H. (2018, Aug 14). The HAM10000 dataset, a large collection of multi-source dermatoscopic images of common pigmented skin lesions. *Scientific Data, 5*(1), 1–9
8. Wolberg, W. H., Street, W. N., & Mangasarian, O. L. (1994, Mar 15). Machine learning techniques to diagnose breast cancer from image-processed nuclear features of fine needle aspirates. *Cancer Letters, 77*(2–3), 163–71. doi: https://doi.org/10.1016/0304-3835(94)90099-x
9. BACH, ICIAR. (2018). *Grand challenges on breast cancer histology images*. https://iciar2018-challenge.grand-challenge.org
10. Spanhol, F., Oliveira, L. S., Petitjean, C., & Heutte, L. (2016). A dataset for breast cancer histopathological image classification. *IEEE Transactions on Biomedical Engineering (TBME), 63*(7), 1455–1462.
11. Zou, L., Yu, S., Meng, T., Zhang, Z., Liang, X., & Xie, Y. (2019). A technical review of convolutional neural network-based mammographic breast cancer diagnosis. *Computational and Mathematical Methods in Medicine, 2019*, 1–16. https://doi.org/10.1155/2019/6509357
12. Zou, L., Yu, S., Meng, T., Zhang, Z., Liang, X., & Xie, Y. (2019). A technical review of convolutional neural network-based mammographic breast cancer diagnosis. *Computational and Mathematical Methods in Medicine*, 1–16. doi:https://doi.org/10.1155/2019/6509357
13. Yi, F. L., Yang, L., Wang, S. D., Guo, L., Huang, C. L., Xie, Y., & Xiao, G. H. (2018). Microvessel prediction in H&E Stained Pathology Images using fully convolutional neural networks. *BMC Bioinform, 19*, e64.
14. Brinker, T. J., Hekler, A., Utikal, J. S., Grabe, N., Schadendorf, D., Klode, J., Berking, C., Steeb, T., Enk, A. H., Von Kalle, C. (2018, Oct 17). Skin cancer classification using convolutional neural networks: Systematic review. *Journal of Medical Internet Research, 20*(10), e11936.
15. de Groot, P. M., Wu, C. C., Carter, B. W., & Munden, R. F. (2018). The epidemiology of lung cancer. *Translation Lung Cancer Research, 7*, 220–233.
16. Raza, K., & Singh, N. (2021). A tour of unsupervised deep learning for medical image analysis. *Current Medical Imaging, 17*(9), 1059–1077. https://doi.org/10.2174/1573405617666210127154257

Automatic Cancer Detection Using Probabilistic Convergence Theory

Arif Md.Sattar and Mritunjay Kr. Ranjan

Abstract The work is to design an automatic cancer detection computational intelligence (CI) model using Machine Learning by applying the concept of Probabilistic Convergence theorem on homogeneous and heterogeneous datasets. This model also displays the intensity of cancer patients. The model is for cancer detection, which is automatic and can send data values generated during testing and propagate to the next step to create a dataset that can be homogeneous and heterogeneous depending on the test. As per the "Testing Model" developed by researchers, Galleri is a new blood test that can detect more than 50 types of cancer through a single blood drop. Out of which, a heterogeneous dataset can arise. However, the homogeneous dataset is straightforward to handle. So, it is necessary to decompose the dataset categorically for each category of cancer. After decomposition, the dataset can be of type homogeneous as well as heterogeneous. If we use the current testing tools as Computerized Tomography (CT) scan, Magnetic Resonance Imaging (MRI), Positron Emission Tomography (PET), Ultrasound, X-ray, Biopsy, etc., then we can get heterogeneous datasets directly. Here machine learning is used on the heterogeneous datasets to analyse the dataset to get Fuzzy probabilistic data values. Applying the Fuzzy Probabilistic theorem, a more accurate dataset can be derived. Further, comparing the dataset with various cancer databases such as CGA, GLOBOCAN2020, NCDB, CGAP, COSMIC, TCGA, and CGHub to get the intensity of cancer of a patient. The model can detect cancer using the concept of computer vision (edge detection process). The model used two edge detection processes "Sobel operator" and "Laplacian matrix".

Keywords Machine learning · Probabilistic · Edge detection process · Sobel operator · Laplacian matrix · Convergence

---

A. Md.Sattar (✉)
Department of Computer Science, Anugrah Memorial College, Gaya, India

M. Kr. Ranjan
Department of Computer Science, Magadh University, Bodh Gaya, India

K. Raza (ed.), *Computational Intelligence in Oncology*, Studies in Computational Intelligence 1016, https://doi.org/10.1007/978-981-16-9221-5_6

1 Introduction

Cancer is one of the gravest issues for humanity concerning healthiness. The different forms and shapes acclimatize on the root of cell origin, place, and ancestral alterations. The disease has affected human creation. Treating cancer has become a little smooth compared to early days because of the progression in the cancer detection process and techniques. Machine learning algorithms have the potential to be invested deeply in all fields of diagnosis of disease and making a decision regarding the intensity of the disease and also other clinical actions. As per medical science, a single blood test predicts fifty types of cancer, but the issue is that the test is not concrete [8]. Medical science says that biopsy is the most reliable test by which cancer detection is almost accurate (Cancer.Net).

A Biopsy has been one of the most promising techniques for detecting cancer for the last couple of decades due to its most advantageous diagnostic methods, such as (i) no tissues removal, (ii) minimal invasiveness, and (iii) less time consumption and reproducibility.

2 Literature Survey

The term "cancer" was first used in 1984 by Alfano et al. [1]. First time [2, 3] has identified as the measurement of (NF) Native fluorescence.

The human body's tissues are mainly serene of an extracellular matrix that contain fibre, fat, proteins, water, and collagen epithelial cells. As per [12, 15], tissues have multiple key fingerprints: porphyrins, flavin adenine dinucleotide (FAD), collagen, reduced nicotinamide adenine dinucleotide hydrogen (NADH), elastin, tryptophan, and native endogenous fluorophore molecules. As per [14], tryptophan is a type of amino acid required by all forms of life for protein synthesis and other essential metabolic functions, accounting for the majority of protein fluorescence. FAD and NADH are presented in the oxidation of fuel molecules, and 326 Lasers for medical applications can be used to probe changes in cellular metabolism [15].

As per [9], NADH fluorescence dynamically interprets the metabolic activity within the cell. It came in to picture through several studies that abnormalities in metabolic activity precede the onset of many diseases: carcinoma, diabetes mellitus, atherosclerosis, Alzheimer's, and Parkinson's illness, etc. As per [18]. Possibly the morphologic changes or biochemical roots the spectral variations would seem earlier than the histological aberration. Hence, biopsy is one of the great promising tools for the clinical detecting initial stages of carcinomas and other diseases in connection with existing technology. (e.g., fibre spectroscopic radiometer, fibre optic end microscope and nasopharyngoscopy) for in vivo use.

Using UV excitation [3]. The work was prolonged to segregate human malignant breast tissues from benign and normal tissue types. As per [6, 17], the work extended on prostate tissues [7] showed the diagnostic potential of fluorescence spectroscopy for cancer and other diseases in, unlike organs. This very procedure can be used to extract intrinsic (undistorted) tissue fluorescence spectra during the induction of morphological and molecular changes in human tissue in vivo by combining it with the Nonnegative Constraint Blind Source Separate mathematical tools [11]. Accordingly, the key fluorescent biomolecules can serve as in vivo biomarkers of malignant change without tissue removal. Several groups have inspected several promising methods using optical spectroscopy with high sensitivity and specificity [1, 3, 6, 7, 10–12, 15–17, 19].

As per [13], Alternative spectral tactic, called Stokes Shift Spectra (S3), offers a novel and more simple way of speedily measuring spectral fingerprints of complex mixtures in tissue. S3 combines both absorption and emission spectral features of molecules and therefore offers a more accurate tactic. It can be used to obtain enough evidence on different key fluorophores in one spectrum to speed up spectral procurement time. It is required to employ a single scan to obtain the most critical data on the fingerprint of the main fluorophores, which are valuable for the detection of cancer. The Stokes Shift Spectra modality was the first optical biopsy for cancer detection proposed and used by [4] for cancer detection and later for biochemical analysis and detection of breast cancer [5].

3 Proposed Work

Detection of cancer is a multi-stage process. During this process, the patient consults the doctor because of some symptoms or complications. Sometimes cancer is discovered by chance or through screening. The detection of the first stage begins with analysing multiple biopsy images. The specified images accumulated through the process undergo several preprocessing tasks such as noise removal and enhancement (Fig. 1).

A. Cancer Detection Hierarchy: A Training (This is Only for Images)

The above diagram describes the hierarchy of cancer detection:

- The images are generated during biopsy testing are captured, and the features extracted for the next stage.
- The next phase checks the scatteredness and non-proportionality of points of the grey scaled images. If the points are scattered or non-proportional, we need to apply the Naive Bayes algorithm to calculate the accurate probabilistic value of points to produce accurate images. Subsequently, if images are not scattered in the next phase and points are proportional, we may proceed to the next phase directly.
- Now we have to extract features of actual images for the next stage by applying the concept of computer vision, i.e. the edge detection process.
- Thereafter, the new images are compared and classified on the basis of colours, shapes, arrangement of points, and scattered edges. In this stage, edges of images

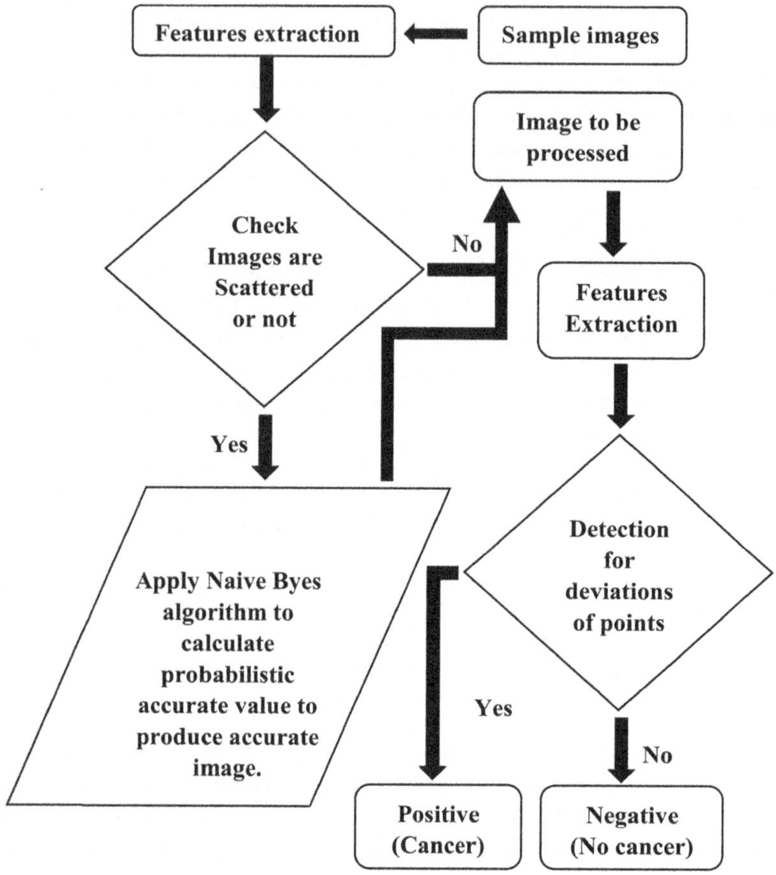

Fig. 1 Cancer Detection Flow-Chart

are detected whether they are scattered or not. If edges of images are scattered, then the value will be positive; otherwise, it will be negative.

- If the result is positive, the cells are cancerous. Otherwise, the cells are non-cancerous (Fig. 2).

B. Detailed Methodology

Here the architectural diagram contains the following steps:

- Tested images can be taken as input after the Biopsy test. Therefore, the images can be enhanced before segmentation to remove noise using an appropriate Naive algorithm.
- Based on inputted images, the task of segmentation could be performed, which may or may not contain nuclei, cytoplasm and other features. After that the images

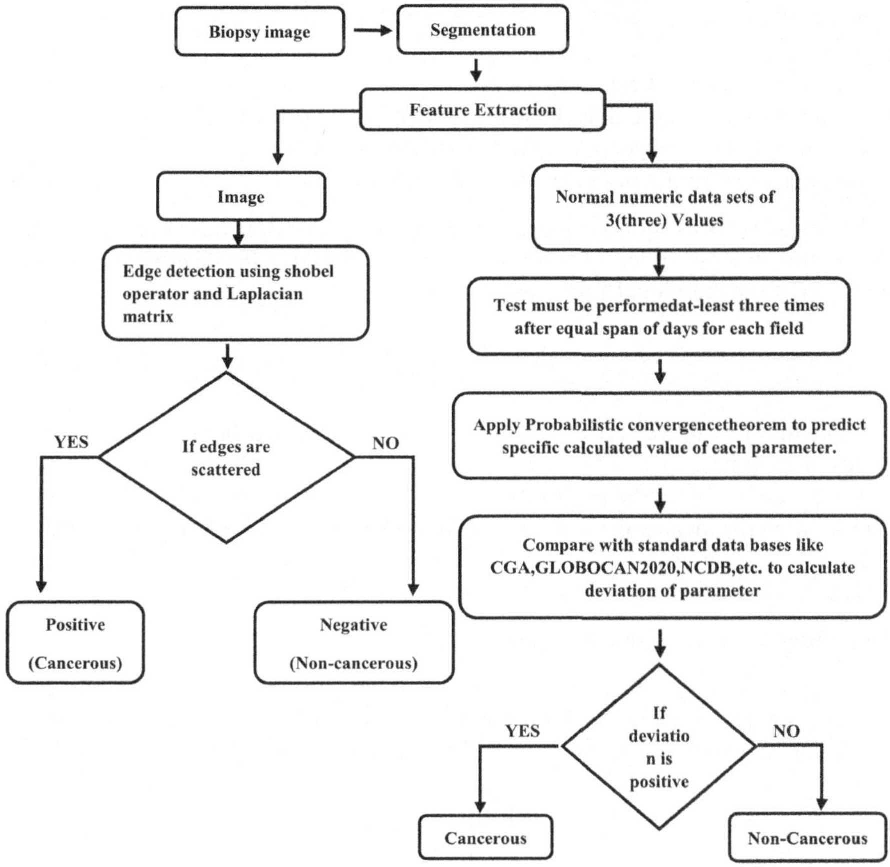

Fig. 2 Cancer detection architecture

can be segmented on the basis of region, threshold or cluster using a particular algorithm.

- Moving forward towards the step of "Features Extraction", various biologically interpretable and clinically notable shapes plus morphology-based image features can be extracted from the segmented images, including grey-scale feature, Law's Texture Energy (LTE)-based, wavelet, and Tamura's features.
- Using the appropriate Naive Bayes (NB) algorithm, images can be appropriately classified, whether scaled or sharp. By applying the alternate appropriate Naive Bayes algorithm, we can sharpen the Grey scaled Image.
- Subsequently, we can apply edge detection methods such as Laplacian matrix and Sobel Operator to identify the scattered images and the cancerous or non-cancerous cells.

Values of the fields that are calculated during biopsy are as follows

- Native fluorescence (NF)
- Tryptophan (An Amino acid)
- Collagen (Protein of cell boundary)
- Nicotinamide adenine dinucleotide hydrogen (NADH), Energy producer
- Flavin adenine dinucleotide (FAD), Breast tumour)
- Porphyrins (Binding protein of Red Blood cells)

During the process of biopsy, the above or more parameters have been calculated. During this process, at least three results must be found. After that we have to find the mean of the individual values as:

$$X1 = \frac{x1 + x2 + x3}{3}$$

After that the above process should be applied for each field to find the mean values of each field as $Y1, Z1\ldots$, etc.

If we want to apply the probabilistic convergence theorem, then we have to find at least three (3) mean values of each field as ($X1$, $X2$, $X3$), ($Y1$, $Y2$, $Y3$), (Z1, Z2, Z3), etc.

The probabilistic convergence theorem is given below.

Probabilistic convergence theorem

Convergence in the probability or stochastic convergence is defined as follows:

A sequence of random variables $X1, X2, \ldots, Xn$ is said to converge in probability to a certain constant a, if for any $\epsilon > 0$(However small it may be)

$$\underset{n \to \alpha}{\mathrm{Lt}}\ p(|X_n - a| < \varepsilon) = 1$$

$$\text{or} \quad \underset{n \to \infty}{\mathrm{Lt}}\ p(|X_n - a| \geq \varepsilon) = 0$$

$$or \quad \underset{inp}{X_n} \to a \quad \text{as} \quad n \to \infty$$

That is speaking practically, as $\boldsymbol{n}$ increases, the probability mass of the distribution of $\boldsymbol{X_n}$ accumulates more and more about pointing $\boldsymbol{a}$. That means the probabilistic convergence value of $X_1, X_2, X_3, \ldots, X_n$ converges to a. Here p is the domain of probability.

If X is a random variable in the probabilistic domain p such that

$$\underset{inp}{Xn - X} \to 0 \quad \text{as} \quad n \to \infty$$

then we can say that the given sequence of probabilistic random variables convergences to the random variable $\boldsymbol{X}$.

If a constants sequence $\boldsymbol{an} \to \boldsymbol{a}$ as $\boldsymbol{n} \to \infty$, then that constant will be having a one-point distribution at that point irrespective of any other probabilistic random variable, and it can be represented as:

$$\boldsymbol{an} \underset{\boldsymbol{inp}}{\to} \boldsymbol{a} \text{ as } \boldsymbol{n} \to \infty$$

The following simple rules hold for convergence in probability:

Let $X_n \underset{inp}{\to} a$ and $Y_n \underset{inp}{\to} b$ as $n \to \infty$

Then,

1. $X_n \pm Y_n \to a \pm b$ as $n \to \infty$
2. $X_n Y_n \to ab$ as $n \to \infty$
3. $X_n / Y_n \to a/b$ as $n \to \infty$

−1	−2	−1
0	0	0
1	2	

−1	0	1
−2	0	2
−1	0	1

When we apply the probabilistic convergence theorem on each field value calculated during biopsy, we can predict a specific fixed value that should be stored in a database of patients as AX, BY, CZ, etc.

We have to use a standard database like CGA (absolute, breakpoint, contest, HAPSEG, MuTect, PathSeq, RNA-seQC, RefSeq), GLOBOCAN2020 (Statistical database of cancer patients of 185 countries and 36 types of cancer), National Cancer database (NCDB maintained by American cancer society and American college of surgeons), CanEvolve (Genes, microRNA, PEP, CAN, PPI) CBioportal (CAN, gene mutation), CGAP(cDNA clone, gene expression, SNP, GVI), Catalogue of Somatic Mutations in Cancer (COSMIC)—tumour database (CAN, methylation, genefusion, SNP, gene expression), The cancer genome Atlas[TCGA—Tumour database (epigenetics, gene expression profiles, miRNAs)], CGHub (This is an extensive database contains 25 types of cancer information in three categories—TCGA, CCLE, and TARGET), etc. to check deviations of calculated value and expected value, as (DBAX-AX), (DBBY-BY), (DBCZ-CZ), etc. According to the deviation, we can predict about the patients. If the deviation is positive, the patient is cancerous. Otherwise, he/she is not cancerous. (DBAX—database value of field ax, AX -calculated value of field ax, DBBY—database value of the field by, BY -calculated value of the field by, DBCZ—database value of the field cz, CZ—calculated value of field cz, and so on).

4 Edge Detection Method—"Sobel Operator"

The Sobel operator performs spatial gradient measurement on an image in a 2-D coordinate form and emphasizes regions of the high spatial frequency of corresponding edges. Typically, it is used on input grayscale images to find the approximate absolute gradient magnitude at each point on the Image [20] (Fig. 3).

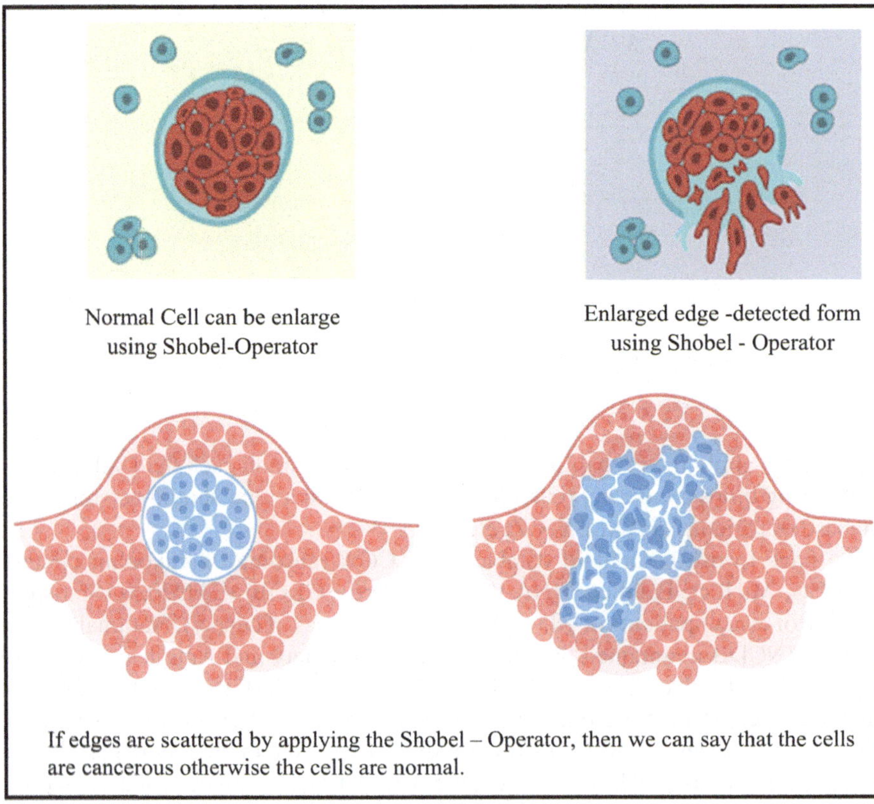

Fig. 3 Sobel operator

4.1 Edge Detection Method—"Laplacian"

Laplacian matrix is one of the best edge detection methods of an image for finding the boundaries of the Image. This method is quite the best among edge detection methods [21].

$$\nabla^2 f = \frac{\partial^2 f}{\partial^2} + \frac{\partial^2 f}{\partial^2}$$

0	−1	0
−1	4	−1
0	−1	0

4.2 Intermediate Laplacian Matrix

To find the location of an edge using zero-crossing property—we need to convolve the Image with Laplacian of a 2-D Gaussian function (Fig. 4).

$$h(x, y) = \exp\left[\frac{x^2 + y^2}{2\sigma^2}\right]$$

Level-3-Laplacian Image is a pixel form illuminated Image and fully certified the Laplacian matrix. If the level-3—image is not certified in the Laplacian matrix, we can say that the ages are scattered, and the cells are cancerous; otherwise, the cells are not cancerous (Table 1, Fig. 5).

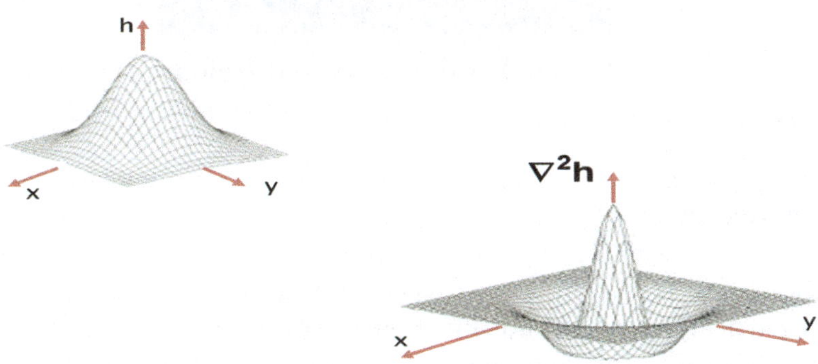

Fig.4 Edge detection—"Laplacian"

Table 1 Final Laplacian matrix

0	0	−1	0	0
0	−1	−2	−1	0
−1	−2	16	−2	−1
0	−1	−2	−1	0
0	0	−1	0	0

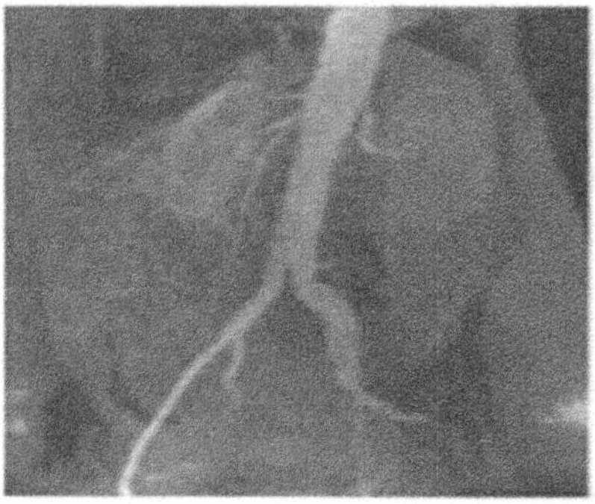

Level -1- Edge -detected Image

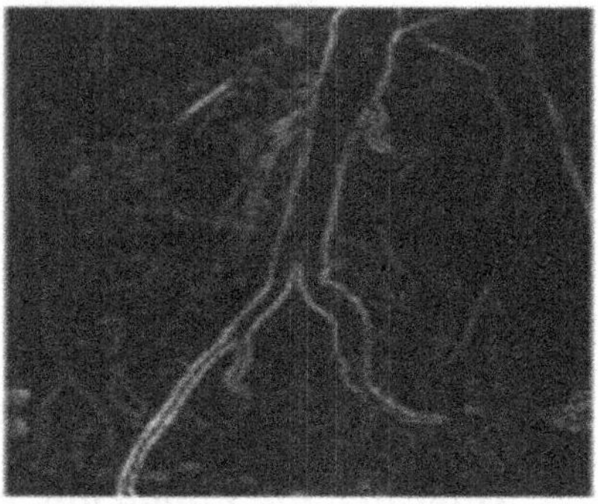

Level -2- Edge -detected Image

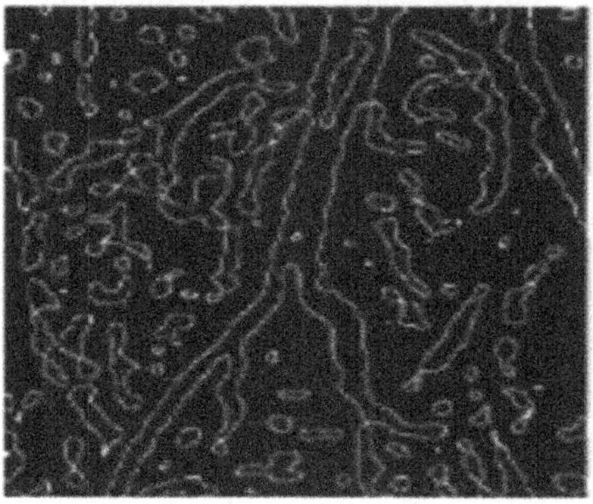

Level -3- Edge -detected Image

Fig. 5 Edge detection—"Laplacian"

5 Conclusion

The above model is perfect for predicting cancerous and non-cancerous patients according to the Biopsy report using Probabilistic Convergence Theorem and Edge Detection of images. The Probabilistic Convergence Theorem is precise for non-uniform discrete values. It is applicable to find specific convergence values using at least three sample values. Edge detection is performed using Sobel operator and

Laplacian—Equation as well as Laplacian matrix. The edge detection methods find the displacement of points of edges. If the points are proportional, then edges are smooth and not cancerous; if points are not proportional, the edges are scattered then cancerous. Using the above two edge detection methods, we can ideally find the cancerous cells of Biopsy images.

5.1 Future Prospects

1. The intensity of propagation of cancer
2. Remaining time to infect the entire body
3. Prescribe the probable medicines
4. Prescribe the diet chart.

References

1. Alfano, R. R., Tata, D., Cordero, J., Tomashefsky, P., Longo, F., et al. (1984). Laser induced fluorescence spectroscopy from native cancerous and normal tissue. *IEEE Journal of Quantum Electronics, 20*, 1507–1511.
2. Alfano, R. R., Tang, G. C., Pradhan, A., Lam, W., Choy, D. S. J., et al. (1987). Fluorescence spectra from cancerous and normal human breast and lung tissues. *IEEE Journal of Quantum Electronics QE, 23*, 1806.
3. Alfano, R. R., Das, B. B., Cleary, J. B., Prudente, R., Celmer, E., et al. (1991a). Light sheds light on cancer. *Bulletin of the New York Academy of Medicine, 67*, 143–150.
4. Alfano, R. R., Yang, Y., et al. (2003). Stokes shift emission spectroscopy of human tissue and key biomolecules. *IEEE Journal of Quantum Electronics, 9*(2), 148–153.
5. Alfano, R. R., & Yang, Y., et al. (2007, March 20). Stokes shift emission spectroscopy for detection of disease and physiological state of specimen. *USA Patent, 7*, 192, 783.
6. Baraga, J. J., Rava, R. P., Taroni, P., Kittrell, C., Fitzmaurice, M., et al. (1990). Laser induced fluorescence spectroscopy of normal and atherosclerotic human aorta using 306–310 nm excitation. *Lasers in Surgery and Medicine, 10*, 245–261.
7. Bigio, I. J., Mourant, J. R., et al. (1997). Ultraviolet and visible spectroscopies for tissue diagnosis. *Physics in Medicine and Biology, 42*, 803–814.
8. Bird, E., et al. (2020, April 9). Blood test can detect 50 different types of Cancer. *Medical News*.
9. Chance, B., Williamson, J. R., Famieson, D., Schoener, B., et al. (1965). Properties and kinetics of reduced pyridine nucleotide fluorescence of the isolated and in vivo rat heart. *Biochemische Zeitschrift, 341*, 357–377.
10. Drezek, R., Sokolov, K., Utzinger, U., Boiko, I., Malpica, A., et al. (2001). Understanding the contributions of NADH and collagen to cervical tissue fluorescence spectra: Modeling, measurements, and implications. *Journal of Biomedial Optics, 6*(4), 385–396.
11. Georgakoudil, J. B. C., Muller, M. G., Sheets, E. E., Badizadegan, K., et al. (2002). NAD(P)H and collagen as in vivo quantitative fluorescent biomarkers of epithelial precancerous changes. *Cancer Research, 62*, 682–687.
12. Heintzelman, D. L., Lotan, R., Richards-Kortum, R. R., et al. (2000). Characterization of the autofluorescence of polymorphonuclear leukocytes, mononuclear leukocytes and cervical

epithelial cancer cells for improved spectroscopic discrimination of inflammation from dysplasia. *Photochemistry and Photobiology, 71*(3), 327–332.
13. Liu, Q., Grant, G., Vo-Dinh, T., et al. (2010). Investigation of synchronous fluorescence method in multicomponent analysis in tissue. *IEEE Journal of Quantum Electronics, 16*(4), 927–940.
14. Moffett, J. R., Namboodiri, M. A., et al. (2003). Review article: Tryptophan and the immune response. *Immunology and Cell Biology, 81*, 247–265.
15. Palmer, G. M., Keely, P. J., Breslin, T. M., Ramanujam, N., et al. (2003). Autofluorescence spectroscopy of normal and malignant human breast cell lines. *Photochemistry and Photobiology, 78*(5), 462–469.
16. PanjehpourM, J. C. E., Phan, M. N., Vo-Dinh, T., Overholt, S., et al. (2002). Laser-induced fluorescence spectroscopy for in vivo diagnosis of non-melanoma skin cancers. *Lasers in Surgery and Medicine, 31*, 367–373.
17. Pu, Y., Wang, W., Tang, G., Alfano, R. R., et al. (2010). Changes of collagen and NADH in human cancerous and normal prostate tissues studied using fluorescence spectroscopy with selective excitation wavelength. *Journal of Biomedical Optics, 15*, 047008-1–47015.
18. Silberberg, M. B., Savage, H. E., Sacks, P. G., Schantz, S. P., Tang, G., et al. (1994). Detecting retinoic acid- induced biochemical alterations in squamous cell carcinoma using intrinsic fluorescence spectroscopy. *The Laryngoscope, 104*(3), 278–282.
19. Villringer, A., Chance, B., et al. (1997). Non- invasive optical spectroscopy and imaging of human brain function. *Trends in Neurosciences, 20*, 435.
20. https://homepages.inf.ed.ac.uk/rbf/HIPR2/sobel.htm
21. https://kalpanileo1996.medium.com/edge-detection-with-laplacianoperator-without-using-opencv-laplacian-inbuilt-function-fa6d4966065f

Computational Intelligence Methods for Cancer Survival Prediction

Abdullahi Isa

Abstract Cancer is one of the deathly diseases that kills millions of people every year around the globe. Recent studies show computational intelligence (CI) methods have gotten perhaps the most prominent and versatile instruments with applications spread across multiple disciplines, including oncology. The presentation of CI has carried extremist changes to the field, particularly in pathology. Current CI-based methods are widely used as an adjunct, along with current methods on oncology to assist human pathologists. This study will focus on the trend of various CI methods being used in cancer survival prediction and explore the effectiveness of previously reported methods. However, this study will guide researchers and the entire community on the cutting-edge CI techniques of cancer survival forecasting application and motivate researchers to develop a cost-effective and user-friendly framework of survival prediction.

Keywords Computational intelligence · Cancer · Survival model · Prediction model · Oncology

1 Introduction

Many developed countries identify cancer as one of the major drivers of illness among humans that cause deaths. Approximately, annual growth of cancer incidence shows 19.3 million patients were diagnosed with an illness and 10 million deaths according to GLOBOCAN 2020 [1]. Also, Fig. 1 represents an estimated of different cases of cancer among females, which shows breast cancer as the most common among females of all ages. And Fig. 2 represents the estimated cases of cancer among males, which indicated lung and prostate cancer as the most common cancer among males of all age. However, improved treatment options, such as metastatic, had improved the survival rates of patients with cancer disease. Prostate, lung, and breast cancer record the highest incidence with a propensity to metastasize to bone [2–4]. Bone

A. Isa (✉)
Department of Mathematical Sciences, Faculty of Science, University of Maiduguri, Maiduguri, Nigeria
e-mail: isaabdullahi@unimaid.edu.ng

K. Raza (ed.), *Computational Intelligence in Oncology*, Studies in Computational Intelligence 1016, https://doi.org/10.1007/978-981-16-9221-5_7

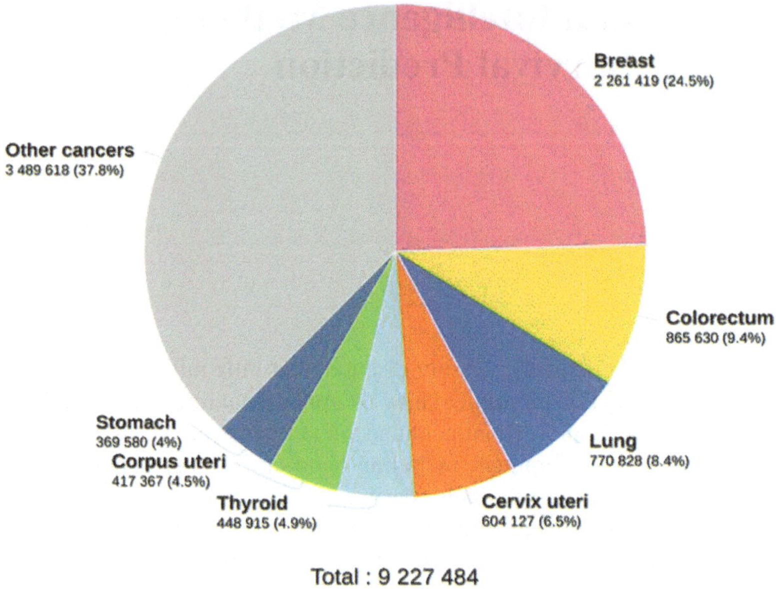

Fig. 1 Cases of cancer among females of all ages [1]

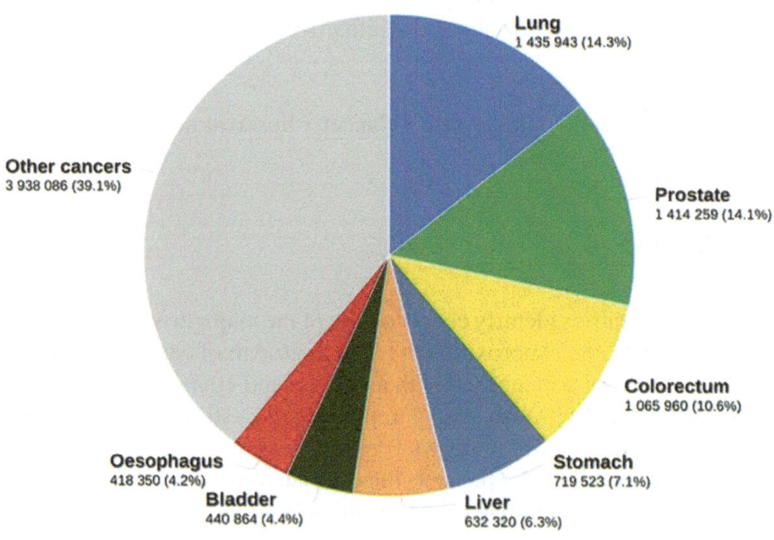

Fig. 2 Cases of cancer among males of all ages [1]

metastases caused immobility of patients, pain, and reduced quality of his/her life because of pathologic fractures [5]. Patients with bone metastases have two survival thresholds of 90 days or 1 year [6]. However, glioblastomas (GBM), a cancer brain tumor, have average survival rates of less than 2 years and under 5% survival rate in 5 years [7].

Several investigations have gathered survival data dependent on longitudinal follow-up for various patient accomplices in the past four decades. However, modeling of survival rate is imperative to precision oncology. Treatment and handling of a cancer patient are personalized to a patient because of his/her genomic characteristics, pathology, demographic, and clinical of that patient [8]. The meta-analysis of the number of research investigations that have been published in this domain from the year 2000 to 2021 presents more than 6000 publications based on the PubMed database using the following search keywords like ["computational intelligence in cancer survival"], ["expert systems in oncology"], and ["intelligent systems in oncology"]. However, several CI methods have been developed and used as an adjunct to the current methods utilized in predicting the rates of survival of patients associated with cancer infection. These CI methods range from basic scoring systems to further advanced computational intelligence (CI) techniques. However, these CI methods perform well, it is significant to continue changing and improving them. This is because new prognostic factors are constantly being investigated and further developed CI strategies have been utilized on detection, diagnoses, and prediction of many infectious diseases, including COVID-19 [9]. Also, a report as shown in Fig. 3 on survival, incidence, and motility rate of lung cancer in five different countries as shown by [10] is very scary.

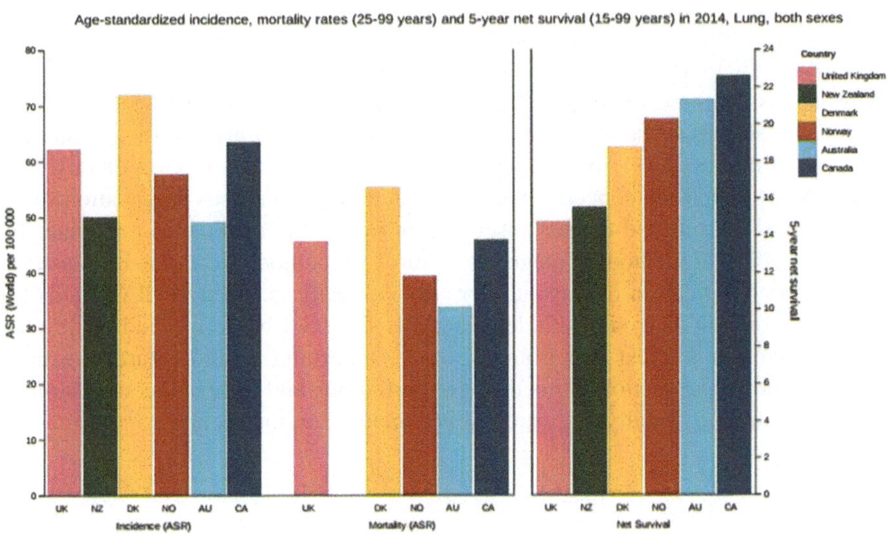

Fig. 3 Mortality incidences and 5-year net survival of lung cancer

Definition of computation intelligence (CI) by [11] "as a set of strong data processing approaches for knowledge-driven and decision-making". CI techniques have been utilized as a device for the improvement of cutting-edge systems with intellectual abilities like learning, adaptation, and development for addressing complex problems [11]. Therefore, cancer survival prediction would not be an exception. CI strategies have the capacity of dealing with a lot of data and perceiving complex mixes of predictors for a specific result by utilizing present-day computational intelligence techniques and mathematic algorithms [12, 13].

Several studies developed and applied survival prediction methods that focus essentially on accuracy throughout the most recent couple of many years. For instance, the Cox model (CoxPH) proposed by [14] is one of the most seasoned and most well-known strategies that was utilized to predict survival. Another method proposed by [15], named multi-task logistic regression (MTLR) as an improvement to the model in [14], which incited expanded prediction exactness over CoxPH. MTLR utilizes various task regression and joint probability minimization to display log risk in a time frame as a direct blend of the covariates. Also, a study by [16] proposed neural-MTLR that to improve precision over MTLR. Neural-MTLR models nonlinear coordinated efforts among covariates as provisions extricated by the lower layers of a neural network, whose last layers are comparable to that of an MTLR model.

Therefore, this investigation will focus on the trend of various CI methods being used in cancer survival prediction and explore the effectiveness of previously reported methods. However, this study will guide researchers and the entire community on the state-of-the-art CI methods of cancer survival prediction application and motivate researchers to develop a cost-effective and user-friendly framework of survival prediction.

The outline of this study is section survival models in predicting outcomes describe the model and algorithms behind survival models. Description of concepts survival analysis was captured in section basic concepts of survival model analysis. Also, concepts examples of how CI survival prediction methods are used to predict the outcome of interest in various domains discussed in the section CI methods used in survival prediction: concept examples. Section CI methods application challenges based on survival dataset discussed missing data challenges encounter by survival prediction methods. Categories of survival methods were also discussed in the section classification of methods for survival analysis. Section CI methods for survival prediction analysis were dedicated strictly to CI-based methods of prediction of events of interest at a point in time. Opportunities and future directions are discussed in the section CI methods opportunities and future direction towards survival prediction. Finally, the article was concluded in the section conclusions.

2 Survival Models in Predicting Outcomes

Survival models have been used in various domains, similar to the medical industry, to predict the danger of fostering a specific outcome of interest. The survival models are equivalent to "time-to-occasion" as characterized by [17] as the amount of time to an event of interest, like time-to-death, time-to-repeat, and time-to-employment. One significant trait of survival data is that they are consistently censored, which prompts lacking sufficient outcomes. Statistical analysis of survival data is usually much more complicated than regular statistical analysis, because of the presence of censoring [18]. However, survival models are commonly created based on Cox model methodologies, and simulations of the model were utilized in the [5, 19]. Equation (1) represents the Cox model.

$$D(t|x) = D_0(t) \times \exp(\mu) \tag{1}$$

From Eq. (1), $D(t|x)$ refers to hazard at a given period t, as a product of $D_0(t)$ (i.e., hazard baseline of a nonparametric) and $\mu = B_1x_1 + \cdots + B_px_p = B^Tx$ as the exponential of the prognostic index. The former linearly consolidates p indicator values with coefficients of regression B_1, $B2\ldots$, B_p giving weights. The predictive form of this model can be written as far as survival function as

$$Q(t|x) = Q_0(t)^{\exp(n)} \tag{2}$$

where $Q(t|x)$ is the likelihood of surviving beyond period t given estimator x, and $Q_0(t)$ is the survival function baseline at period t, where $Q_0(t) = \exp\left[-\int_0^t h_0(u)\mathrm{d}u\right]$]. To make forecasts at a particular time point T, one requires estimates of $\widehat{B}$ and $\widehat{Q}_0(T)$.

Several kinds of research have shown the significance of survival prediction models in guiding patients' clinical management and health institutions on performance monitoring [20, 21]. For instance, models for estimating the danger of heart valve surgery mortality in hospitals have been created, in addition, for estimating the risk of developing cardiovascular disease within the ranged of 5–10 years as shown by [19, 22]. Because of the significant role of CI methods in health research, it is important to assess the survival prediction model performance, using appropriate statistical methods, in data that were not used during the development of the model [23, 24]. The term "model validation" refers to evaluating a model [25, 26]. Studies in [23–26] discussed two different validation processes which include internal and external validation. The former divides the single dataset into two, based on time or random selection. One is used during model development and the other is utilized during validation. While external validation gathers new datasets from a patient in various focus or distinct centers or different demographic areas, for testing the model generality or transportability to new patients.

3 Survival Model Analysis: Basic Concepts

In many investigations, the chance to an occasion of interest was the essential outcome under assessment. The survival time was the conventional name for the time, although it could apply to the time to survive from diagnoses of illness to death, and a temporary remission of symptoms or relapse of symptoms. Many strategies of analysis would apply if the occasion happened to all people. It is generally expected that around the completion of follow-up, a part of the people has not had the occasion of interest, and thusly their real exact time to the occasion is obscure. Further, survival data are skewed, they are seldom normally distributed and include consistently numerous early occasions and moderately scarcely any late ones. It is these provisions of the data that make the exceptional strategies called survival analysis investigation vital [27].

However, there are many types of "events" in clinical investigations. The event of interest is usually time-to-death. In cancer, is entirely different, it has the time between response to treatment and repeat or ailment-free survival time. It is basic to state what the occasion is and when the time of observation starts and wraps up. For instance, we might be interested in a relapse in the interval of time between an affirmed reaction and the initial relapse of malignancy [27].

However, survival data are portrayed and modeled similarly to two-related probabilities, explicitly "survival and hazard". The survival likelihood also refers to as "survivor function" $S(t)$ is the likelihood of survives time of a person, from the (initial time) diagnosed with cancer to a predetermined future period t. It is fundamental for survival analysis since survival likelihood for different values of time (t) gives imperative information in summary from time to occasion data. These qualities depicted review partner survival experience straightforwardly. The $h(t)$ or $l(t)$ represents the hazard that is the likelihood at a time t that an occasion happens for a person under perception. All in all, it addresses an individual momentary occasion rate, who survived throughout a period t. Note, this is not the same as the survivor function which focuses on not having an occasion, the hazard function focus on occasions occurring. Also, it is of interest, since it gives a comprehension of the restrictive failure rates and gives a vehicle for deciding a survival model. More or less, the hazard identifies with the episode occasion happens rate, while survival reflects entirely non-occasion [27, 28].

4 CI Methods Utilized in Survival Prediction: Concept Examples

Several studies have shown survival models have been used in various domains, to predict the outcome of interest. In several applications, the result is estimated as a chance to an occasion of interest. For example, a study by [28] models, the career paths based on talents, with an emphasis on two basic issues in the talents board, particularly turnover and career progression. Their study approach was assessed, with a few cutting-edge standard techniques on a certifiable talent dataset. The outcome of the study reveals powerful anticipating turnover and professional progression of talents. A similar study by [14, 29] also, modeled career path by foreseeing worker's survival time at an occasion of interest.

Another study by [30] modeled perhaps the most challenging issue in contemporary medication that is the survival of patients after liver transplantation. The researchers compared machine learning models' techniques with the traditional Cox models. A dataset of 62,294 patients from the United States, including (97 predictors and more than 600 chosen based on clinical/factual grounds), to foresee survival from transplantation. Three various Cox models and machine learning techniques were each applied to the dataset. The outcomes show random survival forests perform better than the Cox models based on the C-index. In light of this, the research results show machine learning techniques can be applied as an instrument for both prediction and understanding in the survival setting.

Also, an investigation by [31] developed a changed version of the CoxPH model using deep learning techniques that use images with survival data to predict the outcome. The developed model presents the architecture of the neural network for the survival prediction using images. The model was simulated with the MNIST dataset. Because of the small-sized MNIST dataset of the gray-scale image, transfer learning with state-of-the-art networks used by the model decrease substantially, the computing time. However, the minimalist network for net shows high performance than the state-of-the-art EfficientNet.

Another study by [32] modeled a mobile app survival prediction that shows which application will kick the bucket? utilizing multi-task learning. However, modeling the survival of mobile applications contrasts from existing predictions undertakings in two unique ways. In the first place, patient's survival probabilities decay similarly in bioinformatics survival prediction, whereas mobile app survival pattern varies. Second, mobile app popularity varies with time which is affected by numerous factors, for example, suggestion records from the application market, versions upgrades, surveys in-application market, social impacts, which hence is hard to give an exact prediction. These factors, however, make the existing short-term prediction strategies not directly versatile in long haul forecast since the estimation error amasses after some time truly. Those features make mobile app survival prediction difficult. The researchers create an AppLife system model utilizing multi-task learning (MTL) that joins the state data of mobile applications for survival forecast. A huge scope dataset of 35,000 mobile apps was used to simulate the proposed system AppLife. Based on the evaluation of the system, the results presented a high performance of the proposed system model over the seven state-of-the-art system models that were compared.

5 Classification of CI Methods and Application Challenges Based on Survival Dataset

A study by [33, 34] classified methods for survival analysis in two major categories: conventional statistical techniques and CI-based approaches. Both offer a similar objective of predicting outcome within the range of a survival time and assess the likelihood of survival at the predicted survival time of the event of interest, for instance, "death" in the biomedical domain. Statistical methods center more on describing the distributions of the occasion times and the properties of the statistical parameter assessment, by assessing the survival curves. However, statistical techniques are partitioned into three significant classes, for example, (parametric, nonparametric, and semi-parametric strategies).

The parametric strategy utilized the following distributions like exponential, logistic, Weibull, normal, log-logistic, and log-normal. The strategy tolerating that the survival period or the logarithm of the survival period of all cases in the data follow these distributions [35]. A few areas utilized this strategy as an option in contrast to the cox-based semi-parametric technique because of its efficiency, effectiveness, and simplicity, in foreseeing the chance to occasion of interest utilizing parametric strategies. It generally gets the survival gage that is harmonious with these theoretical distributions. Expecting all cases of the survival time followed these distributions, the case can be inspected utilizing the accelerate failure time model, in which we acknowledge the variable can influence the period to the occasion of interest of a case by some consistent factors [35]. However, note the accompanying, nonparametric strategies are more productive if no equivalent hypothetical distribution is known.

The nonparametric method is a widely used method among all the methods. If the theoretical distributions are unknown, the nonparametric method is more efficient. A study by [36] fostered the Kaplan–Meier (KM) curve to gage the survival function utilizing the genuine length of the noticed time. This technique is the most broadly utilized for assessing survival function. Coming up next are strategies applied in nonparametric, for example, Kaplan–Meier [37], Nelson-Aalen [38, 39], life-table [40]. However, note, nonparametric strategies are less productive contrasted with the parametric techniques, when the period to the occasion of interest follows a particular distribution like exponential, logistic, Weibull, normal, and so forth.

The semi-parametric method can be described as parametric and nonparametric hybrid approaches. Under a more extensive scope of conditions, the semi-parametric technique can get a more predictable assessor than parametric technique, and an accurate assessor than the nonparametric strategy [37]. However, here, the characteristics are expected to impact the result, however, information on the fundamental distribution of survival times is not needed. The most utilized survival investigation technique in this classification was the Cox model [14]. Nonetheless, there are augmentations and various variations of the Cox model like regularized, boost, and time-dependent Cox methods.

The survival prediction model has been used widely not only in the biomedical field but in almost every domain since data structures that apply to the models are available in those domains [33]. Recent investigation has described survival prediction methods as a powerful tool in risk awareness of events of interest, for instance, "death" in biomedical application [31]. However, survival prediction models face a lot of challenges, such as an incomplete observation, because of the presence of censoring [34]. Censorship is the same as the missing data problem. For instance, in clinical investigation, collection of data for various reasons might face some challenges like the duration for data collection might take several months or years to complete and would require participants under investigation consistency to keep track of their data. It is possible some instances of the event of interest cannot be observed by some participants. Therefore, a traditional regression model cannot be fitted for making predictions using such data [38].

The concentrate by [27, 35] sorted blue penciling into three distinct sorts: first, left-editing, which is depicted as a noticed endurance season of the occasion of revenue, is more than or same as the specific endurance time. Second, right-blue penciling, which is portrayed as exceptionally normal, happened when the noticed endurance season of an occasion of interest is not exactly or equivalent to the specific endurance time. Last, span controlling just recognizes that the occasion of interest occurred inside the scope of a period stretch. Nonetheless, when utilizing controlled information during endurance investigation, the main objective variable was "the ideal opportunity for the occasion of revenue". We can just recognize those occurrences from members who encountered the occasion inside the examination time frame. For additional subtleties, see the idea of editing in [34] given this fractional.

The study by [27, 34] categorized censoring into three different types: first, left-censoring, which is described as an observed survival time of the event of interest, is more than or same as the exact survival time. Second, right-censoring, which is described as very common, happened when the observed survival time of an event of interest is not exactly or equivalent to the exact survival period. Last, interval censoring only acknowledges that the event of interest happened within a range of a time interval. However, when using censored data during survival analysis, the only target variable was the "time" for the occasion of interest. We can only acknowledge those occurrences from members who encountered the occasion within the examination time frame. For more details, see the concept of censoring in [33]. Because of this partial information, typical CI algorithms are incapacitated to use such information effectively, there is a need to create survival prediction algorithms to accommodate censoring [39]. Another study by [40] mentions two other challenges face by survival prediction models like multi-modality of the datasets used and small size sample of the dataset available.

Despite this censoring data handling issue, there is also a particular challenge of apply survival models algorithms with such censored data. However, several investigations recently developed traditional statistical methods for handling such complex, challenging issues. In addition, to address such a practical problem at hand, some CI researchers have developed and applied several sophisticated CI techniques to either complete or complement statistical methods [34].

6 CI Methods for Survival Prediction Analysis

CI methods are used in high-dimensional cases. Also, CI methods center more on the predicting occurrence of the event of interest at a particular period by absorbing the conventional survival investigation strategies with different CI procedures. In addition, CI techniques proffer more successful algorithms engrossing survival cases with both statistical strategies and CI techniques. Exploiting the new advancement of CI techniques to get familiar with the dependencies among covariates and survival times in various ways. Recent popular CI methods used in survival prediction analysis like neural networks, Bayesian techniques, support vector machines, and survival trees. There are many advanced CI strategies, for example, active, ensemble, multi-task, and transfer learning techniques. In addition, other related CI methods for survival prediction analysis include data transformation, complex events, and early prediction. However, CI methods have been used in different practical domains and achieved significant success. The key challenge of CI methods remains a difficulty in handling censored data and the time estimation of the models [34]. A study by [41] shows that, when there is a large dataset of instances, CI methods are very effective. However, this is not the same in certain problems in survival analysis. The following is the highlight of a portion of the utilized and further developed CI strategies in survival investigation.

6.1 Survival Trees Method

Survival trees are one sort structured like tree algorithms that are fitted to oversee censored data. An investigation by [42] was the first to have discussed the development of survival trees. The survival tree differs from the normal decision tree based on the splitting criterion. The survival trees strategy dividing models into two unique methodologies, for example, (augmenting between-node heterogeneity and limiting inside-node homogeneity). Utilizing the inside-note homogeneity measure, the first methodology limits the loss function. In the second methodology of dividing criteria, the study by [43] utilized log-rank test statistics for between-node heterogeneity measures. Also, after two years, the authors in [44] proposed a probability ratio measurement to measure the divergence between two nodes. However, the capacity to deal with censored data by the survival tree strategy, utilizing the tree structure, was a significant improvement over the standard choice tree. Furthermore, the choice of the last tree is one of the imperative parts of developing a survival tree. Nonetheless, reverse determination and forward choice methodologies can be applied while looking for the ideal tree [45]. However, when searching for the optimal tree, backward and forward selection methodologies can be applied [46]. A study by [47] compared survival trees with Cox proportional hazards (CoxPH) on predicting the incident of coronary heart disease (CHD), using a dataset of Tehran Lipid and Glucose Study (TLGS) of 8279 participants. The study results show survival trees outperform

Cox proportional hazards (CoxPH). For more details, see [47]. Another study by [48] applied the survival trees technique to predict the development of hypothyroidism in patients undergo radiotherapy nasopharyngeal cancer (NPC). Used a dataset of 97 patients from Jakarta hospital that have undergone radiotherapy. The study investigated the post-radiated NPC patients, to distinguish subgroups of patients with an alternate hazard rate of development of hypothyroidism.

6.2 *Bayesian Methods*

Bayes' theorem has been described as one of the underlying principles of mathematical statistics and probability theory. Also, Bayes' hypothesis gives a connection between before likelihood and the after likelihood, in other to see the differences in the prior and the posterior probability values on accounting of a specific occasion of interest. The study in [43] classified techniques for applying the Bayes theorem into two, for example, Naïve Bayes and Bayesian network. The two methods are commonly used in the clinical prediction domain, which gives a likelihood of the specific occasion of interest as their results [41, 45, 49]. In any case, utilizing Bayesian techniques for endurance information tests, the outcomes show it has extraordinary qualities of interpretability and vulnerability thinking properties [50]. However, utilizing Bayesian techniques for survival data experiment, the outcomes reveal it has outstanding characteristics of interpretability and uncertainty reasoning properties [51]. While Naïve Bayes (NB) has been described as the effective and simplest prediction algorithm. Even though it has one disadvantage of making an independence assumption, while in survival investigation, this may not be valid on most occasions. An investigation in [52] developed a model that integrates Bayesian techniques with an AFT strategy by extrapolating the earlier occasion probability to implement early phase prediction on survival data for the future period. An investigation by [53] applied the Bayesian method to identify factors that influence the short-term and long-term survival of patients with gastric cancer. For more details on Bayesian methods, see [54]. Also, the authors in [54] discussed some Bayesian R-packages.

6.3 *Artificial Neural Networks Method*

A study in [55] was the first to have described artificial neural network (ANN), which was inspired by the biological neural system. The artificial nodes in the ANN method are denoted by neurons that simulate a biological neural network, which forms a network connection based on a weighted link. However, ANN neuron produces results based on a specific initiation function. The artificial neural network (ANN) has been utilized broadly in survival investigation. For instance, a study by [50] applied an artificial neural network (ANN) to predict survival in bladder cancer patients. A dataset of 161,227 patients from the National Cancer Institute's surveillance, epidemiology, and end results (SEER) was used in the study. The investigation results show artificial neural network (ANN) outperforms a Cox proportional hazards (CPH) model. Also, the model shows the ability to the interpretation of the complex data it contains. For more details on artificial neural networks (ANNs), see investigations that applied it, like [50, 56].

6.4 Support Vector Machines Method

A study by [57] described support vector machines (SVMs) as mostly used in classification cases, even though it has also been changed for regression cases successfully. Also, it is a supervised learning method. In addition, it has been applied in survival analysis cases successfully. For instance, a study in [58] applied a support vector machine in predicting treatment response to neoadjuvant chemoradiotherapy (nCRT) in rectal cancer patients. 428 patients' data were used in the study and divided for training in a [7:3 ratio] that is (299 patients) in training and (129 patients) for validation. The investigation results show 0.834 in the training cohort and 0.854 in the area under the receiver operating characteristic curves (AUROCs). Another investigation by [59] compared CT methods which include random survival forests, survival support vector machines, and extreme gradient boosting [XGB] with Cox proportional hazards (CPH). Also, the study used shapley additive explanation (SHAP) values to explain the method's predictions. The CI methods not only outperform Cox proportional hazards (CPH) but tells how methods make their predictions, which increase adoption and trusting CI methods as an adjunct to traditional methods in the oncology and healthcare domain at large. For more details in support vector machines, see investigations, like [58–60].

However, there are other advanced methods that have unique advantages over the methods discussed above like ensemble, active, transfer, and multi-task learning. Nonetheless, Table 1 provides highlights of the strengths and weaknesses of some CI models.

CI helps researchers and medical practitioners in many ways, like image interpretation during diagnosis is perform by computer with help of computational intelligence techniques [62]. Also, CI has been applied in cancer detection, prognosis, and therapy application [63]. The abundant clinical dataset collected in recent decades, and the availability of a low-cost computer with high computing power processing large data has to reshape how researchers conducted their research in the various medical fields [64]. Also, an investigation by [65] shows how computer technologies advancement increases CI application in a medical domain like radiology, pathology, ophthalmology, and cardiology received positive impact. Also using various computational intelligence approaches to manage data over the cloud and connects the doctors, patients, and nurses through smart intelligent sensor devices at low cost with high bandwidth networks.

Table 1 Summary of strengths and weaknesses of various CI models

S. No.	Model	Strength(s)	Weakness(s)
1	Survival trees	Capability to manipulate censored data utilizing the tree structure	The problem of choosing an optimal tree. Also, no widely acceptable evaluation of the fit quality of the model like (accuracy and explainable variance) see discussion in [61]
2	Bayesian methods	It has good features of both interpretability and uncertainty rationale [51]. It gives a characteristic and principled method of joining earlier data with information, inside a strong choice hypothetical system. Its ability to predict any function without utilizing the plug-in method	Independence assumption between all the features, which may not be valid for some issues in survival examination. Bayesian inferences require skills to translate subjective prior beliefs into a mathematically formulated prior. Which can create a misleading result. It can produce posterior distributions that are intensely affected by the priors which may disagree with the legitimacy of the chosen prior
3	Artificial neural networks	All information is stored in the network. Capability to work with incomplete data. It has features of fault-tolerant, parallel processing ability, and making a decision based on a similar event	Required processor with high processing power. It does not give information on why or how it arrived at a given solution. Duration and determination of the appropriate network structure are unknown
4	Support vector machines	Memory is efficient and works effectively on high-dimensional data. Over-fitting risk is very minimal	Difficult to work with a large dataset. Underperformance when the features of the training data are less than the sample data. No explanation by the model on why or how it arrived at a particular solution

7 CI Techniques Opportunities and Future Direction Toward Survival Prediction

The aim of CI survival prediction methods is to predict the occurrence of the occasion of interest, for example, a death in bioinformatics, at a future time point. However, because of the widespread availability of a dataset for survival analysis from various domains, CI methods have been used to model real-world applications from various domains. Recent advances of many CI methods in cancer survival prediction application have involved CI-based methods as an adjunct to the traditional statistical methods used in survival prediction. This, therefore, increasing demand for improving and understanding of CI-based methods for handling survival data analysis effectively. However, many bodies of kinds of literature have shown a different application of survival prediction methods in various domains like healthcare [66], Reliability [67], crowdfunding [68], bioinformatics [69, 70], student dropout [71], customer lifetime value [72], click-through rate [73], duration modeling in economics [74]. Many bodies of pieces of literature proved beyond reasonable doubt not only cancer befitted from survival prediction methods, but various domains.

However, future directions toward CI methods of survival prediction are proving the performance of CI methods via applying multiple external validation sets may be required [75], limitations of the data access and equity are also one obstacle to CI survival prediction methods. The authors [76, 77] proposed strategies for findable, accessible, interoperable, reusable (FAIR) data use and researchers to publish their dataset used. In addition, CI survival methods proved a success and high performance in pieces of literature, however, how do the methods make their prediction? This referred to the "black box" problem [78]. There is a need for further research on interpretability and the black box problem of CI survival prediction methods, because of its implication for the adoption of CI survival prediction methods by various domains, including healthcare by both practitioner and regulatory agency [79–81]. Also, collaboration among CI researchers and experts from various domains would bring an understanding of CI methods and the adoption of CI survival methods.

8 Conclusions

Recent literature shows CI survival prediction methods have been used not only in cancer survival prediction but in almost every domain, since there is an available dataset relevant to those areas. Even though, there are various published kinds of literature applying CI methods to predict time to an event of interest which proved successful and excellent performance. However, obstacles still exist based on the application of CI methods because of censoring, small size dataset, data access and quality, and interpretability of the challenges of the method. Despite these challenges, CI methods are poised to make practice-changing effects on the survival prediction analysis arena. CI methods, at presents, have shown promising results in cancer survival prediction, as shown on others domain. Cancer survival prediction based on CI methods is the future of survival analysis techniques toward the accurate determining time of occurrence of an event of interest. By utilizing CI-based system methods, researchers can collaborate in real-time to shared outcomes electronically of time of the event of interest.

References

1. GLOBOCAN 2020: New Global Cancer Data|UICC. Retrieved on September 30, 2021, from https://www.uicc.org/news/globocan-2020-new-global-cancer-data
2. Roodman, G. D. (2004). Mechanisms of bone metastasis. *New England Journal of Medicine, 350*(16), 1655–1664. https://doi.org/10.1056/nejmra030831
3. D'Oronzo, S., Coleman, R., Brown, J., & Silvestris, F. (2019, April 01). Metastatic bone disease: Pathogenesis and therapeutic options: Up-date on bone metastasis management. *Journal of Bone Oncology, 15*. Elsevier GmbH, p. 004. https://doi.org/10.1016/j.jbo.2018.10.004
4. Coleman, R. E. (2001). Metastatic bone disease: Clinical features, pathophysiology and treatment strategies. *Cancer Treatment Reviews, 27*(3), 165–176. https://doi.org/10.1053/ctrv.2000.0210
5. Coleman, R. E., Roodman, S., Body, S., & Vessella. (2006, October 15). Clinical features of metastatic bone disease and risk of skeletal morbidity. *Clinical Cancer Research, 12*(20), PART 2. https://doi.org/10.1158/1078-0432.CCR-06-0931
6. Forsberg, J. A., Eberhardt, J., Boland, P. J., Wedin, R., & Healey, J. H. (2011). Estimating survival in patients with operable skeletal metastases: An application of a Bayesian belief network. *PLoS One, 6*(5). https://doi.org/10.1371/journal.pone.0019956
7. Poon, M. T. C., Sudlow, C. L. M., Figueroa, J. D., & Brennan, P. M. (2020, December). Longer-term ($\geq$2 years) survival in patients with glioblastoma in population-based studies pre- and post-2005: A systematic review and meta-analysis. *Scientific Reports, 10*(1). https://doi.org/10.1038/s41598-020-68011-4
8. Loya, H., Poduval, P., Anand, D., Kumar, N., & Sethi, A. (2020) Uncertainty estimation in cancer survival prediction (pp. 1–6) [Online]. http://arxiv.org/abs/2003.08573
9. Isa, A. (2021). Computational intelligence methods in medical image-based diagnosis of COVID-19 infections. In *Studies in Computational Intelligence* (Vol. 923, pp. 251–270). Springer Science and Business Media Deutschland GmbH.
10. SURVMARK-2—viz1. Retrieved on September 30, 2021, from https://gco.iarc.fr/survival/survmark/visualizations/viz1/?groupby=%22country%22&period=%225%22&cancer_site=%22Colon%22&country=%22Australia%22&year=%222014%22&gender=%22All%22&sorting=%220%22
11. Cuevas, E., Zaldívar, D., Pajares, G., Perez-Cisneros, M., & Rojas, R. (2018). Computational intelligence in image processing 2018. *Mathematical Problems in Engineering*, Hindawi Limited. https://doi.org/10.1155/2018/6952803
12. Obermeyer, Z., & Emanuel, E. J. (2016). Predicting the future—Big data, machine learning, and clinical medicine. *New England Journal of Medicine, 375*(13), 1216–1219. https://doi.org/10.1056/nejmp1606181
13. Deo, R. C. (2015). Machine learning in medicine. *Circulation, 132*(20), 1920–1930. https://doi.org/10.1161/CIRCULATIONAHA.115.001593
14. Cox, D. R. (1972). Regression models and life-tables
15. Yu, C.-N., Greiner, R., Lin, H.-C., & Baracos, V. (2011). Learning patient-specific cancer survival distributions as a sequence of dependent regressors.
16. Fotso, S. (2018, January). Deep neural networks for survival analysis based on a multi-task framework. Retrieved on July 04, 2021, from http://arxiv.org/abs/1801.05512
17. Hao, L., Kim, J., Kwon, S., & Do Ha, I. (2021). Deep learning-based survival analysis for high-dimensional survival data (pp. 1–18)
18. Do Ha, I., Jeong, J.-H., & Lee, Y. (2017). *Statistical modelling of survival data with random effects*. Springer.
19. Hippisley, J. Predicting cardiovascular risk in England and Wales: Prospective derivation and validation of QRISK2. https://doi.org/10.1136/bmj.39609.449676.25
20. Omar, R. Z., Ambler, G., Royston, P., Eliahoo, J., & Taylor, K. M. (2004). Cardiac surgery risk modeling for mortality: A review of current practice and suggestions for improvement. *Annals of Thoracic Surgery, 77*, 2232–2239. https://doi.org/10.1016/j.authoracsur.2003.10.032

21. Moons, K. G. M., Royston, P., Vergouwe, Y., Grobbee, D. E., & Altman, D. G. (2009, May 30). Prognosis and prognostic research: What, why, and how? *BMJ (Online), 338*(7706). British Medical Journal Publishing Group, 1317–1320. https://doi.org/10.1136/bmj.b375
22. Ambler, G., Omar, R. Z., Royston, P., Kinsman, R., Keogh, B. E., & Taylor, K. M. (2005). Generic, simple risk stratification model for heart valve surgery. *Circulation, 112*(2), 224–231. https://doi.org/10.1161/CIRCULATIONAHA.104.515049
23. Royston, P., & Altman, D. G. (2013). External validation of a Cox prognostic model: Principles and methods. *BMC Medical Research Methodology, 13*(1), 33. https://doi.org/10.1186/1471-2288-13-33
24. Collins, G. S., et al. (2014, March 19). External validation of multivariable prediction models: A systematic review of methodological conduct and reporting. *BMC Medical Research Methodology, 14*(1). BioMed Central Ltd., 40. https://doi.org/10.1186/1471-2288-14-40
25. Steyerberg, E. W. (2009). Clinical prediction models: A practical approach to development, validation, and updating. *International Statistical Review, 77*(2), 320–321. https://doi.org/10.1111/j.1751-5823.2009.00085_22.x
26. Harrell, F. E., & Levy, D. G. Regression modeling strategies.
27. Clark, T. G., Bradburn, M. J., Love, S. B., & Altman, D. G. (2003). Survival analysis part I: Basic concepts and first analyses. *British Journal of Cancer, 89*(2), 232–238. https://doi.org/10.1038/sj.bjc.6601118
28. Li, H., Ge, Y., Zhu, H., Xiong, H., & Zhao, H. (2017). Prospecting the career development of talents: A survival analysis perspective. In *Proceedings of ACM SIGKDD international conference on knowledge discovery data mining* (Vol. Part F1296, pp. 917–925). https://doi.org/10.1145/3097983.3098107
29. Li, Y., Wang, J., Ye, J., & Reddy, C. K. A multi-task learning formulation for survival analysis KDD '16. https://doi.org/10.1145/2939672.2939857
30. Kantidakis, G., Putter, H., Lancia, C., de Boer, J., Braat, A. E., & Fiocco, M. (2020). Survival prediction models since liver transplantation—Comparisons between Cox models and machine learning techniques. *BMC Medical Research Methodology, 20*(1), 1–19. https://doi.org/10.1186/s12874-020-01153-1
31. Tarkhan, A., Simon, N., Bengtsson, T., Nguyen, K., & Dai, J. (2021). Survival prediction using deep learning. *Journal of Machine Learning Research, 1*(1), 1–8.
32. Guo, B., Zhang, Y., Liu, J., Guo, T., Ouyang, Y., & Yu, Z. (2020). Which app is going to die? A framework for app survival prediction with multi-task learning. *IEEE Transactions on Mobile Computing*, 1–1. https://doi.org/10.1109/tmc.2020.3012767
33. Marinos, G. D. K. (2021). A survey of survival analysis techniques. In *Proceedings of the 14th international joint conference on biomedical engineering systems and technologies (BIOSTEC 2021)* (Vol. 5, no. Biostec, pp. 716–723). https://doi.org/10.5220/0010382307160723
34. Wang, P., Li, Y. A. N., & Reddy, C. K. (2017). Machine learning for survival analysis: A survey (Vol. X, No. X, pp. 1–39). arXiv:1708.04649v1 [cs.LG].
35. Lee, E. T., & Wenyu Wang, J. Statistical methods for survival data analysis. In *Wiley Series in Probability and Statistics* (3rd ed.).
36. Kaplan, E. L., & Meier, P. (1958). Nonparametric estimation from incomplete observations nonparametric estimation from incomplete observations.
37. Powell, J. L. (1994, January 01). Estimation of semiparametric models. In *Handbook of econometrics* (Vol. 4, pp. 2443–2521), Elsevier. https://doi.org/10.1016/S1573-4412(05)80010-8
38. Prinja, S., Gupta, N., & Verma, R. (2010, April 01). Censoring in clinical trials: Review of survival analysis techniques. *Indian Journal of Community Medicine, 35*(2), 217–221. Wolters Kluwer—Medknow Publications. https://doi.org/10.4103/0970-0218.66859
39. Sloma, M., & Xu, K. S. (2021). Empirical comparison of continuous and discrete-time representations for survival prediction. *Proceedings of Machine Learning Research, 1*, 1–14.
40. Huang, C., Zhang, A., & Xiao, G. (2018). Deep integrative analysis for survival prediction. In *Pacific symposium on Biocomputing* (pp. 343–352)

41. Zupan, B., Demšar, J., Kattan, M. W., Beck, J. R., & Bratko, I. (2000). Machine learning for survival analysis: A case study on recurrence of prostate cancer. *Artificial Intelligence in Medicine, 20*(1), 59–75. https://doi.org/10.1016/S0933-3657(00)00053-1
42. Gordon, L., & Olshen, R. A. (1985). Tree-structured survival analysis. *Cancer Treatment Report, 69*(10), 1065–1068. Retrieved on August 15, 2021 from https://pubmed.ncbi.nlm.nih.gov/4042086/
43. Friedman, N., Geiger, D., & Goldszmidt, M. (1997). Bayesian network classifiers. *Machine Learning, 29*(2–3), 131–163. https://doi.org/10.1023/a:1007465528199
44. Ciampi, A., Chang, C.-H., Hogg, S., & McKinney, S. (1987). Recursive partition: A versatile method for exploratory-data analysis in biostatistics. In *Biostatistics* (pp. 23–50). Springer Netherlands.
45. The Statistical Evaluation of Medical Tests for Classification and Prediction ... von Margaret Sullivan Pepe—Portofrei bei bücher.de. Retrieved on August 15, 2021, from https://www.buecher.de/shop/mund/the-statistical-evaluation-of-medical-tests-for-classification-and-prediction-ebook-pdf/pepe-margaret-sullivan/products_products/detail/prod_id/40069258/
46. Bou-Hamad, I., Larocque, D., & Ben-Ameur, H. (2011, January). A review of survival trees. *Statistical Survey, 5*, 44–71. https://doi.org/10.1214/09-SS047
47. Ramezankhani, A., Bagherzadeh-Khiabani, F., Khalili, D., Azizi, F., & Hadaegh, F. (2017). A new look at risk patterns related to coronary heart disease incidence using survival tree analysis: 12 years longitudinal study. *Science and Reports, 7*(1), 1–11. https://doi.org/10.1038/s41598-017-03577-0
48. George, P. M. A., Abdullah, S., & Rachman, A. (2021). Analysis of hypothyroidism development in post-radiotherapy nasopharyngeal cancer patients using survival trees. *Journal of Physics*, 12095. https://doi.org/10.1088/1742-6596/1722/1/012095
49. Kononenko, I. (1993). Inductive and Bayesian learning in medical diagnosis. *Applied Artificial Intelligence, 7*(4), 317–337. https://doi.org/10.1080/08839519308949993
50. Bhambhvani, H. P., et al. (2021). Development of robust artificial neural networks for prediction of 5-year survival in bladder cancer. *Urologic Oncology: Seminars and Original Investigations, 39*(3), 193.e7-193.e12. https://doi.org/10.1016/j.urolonc.2020.05.009
51. Raftery, A., Raftery, A., Madigan, D., & Volinsky, C. T. (1995). Accounting for model uncertainty in survival analysis improves predictive performance. *BAYESIAN Statistics, 5*, 323–349. Retrieved on August 15, 2021, on http://citeseerx.ist.psu.edu/viewdoc/summary?doi=10.1.1.40.8597
52. Fard, M. J., Wang, P., Chawla, S., & Reddy, C. K. (2016). A Bayesian perspective on early stage event prediction in longitudinal data. *IEEE Transactions on Knowledge and Data Engineering, 28*(12), 3126–3139. https://doi.org/10.1109/TKDE.2016.2608347
53. Karamoozian, A., Baneshi, M. R., & Bahrampour, A. (2021). Short-term and long-term survival of patients with gastric cancer. *Gastroenterology Hepatology from bed to bench, 14*(2), 115–122. Retrieved on August 18, 2021, from http://www.ncbi.nlm.nih.gov/pubmed/33968338
54. Alvares, D., Lázaro, E., Gómez-Rubio, V., & Armero, C. (2021). Bayesian survival analysis with BUGS. *Statistics in Medicine, 40*(12), 2975–3020. https://doi.org/10.1002/sim.8933
55. Rosenblatt, F. (1958). The perceptron: A probabilistic model for information storage and organization in the brain. *Psychological Review, 65*(6), 386–408. https://doi.org/10.1037/h0042519
56. Wang, J., Chen, N., Guo, J., Xu, X., Liu, L., & Yi, Z. (2021). SurvNet: A novel deep neural network for lung cancer survival analysis with missing values. *Frontiers in Oncology, 10*, 3128. https://doi.org/10.3389/fonc.2020.588990
57. Smola, A. J., Sch¨olkopf, B., & Sch¨olkopf, S. (2004). A tutorial on support vector regression, Kluwer Academic Publishers.
58. Jiang, W., et al. (2021, June). A nomogram based on a collagen feature support vector machine for predicting the treatment response to neoadjuvant chemoradiotherapy in rectal cancer patients. *Annual Surgical Oncology*, 1–14. https://doi.org/10.1245/s10434-021-10218-4
59. Moncada-Torres, A., van Maaren, M. C., Hendriks, M. P., Siesling, S., & Geleijnse, G. (2021). Explainable machine learning can outperform Cox regression predictions and provide insights

in breast cancer survival. *Science and Reports, 11*(1), 1–13. https://doi.org/10.1038/s41598-021-86327-7
60. Sadhu, A. (2021). Prediction of breast cancer using support vector machines. *International Research on Journal of Engineering and Technology*. Retrieved on August 19, 2021, from www.irjet.net
61. Schemper, M., & Stare, J. (1996). Explained variation in survival analysis. *Statistics in Medicine, 15*(19), 1999–2012. https://doi.org/10.1002/(SICI)1097-0258(19961015)15:19%3c1999::AID-SIM353%3e3.0.CO;2-D
62. Raza, K., & Singh, N. K. (2021, January). A tour of unsupervised deep learning for medical image analysis. *Current Medical Imaging. Formerly: Current Medical Imaging Review, 17*. https://doi.org/10.2174/1573405617666210127154257
63. Qazi, S., Raza, K., & Iqbal, N. (2021). 5 Artificial intelligence in medicine (AIM): Machine learning in cancer diagnosis, prognosis and therapy. In *Artificial intelligence for data-driven medical diagnosis*, De Gruyter (pp. 103–126).
64. Bhinder, B., Gilvary, C., Madhukar, N. S., & Elemento, O. (2021, April 01). Artifi Cial intelligence in cancer research and precision medicine. *Cancer Discovery, 11*(4), 900–915. American Association for Cancer Research Inc. https://doi.org/10.1158/2159-8290.CD-21-0090
65. Alam, A., Qazi, S., Iqbal, N., & Raza, K. (2020). Fog, edge and pervasive computing in intelligent internet of things driven applications in healthcare: Challenges, limitations and future use. In *Fog, edge, and pervasive computing in intelligent IoT driven applications* (pp. 1–26), Wiley.
66. Miller, R. G. (2011). *Survival analysis*. Wiley.
67. Mohammad, V. K., Modarres, & Mark, P. (2009). *Reliability engineering and risk analysis, 43*(1). CRC Press.
68. Li, Y., Rakesh, V., & Reddy, C. K. Project success prediction in crowdfunding environments. Retrieved on August 24, 2021, from https://doi.org/10.1145/2835776.2835791
69. Li, Y., Wang, J., Ye, J., & Reddy, C. K. (2016, August). A multi-task learning formulation for survival analysis. In *Proceedings of the ACM SIGKDD international conference on knowledge discovery and data mining* (Vol. 13–17, pp. 1715–1724). https://doi.org/10.1145/2939672.2939857
70. Antonov, A. V., Krestyaninova, M., Knight, R. A., Rodchenkov, I., Melino, G., & Barlev, N. A. (2014). PPISURV: A novel bioinformatics tool for uncovering the hidden role of specific genes in cancer survival outcome. *Oncogene, 33*(13), 1621–1628. https://doi.org/10.1038/onc.2013.119
71. Ameri, S., Fard, M. J., Chinnam, R. B., & Reddy, C. K. (2016, October). Survival analysis based framework for early prediction of student dropouts. In *International conference on information and knowledge management, proceedings* (Vol. 24–28, pp. 903–912). https://doi.org/10.1145/2983323.2983351
72. Rosset, S. (2003). Customer lifetime value models for decision support.
73. Barbieri, N., Silvestri, F., & Lalmas, M. (2016, April). Improving post-click user engagement on native ads via survival analysis. In *25th international world wide web conference, WWW 2016* (pp. 761–770). https://doi.org/10.1145/2872427.2883092
74. Kiefer, N. M., Kiefer, & Nicholas. (1988). Economic duration data and hazard functions. *Journal of Economic Literature, 26*(2), 646–79. Retrieved on August 24, 2021, from https://econpapers.repec.org/RePEc:aea:jeclit:v:26:y:1988:i:2:p:646-79
75. Zech, J. R., Badgeley, A., Liu, M., Costa, A. B., Titano, J. J., & Oermann, E. K. (2018, November). Variable generalization performance of a deep learning model to detect pneumonia in chest radiographs: A cross-sectional study. *PLOS Medicine, 15*(11), e1002683. https://doi.org/10.1371/journal.pmed.1002683
76. Wilkinson, M. D., et al. (2016). The FAIR guiding principles for scientific data management and stewardship. *Scientific Data, 3*(1), 1–9. https://doi.org/10.1038/sdata.2016.18
77. Chavan, V., & Penev, L. (2011). The data paper: A mechanism to incentivize data publishing in biodiversity science. *BMC Bioinformatics, 12*(Suppl 15). https://doi.org/10.1186/1471-2105-12-S15-S2

78. Castelvecchi, D. (2016). Can we open the black box of AI? *Nature, 538*(7623), 20–23. https://doi.org/10.1038/538020a
79. Towards trustable machine learning. *Nature Biomedical Engineering, 2*(10), 709–710 (2018, October 01). Nature Publishing Group. https://doi.org/10.1038/s41551-018-0315-x
80. Can A.I. Be Taught to Explain Itself?—The New York Times. Retrieved on August 24, 2021, from https://www.nytimes.com/2017/11/21/magazine/can-ai-be-taught-to-explain-itself.html
81. EU General Data Protection Regulation—Key changes|DLA Piper Global Law Firm. Retrieved on August 24, 2021, from https://www.dlapiper.com/en/us/focus/eu-data-protection-regulation/key-changes/

Breast Cancer Survival Prediction Using Machine Learning

Parul Tiwari, Piyush Bhardwaj, Arvind Keprate, and Ashish Tyagi

Abstract Breast cancer is one of the most prevalent cancers in women, and recent breakthroughs in data mining have provided more insight into the disease and its prognosis. We offer a set of machine learning models for predicting breast cancer survival in this chapter. There are 272 occurrences, 1564 characteristics, and a target variable in the original data, which were obtained from the data world Website (195 not survived, 77 survived). Out of 1564 features, the top ten features were selected using the extreme gradient boosting (XGB) method. 5-fold and 10-fold stratified cross-validation were used to extract the average results and accuracy for both methods is compared. The outcomes of six machine learning classifiers were compared and rated using a variety of statistical rates (accuracy, precision, true positive rate, true negative rate, F1-score, ROC–AUC score). We offer random forest (RFC) and XGB as the top classifiers after evaluating the models, with overall testing accuracy of 78% and 77.2%, respectively. However, all the classifiers performed well in predicting label 0 (high true negative rate) as compared to label 1 (low true positive rate).

Keywords Breast cancer · Machine learning · Feature selection · Classification

---

P. Tiwari (✉) · P. Bhardwaj
Centre for Advanced Computational Solutions (C-fACS), Lincoln University, Lincoln, New Zealand

A. Keprate
Department of Mechanical, Electronics and Chemical Engineering, Oslo Metropolitan University, Oslo, Norway
e-mail: arvind.keprate@oslomet.no

A. Tyagi
Department of Forensic Medicine and Toxicology, SHKM Govt. Medical College, Nalhar, Haryana, India

K. Raza (ed.), *Computational Intelligence in Oncology*, Studies in Computational Intelligence 1016, https://doi.org/10.1007/978-981-16-9221-5_8

1 Introduction

Cancer is a destructive disease, and breast cancer is one of the most common cancers affecting the health of women globally [1]. It has a high mortality rate all around the world. Though recent technical advances reduce the mortality rate up to some extent, still there is an immediate need to design such predictive models which can detect the occurrence as well as recurrence of breast cancer at early stages [2]. In this way, these models will help in setting up more effective treatment and will escort the clinicians and doctors in identifying important responsible factors for breast cancer.

Traditional statistical methods and software packages are being used for a long time to determine the factors responsible for breast cancer survival rate. Though these conventional methods serve their purpose up to some extent but are not flexible and robust in terms of adaptability to the presence of new variables [3]. Thus, developing fast computing robust models are on the top-priority list of researchers and scientists. The survival rate in breast cancer is higher as compared to other neoplasms because human survival is possible without the breast tissue [4]. It is necessary to understand the factors responsible for cancer survival and artificial intelligence (AI)-based algorithms can assist in uncovering the mysteries behind cancer. Not only cancer, machine learning (ML) algorithms have been used in various studies in order to understand other medical conditions such as heart disease, and ML was also found successful with genomics data [5–7].

In [8], a predictive model for the recurrence of breast cancer using a recurrence neural network (RNN) was developed. The authors compared the ML models with deep learning models and achieved higher accuracy in terms of area under the curve (AUC) score. Different pathological characteristics such as hormone receptors, tumor size, and nuclear grade have been used in traditional methods [9]. However, the use of robust and efficient computational algorithms allowed the researchers to test high-dimensional parameters and to select important features [10, 11]. Gene signature panels are utilized in [8] for the prognosis of breast cancer patients in place of clinical-pathological features. Recently, authors in [12] compared the performance of three ML models with OADICEA model. The authors reconnoitered the differences in reclassification and discussed its significance in clinical decision-making for the initial screening of breast cancer patients.

There are several research articles that exist in the literature that mark of the importance of ML algorithms. An artificial intelligence study predicted breast cancer survivals using a dataset containing information of 900 patients and provided outcomes with 96% accuracy and showed an accuracy of 93% for ROC-AUC [10]. Based on the methods used in [11], 77% classification accuracy was predicted using a backpropagation neural network for breast cancer patients. Mortality rate was predicted for Ireland's colorectal cancer patients using a large size of data from the World Health Organization (WHO) for the period 1950–2002 [12].

In recent years, [13] marked the capability of ML techniques and predicted breast cancer survivals with 82.7% accuracy after investigating breast cancer dataset of 8066 records from the University Malay Medical Center (Kuala Lumpur, Malaysia).

A retrospective study using electronic administrative records has been carried out and tested the hypothesis for improving the performance of conventional methods [14]. All the ML algorithms are famous among the scientific fraternity for their potential to solve classification problems (survived or not survived, men or women, 0 or 1, malignant or benign) in machine learning.

Nevertheless, achieving 100% accuracy in survival prediction for cancer patients remains a challenge due to the immunity of the individuals, mushrooming the heterogeneity and complexity of the disease and various treatment therapies. However, if anyhow we get high prediction accuracy, the patient can get individualized care and treatment. The idea of using ML approaches for clinical trials is not new [15]. In addition, with the emergence of more polished and validated algorithms, prediction accuracy is improved and the inclusion of a broad range of heterogeneous data is possible [15–17].

In this chapter, we are using the Netherlands Cancer Institute (NKI) breast cancer dataset to identify the important features responsible for breast cancer using machine learning algorithms and utilizing these features to predict mortality rates. This analysis intentions to assess the performance of various ML algorithms using a large dataset. Further sections of the chapter are as follows: Next section describes for a method for data acquisition and a small description of the methods applied and how the machine learning analysis is done. The results obtained from ML models are summarized subsequent Sect. 3 with 5-fold and 10-fold cross-validation results. Section 4 is all about the discussion of key features which are obtained through the analysis and contribute directly or indirectly to diagnosing breast cancer. This section also discusses key findings from related studies, and noteworthy findings from the current study are compared to the published articles. The authors discussed how the present analysis could be used in clinical research. The conclusion and practicality of the current study are highlighted in the last section.

2 Methodology and Data Acquisition

2.1 Data Comprehension

This study's NKI dataset was obtained from the data world Website (https://data.world/datasets/breast-cancer). This dataset comprises gene expression profiling and clinical information for breast cancer patients between the ages of 28 and 53. The original dataset has 1570 columns and 272 rows. Five columns: patients, id, barcode, event death, and time recurrence were removed. The dataset now comprises 272 occurrences with 1565 variables, one of which is a response variable (survived/not survived). Out of 1564 independent variables, 10 contain data on age, chemotherapy, hormonal treatment, amputation treatment, histological type, tumor diameter, number of nodes, cancer grade, lymphocytic infiltration, and gene expression profiling. Table 1 shows the treatment given to 272 patients.

Table 1 Treatment type received by all patients

No. of patients	Type of treatment			
	No treatment	Chemotherapy	Amputation treatment	Hormonal therapy
87	✓			
48		✓		
101			✓	
9				✓
8		✓		✓
11		✓	✓	✓

2.2 *Preparation of Data*

2.2.1 Pre-processing

Raw data were verified for missing values within the dataset before being subjected to any analysis, and none were identified. Label 0 (not survived) and label 1 (survived) were used to categorize mortality. The standard scaler technique was used to scale the columns using gene expression profiling.

2.2.2 The XGB Technique to Determine the Significant Features

In machine learning, feature selection is extremely important. High-dimensional data increase the distance between variables, making it more difficult to anticipate proper outcomes [18]. The goal of feature selection is to eliminate non-essential characteristics in order to create models that are quicker, more stable, and more accurate. Irrelevant and undesired characteristics might impair the algorithms' capacity to accurately distinguish between labels, increasing the modeling error. The removal of features decreases the noise in the data and improves the performance of the models [19]. The XGB method was used to identify features, and the top 10 rated features were chosen for further research based on their significance score. The dataset now comprises 272 samples with the top 10 characteristics (195-label 0, 77-label 1). Table 2 shows the descriptive analysis of data post feature selection. Because of its default use of the Gini index as an internal feature significance score and its reputation in machine learning contests, the XGB method was chosen. Individual trees are created by XGB utilizing several cores, and data are arranged to reduce lookup times [20].

Table 2 Descriptive analysis of data after feature selection

Selected variables	Number	Average	Standard deviation	Minimum	1st quartile	Median	3rd quartile	Maximum
NM_003287	272	−0.12639	0.334972	−1.26505	−0.28836	−0.09242	0.085273	0.64372
Contig55725_RC	272	−0.27040	0.41109	−1.05267	−0.5789	−0.3468	−0.01759	0.889981
Contig43639_RC	272	−0.06039	0.24237	−0.83006	−0.198	−0.09614	0.054724	0.789322
NM_001677	272	−0.09010	0.263588	−0.88008	−0.25794	−0.07209	0.087963	0.552245
NM_001448	272	−0.09030	0.297223	−0.87798	−0.30221	−0.07782	0.114648	0.805414
NM_005940	272	−0.13275	0.363215	−1.01606	−0.42842	−0.12393	0.141145	0.956928
NM_000826	272	−0.28510	0.37686	−1.03486	−0.48073	−0.38000	−0.24403	1.244715
Contig22685_RC	272	0.026887	0.286426	−2.0000	−0.04807	0.04634	0.142145	0.878141
NM_000903	272	−0.12346	0.297391	−0.80991	−0.31877	−0.11441	0.062673	0.722897
AL049265	272	−0.15527	0.365423	−1.11636	−0.43231	−0.12789	0.107949	0.747609

2.3 Machine Learning Analysis

The models are trained using a training dataset, and the testing dataset was utilized to test them. To solve underfitting and overfitting issues, 5-fold and 10-fold stratified cross-validation were used. This topic is classified as a classification problem since the major goal of this study is to estimate patients' survival from breast cancer.

In stratified V-fold cross-validation, the output variable is initially stratified, and the dataset is then pseudo-randomly divided into V-folds (5-folds and 10-folds in this study), with each fold containing about the same percentage of various strata. When building cross-validation folds in the case of classification problems, stratification is typically a suitable technique [21]. Repeatedly doing cross-validations, the problem of stratification becomes superfluous while picking a model but stratified cross-validation is recommended for evaluating the model.

Support vector machines (SVMs), XGB, stochastic gradient decision classifier (SGDC), adaptive boosting (AdaBoost), Gaussian Naive Bayes (GNB), and random forest (RFC) are five supervised machine learning methods utilized to complete the machine learning analysis. A support vector machine finds natural divisions in data that enable the biggest consistent margin from the selected function's route. In terms of adopting alternative kernels to modify the kind of discriminating function, a support vector machine offers more versatility. Kernels specify how the data should be separated by the support vector machine. A linear kernel (like logistic regression) seeks to separate data using a straight line, but a Gaussian kernel allows for more complicated, organic data patterns to be separated. A researcher must utilize one vs all technique, same as logistic regression [22], to apply a support vector machine for multiclass classification. Equation (1) gives the kernel function $K(x, y)$ with n-dimensional inputs x, y and the map function f from n-dimensional to m-dimensional space. $<x, y>$ denotes the dot product. Note that, in general $n < m$(22).

$$K(x, y) = <f(x), f(y)> \tag{1}$$

The Bayes theorem is used by GNB to calculate the occurrence of an event on the basis of the probability of an already existing event. In the absence of evidence, $P(A)$ is the prior probability of an event A and $P(B)$ is of event B. The mathematics underpinning the Bayes theorem is represented by Eq. (2), in which the probability of an event A when evidence B is known is represented by $P(A|B)$ [23] and is given by

$$P(A|B) = \frac{P(B|A)P(A)}{P(B)} \tag{2}$$

An ensemble of decision trees is known as RF. It employs the bagging technique. Bagging is a machine learning ensemble meta-algorithm that aims to increase the model's stability. It also lowers the variance. Ensembles are a divide-and-conquer strategy for increasing performance. Ensemble techniques work on the idea on a collection of weak learners might come together to generate a strong learner. Each classifier is a poor learner on its own, but the classifiers as a whole are powerful learners. As a result, ensemble techniques lower variance and enhance model performance. While developing trees, RF adds more randomization and seeks the greatest feature from a random collection of features [24]. The RF classifier is explained by Eq. (3), where θ_k is the identically distributed random vector. The most popular class is voted by the tree at the input x.

$$\{h(x, \theta_k), k = 1\} \tag{3}$$

The XGB method is a well-known method [25] and it controls the problem of overfitting by adding regularization in the objective function O (Eq. 4) at k time iterations $R(f_k)$, where C is a constant. Individually, $R(f_k)$ is defined in Eq. (5) in which H leaves are with complexity rate α, the output of the node j is w_j, and penalty parameter is η [25].

$$O = \sum_{i=1}^{n} L(y_i, F(x_i)) + \sum_{k=1}^{t} R(f_k) + C \tag{4}$$

$$R(f_k) = \alpha H + \frac{1}{2}\eta \sum_{j=1}^{H} w_j^2 \tag{5}$$

The objective (loss) function in XGB is obtained using the second-order Taylor series and minimizing the square error as defined in Eq. (6). Here, $q(x_i)$ is the function that assigns data points to the inputs. The sum of all loss values is used to calculate the final loss value as mentioned in Eq. (7), where $P_j = \sum_{i \in I_j} p_i$, $Q_j = \sum_{i \in I_j} q_i$ and I_j are denoted to all the samples in leaf node j [25].

$$O = \sum_{i=1}^{n} \left[p_i w_{q(x_i)} + \frac{1}{2}\left(q_i w_{q(x_i)}^2\right) \right] + \alpha H + \frac{1}{2}\eta \sum_{j=1}^{H} w_j^2 \tag{6}$$

$$O = \sum_{j=1}^{T} \left[p_j w_j + \frac{1}{2}(Q_j + \eta) w_j^2 \right] + \alpha H \tag{7}$$

The cost function in logistic regression (LR) is restricted between 0 and 1 [24]. The estimated probability P given by the sigmoid function σ is calculated by Eq. (8) and Eq. (9) with model parameter vector θ, hypothesis function *h*, and the instance feature vector x.

$$P = h_\theta(x) = \sigma(\theta^T.x) \tag{8}$$

$$\sigma(t) = \frac{1}{1 + e^{-(t)}} \tag{9}$$

AdaBoost is used to boost the performance of decision trees with the help of weak learners, also known as stumps, each with one node and two leaves [26]. AdaBoost combines various stumps to accomplish classification. Every stump learns from the previous stump's mistakes. Every sample within the dataset is assigned a sample weight. In the beginning, the sample weight will be the same (Eq. 10). Later, after creating the first stump, this weight will change to direct how the next stump will be created.

$$\text{Sample weight} = \frac{1}{\text{Total Number of Samples}} \tag{10}$$

2.4 *Evaluation of the Model*

The performance of each machine learning model was assessed using a set of evaluators. These assessors are commonly used to assess a model's ability to predict a result. Accuracy (Eq. 11), precision (Eq. 12), true positive rate (TPR) (Eq. 13), true negative rate (TNR) (Eq. 14), F1-score (Eq. 15), and receiver operating characteristics—area under the curve (ROC-AUC). TP, TN, FP, and FN stand for true positives, true negatives, false positives, and false negatives, respectively. For accurate results, TP must be predicted properly by the model. TN, on the other hand, is a result for which the model accurately predicts the negative class of outcomes. FP is when the model forecasts the wrong class as being positive. On the other hand, FN occurs when the model predicts the negative class erroneously. In this study, survived instances (label 1) were considered as positive, and not survived instances were considered as negative (label 0). To put it another way, precision shows how well the classifier is able to avoid labeling an instance as positive if the classifier accurately predicts that it will be negative (Eq. 12). When it comes to the TPR, the model's capacity to identify all occurrences of true positives and false negatives (Eq. 13) is known as the sensitivity or true positive rate [27, 28]. Whereas TNR is a measure of how well a model predicts all of the negative classifications that are present in a dataset (Eq. 14). If one knows the precision/recall/support and F1-score, then decision-maker will have a good idea of how accurate your model is (Eq. 15). As an alternative to the aforementioned model evaluators, all classifier's TPR versus FPR are plotted to derive ROC-AUC scores. Classifiers are used to plot ROC curves to figure out which variables are most important, and the curves closest to the top left corner are treated as the most accurate [29].

$$\text{Accuracy} = \frac{\text{count of accurate predictions}}{\text{Total count of predictions}} \tag{11}$$

$$\text{Precision} = \frac{\text{True Positive}}{\text{True Positive} + \text{False Positive}} \tag{12}$$

$$\text{TPR/recall} = \frac{\text{True Positive}}{\text{True Positive} + \text{False Negatives}} \tag{13}$$

$$\text{TNR} = \frac{\text{TN}}{\text{TN} + \text{FP}} \tag{14}$$

$$\text{F1} - \text{measure} = 2 * \frac{\text{Precision} * \text{Recall}}{\text{Precision} + \text{Recall}} \tag{15}$$

3 Results

In this section, we are demonstrating the machine learning capability to predict whether patients suffering from breast cancer with survival (label 1) or not (label 0). After training on the training dataset, five machine learning algorithms (SVM, RFC, AdaBoost, XGB, GNB, and LR) were evaluated based on their performance on the testing dataset. Training and testing of machine learning algorithms were done using 5-fold and 10-fold stratified cross-validation. Performance from each fold was considered, and the average was calculated. According to the results as illustrated in Fig. 1, in both of the cross-validations, RFC and XGB classifiers outperform other classifiers by achieving the highest accuracy in both cases. In the case of 5-fold stratified cross-validation, the RFC classifier achieved the highest accuracy of 78% followed by XGB (77.2%). However, during 10-fold stratified cross-validation, XGB performed well with the highest accuracy of 78.3% followed by RFC (76.4%).

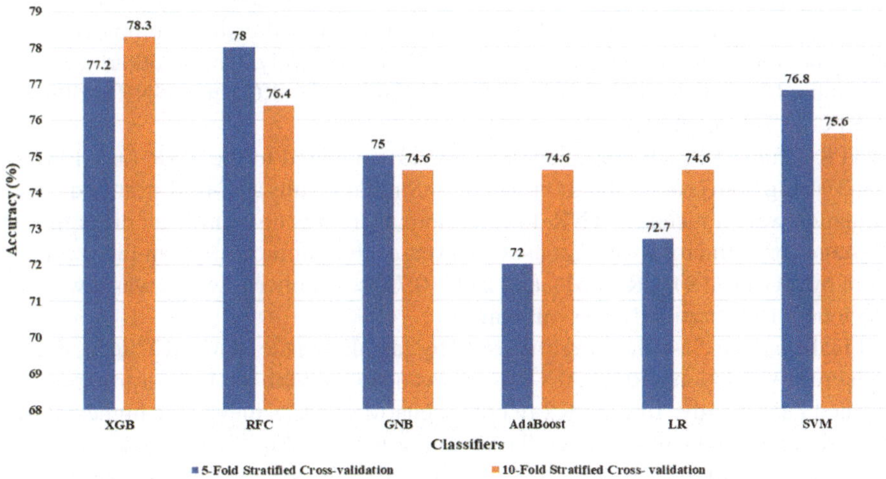

Fig. 1 Classifiers' performance based on accuracy

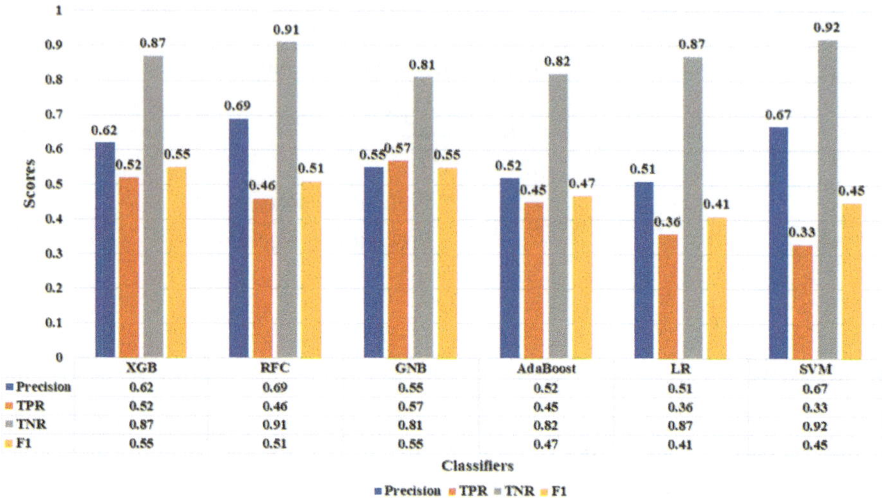

Fig. 2 Classifiers' performance based on the TNR, TPR, precision, and F1-score with 5-fold stratified cross-validation

In terms of TPR (ability to predict label 1), all the classifiers performed at extremely low with the highest and minimum score of 0.57 by GNB and 0.33 by SVM, respectively, (as shown in Fig. 2). On the other hand, the ability of the algorithms to predict label 0 was exceptionally well with the highest TNR of 0.92 by SVM. Moreover, the minimum TNR achieved by any classifiers was 0.81 by GNB (as shown in Fig. 2). As demonstrated in the results, the performance of all classifiers in predicting the not survived instances (label 0) was better as compared to label 1, it could be because of the imbalance in the outcome variables (label 0–195, label 1–77). In the case of precision, XGB and SVM performed well as compared to the other classifiers with a score of 0.69 and 0.67, respectively. On the other hand, the maximum F1-score achieved by any classifiers was 0.55 (XGB and GNB), followed by RFC (0.51) (as shown in Fig. 2).

TPR achieved by all classifiers was low as compared to the TNR (as shown in Fig. 3) using both cross-validation schemes. Similar results as 5-fold stratified cross-validation were noticed for TNR. Furthermore, there was no significant difference in F1-score for both cross-validations. However, a slight improvement in the precision score by XGB (0.69), LR (0.61), and RFC (0.75) was noticed, which was low in the previous 5-fold stratified cross-validation.

Finally, all the classifiers were assessed by calculating the ROC-AUC score during both cross-validations. ROC-AUC score was obtained with the help of true positive rate and false positive rate (FPR). In both scenarios, RFC achieved the highest ROC-AUC score as compared to other classifiers as shown in Fig. 4. In the case of 5-fold stratified cross-validation, after RFC, XGB, and SVM achieved the second highest score (0.77), as shown in Fig. 4a. During 10-fold stratified cross-validation, RFC still attained highest score, however, SVM (0.77) outperformed XGB (0.74).

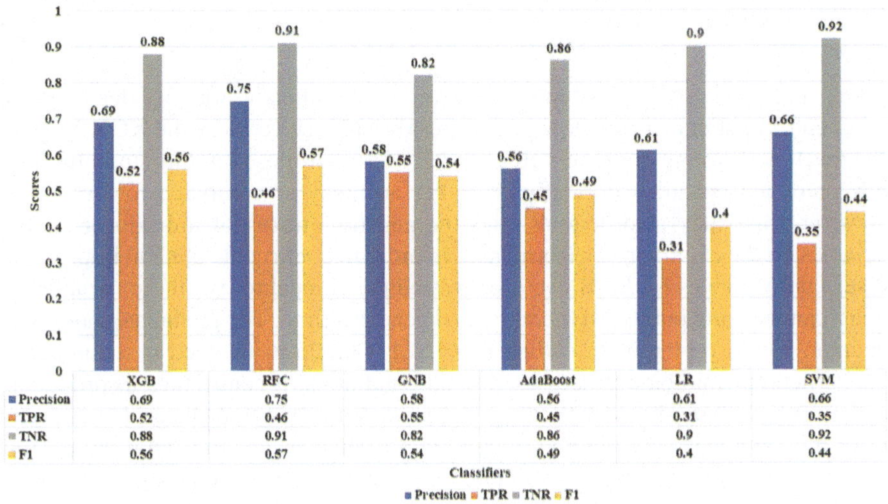

Fig. 3 Classifiers performance based on the TNR, TPR, precision, and F1-score with 10-fold stratified cross-validation

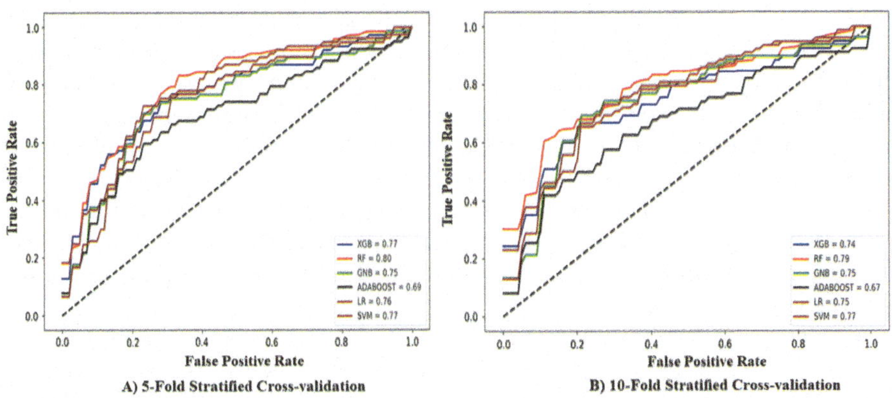

Fig. 4 ROC-AUC score by classifiers

After running all the machine learning experiments using two cross-validations and based on the average scores of different classifiers, we can propose RFC and XGB classifiers as better classifiers as compared to the others.

4 Discussion

In this study, we used several machine learning classifiers to identify death risk in breast cancer patients using the top ten input variables selected by the XGB method. The machine learning classifiers RFC and XGB are proposed in this study because they predicted instances correctly at higher accuracy as compared to the others. However, this study also demonstrates the negative impact of imbalanced output variables on the classifiers' performance. In order to confirm the clinical importance of selected variables by XGB, we investigated the clinical role of these variables in breast cancer using published literature and gene profiling. The glutamate ionotropic receptor AMPA type protein-coding gene NM 000,826 is involved in a number of typical neurophysiologic processes. In odd conditions, it contributes to producing breast cancer cells. The AL049265 gene encodes a signal transducer that is found in several cytokines. The binding of cytokines to their receptors is required for this protein's activity. In the breast cancer cell line MCF-7, it is linked to IL6ST—endoplasmic reticulum membrane-associated genes [30]. Another important feature is Contig55725_RC, an Oncorhynchus mykiss mRNA that is related to the Ras homologous family member. A (RhoA) gene which participates in the pathologic processes of cancer including breast cancer. Gene type NM_003287 is protein-coding. This gene is highly expressed in prostate cancer cells and could be used to predict the risk of prostate cancer. NM_005940 is RNA binding motif protein. This protein is thought to function as a splicing regulator during spermatogenesis. Another variable (NM_000903) is observed as significant by the XGB algorithm and is linked with a peptide (neuropeptide 7) which is broadly distributed in the central nervous system and found over-expressed in a variety of human cancers such as breast carcinomas. NM_001448 is fibromodulin and a proteoglycan that plays an important role in the start and advancement of a variety of cancers [31]. In this research, the authors considered all the important features suggested by the XG boost algorithm for further ML analysis.

Various research groups attempted to predict breast cancer survival using machine learning, similar to the current work. In a study conducted by [10], artificial intelligence techniques are applied to predict breast cancer survival using a dataset including information from 900 patients, and the results had in total 96%accuracy and a ROC-AUC curve with 93%. Kalafi and colleagues looked at the records of 4902 patients and came up with a model that predicted survival with an accuracy of 88.2%, with tumor size being the most important variable among all characteristics [32]. After analyzing a breast cancer dataset of 8066 records from the University Malay Medical Center, [6] showed the potential of machine learning algorithms to predict breast cancer survival with 82.7% accuracy (Kuala Lumpur, Malaysia). Furthermore, Boeri et al. (2020) created two models for breast cancer prognosis prediction, with overall accuracy ranging from 95.29 to 96.86% [27]. Class-imbalanced data, according to the literature, are more prone to bias toward the majority class (label 0 in our investigation) [28]. The current study, which used machine learning to predict label 0 with more accuracy than label 1, totally supports the previous conclusion (Fig. 2). In addition, feature selection is important in machine learning. High-dimensional data increase the distance between variables, making it more difficult to anticipate proper outcomes [31]. The goal of feature selection is to eliminate non-essential characteristics in order to create models that are quicker, more stable, and more accurate. Irrelevant and undesired variables might impair the algorithms' capacity to distinguish between classes, increasing the modeling error. In the presence of irrelevant variables, for example, the KNN algorithm does not work with stability since their existence exponentially increases sample complexity [33]. The reduction of variables minimizes the noise in the data and improves the performance of the models. The effects of feature selection on machine learning models were proven. As per the findings, feature selection, the SVM classifier produced higher classification results [34]. All of the research listed above had greater levels of accuracy than the current study, which might be due to the quantity of the data they utilized; in general, models trained on larger datasets produce more accurate findings.

5 Conclusion

Breast cancer is highly treatable in the early stages of the condition before it spreads to other parts of the body. Therefore, early prognosis is important to support the patients with the best possible care, medications, and therapies. A specific and precise prediction of mortality rates with a large data size can bring forth relevant information in terms of pervasiveness and public awareness. Different commercial organizations applied artificial intelligence (AI) and ML algorithms along with various independent research groups to manifest the ability of computational intelligence and to assist medical experts in the diagnosis and prediction of cancer risk. One of the major hitches of computational intelligence in clinical medicine is the constraint of complex algorithms in handling multivariable data that strongly affect the decision-making process. AI and ML algorithms can be utilized in a smart way that optimizes the impact in a much-supervised way, and future challenges are not limited to only one solution but require multitudinous ways of training, testing, and validating the models. It will provide more flexibility to the researcher and experts for the integration of these approaches into breast cancer prediction.

In this chapter, the authors used different machine learning algorithms for breast cancer patients' datasets and compared their performance based on a ROC-AUC score. ML classifiers are also examined on the basis of accuracy, precision, true positives, true negatives, ROC-AUC, and F1-score. The advancement in basic concepts and technological progress in these ML approaches helps the researchers to make decisions and spread public awareness at the very early stage of breast cancer.

References

1. Sharma, G. N., Dave, R., Sanadya, J., Sharma, P., & Sharma, K. K. (2010, April). Various types and management of breast cancer: An overview. *Journal of Advanced Pharmaceutical Technology & Research [Internet]* [cited 2021 Aug 31] *1*(2), 109. Available from: /pmc/articles/PMC3255438/
2. Boyle, P. (2012, August 1). Triple-negative breast cancer: Epidemiological considerations and recommendations. *Annals of Oncology* [Internet] [cited 2021 Aug 31], *23*(SUPPL. 6), vi7–12. Available from: http://www.annalsofoncology.org/article/S0923753419376355/fulltext
3. Vickers, A. J., & Cronin, A. M. (2010). Traditional statistical methods for evaluating prediction models are uninformative as to clinical value: Towards a decision analytic framework. *Seminars in Oncology., 37*(1), 31–38.
4. Feng, Y., Spezia, M., Huang, S., Yuan, C., Zeng, Z., Zhang, L., et al. (2018). Breast cancer development and progression: Risk factors, cancer stem cells, signaling pathways, genomics, and molecular pathogenesis [Internet]. In *Genes and diseases*. Chongqing yi ke da xue, di 2 lin chuang xue yuan Bing du xing gan yan yan jiu suo [cited 2021 Mar 7] (Vol. 5, pp. 77–106). Available from: /pmc/articles/PMC6147049/
5. Qazi, S., Raza, K., & Iqbal, N. (2021). Artificial intelligence in medicine (AIM): Machine learning in cancer diagnosis, prognosis and therapy. *Artificial Intelligence for Data-Driven Medical Diagnosis, 10*, 103–126.
6. Jabeen, A., Ahmad, N., & Raza, K. (2018). Machine learning-based state-of-the-art methods for the classification of RNA-seq data. *Lecture Notes in Computational Vision and Biomechanics [Internet], 26*, 133–172. Available from: https://link.springer.com/chapter/https://doi.org/10.1007/978-3-319-65981-7_6
7. Raza, K. (2019). Improving the prediction accuracy of heart disease with ensemble learning and majority voting rule. *U-Healthcare Monitoring Systems, 1*, 179–196.
8. Kim, J.-Y., Lee, Y. S., Yu, J., Park, Y., Lee, S. K., Lee, M., et al. (2021). Deep learning-based prediction model for breast cancer recurrence using adjuvant breast cancer cohort in tertiary cancer center registry. *Frontiers in Oncology, 4*, 655.
9. Ganggayah, M. D., Taib, N. A., Har, Y. C., Lio, P., & Dhillon, S. K. (2019, March 22). Predicting factors for survival of breast cancer patients using machine learning techniques. *BMC Medical Informatics and Decision Making [Internet]*. [cited 2021 Mar 7], *19*(1), 48. Available from: https://bmcmedinformdecismak.biomedcentral.com/articles/https://doi.org/10.1186/s12911-019-0801-4
10. Genuer, R., Poggi, J.-M., & Tuleau-Malot, C. VSURF: An R package for variable selection using random forests [cited 2021 Aug 31]. Available from: http://CRAN.R-project.org/package=VSURF
11. Kourou, K., Exarchos, T. P., Exarchos, K. P., Karamouzis, M. V., & Fotiadis, D. I. (2015, January 1). Machine learning applications in cancer prognosis and prediction. *Computational and Structural Biotechnology Journal, 13*, 8–17.
12. Ming, C., Viassolo, V., Probst-Hensch, N., Dinov, I. D., Chappuis, P. O., & Katapodi, M. C. (2020, June 22). Machine learning-based lifetime breast cancer risk reclassification compared with the BOADICEA model: Impact on screening recommendations. *British Journal of Cancer 2020* [Internet]. [cited 2021 Aug 31], *123*(5), 860–867. Available from: https://www.nature.com/articles/s41416-020-0937-0
13. Montazeri, M., Montazeri, M., Montazeri, M., & Beigzadeh, A. (2016). Machine learning models in breast cancer survival prediction. *Technology and Health Care., 24*(1), 31–42.
14. Sekeroglu, B., & Tuncal, K. (2021, January 28). Prediction of cancer incidence rates for the European continent using machine learning models [Internet] [cited 2021 Aug 31], *27*(1). Available from: https://journals.sagepub.com/doi/full/https://doi.org/10.1177/1460458220983878
15. O'Lorcain, P., Deady, S., & Comber, H. (2006, June 1). Mortality predictions for colon and anorectal cancer for Ireland, 2003–17. *Colorectal Disease* [Internet] [cited 2021 Aug

31], *8*(5), 393–401. Available from: https://onlinelibrary.wiley.com/doi/full/https://doi.org/10.1111/j.1463-1318.2006.00951.x

16. Ganggayah, M. D., Taib, N. A., Har, Y. C., Lio, P., & Dhillon, S. K. (2019, March 22). Predicting factors for survival of breast cancer patients using machine learning techniques. *BMC Medical Informatics and Decision Making, 19*(1).
17. Gupta, S., Tran, T., Luo, W., Phung, D., Kennedy, R. L., Broad, A., et al. (2014, March 1). Machine-learning prediction of cancer survival: A retrospective study using electronic administrative records and a cancer registry. *BMJ Open* [Internet]. [cited 2021 Aug 31], *4*(3), e004007. Available from: https://bmjopen.bmj.com/content/4/3/e004007
18. Chang, C.-M., Su, Y.-C., Lai, N.-S., Huang, K.-Y., Chien, S.-H., Chang, Y.-H., et al. (2012, August 30). The combined effect of individual and neighborhood socioeconomic status on cancer survival rates. *PLOS ONE* [Internet] [cited 2021 Aug 31], *7*(8), e44325. Available from: https://journals.plos.org/plosone/article?id=https://doi.org/10.1371/journal.pone.0044325
19. Woojae, K., Ku Sang, K., Jeong Eon, L., Don-Yong, N., Sung-Won, K., Yong Sik, J., et al. (2012, June). Development of novel breast cancer recurrence prediction model using support vector machine. *Journal of breast cancer* [Internet]. [cited 2021 Aug 31], *15*(2), 230–238. Available from: https://pubmed.ncbi.nlm.nih.gov/22807942/
20. Manilitch, E. A., Kiran, R. P., Tomas, R., Ian, L., Fazio, V. W., & Remzi, F. H. (2011). A novel data-driven prognostic model for staging of colorectal cancer. *Journal of the American College of Surgeons* [Internet] [cited 2021 Aug 31], *213*(5), 579–588.e2. Available from: https://pubmed.ncbi.nlm.nih.gov/21925905/
21. Keogh, E., & Mueen, A. (2017). Curse of dimensionality. In: *Encyclopedia of machine learning and data mining* [Internet]. Springer US; [cited 2021 Jan 13], pp. 314, 315. Available from: https://link.springer.com/referenceworkentry/https://doi.org/10.1007/978-1-4899-7687-1_192
22. Albattah W, Khan RU, Khan K (2020, July 17). Attributes reduction in big data. *Applied Sciences* [Internet] [cited 2021 Jan 13], *10*(14), 4901. Available from: https://www.mdpi.com/2076-3417/10/14/4901
23. Liu, L., Yu, Y., Fei, Z., Li, M., Wu, F.-X., Li, H.-D., et al. (2018, November 22). An interpretable boosting model to predict side effects of analgesics for osteoarthritis. *BMC Systems Biology* [Internet]. [cited 2021 Jul 14], *12*(6), 29–38. Available from: https://bmcsystbiol.biomedcentral.com/articles/https://doi.org/10.1186/s12918-018-0624-4
24. Krstajic, D., Buturovic, L. J., Leahy, D. E., & Thomas, S. (2014, March 29). Cross-validation pitfalls when selecting and assessing regression and classification models. *Journal of Cheminformatics 2014* [Internet] [cited 2021 Aug 31], *6*(1), 1–15. Available from: https://jcheminf.biomedcentral.com/articles/https://doi.org/10.1186/1758-2946-6-10
25. Battineni, G., Chintalapudi, N., & Amenta, F. (2019, January 1). Machine learning in medicine: Performance calculation of dementia prediction by support vector machines (SVM). *Informatics in Medicine Unlocked, 16*, 100200.
26. Fahidy, T. Z. (2011). Some applications of Bayes' rule in probability theory to electrocatalytic reaction engineering. *International Journal of Electrochemistry., 2011*, 1–5.
27. Haury, A.-C., Gestraud, P., & Vert, J.-P. (2011, December 21). The influence of feature selection methods on accuracy, stability and interpretability of molecular signatures. In M.-T. Teh (Ed.) *PLoS ONE* [Internet] [cited 2021 Feb 11], *6*(12), e28210. Available from: https://dx.plos.org/https://doi.org/10.1371/journal.pone.0028210
28. Lai, C., Reinders, M. J. T., van't Veer, L. J., Wessels, L. F. A. (2006, May 2). A comparison of univariate and multivariate gene selection techniques for classification of cancer datasets. *BMC Bioinformatics* [Internet] [cited 2021 Feb 11], *7*(1):235. Available from: http://bmcbioinformatics.biomedcentral.com/articles/https://doi.org/10.1186/1471-2105-7-235
29. Tyagi, A., Tiwari, P., Bhardwaj, P., & Chawla, H. (2021, October 6). Prognosis of sexual dimorphism with unfused hyoid bone: Artificial intelligence informed decision making with discriminant analysis. *Science & Justice* [Internet] [cited 2021 Oct 18]. Available from: https://linkinghub.elsevier.com/retrieve/pii/S1355030621001283

30. Futreal, P. A., Coin, L., Marshall, M., Down, T., Hubbard, T., Wooster, R., et al. (2004). A census of human cancer genes. *Nature Reviews Cancer* [Internet] [cited 2021 Sep 2], *4*(3), 177–183. Available from: https://www.nature.com/articles/nrc1299
31. Nicolau, M., Levine, A. J., & Carlsson, G. (2011, April 26). Topology based data analysis identifies a subgroup of breast cancers with a unique mutational profile and excellent survival. In *Proceedings of the national academy of sciences* [Internet] [cited 2021 Sep 2], *108*(17), 7265–7270. Available from: https://www.pnas.org/content/108/17/7265
32. Wang, R. (2012). AdaBoost for feature selection, classification and its relation with SVM. *A Review. Physics Procedia, 1*(25), 800–807.
33. Kalafi, E. Y., Nor, M., Taib, N. A., Ganggayah, M. D., Town, C., Dhillon, S. K., et al. (2019). Original article machine learning and deep learning approaches in breast cancer survival prediction using clinical data (breast cancer/survival prediction/deep learning/machine learning) (Vol. 65), Folia Biologica (Praha).
34. Boeri, C., Chiappa, C., Galli, F., de Berardinis, V., Bardelli, L., Carcano, G., et al. (2020, May 10). Machine learning techniques in breast cancer prognosis prediction: A primary evaluation. *Cancer Medicine* [Internet] [cited 2021 Mar 7], *9*(9), 3234–3243. Available from: https://onlinelibrary.wiley.com/doi/abs/https://doi.org/10.1002/cam4.2811

Deep Learning Models for Classification of Brain Tumor with Magnetic Resonance Imaging Images Dataset

L. J. Muhammad, Ibrahim Badi, Ahmed Abba Haruna, I. A. Mohammed, and O. S. Dada

Abstract Brain tumor is known among the most aggressive diseases among adults and children around the world. It is estimated that every year, more than 11,700 people around the world are being diagnosed with the disease. Moreover, brain tumor has also been among the most common cancers affecting people in Nigeria. In fact, in the year 2018, according to WHO, Nigeria has 2.1% incidence cases and a 2.7% mortality rate, respectively. Consequently, many ways and techniques are being used for classifying and detecting brain tumors; however, the most common non-invasive technique is called MRI. Nowadays, many MRI images dataset of brain tumors is being generated and examined by radiologists for the classification of the brain tumor as either benign or malignant. Nevertheless, the manual examination and classification of the MRI images dataset are prone to errors due to complexities and uncertainty that are often associated with the examination and classification, respectively. Therefore, a deep learning technique, which is an applied artificial technique, is used to develop a system or model that trains itself automatically or learns sensible features from the dataset. Hence, this technique has been harnessed in this work to develop the classification models of the brain tumors with MRI images dataset. VGG16 and ResNet50 deep learning algorithms were used in developing the models, and each model was evaluated based on accuracy, sensitivity, specificity, and area under the ROC curve evaluations metrics. The VGG16 classification model has comparatively outperformed the ResNet50 model for being able to classify the brain tumor as either benign or malignant with 96% accuracy and for the ability to correctly classify

L. J. Muhammad (✉) · O. S. Dada
Computer Science Department, Federal University of Kashere, Gombe, Nigeria
e-mail: lawan.jibril@fukashere.edu.ng

I. Badi
Libyan Academy, Misrata, Libya
e-mail: i.badi@lam.edu.ly

A. A. Haruna
College of Computer Science & Engineering, University of Hafr Al Batin, Al Jamiah, Hafar Al Batin 39524, Saudi Arabia

I. A. Mohammed
Department of Computer Science, Yobe State University, Damaturu, Yobe, Nigeria

K. Raza (ed.), *Computational Intelligence in Oncology*, Studies in Computational Intelligence 1016, https://doi.org/10.1007/978-981-16-9221-5_9

malignant cases with 94.30% accuracy. However, for the ability to correctly classify benign cases of brain tumors, ResNet50 has comparatively outperformed the VGG16 classification model with 93.10% accuracy. Yet, in terms of how much the model differentiates between malignant cases against benign cases, the model developed with the ResNet50 deep learning algorithm comparatively outperformed the VGG16 classification model with 91.20% accuracy. Therefore, the VGG16 classification model which has the highest sensitivity of 94.30% could be used for the classification of the brain tumor and could also be used as an adjuvant tool in radiology departments in various hospitals in Nigeria.

Keywords Brain tumor · MRI dataset · Deep learning · VGG16 · ResNet50 · Disease

1 Introduction

Nowadays, various diseases are affecting human beings across the globe. Unfortunately, brain tumor happens to be one of them [1, 2]. The brain tumor is an uncontrolled and unnatural growth of brain cells in the human skull [3]. The skull of human beings is very rigid with a limited volume of the body and any growth in the skull affects its smooth functions and even other parts of the human brain involved [4, 5]. Moreover, brain tumor is very complicated in nature and has severe morbidity according to World Health Organization (WHO), even though it accounts for less than 2% of all human cancers [6]. In Nigeria, brain tumor is known among the most common cancers. According to WHO, Nigeria has 2.1% incidence cases and a 2.7% mortality rate, respectively, of the brain tumor in the year 2018 [7].

A brain tumor can be divided into primary and secondary brain tumors [3]. The primary brain tumor constitutes about 70% of all brain tumor cases, while the secondary brain tumor constitutes 30%, which are residuals. The classification of the brain tumor is determined based on, where the tumor originated, the tumor that is being originated from the brain is called a primary brain tumor, whereas the tumor that is being originated from other parts of the human body and then transferred to the brain is called a secondary brain tumor [8, 9]. Hence, brain tumor is being classified as benign or malignant, where malignant brain tumor is harmful while benign one is not harmful [3, 10], but most of the secondary tumors are malignant brain tumors [11].

Consequently, there are many ways and techniques that are being used to classify and detect brain tumors, but the most common non-invasive technique is called magnetic resonance imaging (MRI) [12]. The scan and create imagery details of the human organs and tissues using magnetic fields and radio waves generated with a computerized system [13, 14]. What makes the technique popular, its ability to use non-ionizing radiation techniques during the scanning process of the human organs, it is the ability to produce a high-resolution soft tissue and get images with many contrast advanced agents or imaging parameters [5]. Hence, effective handling of brain tumors is highly needed and critical which depends on its timely and accurate detection and classification [2]. The best conventional method for classification of the brain tumor is through MRI; and nowadays, huge MRI images dataset of brain tumors is being generated and examined by radiologists in order to classify brain tumors as either benign or malignant. However, the manual examination of the brain tumor MRI images is prone to error dues to complexities and uncertainty that are often associated with examinations [15]. Therefore, a deep learning technique which is an applied artificial technique that enables a system or model to train itself automatically or learn sensible features from data has been used in this research work. This technique is used for the development of classification models of brain tumors with an MRI dataset. Specifically, VGG16 and ResNet50 deep learning algorithms were used to develop the classification models of brain tumors with an MRI images dataset.

2 Deep Learning

Deep learning (DL) is an AI function that operates like the human brain with respect to data processing and formulating patterns to be used in decision-making [16–18]. DL is also a field in machine learning with networks that are able to learn from unstructured or unlabeled data without supervision [19, 20]. DL algorithms are designed to make the same conclusions as humans by consistently evaluating data using a specific logical structure [21, 22]. To attain the same, DL makes use of a multi-layered algorithm structure known as neural networks [23, 24]. The neural network's structure is similar to the human brain's structure; just as the human brain is structured to identify patterns and classify a range of information; neural networks are also taught to execute similar tasks on a range of data [25]. They are structured to receive new information and compare such information against known objects. Neural networks enable individuals to perform different tasks like regression, classification, and clustering [26, 27]. With neural networks, it is possible to sort or group unlabeled data in line with the similarities between data samples. Furthermore, in line with [28], DL approaches have, to a great extent, outperformed modern approaches in several fields like object, speech, and character recognition, computer vision, natural language processing, and signature verification [29]. Literature has also documented various types of DL architectures, for example, recurrent neural network (RNN), deep belief network (DBN), convolutional neural network (CNN), deep neural network (DNN), and sparse auto-encoder (SAE) [23, 30, 31]. The ResNet50 and VGG16 models are classified as CNN DL architectures. In this work, ResNet50 and VGG16 deep learning algorithms were used to develop the classification models of brain tumors with MRI images dataset.

2.1 ResNet50

Residual network (ResNet) became popular post-2012, turning out to be the most interesting thing that the DL world witnessed [32–34]. ResNet's framework made it possible to train networks with thousands of layers without compromising performance. The ResNet model was initially used in image recognition. However, over time, the model has been applied in non-computer vision tasks to enhance accuracy [25, 35]. Specifically, ResNet50 is a ResNet variant with 48 convolution layers alongside 1 average pool layer, 1 Maxpool and it has 3.8×10^9 floating points operations [36]. In line with [36] this, the ResNet variant is broadly used. ResNet50 makes it possible to load a pre-trained network version that is trained on over 1 million images from the ImageNet database [37, 38]. The pre-trained network is capable of classifying images into 1000 object groups, for instance, pencil, mouse, keyboard, and several animals. Consequently, ResNet50 learns feature representation for a wide range of images and accepts sizes 224 by 224 images [25].

ResNet model suggested two types of mapping: residual mapping and identity mapping. As represented in Fig. 1, the "curved curve" is the identity mapping, whereas the part other than the "curved curve" is the residual mapping [36, 39]. Therefore, the final output may be represented as $y = F(x) + x$. Identity mapping is represented by x. On the other hand, residual mapping is the difference, which is expressed as y-x, so the residual is $F(x)$.

ResNet50 has 48 convolutional layers, 1 Maxpool, and average pool layers, respectively. As outlined by [36], ResNet50 performs a convolution operation on the input, and then on 4 residual blocks, before finally performing a full connection operation to accomplish the classification task at hand [55]. ResNet50's network structure is represented in Fig. 2, which consists of 50 convolution operations.

As mentioned by [36], a fully connected layer comes up at CNN's end as a summary of the previous layers' features. Some of the documented uses of the ResNet50 variant include its application on computer vision tasks like detecting objects, localizing objects, and classifying images [40, 41]. This variant may also be

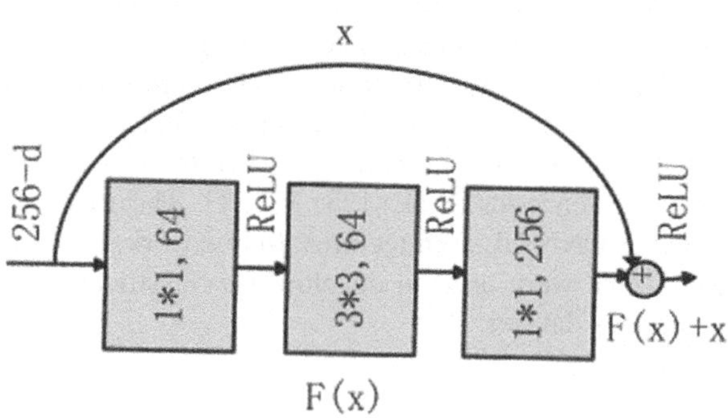

Fig. 1 Residual block [36]

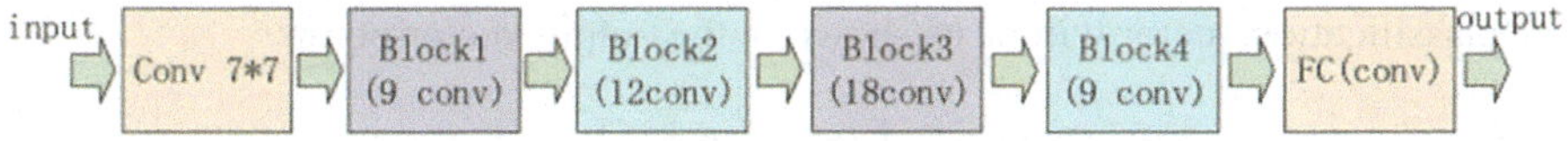

Fig. 2 ResNet50 [36]

used in non-computer vision tasks to realize the benefit of depth and cut computational expenses [36, 42]. In this work, ResNet50 is one of the deep learning algorithms used to develop the classification models of brain tumors with an MRI images dataset.

2.2 *VGG16*

VGG is an acronym for visual geometry group, which is a group of Oxford researchers who invented this architecture. The VGG architecture is made up of blocks, whereby every block has 2D convolution and Max pooling layers [15, 43]. VGGNet comes in two variants: VGG19 and VGG16, where 19 and 16 represent the number of layers in each of them, respectively. VGG16 was proposed in 2014 by Andrew and Karen, both are members of VGG [15]. Their model won first and second place in the ImageNet large scale visual recognition challenge (ILSVRC) of 2014. The ILSVRC is an annual computer vision competition in which teams compete on two fronts: landscape design (finding objects with an image from 200 classes, and image classification (image classification, in which each image is labeled in 1 of 1000 categories) [15].

The ImageNet dataset consists of images with a specific size of 224 by 224 and RGB channels [44]. Thus, the input is given as (224, 224). VGG16 accepts images as an input and gives the output as a vector with 100 values, shown as the following vector.

$$\hat{y} = \begin{bmatrix} \widehat{y_0} \\ \widehat{y_1} \\ \widehat{y_2} \\ \widehat{y_3} \\ . \\ . \\ . \\ \widehat{y_{999}} \end{bmatrix} \quad (1)$$

The vector is a representation of the probability of the classified respective classes. Let for example, a model predicts that the image is a member of class 0 with 0.1 as its probability, class 1 with 0.05 as its probability, class 2 with 0.05 as its probability, class 3 with 0.03 as its probability, class 780 with 0.72 as its probability, class 999 with 0.05 as its probability, and all the other classes with 0.0 as their probabilities.

The classification vector will be as shown in the output vector below.

$$\hat{y} = \begin{bmatrix} \widehat{y_0} = 0.1 \\ 0.05 \\ 0.05 \\ 0.03 \\ . \\ . \\ . \\ \widehat{y_{780}} = 0.72 \\ . \\ . \\ \widehat{y_{999}} = 0.05 \end{bmatrix} \tag{2}$$

To ensure that the probabilities all add to 1, the VGG16 model uses the softmax function, which is as shown in the equation below.

$$P\left(y = j|\theta^{(i)}\right) = \frac{e^{\theta^{(i)}}}{\sum_{j=0}^{k} e^{\theta_k^{(i)}}} \tag{3}$$

$$\text{Where } \theta = w_0 x_0 + w_1 x_1 + \ldots w_k x_k = \sum_{i=0}^{k} w_i x_i = W^T X$$

The next step in the model involves taking the five most probable candidates into the vector, as represented in the Eq. 4.

$$C = \begin{bmatrix} 780 \\ 0 \\ 1 \\ 2 \\ 999 \end{bmatrix} \tag{4}$$

Thus, the ground vector will be defined as shown in the Eq. 5:

$$G = \begin{bmatrix} G_0 \\ G_1 \\ G_2 \end{bmatrix} = \begin{bmatrix} 780 \\ 2 \\ 999 \end{bmatrix} \tag{5}$$

Using the error function defined in Eq. (6), the loss function of the example, using the VGG16 model, is shown in Eq. (7). Every category in the ground truth falls in the predicted top 5 matrices; thus, the loss is given as 0.

$$E = \frac{1}{n}\sum\nolimits_k \min_i d(c_i, G_K) \tag{6}$$

$$\text{Where } d = 0 \; if \; c_i = G_k \text{ else } d = 1$$

$$E = \frac{1}{3}(\min_i d(c_i, G_1) + \min_i d(c_i, G_2) + \min_i d(c_i, G_3)),$$

$$\text{So } E = \frac{1}{3}(0 + 0 + 0) = 0 \tag{7}$$

Despite the minimal loss function, literature has identified some challenges related to the VGG16 model. For the training with the initial VGG to be trained on Nvidia GPU for like two to three weeks, the VGG15 is quite very slow[15, 45]. Also, the size of VGG16 trained ImageNet is about 528 megabytes. This means it consumes a lot of bandwidth and disk space, which makes it inefficient [46]. In other words, the weights of the network architecture are themselves very large [15]. Owing to its depth and the number of nodes that are fully connected, VGG16 has to consume around half a gigabyte of space. As a result, it is tiresome to deploy. Despite such challenges, VGG16 is applied in several DL image classification tasks. Notwithstanding, smaller network architectures are commonly more desirable, for example, SqueezeNet, GoogleNet, among others [47, 48]. Overall, it is a great building block for learning purposes due to its ease of implementation. In this work, VGG16 is one of the deep learning algorithms used to develop the classification models of brain tumors with MRI images dataset.

3 Related Work

Many works have been done and these works have shown the significant use of deep learning algorithms for the classification, diagnosis, and prediction of brain tumors. Hence, this research work used a free search engine for the MEDLINE database for its review. The review and gap of this research were identified based on the meta-analysis of the published papers on the deep learning classification models of the brain tumor with MRI dataset and PubMed. Sixty-two published papers were found on the search engine but only ten papers were found to be relevant and used in this work.

Deep learning models based on concatenation techniques for brain tumor diagnosis were proposed in the work of [4]. The models got 99.34% and 99.51% accuracy, respectively, for Inception-v3 and DensNet201 deep learning algorithm-based models. On the other hand [5], a multi-classification deep learning model of brain tumor was developed and the model achieved significant accuracy of 96.13%. Deep learning and generic algorithm-based classification model for brain tumors with MRI were developed in another work [49] and the model achieved 94.2% accuracy.

Convolutional deep learning neural network classification model with deeper architecture design and small kernels for brain tumor was proposed in the study of [15] and model achieved 97.5% accuracy. Artificial intelligence paradigm multi-classification models for the brain tumor with MRI dataset were developed in the work [10], and the performance of the models showed a significant improvement of 96% accuracy. Deep learning was used to develop an automated model for the classification of brain tumor with MRI dataset that was used in another work [13], and the best model has shown an accuracy of 98.2%. Deep learning was used to develop a Web-based brain tumor classification model with MRI images was developed with convolutional neural network deep learning techniques in the study of [50], and the result of the study showed that the model was proved to be able to detect and diagnose the type of brain tumor accurately with minimal error. A differential model based on deep learning models for the classification of brain tumors was designed in yet another study [9]. Consequently, the experimental result of the study showed that the model significantly achieved 99.25% accuracy. An efficient deep learning model for the classification of brain tumors with MRI image dataset was developed in the work of [51], and a convolutional neural network deep learning algorithm was used for the development of the model. Hence, the issue of brain tumor subtype classification with MRI dataset was addressed in the study of [8], and the result of the study showed that the developed model has shown a good accuracy of 88.82%.

Despite the fact that many works have been done using deep learning algorithms for the development of classification, diagnosis, and prediction of brain tumor models. But most of the proposed models were neither nor evaluated based on accuracy, sensitivity, specificity, and area under the ROC curve (AUC) evaluations metrics. Table 1 shows the summary of the weaknesses and strengths of all the published papers reviewed in this work.

In this work, VGG16 and ResNet50 deep learning algorithms would be used to develop the classification models of brain tumors with MRI images dataset. The developed algorithms would be evaluated based on accuracy, sensitivity, and specificity, and area under the ROC curve (AUC) evaluations metrics.

4 Methods and Material

This section provides dataset description and dataset argumentation and development of VGG16 and ResNet50 models for classification of brain tumor with brain magnetic resonance imaging dataset. Figure 3 shows the methodology adopted for the work.

4.1 Dataset

Public MRI images for brain tumor used in this study which is available on https://www.kaggle.com/navoneel/brain-mri-images-for-brain-tumor-detection [52]. The

Table 1 Summary of the weaknesses and strengths of the published papers reviewed

References	Weakness	Strength
[4]	The performance of the model based on sensitivity, specificity, and AUC was not determined	The performance of the model based on accuracy was determined
[5]	The performance of the model based on sensitivity, specificity, and AUC was not determined	The performance of the model based on accuracy was determined
[49]	The performance of the model based on sensitivity, specificity, and AUC was not determined	The performance of the model based on accuracy was determined
[15]	The performance of the model based on sensitivity, specificity, and AUC was not determined	The performance of the model based on accuracy was determined
[10]	The performance of the model based on sensitivity, specificity, and AUC was not determined	The performance of the model based on accuracy was determined
[13]	The performance of the model based on sensitivity, specificity, and AUC was not determined	The performance of the model based on accuracy was determined
[50]	The accuracy, specificity, sensitivity, and AUC of the models were not determined	The classification error of the model was determined
[9]	The performance of the model based on sensitivity, specificity, and AUC was not determined	The performance of the model based on accuracy was determined
[51]	The performance of the model based on accuracy, sensitivity, specificity, and AUC was not determined	The classification error of the model was determined
[8]	The performance of the model based on sensitivity, specificity, and AUC was not determined	The performance of the model based on accuracy was determined

dataset has 3762 instances, with two classes labeled "1" and labeled "0", respectively. Class 1 has 1683 instances, while class 0 has 2079 instances. Figure 4 shows the frequency of each class of the dataset, respectively, and Fig. 5 shows the sample of the dataset.

4.2 Dataset Argumentation

The accuracy of deep learning models is heavily depending on the quality of the training sample of the imagery dataset [53, 54]. Therefore, to achieve a significant accuracy in the course of the classification of the brain tumor in this study, a contrast limited adaptive histogram equalization (CLACHE) technique was employed to

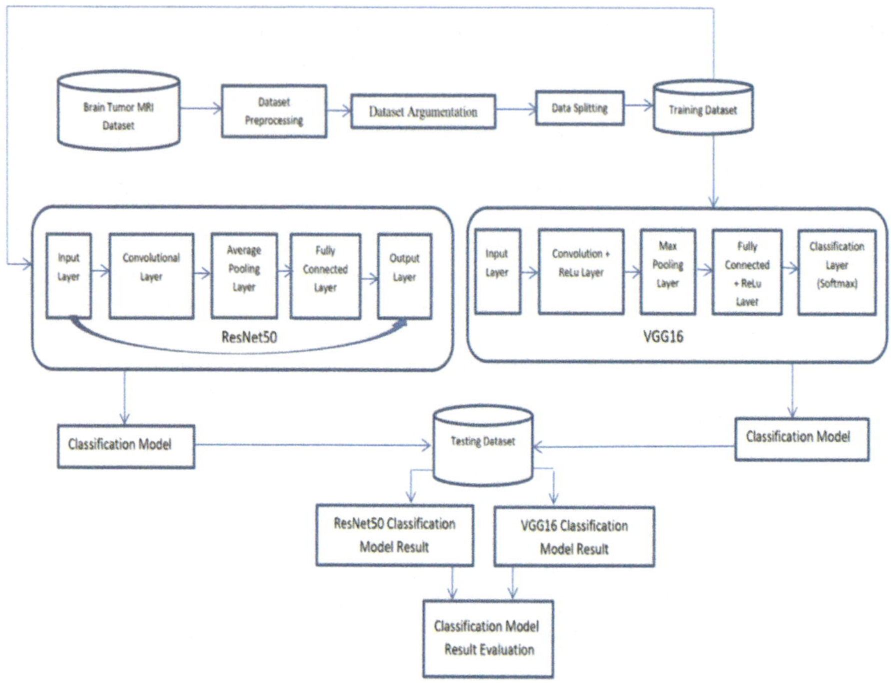

Fig. 3 Methods and material

Fig. 4 Frequency of the classes of the dataset

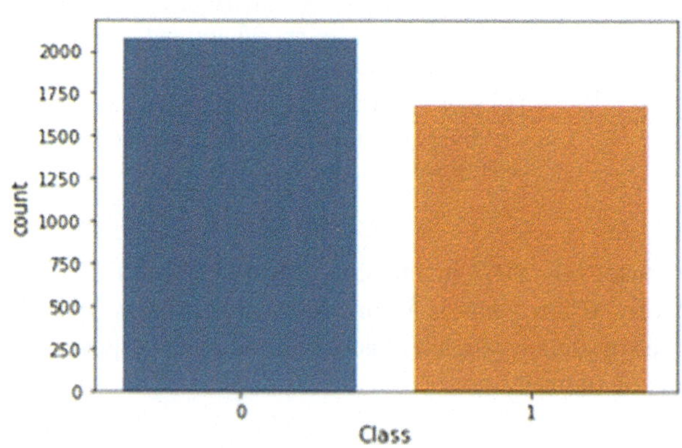

reduce the noise and improve the visibility level of the foggy areas of the images, respectively. Figure 6 shows the sample of the image that has been augmented with CLACHE technique.

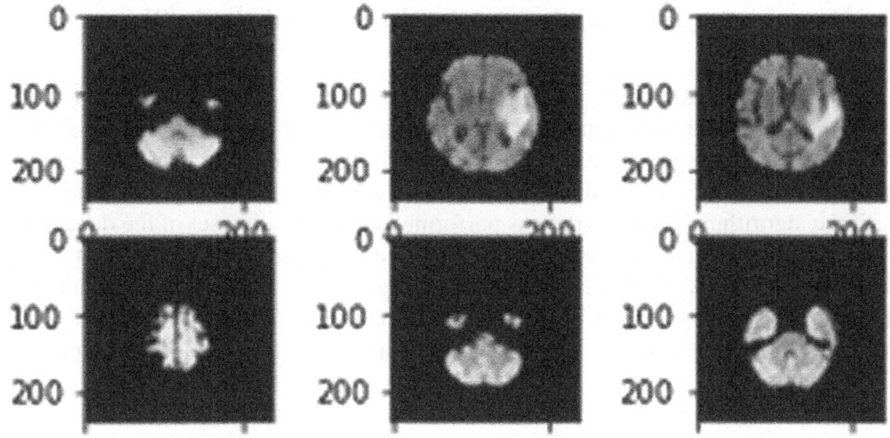

Fig. 5 Sample of the dataset

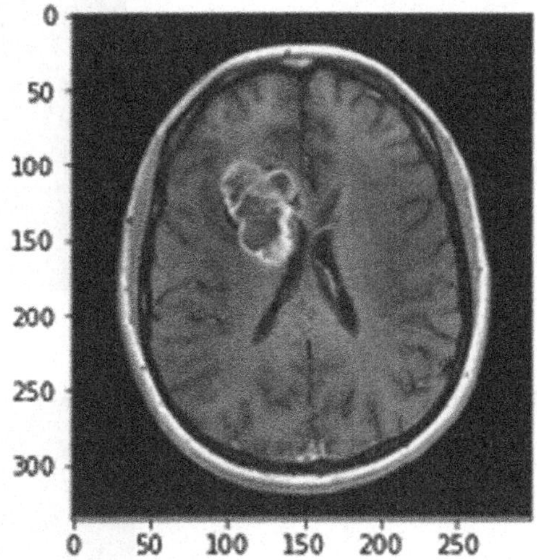

Fig. 6 Sample of the image augmented with CLACHE technique

4.3 *Environmental Setup*

An open-source programming language which is called Python was used for the development of the deep learning models for classification of brain tumor with brain magnetic resonance imaging images dataset using Corei7, GTX1060 6 GB GPU computer system. Python Notebook was used as the development environment and all the necessary libraries were installed such as Keras, Tensor, NumPy, Pandas, Matplotlib, Seaborn, TensorFlow among others.

5 Deep Learning Models for Classification of Brain Tumor

The VGG16 and ResNet50 deep learning algorithms were used to develop the models with MRI images dataset, respectively. The dataset was split into 80% training set and 20% testing set, respectively. Therefore, each deep learning algorithm was trained on an 80% training set, and the remaining 20% was used for testing the model built with the algorithm. The training was performed on the training set of the dataset for 10 epochs and for each epoch, the models were validated using the test set of the dataset. The VGG16 and ResNet50 deep learning-based models were able to classify the brain tumor classified as either benign or malignant. Figure 7 and Fig. 8 show the sample of images of the classified brain tumor as either malignant or benign, respectively.

Fig. 7 Malignant

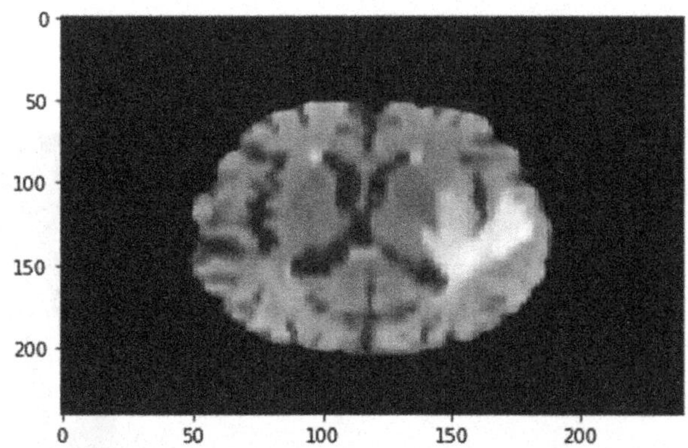

Fig. 8 Benign

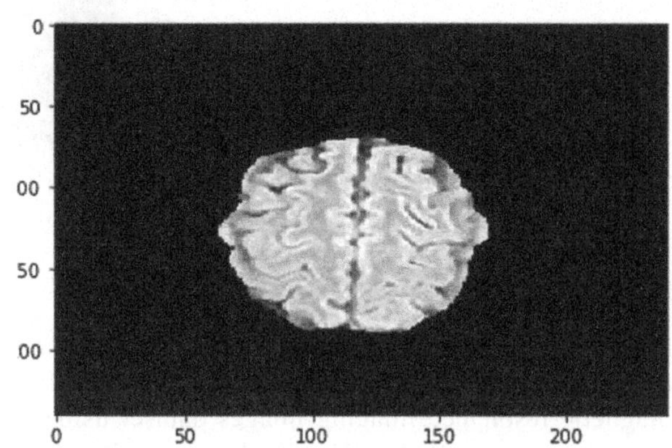

6 Performance Evaluation of Deep Learning Models for Classification of Brain Tumor

The VGG16 and ResNet50 models were evaluated based on the following performance evaluation metrics for deep learning algorithms:

i. Accuracy is the learning evaluation metric that is used to determine or measure the percentage of the instances of the brain tumor MRI images of the dataset that were correctly classified with the models. Accuracy is defined using the Eq. 8:

$$\text{Accuracy} = \frac{\text{tp} + \text{tn}}{\text{tp} + \text{tn} + \text{fn} + \text{fp}} \tag{8}$$

ii. Sensitivity is the learning evaluation metric that is used to determine or measure the percentage of the classified malign cases that were correctly classified with the models. The sensitivity is defined using the Eq. 9:

$$\text{Sensitivity} = \frac{\text{tp}}{\text{tp} + \text{fn}} \tag{9}$$

iii. Specificity is the learning evaluation metric that is used to determine or measure the percentage of the classified benign cases that were correctly classified with the models. The specificity is defined using the Eq. 10:

$$\text{Specificity} = \frac{\text{tp}}{\text{tn} + \text{fp}} \tag{10}$$

iv. The area under the curve (AUC) is the learning evaluation metric that is used to determine the percentage or measure the score of how much the model differentiates between malign or benign classified cases. The AUC is defined using the Eq. 11:

$$\text{AUC} = \frac{\text{fp}}{\text{tn} + \text{fp}} \tag{11}$$

Note: tp stands for true positive, tn stands for true negative, fp stands for false positive, and fn stands for false negative.

Each of the brain tumor classification models in this study was evaluated based on accuracy, sensitivity, and specificity and AUC evaluations metrics as shown in Table 2 and Fig. 9, respectively. VGG16 classification model has comparatively outperformed the ResNet50 model for being able to classify brain tumors as either benign or malign with 96% accuracy and the ability to correctly classify malignant cases with also 94.30% accuracy. However, for the ability to correctly classify benign cases of brain tumors, ResNet50 has comparatively outperformed

Table 2 Performance evaluation results of the models

S/N	Model	Accuracy (%)	Sensitivity (%)	Specificity (%)	AUC (%)
1	VGG16	96.00	94.30	91.20	89.50
2	ResNet50	94.00	92.40	93.10	91.20

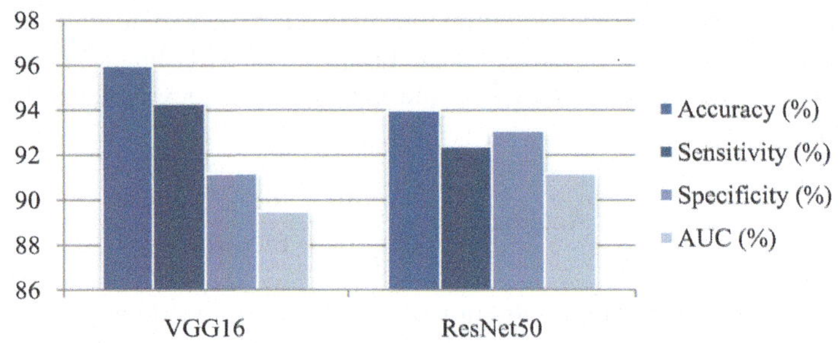

Fig. 9 Chart presentation of the performance evaluation results of the models

the VGG16 classification model with 93.10% accuracy. Moreover, in terms of how much the model differentiates between brain malign cases against benign cases, the model developed with ResNet50 deep learning network comparatively outperformed the VGG16 classification model with 91.20% accuracy. Therefore, the VGG16 classification model which has the highest sensitivity of 94.30% could be used for the classification of the brain tumor and also used as an adjuvant tool in the radiology department in Nigeria's hospitals.

7 Future Prospects and Current Limitations

A brain tumor is very complicated in nature and has severe morbidity. Therefore, effective handling of brain tumors is highly needed and critical, which really depends on its timely and accurate detection and classification. Hence, deep learning techniques have been playing a very important role in the classification of brain tumors with MRI datasets. Even though, brain tumor is very complicated in nature and has severe morbidity. But deep learning techniques and algorithms are being able to learn MRI datasets of the disease without supervision in order to classify it as either malignant or benign brain tumor, respectively. However, the development and implementation of deep learning techniques and algorithms for the classification of brain tumors have many unique challenges due to the inadequate available large MRI training dataset. Therefore, the inadequate available large MRI training dataset is a challenging obstacle for the development and implementation of deep learning techniques and algorithms for the classification of brain tumors. Consequently, this work has so far proved that there is a need to have an adequate and large MRI training dataset for the development and implementation of deep learning techniques and algorithms for the classification of brain tumors. In future work, a large MRI training dataset would be sourced and used to develop and implement new novel deep learning techniques and algorithms for the classification of brain tumors.

8 Conclusion

Brain tumor, which is an uncontrolled and unnatural growth of brain cells in the human skull, is among the most common cancers and it accounts for less than 2% of human cancer across the globe. According to WHO, brain tumor is very complicated in nature and has severe morbidity. In this work, deep learning models for classification of brain tumor with limited magnetic resonance imaging images dataset are used. The models are able to classify the brain tumor as either benign or malignant, respectively. The MRI images dataset was split into 80% training set and 20% testing set, respectively. Additionally, CLACHE technique was employed to reduce the noise and improve the visibility level of the foggy areas of the MRI images dataset. Hence, the models were developed with the VGG16 and ResNet50 deep learning algorithms and accuracy, sensitivity, specificity. Furthermore, AUC evaluations metrics were used to determine the performance of the models. Consequently, the model developed with VGG16 has shown the highest accuracy of 96% and 94.30% sensitivity, respectively, while the model developed with ResNet50 has shown the highest specificity of 93.10% and 91.20% AUC, respectively. Subsequently, the models would be used as assistive tools to radiologists in various hospitals in Nigeria. In future works, a large MRI training dataset would be sourced and used to develop and implement new novel deep learning techniques and algorithms for the classification of brain tumors.

References

1. Muhammad, L. J., Garba, A., & Abba, G. (2015). Security challenges for building knowledge based economy in Nigeria. *International Journal of Security and Its Applications, 9*, 1.
2. Rozita, J., Elham, B., Daniel, R., Licia, P. L., et al. (2021). Role of functional magnetic resonance imaging in the presurgical mapping of brain tumors. *Radiologic Clinics of North America, 59*(3), 377–393. https://doi.org/10.1016/j.rcl.2021.02.001
3. Iqbal, S., Khan, MUG, Saba, T., et al. (2018) Computer-assisted brain tumor type discrimination using magnetic resonance imaging features. *Biomedical Engineering Letters, 8*, 5–28. https://doi.org/10.1007/s13534-017-0050-3
4. Noreen, N., Palaniappan, S., Qayyum, A., et al. (2020). A deep learning model based on concatenation approach for the diagnosis of brain tumor. *IEEE Access, 8*, 55135–55144. https://doi.org/10.1109/ACCESS.2020.2978629
5. Sultan, H. H., Salem, N. M., & Al-Atabany, W. (2019). Multi-classification of brain tumor images using deep neural network. *IEEE Access, 7*, 69215–69225. https://doi.org/10.1109/ACCESS.2019.2919122

6. Stewart, B. W., & Wild, C. P. (2014). *World Cancer Report 2014.* Lyon, France: IARC.
7. World Health Organization (WHO), BURDEN OF CANCER, Cancer Country Profile 2020, https://www.who.int/cancer/country-profiles/NGA_2020.pdf
8. Ge, C., Gu, I. Y., Jakola, A. S. (2020). Enlarged training dataset by pairwise GANs for molecular-based brain tumor classification. In *IEEE Access* (Vol. 8, pp. 22560-22570). https://doi.org/10.1109/ACCESS.2020.2969805
9. Isselmou, A. E., Guizhi, X., Zhang, S., et al. (2021). Differential deep convolutional neural network model for brain tumor classification. *Brain Sciences, 11*(3), 352. https://doi.org/10.3390/brainsci11030352
10. Gopal, S. T., Balestrieri, A. B., Tanay, J., et al. (2020). Multiclass magnetic resonance imaging brain tumor classification using artificial intelligence paradigm. *Computers in Biology and Medicine, 122*, 103804. https://doi.org/10.1016/j.compbiomed.2020.103804
11. Seetha, J., & Selvakumar Raja, S. (2018, September). Brain tumor classification using convolutional neural networks. *Biomedical & Pharmacology Journal, 11*(3), 1457–1461. https://doi.org/10.13005/bpj/1511
12. Singh, N. K., & Raza, K. (2021). Medical image generation using generative adversarial networks: A review. In: R. Patgiri, A. Biswas, P. Roy (Eds.), *Health informatics: A computational perspective in healthcare. Studies in computational intelligence* (Vol. 932). Springer. https://doi.org/10.1007/978-981-15-9735-0_5
13. Ali, N. A., Syafeeza, A. R., Geok, L. J., et al. (2019). Design of automated computer-aided classification of brain tumor using deep learning. In V. Piuri, V. Balas, S. Borah, S. Syed Ahmad (Eds.), *Intelligent and interactive computing. Lecture notes in networks and systems* (Vol. 67). Springer. https://doi.org/10.1007/978-981-13-6031-2_11
14. Yamashita, R., Nishio, M., Do, R. K. G., et al. (2018). Convolutional neural networks: An overview and application in radiology. *Insights Into Imaging, 9*, 611–629. https://doi.org/10.1007/s13244-018-0639-9
15. Simonyan, K., & Zisserman, A. (2014). Very deep convolutional networks for large-scale image recognition. arXiv:1409.1556
16. Alom, M. Z., Taha, T. M., Yakopcic, C., et al. (2019) A state-of-the-art survey on deep learning theory and architectures. *Electronics, 8*, 292.
17. Alghyaline, S., Hsieh, J. W., Chuang, C. H. (2017). Video action classification using symmelets and deep learning. In *2017 IEEE international conference on systems, man, and cybernetics (SMC)* (pp. 414–419). IEEE. https://doi.org/10.1109/SMC.2017.8122640
18. Muhammad, L. J., Algehyne, E. A., & Usman, S. S. (2020). Predictive supervised machine learning models for diabetes mellitus. *SN Computer Science, 1*, 240.
19. Chen, M. C., Ball, R. L., Yang, L., et al. (2018). Deep learning to classify radiology free-text reports. *Radiology, 286*, p845-852.
20. Islam, M., Mahmud, S., Muhammad, L. J., et al. (2020). Wearable technology to assist the patients infected with novel coronavirus (COVID-19). *SN Computer Science, 1*, 320. https://doi.org/10.1007/s42979-020-00335-4
21. Haruna, A. A., Muhammad, L. J., Yahaya, B. Z., et al. (2019). An improved C4.5 data mining driven algorithm for the diagnosis of coronary artery disease. In *International conference on digitization (ICD)* (pp. 48–52). Sharjah, United Arab Emirates.
22. Hussain, S., et al. (2019). Performance evaluation of various data mining algorithms on road traffic accident dataset. In S. Satapathy, A. (Eds.), *Information and communication technology for intelligent systems* (p. 106). Smart Innovation, Systems and Technologies.
23. Tayeb, S., Pirouz, M., Cozzens, B., et al. (2017, December). Toward data quality analytics in signature verification using a convolutional neural network. In *2017 IEEE international conference on big data (Big Data)* (pp. 2644–2651). IEEE. https://doi.org/10.1109/BigData.2017.8258225
24. Sadiq, H., Muhammad, L. J., & Yakubu, A. (2018). Mining social media and DBpedia data using Gephi and R. *Journal of Applied Computer Science & Mathematics, 12*(1), 14–20.
25. He, K., Zhang, X., Ren, S., et al. (2016). Deep residual learning for image recognition. In *Proceedings of the IEEE conference on computer vision and pattern recognition* (pp. 770–778).https://doi.org/10.1109/CVPR.2016.90

26. Muhammad, L. J., Islam, M. M., Usman, S. S., et al. (2020). Predictive data mining models for novel coronavirus (COVID-19) infected patients' recovery. *Springer Nature Computer Science, 1*. https://doi.org/10.1007/s42979-020-00216-w
27. Muhammad, L. J., Algehyne, E. A., Usman, S. S., et al. (2020). Supervised machine learning models for prediction of COVID-19 infection using epidemiology dataset. *Springer Nature Computer Science*. https://doi.org/10.1007/s42979-020-00394
28. Yapici, M. M., Tekerek, A., & Ti, N. (2019). Literature review of deep learning research areas. *GaziMühendislikBilimleriDergisi (GMBD), 5*(3), 188–215. https://doi.org/10.30855/gmbd.2019.03.01
29. Muhammad, L. J., Garba, E. J., Oye, N. D., et al. (2018). On the problems of knowledge acquisition and representation of expert system for diagnosis of coronary artery disease (CAD). *International Journal of u- and e-Service, Science and Technology, 11*(3), 50–59.
30. Kwon, H., Pellauer, M., Parashar, A., et al. (2020). Flexion: A quantitative metric for flexibility in DNN accelerators. *IEEE Computer Architecture Letters, 20*(1), 1–4. https://doi.org/10.1109/LCA.2020.3044607
31. Zhang, Y. D., Satapathy, S. C., Zhu, L. Y., et al. (2020). A seven-layer convolutional neural network for chest CT based COVID-19 diagnosis using stochastic pooling. *IEEE Sensors Journal*. https://doi.org/10.1109/JSEN.2020.3025855
32. Ishaq, F. S., Muhammad, L. J., Yahaya, B. Z., et al. (2020). Fuzzy based expert system for diagnosis of diabetes mellitus. *International Journal of Advanced Science and Technology., 136*, 39–50.
33. Ishaq, F. S., Muhammad, L. J., Yahaya, B. Z., et al. (2018). Data mining driven models for diagnosis of diabetes mellitus: A survey. *Indian Journal of Science and Technology, 11*, 42.
34. Muhammad, L. J., et al. (2019). Performance evaluation of classification data mining algorithms on coronary artery disease dataset. In *IEEE 9th international conference on computer and knowledge engineering (ICCKE 2019)*, Ferdowsi University of Mashhad.
35. Muhammad, L. J., Besiru, M. J., Yahaya, B. Z., et al. (2020). An improved C4.5 algorithm using principle of equivalent of infinitesimal and arithmetic mean best selection attribute for large dataset. In *2020 10th international conference on computer and knowledge engineering (ICCKE)* (pp. 006–010). Mashhad, Iran.
36. Li, B., & Lima, D. (2021). Facial expression recognition via ResNet-50. *International Journal of Cognitive Computing in Engineering, 2*, 57–64. https://doi.org/10.1016/j.ijcce.2021.02.002
37. Muhammad, L. J., Garba, E. J., Oye, N. D., & Garko, A. B. (2021). Fuzzy rule-driven data mining framework for knowledge acquisition for expert system. In *Translational bioinformatics in healthcare and medicine* (pp. 201–214). Elsevier, Academic Press.
38. Muhammad, L. J., Al-Shourbaji, I. A., Haruna, A. A., et al. (2021). Machine learning predictive models for coronary artery disease. *SN Computer Science, 2*, 350.
39. Muhammad, L. J., Algehyne, E. A., & Usman, S. S. (2020). Predictive supervised machine learning models for diabetes mellitus. *SN Computer Sciene, 1*, 240. https://doi.org/10.1007/s42979-020-00250-8
40. Ouyang, W., Chu, X., & Wang, X. (2014). Multi-source deep learning for human pose estimation. In *Proceedings of the IEEE conference on computer vision and pattern recognition* (pp. 2329–2336). https://doi.org/10.1109/CVPR.2014.299
41. Sarumi, O. A., Aouedi, O., & Muhammad, L. J. (2022). Potential of deep learning algorithms in mitigating the spread of COVID-19. In J. Nayak, B. Naik, & A. Abraham (Eds.), *Understanding COVID-19: The role of computational intelligence. Studies in computational intelligence* (Vol. 963). Springer, Cham. https://doi.org/10.1007/978-3-030-74761-9_10
42. Afroj, A., Sahar, Q., Naiyar, I., & Khalid, R. (2020). Fog, edge, and pervasive computing in intelligent IoT driven applications. In *Fog, edge and pervasive computing in intelligent internet of things driven applications in healthcare: Challenges, limitations and future use*. https://doi.org/10.1002/9781119670087.ch1
43. Gupta, T. K., & Raza, K. (2020). Optimizing deep feedforward neural network architecture: A Tabu search based approach. *Neural Processing Letters, 51*, 2855–2870. https://doi.org/10.1007/s11063-020-10234-7

44. Wang, A., Lu, J., Cai, J., Cham, T. J., et al. (2015). Large-margin multi-modal deep learning for RGB-D object recognition. *IEEE Transactions on Multimedia, 17*(11), 1887–1898. https://doi.org/10.1109/TMM.2015.2476655
45. Muhammad, L. J., & Algehyne, E. A. (2021). Fuzzy based expert system for diagnosis of coronary artery disease in Nigeria. *Health Technology, 11*, 319–329.
46. Kaiming, H., Xiangyu, Z., Shaoqing, R., et al. (2015). *Deep residual learning for image recognition*. arXiv:1512.03385 [cs.CV].
47. Al-Qizwini, M., Barjasteh, I., Al-Qassab, H., et al. (2017, June). Deep learning algorithm for autonomous driving using GoogLeNet. In *2017 IEEE intelligent vehicles symposium (IV)* (pp. 89–96). IEEE. https://doi.org/10.1109/IVS.2017.7995703
48. Tang, H., Ni, R., Zhao, Y., & Li, X. (2018). Median filtering detection of small-size image based on CNN. *Journal of Visual Communication and Image Representation, 51*, 162–168. https://doi.org/10.1016/j.jvcir.2018.01.011
49. Amin, K. A., Moosa, A., & Foad, K. (2019). Magnetic resonance imaging-based brain tumor grades classification and grading via convolutional neural networks and genetic algorithms. *Biocybernetics and Biomedical Engineering, 39*(1), 63–74. https://doi.org/10.1016/j.bbe.2018.10.004
50. Ucuzal, U., Yaşar, S., & Çolak, C. (2019). Classification of brain tumor types by deep learning with convolutional neural network on magnetic resonance images using a developed web-based interface. In *2019 3rd international symposium on multidisciplinary studies and innovative technologies (ISMSIT)* (pp. 1–5). https://doi.org/10.1109/ISMSIT.2019.8932761
51. Revathi, S., & Ahilan, A. (2021). *Biomedical and Physics Engineering Express, 7*, 055007.
52. Brain Tumor MRI Dataset. Retrieved on April 8, 2021, from https://www.kaggle.com/navoneel/brain-mri-images-for-brain-tumor-detectionaccessed
53. Suhartono, D., Gema, A. P., Winton, S., et al. (2020). Argument annotation and analysis using deep learning with attention mechanism in Bahasa Indonesia. *Journal of Big Data, 7*, 90. https://doi.org/10.1186/s40537-020-00364-z
54. Yadav, G., Maheshwari, S., & Agarwal, A. (2014). Contrast limited adaptive histogram equalization based enhancement for real time video system. In *2014 international conference on advances in computing, communications and informatics (ICACCI)* (pp. 2392–2397). https://doi.org/10.1109/ICACCI.2014.6968381

Predicting the Cancer Recurrence Using Artificial Neural Networks

Mohamed Soudy, Afroz Alam, and Obiadul Ola

Abstract In the early 1900s, multiple significant studies showed high incidences of cancer. During this period, study with infectious agents produced only modest results which looked irrelevant to people. Then, in the 1980s, groundbreaking evidence that a number of viruses can cause cancer in people began to emerge. Machine learning and deep learning techniques have been widely employed in cancer detection and classification that include support vector machines (SVMs), artificial neural networks (ANNs), and conventional neural networks (CNNs). The recurrence of cancer is also an important issue that needs to be predicted with significant accuracy. This chapter reviews current state-of-the-art of ANNs model in the prediction of cancer recurrence.

Keywords Cancer · Cancer recurrence · Machine learning · Artificial neural networks (ANN)

1 Introduction

Cell division is the process by which a parent cell divides into two or more daughter cells, with enzymatic and catalytic processes orchestrating the process [1]. Furthermore, the alternation between DNA duplication and cell division cycles ensures cellular proliferation. Cancer is the unregulated cell division caused by enzymatic dysregulation, which can result in mutations and illnesses [2]. According to World Health Organization (WHO) reports, cancer, the world's second-biggest cause of death, has been the subject of numerous attempts to treat it. Despite treatment efforts such as surgery, chemotherapy, and hormone therapy, cancer has the potential to reoccur [3, 4].

M. Soudy (✉)
Bioinformatics Program, Faculty of Computer Science and Information Technology, Ain Shams University, Cairo, Egypt

A. Alam
Department of Computer Application, Integral University, Lucknow, India

O. Ola
Maulana Mazharul Haque Arabic and Persian University, Patna, India

K. Raza (ed.), *Computational Intelligence in Oncology*, Studies in Computational Intelligence 1016, https://doi.org/10.1007/978-981-16-9221-5_10

The process of cancer recurrence occurs when a patient completes cancer therapy, and cancer is diagnosed again after a while as cancer recurrence can occur in the same location or a different location. Recurrent cancer begins with cancer cells that were not completely removed or destroyed after the initial treatment [5]. This isn't to say that the treatment you received was ineffective. It simply means that approximately several cancer cells survived therapy but were too small to be detected in subsequent testing. These cells grow into tumors or cancer over time, which your specialist can now diagnose. Cancer recurrence can be categorized into three major types including local recurrence, in which cancer recur in the same place or very close to it, regional recurrence, in which cancer recur or gown in lymph nodes or tissues near to the original region, and distance recurrence in which cancer spread in a place away from the original place that first located in [6]. Researchers made many attempts in vitro to make predictions of the cancer recurrence using wet lab techniques such as the targeted digital sequencing (TARDIS) test that can be tailored to track a patient's cancer progression over time in order to detect tumor recurrence early. Researchers hope that by using a liquid biopsy test, breast cancer patients may be able to prevent unneeded procedures. The cost of the wet lab experiments and the limitations of regular sample collection of patients led the scientists to the in silico prediction and open a wide room of research on this point.

Machine learning, the process in which humans try to make the computer mimic the ability of the human to learn is widely employed in the classification, prediction, and early prediction of cancer [7]. Algorithms such as Support Vector Machines (SVMs) [8], Naive Bayes [9], Decision Tree (DT) [10], and Artificial Neural Networks (ANNs) [11] are widely used in the classification and prediction of cancer recurrence.

2 Artificial Neural Networks

The structure of neural networks is inspired by the structure of the human brain as the interconnected neurons store and process the input data as a biological system [12]. Furthermore, the input layer that is composed of input neurons takes the input from the user and pass the input through the connections 'weights' to the hidden layers to process the input, and finally, the output layer returns the processed data 'output' to the user as shown in Fig. 1.

The formula is to compute the output of a single neuron is represented as,

$$z = g(\mathbf{w}^{\mathrm{T}}\mathbf{x} - b) = g\left(\sum_{i=1}^{d} w_i x_i - b\right)$$

where: $x = (x_1, x_2, x_d)\, T$ be an input vector and $w = (w_1, w_2, w_d)$, T the weight vector, and z is the output of a single neuron. The relapse of cancer occurs in different types

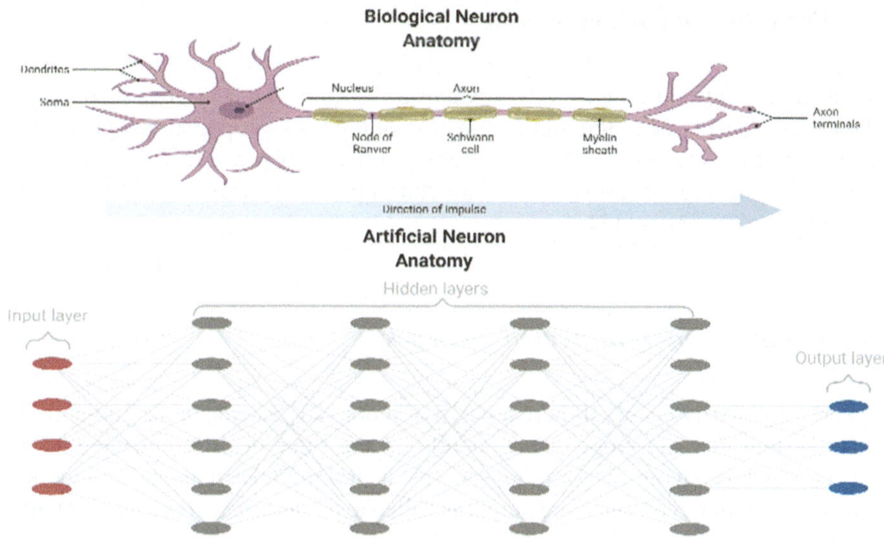

Fig. 1 The architecture of neural networks

of cancers as breast, colorectal, and prostate cancers; many attempts have been made on the prediction of cancer relapse from different types of data achieving optimal performance.

Nowadays, ANN approaches are effectively used for monitoring and detection of recurrence of cancer. Sometimes, ANNs are explained by their depth, i.e., having many layers, which are also called hidden layers in between input and output. Deep learning is described by larger numbers of hidden layers in the ANN architecture. Some of the general types of ANNs used to predict cancer recurrence are as follows [13–15].

2.1 Convolutional Neural Networks

For multidimensional datasets having a large number of attributes, like cancer healthcare datasets, CNN plays a good role in predicting cancer recurrence. With the help of error propagation, CNN can update the weights of input and their output nodes with the help of multilayer architecture. This CNN is a two-stage approach. In the first step, CNN will identify the nuclei in a given tissue or cell, and in the next stage, CNN detects the nuclear centers to predict the problem of input that belongs to a case of cancer recurrence [16].

2.2 Periodic Neural Networks

It is an important sub-type of ANN where a directed graph is generated by the linked nodes. Also, due to the implementation of the back-propagation algorithm in recurrent neural network (RNN), nodes are dominant for predicting the outcomes. With the help of the evolution matrix, we can improve the accuracy for predicting the recurrence of cancer [17].

2.3 Modular Interconnected Network

Network modularity occurs if there are two or more sub-systems in a computational logical system that can work independently on the same or different input so the network which is having two or more separate neural modules that can act independently on the input to produce the output is called a *modular neural network*. Hence, a modular neural network has a lot of advantages due to its divide and conquer strategies. By this strategy, we can reduce the complexity, and achieve the scalability of the module. For modeling a problem efficiently and easy way manner for high dimensional data, this divide and conquer strategies are very efficient while using modularity [18].

3 ANN in Breast, Ovarian, and Lung Cancer

The ANN has been extensively applied in the various aspects of cancer studies including its early detection, diagnosis, recurrence prediction, survival prediction, and so on [19]. This section highlights some brief accounts of ANN applications.

3.1 Breast Cancer

Breast cancer is the most frequent malignancy in women that causes high mortality. Classical methods used for its diagnosis and staging require expertise from the oncologist who examines the breast lesions, which is time-consuming, and sometimes inefficient [20]. The ANN has been previously applied for analyzing the complex breast cancer dataset for its diagnosis [21, 22], early detection [23], and assessing breast cancer risk [24].

3.2 *Ovarian Cancer*

Ovarian cancer is one of the lethal and highly prominent gynecological malignancies after breast cancer, having a 5-years survival rate of 50% [25–27]. Ghoniem et al. [15] proposed a hybrid evolutionary deep learning model using multi-modal data for the ovarian cancer diagnosis, while Kappen and Neijt [28] developed an ANN-based model for the prediction of treatment outcome of advanced ovarian cancer.

3.3 *Lung Cancer*

Lung cancer is a malignancy of the lung due to the growth of lung tissues, which is a primary cause of cancer-related death worldwide. ANNs have also been applied in the detection and diagnosis of lung cancer [29] using various clinical symptoms such as yellow fingers, anxiety, fatigue, allergy, coughing, wheezing, shortness of breath, difficulty in swallowing and chest pain [30, 31], and sputum color images [32]. A multi-parameterized ANN has been proposed for lung cancer risk prediction by Hart et al. [33]. Adetiba and Olugbara [34] developed ANN and SVM-based ensembles to predict lung cancer using genomics data from nucleotides having mutations in the epidermal growth factor receptor (EGFR), Kirsten rat sarcoma (KRAS) viral oncogenes, and tumor suppressor p53, which achieves an accuracy of 95.90%.

4 ANNs in Cancer Recurrence Prediction

We collected published literature from the PubMed database using various search queries related to cancer recurrence prediction and ANNs. The research attempts made in predicting the cancer recurrence using ANNs rely on the theory that the ANNs can classify the input data into two main classes (Recurrence; No-recurrence) based on either pathological or clinical features as annotated in Table 1.

Most of the data used in the cancer recurrence were clinical features (including age, gender, WHO grade, tumor budding, and depth of invasion) mixed with pathological or image datasets, and some researchers use the gene expression data. Researchers that use the gene expression data rely on the theory that the biological biomarkers will have a significant role in the model construction as a core feature, as evidenced that the estrogen receptors (ER) and progesterone receptors (PR) are critical biomarkers for the prognosis of endocrine therapy of breast cancer. Furthermore, the carcinoembryonic antigen (CEA), a high-molecular weight glycoprotein produced in embryonic tissue and colorectal cancers, is the most commonly utilized prognostic biomarker in clinical practice. These biological markers combined with the clinical features will lead to a robust classification model [53]. The usage of ANNs over other methods as SVMs is that the neural networks outperform the SVM in the prediction time for

Table 1 Summary of ANN-based methods for cancer recurrence prediction

Cancer type	Data type	Number of samples	Reported accuracy (%)	References
Bladder cancer	Clinico-pathological and molecular characteristics	201 patients	82	Qureshi et al. [35]
Bladder cancer	Clinico-pathological	109 patients	88	Catto et al. [36]
Breast cancer	Clinico-pathological	2842 patients	80	Lundin et al. [37]
Breast cancer	Clinico-pathological	1035 patients	82	Jerez-Aragonés, et al. [38]
Breast cancer	Clinico-pathological	679 patients	80	Kim et al. [39]
Breast cancer	Ultrasound imaging	100 patients	96	Tadayyon et al. [40]
Head and neck cancer	CT scan	188 patients	93.2	Tang et al. [41]
Hepatocellular cancer	Undergone primary LT	19 patients	89.5	Rodriguez-Luna et al. [42]
Lung cancer	Gene expression	280 patients	65.71	Chen et al. [43]
Oral tongue cancer	Clinico-pathological	311 patients	92.7	Alabi et al. [44]
Ovarian cancer	Laparotomy	242 patients	90	Snow et al. [45]
Ovarian cancer	CT scan	245 patients	82.5	Wang et al. [46]
Prostatic cancer	Histopathological	20 patients versus 20 control	85	Mattfeldt et al. [47]
Prostatic cancer	Pathological and clinical	564 patients	78	Han et al. [48]
Prostatic cancer	Pathological (radical prostatectomy)	309 patients	80	Ziada et al. [49]
Prostatic cancer	Gene expression	597 patients	95.3	Hou et al. [50]
Squamous cancer	Clinico-pathological	79 patients	91.7	Damiani et al. [51]
Urothelial cancer	Clinico-pathological	2111 patients	76	Buchner et al. [52]

most of the datasets, so when we need to make a rapid prediction, we use the ANNs [54], Moreover, the ANNs are better than the random forest (RF) a type of decision trees as the ANNs perform well when the complexity of data increased compared to the RFs [55, 56]. The optimal performance of ANNs led to massive usage in a critical problem such as cancer recurrence prediction.

5 Discussion

Cancer relapse is documented in 10–15% of cancer cases; this relapse may occur at any time, so the prediction of cancer recurrence or relapse may save thousands or millions of lives [38]. The early prediction will help the doctors to make a decision on the cancer cases whether surgery, chemotherapy, biological and hormonal therapies, and radiotherapy. The attempts made for the prediction of cancer relapse in a wet lab include many methods such as the targeted digital sequencing with common limitations regarding the time, cost, and regular sample collection. Therefore, the need for computational resources increased and many attempts have been made in silico to make a prediction of cancer relapse. The attempts use the different types of available data to make a good prediction including the clinical data, clinical data combined with pathological data, gene expression data with previous knowledge of progression or relapse biomarkers, and image data [57]. The variety and availability of the data sets led to the usage of various machine learning models, and we selected the ANNs as it outperforms the other models. The average accuracy on the different cancer types is 82–90% which is a fair accuracy in the biological field. However, the optimal performance of the ANNs in predicting the cancer recurrence still needs further improvement, and we have some obstacles and limitations to overcome. All the machine learning models are data dependent, and we can't generalize the model output to any other type of data, and there are no models that combine or integrate the cancer cases together into one dataset ignoring the cancer type to generalize the cancer prediction.

6 Conclusion

Cancer recurrence is considered the biggest fear in cancer treatment and therapy. Many attempts are made to predict the recurrence of different cancer types and various datasets to optimize the prediction accuracy and contribute to saving human lives. The performance of ANNs in cancer recurrence led to the popularity of its usage in other tasks such as cancer metastasis. The overall comparison performed from the collected literature showed that although the ANNs require large time for training, it outperforms other models in terms of prediction time and performance.

References

1. Donachie, W. D., Begg, K. J., & Vicente, M. (1976). Cell length, cell growth and cell division. *Nature, 264*(5584), 328–333.
2. Cairns, R. A., Harris, I. S., & Mak, T. W. (2011). Regulation of cancer cell metabolism. *Nature Reviews Cancer, 11*(2), 85–95.

3. Jemal, A., Bray, F., Center, M. M., Ferlay, J.,Ward, E., & Forman, D. (2011). Global cancer statistics. *CA: A Cancer Journal for Clinicians, 61*(2), 69–90.
4. Jemal, A., Siegel, R., Ward, E., Hao, Y., Xu, J., & Thun, M. J. (2009). Cancer statistics. *CA: A Cancer Journal for Clinicians, 59*(4).
5. Warnakulasuriya, S., & Greenspan, J. S. (Eds.) (2020). *Textbook of oral cancer: prevention, diagnosis and management*. Springer Nature.
6. Moschini, M., Sharma, V., Zattoni, F., Quevedo, J. F., Davis, B. J., Kwon, E., & Karnes, R. J.: Natural history of clinical recurrence patterns of lymph node–positive prostate cancer after radical prostatectomy. *European Urology, 69*(1), 135–142.
7. Burki, T. K. (2016). Predicting lung cancer prognosis using machine learning. *The Lancet Oncology, 17*(10), e421.
8. Noble, W. S. (2006). What is a support vector machine? *Nature Biotechnology, 24*(12), 1565–1567.
9. Rish, I. (2001). An empirical study of the naive Bayes classifier. In IJCAI 2001 Workshop on Empirical Methods in Artificial Intelligence (Vol. 3, No. 22, pp. 41–46).
10. Safavian, S. R., & Landgrebe, D. (1991). A survey of decision tree classifier methodology. *IEEE Transactions on Systems, Man, and Cybernetics 21*(3), 660–674.
11. Sarle, W. S. (1994). Neural networks and statistical models.
12. Yegnanarayana, B. (2009). Artificial neural networks. PHI Learning Pvt. Ltd.
13. MmmBakr, M. A. H. A., Al-Attar, H. M., Mahra, N. K., & Abu-Naser, S. S. (2020). Breast cancer prediction using JNN. *International Journal of Academic Information Systems Research (IJAISR), 4*(10).
14. Setiono, R. (2000). Generating concise and accurate classification rules for breast cancer diagnosis. *Artificial Intelligence in Medicine, 18*(3), 205–219.
15. Ghoniem, R. M., Algarni, A. D., Refky, B., & Ewees, A. A. (2021). Multi-modal evolutionary deep learning model for ovarian cancer diagnosis. *Symmetry, 13*(4), 643.
16. Kumar, N., Verma, R., Arora, A., Kumar, A., Gupta, S., Sethi, A., & Gann, P. H. (2017, March). Convolutional neural networks for prostate cancer recurrence prediction. In *Medical Imaging 2017: Digital Pathology* (Vol. 10140, p. 101400H). International Society for Optics and Photonics.
17. Shiva Shankar, R., Murthy, K. V. S., & Someswara Rao, C. (2020). Breast cancer disease prediction with recurrent neural networks (RNN). *International Journal of Industrial Engineering & Production Research, 31*(3), 379–386.
18. Pandey, B., Jain, T., Kothari, V., & Grover, T. (2012). Evolutionary modular neural network approach for breast cancer diagnosis. *International Journal of Computer Science Issues, 9*(1), 219–225.
19. Qazi, S., Iqbal, N., & Raza, K. (2021). *Artificial intelligence in medicine (AIM): Machine learning in cancer diagnosis* (pp. 103–126). De Gruyter.
20. Sandhu, I. K., Nair, M., Shukla, H., & Sandhu, S. S. (2015). Artificial neural network: As emerging diagnostic tool for breast cancer. *International Journal of Pharmacy and Biological Sciences, 5*(3), 29–41.
21. Jafari-Marandi, R., Davarzani, S., Gharibdousti, M. S., & Smith, B. K. (2018). An optimum ANN-based breast cancer diagnosis: Bridging gaps between ANN learning and decision-making goals. *Applied Soft Computing, 1*(72), 108–120.
22. Ortiz-Rodriguez, J. M., Guerrero-Mendez, C., Martinez-Blanco, M. D., Castro-Tapia, S., Moreno-Lucio, M., Jaramillo-Martinez, R., & Garcia, J. A. (2018). Breast cancer detection by means of artificial neural networks. *Advanced Applications for Artificial Neural Networks, 28*, 161–179.
23. Mehdy, M. M., Ng, P. Y., Shair, E. F., Saleh, N. I., & Gomes, C. (2017). Artificial neural networks in image processing for early detection of breast cancer. *Computational and Mathematical Methods in Medicine, 3*, 2017.
24. Sepandi, M., Taghdir, M., Rezaianzadeh, A., & Rahimikazerooni, S. (2018). Assessing breast cancer risk with an artificial neural network. *Asian Pacific Journal of Cancer Prevention: APJCP, 19*(4), 1017.

25. Zhang, Y., Qazi, S., & Raza, K. (2021). Differential expression analysis in ovarian cancer: A functional genomics and systems biology approach. *Saudi Journal of Biological Sciences, 28*(7), 4069–4081.
26. Qazi, S., & Raza, K. (2021). Phytochemicals from Ayurvedic plants as potential medicaments for ovarian cancer: An in silico analysis. *Journal of Molecular Modeling, 27*, 114. https://doi.org/10.1007/s00894-021-04736-x
27. Qazi, S., Sharma, A., & Raza, K. (2021). The role of epigenetic changes in ovarian cancer: A review. *Indian J Gynecol Oncolog, 19*, 27. https://doi.org/10.1007/s40944-021-00505-z
28. Kappen, H. J., & Neijt, J. P. (1993). Neural network analysis to predict treatment outcome. *Annals of Oncology, 1*(4), S31–S34.
29. Kweik, O. M. A., Hamid, M. A. A., Sheqlieh, S. O., Abu-Nasser, B. S., & Abu-Naser, S. S. (2020). Artificial neural network for lung cancer detection. *International Journal of Academic Engineering Research (IJAER), 4*(11).
30. Bertolaccini, L., Solli, P., Pardolesi, A., & Pasini, A. (2017). An overview of the use of artificial neural networks in lung cancer research. *Journal of Thoracic Disease, 9*(4), 924.
31. Nasser, I. M., & Abu-Naser, S. S. (2019). Lung cancer detection using artificial neural network. *International Journal of Engineering and Information Systems (IJEAIS), 3*(3), 17–23.
32. Taher, F., & Sammouda, R. (2011). Lung cancer detection by using artificial neural network and fuzzy clustering methods. In 2011 IEEE GCC Conference and Exhibition (GCC), 2011 Feb 19 (pp. 295–298). IEEE.
33. Hart, G. R., Roffman, D. A., Decker, R., & Deng, J. (2018). A multi-parameterized artificial neural network for lung cancer risk prediction. *PLoS One, 13*(10), e0205264.
34. Adetiba, E., & Olugbara, O. O. (2015). Lung cancer prediction using neural network ensemble with histogram of oriented gradient genomic features. *The Scientific World Journal, 1*, 2015.
35. Qureshi, K. N., Naguib, R. N. G., Hamdy, F. C., Neal, D. E., & Kilian Mellon, J. (2000). Neural network analysis of clinicopathological and molecular markers in bladder cancer. *The Journal of Urology, 163*(2), 630–633.
36. Catto, J. W. F., Linkens, D. A., Abbod, M. F., Chen, M., Burton, J. L., Feeley, K. M., & Hamdy, F. C. (2003). Artificial intelligence in predicting bladder cancer outcome: a comparison of neuro-fuzzy modeling and artificial neural networks. *Clinical Cancer Research, 9*(11), 4172–4177.
37. Lundin, J., Lundin, M., Holli, K., Kataja, V., Elomaa, L., Pylkkänen, L., Turpeenniemi-Hujanen, T., & Joensuu, H. (2001). Omission of histologic grading from clinical decision making may result in overuse of adjuvant therapies in breast cancer: Results from a nationwide study. *Journal of Clinical Oncology, 19*(1), 28–36.
38. Jerez-Aragonés, J. M., Gómez-Ruiz, J. A., Ramos-Jiménez, G., Muñoz-Pérez, J., & Alba-Conejo, E. (2003). A combined neural network and decision trees model for prognosis of breast cancer relapse. *Artificial Intelligence in Medicine, 27*(1), 45–63.
39. Kim, W., Kim, K. S., Lee, J. E., Noh, D.-Y., Kim, S.-W., Jung, Y. S., Park, M. Y., & Park, R. W.(2012). Development of novel breast cancer recurrence prediction model using support vector machine. *Journal of Breast Cancer, 15*(2), 230–238.
40. Tadayyon, H., Gangeh, M., Sannachi, L., Trudeau, M., Pritchard, K., Ghandi, S., Eisen, A., et al. (2019). A priori prediction of breast tumour response to chemotherapy using quantitative ultrasound imaging and artificial neural networks. *Oncotarget, 10*(39), 3910.
41. FH, T., Chu, C. Y. W., & Cheung, E. Y. W. (2021). Radiomics AI prediction for head and neck squamous cell carcinoma (HNSCC) prognosis and recurrence with target volume approach. *BJR*|Open 3 (2021), 20200073.
42. Rodriguez-Luna, H., Vargas, H. E., Byrne, T., & Rakela, J. (2005). Artificial neural network and tissue genotyping of hepatocellular carcinoma in liver-transplant recipients: Prediction of recurrence. *Transplantation, 79*(12), 1737–1740.
43. Chen, Y.-C., Chang, Y.-C., Ke, W.-C., & Chiu, H.-W. (2015). Cancer adjuvant chemotherapy strategic classification by artificial neural network with gene expression data: An example for non-small cell lung cancer. *Journal of Biomedical Informatics, 56*, 1–7.

44. Alabi, R. O., Elmusrati, M., Sawazaki-Calone, I., Kowalski, L. P., Haglund, C., Coletta, R. D., Mäkitie, A. A., Salo, T., Leivo, I., & Almangush, A. (2019). Machine learning application for prediction of locoregional recurrences in early oral tongue cancer: A web-based prognostic tool. *VirchowsArchiv, 475*(4), 489–497.
45. Snow, P. B., Brandt, J. M., & Larry Williams, R. (2001). Neural network analysis of the prediction of cancer recurrence following debulking laparotomy and chemotherapy in stages III and IV ovarian cancer. *Molecular Urology, 5*(4), 171–174.
46. Wang, S., Liu, Z., Rong, Y., Zhou, B., Bai, Y., Wei, W., Wang, M., Guo, Y., & Tian, J. (2019). Deep learning provides a new computed tomography-based prognostic biomarker for recurrence prediction in high-grade serous ovarian cancer. *Radiotherapy and Oncology, 132*, 171–177.
47. Mattfeldt, T., Kestler, H. A., Hautmann, R., & Gottfried, H. W. (1999). Prediction of prostatic cancer progression after radical prostatectomy using artificial neural networks: A feasibility study. *BJU International, 84*, 316–323.
48. Han, M., Snow, P. B., Epstein, J. I., Chan, T. Y., Jones, K. A., Walsh, P. C., & Partin, A. W. (2000). A neural network predicts progression for men with Gleason score 3+ 4 versus 4+ 3 tumors after radical prostatectomy. *Urology, 56*(6), 994–999.
49. Ziada, A. M., Lisle, T. C., Snow, P. B., Levine, R. F., Miller, G., & David Crawford, E. (2001). Impact of different variables on the outcome of patients with clinically confined prostate carcinoma: prediction of pathologic stage and biochemical failure using an artificial neural network. *Cancer, 91*(8), Suppl, 1653–1660.
50. Hou, Q., Bing, Z.-T., Hu, C., Li, M.-Y., Yang, K.-H., Mo, Z., Xie , X.-W., et al. (2018). RankProd combined with genetic algorithm optimized artificial neural network establishes a diagnostic and prognostic prediction model that revealed C1QTNF3 as a biomarker for prostate cancer. *EBioMedicine, 32*, 234–244.
51. Damiani, G., Grossi, E., Berti, E., Conic, R. R. Z., Radhakrishna, U., Pacifico, A., Bragazzi, N. L., Piccinno, R., & Linder, D. (2020). Artificial neural networks allow response prediction in squamous cell carcinoma of the scalp treated with radiotherapy. *Journal of the European Academy of Dermatology and Venereology, 34*(6), 1369–1373.
52. Buchner, A., May, M., Burger, M., Bolenz, C., Herrmann, E., Fritsche, H.-M., Ellinger, J., et al. (2013). Prediction of outcome in patients with urothelial carcinoma of the bladder following radical cystectomy using artificial neural networks. *European Journal of Surgical Oncology (EJSO,) 39*(4), 372–379.
53. Martins, A., Augusto, B., De Bulhões, G. F., Norat Cavalcanti, I., Martins, M. M., de Oliveira, P. G., & Martins, A. M. A. (2019). Biomarkers in colorectal cancer: the role of translational proteomics research. *Frontiers in Oncology 9*, 1284.
54. Ren, J. (2012). ANN vs. SVM: Which one performs better in classification of MCCs in mammogram imaging. *Knowledge-Based Systems, 26*, 144–153.
55. Oshiro, T. M., Perez, P. S., & Baranauskas, J. A. (2012). How many trees in a random forest?. In International Workshop on Machine Learning and Data Mining in Pattern Recognition (pp. 154–168). Springer.
56. Ahmad, M. W., Mourshed, M., & Rezgui, Y. (2017). Trees vs neurons: Comparison between random forest and ANN for high-resolution prediction of building energy consumption. *Energy and Buildings, 147*. 77–89.
57. Raza, K., & Hasan, A. N. (2015). A comprehensive evaluation of machine learning techniques for cancer class prediction based on microarray data. *International Journal of Bioinformatics Research and Applications, Inderscience, 11*(5), 397–416.

Computer Intelligence in Detection of Malignant or Premalignant Oral Lesions: The Story So Far

Astha Singh, Ankita Sahu, and Saurabh Verma

Abstract Cancer is a highly morbid disease affecting 20% of the world population. The third most common type of cancer is oral cancer which develops in the tissues of the mouth and neck and has different survival rates in men and women. Oral squamous cell carcinomas (OSCC), are the most common type of oral cancer and its early detection is key to longevity, successful outcome of treatment, and better quality of life. Computational intelligence (CI) may be a good tool in the detection of lesions in the early stage. The studies based on CI depend on images obtained through various light or resonance-based detection techniques as well as clinical images, while only one study has shown the accuracy of CI in detecting the gene expression patterns. Besides, there are several studies that have shown the efficacy of machine learning and deep learning in the field of radiology and spectroscopy. In totality, CI may be described as an upcoming tool that holds the promising potential to be used for the early diagnosis of malignant or premalignant lesions. The present review work is an attempt to propose a patient workup plan based on the concepts and models designed so far for the early detection of cancerous lesions. Thus, it may then help identify patients for closer follow-up, suggestive behavioral, and lifestyle modification to reduce the incidence of OSCC.

Keywords Computational intelligence · Lesions · Diagnosis · Oral cancer

1 Introduction

Cancer is a highly morbid disease affecting 20% of the world population and there is an increasing burden of this disease on the world population. The third most common type of cancer is oral cancer which develops in the tissues of the mouth and neck and has different survival rates in men and women [1]. Oral squamous cell carcinomas (OSCC), are the most common type of oral cancer and its early detection is key to longevity, successful outcome of treatment, and better quality of life [2]. The detection of cancer is based on its diagnosis based on TNM classification where T

A. Singh · A. Sahu · S. Verma (✉)
Tumor Biology, ICMR-National Institute of Pathology, New Delhi 110029, India

K. Raza (ed.), *Computational Intelligence in Oncology*, Studies in Computational Intelligence 1016, https://doi.org/10.1007/978-981-16-9221-5_11

refers to tumor size, N stands for the number of nodes involved in cancer and M is for metastasis. This TNM classification is based on the decision of a pathologist after observing prepared histopathological slides of the tissue from the affected area. The whole process is known as biopsy [3]. Several studies have been done so far to use artificial intelligence at the histological examination of slides in clinical samples with the orientation revolving around the benefit to patient [4, 5]. Semi-automated detection of tumor stage has been used by Sung et al. [4]. They have proposed a 6 stage grading of tumors based on a descriptive model for semi-automated detection of tumor stage and prediction of survival in OSCC patients (cohort of 256 patients). Another semi-automated detection model has been given for the detection of occult lymph node metastasis. Its efficacy revolved around digital tumor bud count in early OSCC cases (222 patients). Nuclei segmentation leads to enhanced stain-specific color intensity. This parameter was used for automated detection of oral lesions in histological images with great success deploying a multi-scale neural network. The study also claims the accuracy of this method in computer precision medicine to be better than all the other techniques of oral lesion detection [6]. The limitation of this system is its inability to use the prediction quality of all parameters simultaneously on the whole slide which is not the case with CI [4]. Further, this process cannot be done frequently, with new samples at different stages of patient treatment and prognosis. Besides this most of the studies are aimed at proving the effectiveness of computer intelligence in improvising various techniques rather than their refinement for patient-specific intervention. The present chapter summarizes the use of CI in disease prognosis from a patient perspective.

Imaging is the basic principle for diagnosis staging treatment and monitoring of oral cancer like other carcinomas. Along with it, the extent of disease, secondary lesions, and recurrence of cancer is assessed using techniques certain non-invasive techniques that are as follows:

1.1 Computer Tomography (CT) Scan

CT,formerly called computer-assisted tomography was invented by A. M. Cormack and G. N. Hounsfield a brilliant discovery that won them the Nobel prize in medicine that uses X-ray beams for the generation of object images non-invasively. Since then the application of CT scans in the diagnosis of bone defects and mass has been key to the diagnosis of spread and secondary tumors in head and neck cancer. The conventional CT scans use a single X-ray beam rotating around the object on the table for this purpose while the Gunter is fixed with detectors. In spiral or helical variants of CT scans X-ray tubes spin around the object to be scanned. This generates slices of images which are then used to reconstruct the image in coronal, sagittal, and oblique planes. The spiral scanners gave way to multislice scanners which are faster and take better scans owing to the use of multiple detectors and scanners. The latter uses an advanced computer facility to process the CT scan output thus generating more detailed images which seldom miss out on lesions and take much less time. The noise in images is produced by the limitation of CT scanners in processing lower radiation signals producing blurred images. These scanners need a higher dose of radiation for the better quality of images but at the same time, it is harmful to the patient. The use of CI and DL has the capacity to reduce such noise thus allowing lower radiation dose and exposure time of patients that is as low as reasonably attainable (ALARA). A popular phrase used to highlight the importance of low dose exposure of patients to radiation [7].

The use of bone and tissue algorithms in CT scans makes it possible to study bone erosion and lymphadenopathy. One study has recommended the use of the puffed cheek technique ($n = 7$) for CT scans as the air trapped in the oral cavity gives excellent contrast which makes lesions appear clearer [8]. Some medical institutions like MD Anderson Cancer Centre use specific algorithms designed for their patients [8].

1.2 Positron Emission Tomography (PET) Scan

PET scan is another imaging technique that utilizes radiotracers like acetate, choline, FDG (flourodeoxy glucose), etc. non-invasively [6]. FDG is an eminent radio used in oncology. It has fluorine 18 isotopes bound to the analog of glucose. This molecule then interacts in the glucose/hexokinase pathway in place of glucose. The gamma cameras are able to detect this molecule thus generating the details of the metabolic status of the cells. The radiotracers become trapped in the cancer cells owing to their increased glucose uptake thus producing bright spots in PET scans. PET scans are used to find if there is metastasis, cancer treatment outcome monitoring as well as recurrence of cancer. The limitations of a PET scan however may cause false positive or negative results as the radiotracer may get trapped in the site of inflammation. To overcome this CT scan is combined with a PET scan (CT/PET scan) to validate the presence of mass. The combined CT/PET scan is of high importance during the monitoring of cancer treatment and checking recurrence as well as finding secondary lesions. The combined use of CT/PET scans was found to be significant in detecting nasopharyngeal carcinoma [9]. The use of CI in increasing the efficacy of PET/CT in the detection of OC by decreasing the dose and cost to patient was shown by Katsari et al. using 66 samples. A support vector machine (SVM) algorithm was used to detect hyperplastic nasopharyngeal lesions ($n = 20$) successfully using CT/PET scans [10].

1.3 Magnetic Resonance Imaging (MRI)

MRI is based on the principle of non-invasive visualization of the tissue by hydrogen atoms proton nuclear spin. The hydrogen has a single proton which if excited gives a spin. This spin varies under different pulses of radio waves. Most MRI scanners use the hydrogen atoms abundant in the tissues to generate the images based on hydrogen atom polarization under different contrasts. MRI was developed in the late 1970s–1980s and since then it has been used in clinical as well as in other fields. An area of the patient is first subjected to a strong magnetic field under two gradient coils (x and y). The excited tissue then releases a signal which is caught by receiving coil. This signal may be recorded with T1 or T2 weighting. In T1 weighted images, the radio frequency RF is measured in different repetition times while in T2 the RF is measured in changing echo time. These two types of weighing systems have their own advantages and are used for imaging different tissue attributions. The T1W images are suitable for assessing the tumor thickness, invasion, and necrosis of the lymph nodes as well as lymphadenopathy. This is of much importance in tumor staging and grading for preoperative treatment design. MRI is a very powerful tool in finding the tumors in primary stages in the base of the tongue and floor of the mouth. Its use in evaluating the soft tissues makes it more advantageous than the CT scan in assessing the presence and extent of tumor growth and nodal metastasis in the oropharynx with great precision. The occurrence of human error in the evaluation of histological tissue is much higher as compared to MRI scan leading to inaccurate staging of the tumor. The combination of PET and MR images is in the early stage. The differential diagnosis of NPC and benign lesions of the nasopharynx was done using an automated Dense Net model using MRI images from 18 subjects [11]. Considering the limitation in performing the CT or PET scan repeatedly the monitoring of treatment and recurrence is one area where combined PET-MRI can be beneficial to patient care. However, the use of MRI in designing radiotherapy dose and patient workflow makes it much less complicated instead of using CT with MR images for the same purpose. One study was conducted to generate synthetic CT (sCT) scans based on 4100 patient MRIs using a deep convolution neural network (CNN). This study successfully generated the sCT using a deep CNN with accuracy but has not been validated on large samples [12].

1.4 Endoscopy

The endoscopy is the use of a small camera fitted to a tube with a light source to visualize the organs with the cavity. This technique may or may not involve the use of anesthesia depending on the target site and targeted organ. Panendoscopy is the collective name of laryngoscope, bronchoscope, and esophagoscope [13]. In the examination of the oropahrynx and the nasopharynx, this technique helps in the detection and monitoring of primary and secondary malignancies, treatment plan, and evaluation and recurrence. The images from endoscopy have been successfully used to detect nasopharyngeal malignancies using a deep learning model [14]. Patient perspective CI is a highly specialized tool that may be used for patient-specific designing of interventions required for averting the development and progression of the lesion into carcinoma or its treatment. It has been mainly used in the detection of cancer using histological images for diagnosis staging and metastasis [15]. CI including deep learning enabled the development of hardware and software that may perform complex decision-making based on the training of such machines with large datasets ($n = 27{,}536$) [14]. One such study has been done based on the oral images of patients ($n = 1469$). A cascaded CNN algorithm was used for the evaluation of these images. The study claims this algorithm to be equally effective in detecting oral lesions as an expert and better than medical or non-medical students [16].

2 Computational Intelligence and Oral Cancer

There has been a marked increase in the number of studies involving the application of CI in image analysis for the diagnosis and prognosis of oral lesions since 2017 [17–19] as shown in Fig. 1.

Only three studies were done from 2005 to 2015 exploring the applicability of CI in OSCC detection. These studies used ANN algorithms while those which came after 2015 predominantly used CNN-based algorithms [20–54]. Further, the number of samples increased dramatically after 2015 Table 1. This may be due to the availability of enormous data and the use of more sophisticated machinery allowing high throughput image processing. Such evolution of CI in the detection and prognostics of oral lesions using high-resolution images has led to a revolution in the research field. However, the success of CI in the precise diagnosis of OC is far from achieved. The time now demands efforts to use CI for the diagnosis of lesions in the clinical setup.

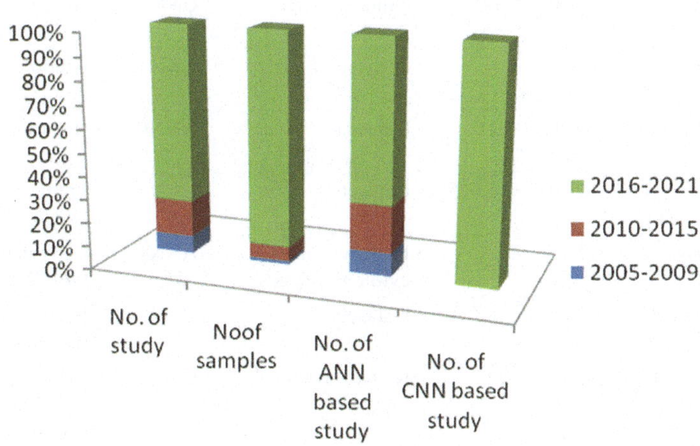

Fig. 1 Graph showing the increase in CNN-based study since 2015

Table 1 Showing the studies on the application of CI to various elements in cancer diagnosis and prognosis

S. No.	Study	Year	Sample size	Modality	Type of CI	Achieved target
1	Nayak et al. [17]	2005	50	Recorded spectra	ANNs	Differentiating premalignant and malignant oral lesions
2	Rosma et al. [18]	2010	191	Datasets	ANNs	Prediction of OC
3	Tseng et al. [19]	2015		Autofluorescence imaging (AFI) and white light imaging (WLI)	ANNs	Prediction of OL and prognosis
4	Uthoff et al. [20]	2017	170	Datasets	CNN	Early detection of OPL and OML
5	Shams et al. [21]	2017	10	Gene expression data	CNN	Predicting the chances of OPL and OML
6	Aubreville et al. [22]	2017	7894	Confocal laser end, microscopy	CNN	Classification of OC
7	Das et al. [23]	2018	126	Histological images	CNN	Classification of OC
8	song et al. [24]	2018	190	Auto florescence images	CNN	Classification of OC
9	Jeyaraj et al. [25]	2019	100	Clinical images	CNN	Automated detection of OC
10	Rathod et al. [26]	2019		Datasets	CNN	Grading of lesions
11	Alabi et al. [27]	2019	311	Datasets	ANNs	Recurrence of OC
12	Karadaghy et al. [28]	2019	33,065	Datasets	CNN	Prediction of OSCC
13	Sunny et al. [29]	2019	82	High-resolution cytology images	ANNs	Early detection of OPL and OML
14	Kim et al. [30]	2019	255	Datasets	CNN	Survival of patients
15	Yan et al. [31]	2019	22	Raman spectra image	CNN	Identify Tounge squamous cell carcinoma
16	Yu et al. [32]	2019	26	Raman spectra image	CNN	Differentiate tongue and non-tongue SCC
17	Chan et al. [33]	2019	80	Raman spectra image	CNN	Detection of OC

(continued)

Table 1 (continued)

S. No.	Study	Year	Sample size	Modality	Type of CI	Achieved target
18	Horie et al. [34]	2019	9546	Endoscopic image	CNN	Detect oral esophageal and distinguish from advanced cancer
19	Das et al. [35]	2019	126	Histological images	CNN	Detection and delineation of nucleus in oral histological images
20	Shaban et al. [36]	2019	70	Clinical image	CNN	Quantify tumor-infiltrating lymphocytes
21	Tamashiro et al. [37]	2020	7312	Endoscopic image	CNN	CNNs detected pharyngeal cancer
22	Panigrahi et al. [38]	2020	150	Histopathological image	CNN	Classify OC
23	Kouznetsova et al. [39]	2020	180	Saliva	Machine learning	Distinguish OC from periodontitis
24	Alhazmi et al. [40]	2020	73	Datasets	ANNs	Prediction of OC
25	Fahed et al. [41]	2020	716	Clinical images	CNN	Detection of OC
26	Ariji et al. [42]	2020	1068	CT image	CNN	Identify extranodal extension of cervical lymph node metastases
27	Xia et al. [43]	2020	24	Fiber optic Raman spectroscopy	CNN	Identify oral tongue squamous cell carcinoma resection margins
28	Fujima et al. [44]	2020	113	CT image	CNN	Predicted the disease-free survival of patients
29	Fu et al. [45]	2020	44,409	Clinical images	CNN	Rapid and non-invasive detection of OCSCC
30	Ding et al. [46]	2020	22	Raman spectral image	CNN	Accurate detection of TSCC

(continued)

Table 1 (continued)

S. No.	Study	Year	Sample size	Modality	Type of CI	Achieved target
31	Das et al. [48]	2020	156	Histopathological image	CNN	Grading of OC
32	Musulin et al. [49]	2021	322	Histological images	ANNs	Detection of OC
33	Kirubabai et al. [50]	2021	160	Oral images	CNNs	Detection of OC
34	Chu et al. [27]	2021	467	Clinicopathological datasets	ANNs	Prediction of OC
35	Welikala et al. [51]	2021	1085	Pathological images	CNN	Early detection of oral lesions
36	Paderno et al. [52]	2021	34	Neoplastic images	CNN	Segmentation of SCC
37	Tomita et al. [53]	2021	320	CT image	CNN	Differentiated benign and metastatic lymph nodes
38	Nanditha et al. [54]	2021	320	Oral lesion images	CNN	Differentiate benign and malignant OL
39	Musulin et al. [55]	2021	322	Histopathological image	CNN	Detection and grading of OSCC
40	Trajanovski et al. [56]	2021	14	Hyperspectral images	CNN	Detection of tongue cancer
41	Kim et al. [57]	2021	173	Clinical data	CNN	Identification of high risk groups

3 Computational Intelligence and the Patient Perspective

The use of CI made it possible to combine different techniques like CT/PET or CT-PET/MRI for the simultaneous diagnosis of primary and secondary lesions as well as lymph node metastasis. The adoption of these CI-based models in clinical practices needs the algorithms to perform better than the panelists for precision in diagnosis or prognosis and should be more time-efficient. These models also need to identify even minor changes in the tissues to be able to differentiate patients with low-grade dysplasia or ulcer from higher grades as the former may revert but the latter may not even after behavioral corrections as in tobacco users the removal of the putative cause may revert the dysplasia to normal tissue [22, 30, 34, 35, 37, 38]. Further, the MRI Scan and PET/CT scan images/output are more robust than their results may be simultaneously analyzed using algorithms that can be used for finalizing the staging and treatment procedure [9]. This would completely reduce the use of biopsies which are invasive, take much time, and are not preferred for treatment monitoring. A database may be created with the decisions of panelists who are highly experienced separately as done by certain agencies [14]. Such a database may be used in future situations when the panelist's expertise may not be available due to human reasons. This would ensure the conservation of expertise in cancer detection which would otherwise be lost with the specialist. This would also ensure the availability of experts to the masses in a time-efficient manner which was otherwise not possible.

4 Computational Intelligence and the Patient Workup Plan

Toluidine blue can be used for monitoring the treatment outcome as well as the aggressiveness of the tumor as highlighted in the previous study by Epstein and Sciubba in 2010 [55]. In a time frame, the change in the number of stain-positive cells can give a fair idea of the tumor growth—algorithm. The binary decision diagram BDD can be used for toluidine positive or negative lesions. The authors believe that more studies on the prognosis of oral premalignant lesions (OPL) to malignant lesions in a time scale manner combined with CI-based on toluidine blue approach will render us a remarkable tool. This tool may be used for the early detection of OPLs so that a patient may be given timely interventions and behavioral correction modules to completely avert or delay the progression of oral lesions to malignancies. The present patient workup plan (PWP) has been thus proposed (Fig. 2). In the existing PWP, the use of toluidine blue is restricted to the initial stage of visual observation.

5 Computational Intelligence and the Future

Computer intelligence application in the field of medicine has been promising and holds tremendous potential as a tool for rendering patient-specific medical interventions [58, 59]. The role of computer intelligence in developing such medical interventions in a time and cost-effective manner is the key to precision medication—an aspect that makes the efforts being put in this field worthy. CI has revolutionized the healthcare system by providing the platform for identifying patients with phenotypes that have the possibility of developing certain diseases including OSCC [41]. This technology also gives the advantage of developing specific treatment modules that may be more suitable for a particular patient by predicting the treatment outcome and disease-free survival. The role of computer intelligence in developing such medical interventions in a time and cost-effective manner is the key to precision medication—an aspect that makes the efforts being put in this field worthy [10]. The use of high throughput next-generation sequencing (NGS) [60] for diagnosing the particular pathways involved in disease progression at the patient level combined with imaging techniques (for tissue level validation) will help in developing patient-specific treatment modules [59, 61, 62]. Such a combination of high throughput imaging and

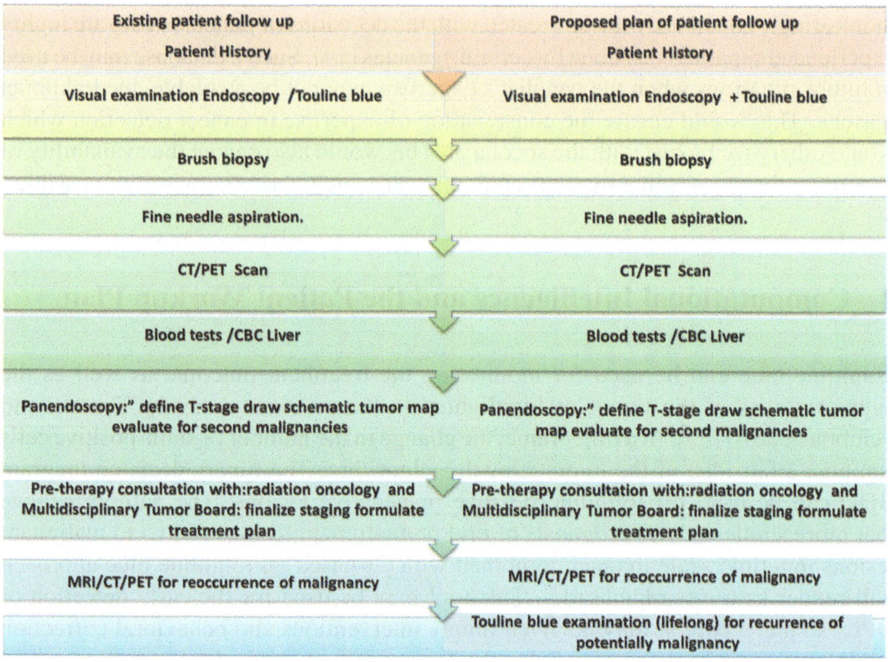

Fig. 2 Existing and proposed patient workup plan. (*Abbreviations* CT: Computer-assisted tomography; PET: Positron emission tomography; MRI: Magnetic resonance tomography; CBC: Complete blood count)

transcriptomics will not only provide better treatment, and increase the chances of patient survival [63–66].

6 Conclusion

Computational Intelligence (CI) holds tremendous potential in the differential diagnosis of benign and malignant lesions. It may again help in designing patient-specific treatment and interventions along with monitoring for detecting tumor recurrence. The different models and approaches of CI magnify the capability of various imaging techniques like CT, PET, MRI, whole slide, and oral images in providing computer precision medicine. A universal approach to using CI at the clinical level needs successful implementation. The authors believe Toulidine blue examination (lifelong) for recurrence of potentially malignant lesion considering its cost-effectiveness and ease of use along with patient comfort must be given its due importance. A novel toluidine blue-based algorithm can be used to identify the probable time needed for a benign lesion to convert into a malignancy. This may be of much importance for early detection, monitoring of lesions, and planning and giving intervention to patients with oral lesions. The use of toluidine blue in this regard has been reiterated by several authors. In the future, more studies need to be done which can implement the present-day techniques in providing medical interventions that are patient-specific rather than disease-specific. This would ensure the effectiveness of precision medicine and elevate the quality of life in patients.

References

1. Rebecca, L., Siegel, M. P. H., Mathieu, L. et al. (2021). Global cancer statistics 2020: GLOBOCAN estimates of incidence and mortality worldwide for 36 cancers in 185 countries (GLOBOCAN 2020).
2. Oral cancer article American oral cancer society. Accessed on 28/08/21, cancer.org.
3. Cancer staging WHO accessed on 25/08/21. https://www.who.int/healthtopics/cancer#tab=tab_1
4. Sung, Y. E., Kim, M. S., Lee, Y. S. (2021). Proposal of a scoring system for predicting pathological risk based on a semiautomated analysis of whole slide images in oral squamous cell carcinoma.
5. Ahmed, S., Mohamed, S., Elgharib, A., et al. (2020). The use of artificial intelligence, machine learning and deep learning in oncologic histopathology. *Journal of Oral Pathology and Medicine, 2020*(49), 849–856.
6. Bera, K., Schalper, K. A., Rimm, D. L., et al. (2019). Artificial intelligence in digital pathology—New tools for diagnosis and precision oncology. *Nature Reviews. Clinical Oncology, 16*, 703–715.
7. Graham, S., Rajpoot, N. M. (2018). SAMS-NET: Stain-aware multi-scale network for instance-based nuclei segmentation in histology images. In *2018 IEEE 15th international symposium on biomedical imaging (ISBI 2018)* (pp. 590–594).
8. Strindlund, M. (2021). The impact of artificial intelligence on CT imaging. *Computed Tomography (CT)*. https://www.itnonline.com/article/impact-artificial-intelligence-ct-imaging
9. Weissman, J. L., & Carrau, R. L. (2001). Puffed-cheek. *CT Improves Evaluation of the Oral Cavity American Journal of Neuroradiology, 22*, 741–744.
10. MD Anderson Cancer Centre (2021). *Cancer treatment algorithm*. Head and Neck Cancer—Oral Cancer. https://www.mdanderson.org/for-physicians/clinical-toolsresources/clinical-practice-algorithms/cancer-treatment-algorithms.html, 28/08/2021.
11. Katsari, K., Penna, D., Arena, V., et al. (2021). Artificial intelligence for reduced dose 18F-FDG PET examinations: A real-world deployment through a standardized framework and business case assessment. *EJNMMI, 8*, 25.
12. Chen, Y. K., Su, C. T., Ding, H. J., et al. (2006). Clinical usefulness of fused PET/CT compared with PET alone or CT alone in nasopharyngeal carcinoma patients. *Anticancer Research, 26*, 1471–1478.
13. Ke, L., Deng, Y., Xia, W. et al. (2020). Development of a self-constrained 3D DenseNet model in automatic detection and segmentation of nasopharyngeal carcinoma using magnetic resonance images. *Oral Oncology, 110*, 104862.
14. Levine, B., Nielsen, E. W. (2017). The justifications and controversies of panendoscopy—A review. *Review of Ear, Nose and Throat Journal, 71(8)*, 335–340, 343.
15. Han, X. (2017). MR-based synthetic CT generation using a deep convolutional neural network method. *Medical Physics, 44*, 1408–1419.
16. Li, C., Jing, B., Ke, L., et al. (2018). Development and validation of an endoscopic images-based deep learning model for detection with nasopharyngeal malignancies. *Cancer Communication (London), 2018*(38), 59.

17. Fu, Q., Chen, Y., Li, Z., et al. (2020). A deep learning algorithm for detection of oral cavity squamous cell carcinoma from photographic images: A retrospective study. *ECinicalMedicine, 27*.
18. Nayak, G. S., Kamath, S., Pai, K. M., et al. (2006). Principal component analysis and artificial neural network analysis of oral tissue fluorescence spectra: Classification of normal premalignant and malignant pathological conditions. *Biopolymers, 82*, 152–166.
19. Rosma, M. D., Sameem, A. K., Basir, A., et al. (2010). The use of artificial intelligence to identify people at risk of oral cancer: Empirical evidence in Malaysian University. *International Journal of Science and Research Education, 3*, 10–20.
20. Tseng, W. T., Chiang, W. F., Liu, S. Y., et al. (2015). The application of data mining techniques to oral cancer prognosis. *Journal of Medical Systems, 39*, 59–66.
21. Uthoff, R. D., Song, B., Sunny, S., et al. (2018). Point-of-care, smartphone-based, dual-modality, dual-view, oral cancer screening device with neural network classification for low-resource communities. *PLoS ONE, 13*, 1–21.
22. Shams, W. K., & Htike, Z. Z. (2017). Oral cancer prediction using gene expression profiling and machine learning. *International Journal of Applied Engineering Research, 12*, 4893–4898.
23. Aubreville, M., Knipfer, C., Oetter, N., et al. (2017). Automatic classification of cancerous tissue in laser endomicroscopy images of the oral cavity using deep learning. *Science and Reports, 7*, 11979.
24. Das, D. K., Bose, S., Maiti, A. K., et al. (2018). Automatic identification of clinically relevant regions from oral tissue histological images for oral squamous cell carcinoma diagnosis. *Tissue and Cell, 53*, 111–119.
25. Song, B., Sunny, S., Uthoff, R. D., et al. (2018). Automatic classification of dual-modality, smartphone-based oral dysplasia and malignancy images using deep learning. *Biomedical Optics Express, 9*, 5318.
26. Jeyaraj, P. R., & Samuel Nadar, E. R. (2019). Computer-assisted medical image classification for early diagnosis of oral cancer employing deep learning algorithm. *Journal of Cancer Research and Clinical Oncology, 145*, 829–837.
27. Rathod, J., Sherkay, S., Bondre, H., et al. (2020). Oral cancer detection and level classification through machine learning. *International Journal of Advanced Research in Computer and Communication Engineering, 9*, 177–182.
28. Alabi, R. O., Elmusrati, M., Sawazaki-Calone, I., et al. (2020). Comparison of supervised machine learning classification techniques in prediction of locoregional recurrences in early oral tongue cancer. *International Journal of Medical Informatics, 136*(1040), 68.
29. Karadaghy, O. A., Shew, M., New, J., et al. (2019). Development and assessment of a machine learning model to help predict survival among patients with oral squamous cell carcinoma. *JAMA Otolaryngology. Head & Neck Surgery, 145*, 1115–1120.
30. Sunny, S., Baby, A., James, B. L., et al. (2019). A smart tele-cytology point-of-care platform for oral cancer screening. *PLoS One, 14*, 1–16.
31. Kim, D. W., Lee, S., Kwon, S., et al. (2019). Deep learning based survival prediction of oral cancer patients. *Science and Reports, 9*, 6994.
32. Yan, H., Yu, M., Xia, J., et al. (2019). Tongue squamous cell carcinoma discrimination with Raman spectroscopy and convolutional neural networks. *Vibrational Spectroscopy, 103*, 102938.
33. Yu, M., Yan, H., Xia, J., et al. (2019). Deep convolutional neural networks for tongue squamous cell carcinoma classification using Raman spectroscopy. *Photodiagnosis and Photodynamic Therapy, 26*, 430–435.
34. Chan, C.-H., Huang, T.-T., Chen, C.-Y., et al. (2019). Texture-map-based branch-collaborative network for oral cancer detection. *IEEE Transactions on Biomedical Circuits and Systems, 13*, 766–780.
35. Horie, Y., Yoshio, T., Aoyama, K., et al. (2019). Diagnostic outcomes of esophageal cancer by artificial intelligence using convolutional neural networks. *Gastrointestinal Endoscopy, 89*, 25–32.

36. Das, D. K., Koley, S., Bose, S., et al. (2019). Computer aided tool for automatic detection and delineation of nucleus from oral histopathology images for OSCC screening. *Applied Soft Computing, 83*, 105642.
37. Shaban, M., Khurram, S. A., Fraz, M. M., et al. (2019). A novel digital score for abundance of tumour infiltrating lymphocytes predicts disease free survival in oral squamous cell carcinoma. *Science and Reports, 9*, 13341.
38. Tamashiro, A., Yoshio, T., Ishiyama, A., et al. (2020). Artificial-intelligence based detection of pharyngeal cancer using convolutional neural networks. *Digestive Endoscopy, 32*, 1057–1065.
39. Panigrahi, S., Das, J., Swarnkar, T. (2020). Capsule network based analysis of histopathological images of oral squamous cell carcinoma. *Journal of Kingdom Saudi Arabia University Computer Information Science*, 1–8.https://doi.org/10.1016/j.jksuci.2020.11.003
40. Kouznetsova, V. L., Li, J., Romm, E., et al. (2020). Finding distinctions between oral cancer and periodontitis using saliva metabolites and machine learning. *Oral Diseases, 27*, 484–493.
41. Alhazmi, A., Alhazmi, Y., Makrami, M. A. et al. (2020). Application of artificial intelligence and machine learning for prediction of oral cancer risk. *Journal of Oral Pathology Medicine, 50*, 444–450.
42. Jubair, F., Al-karadsheh, O., Malamos, D., et al. (2021). A novel lightweight deep convolutional neural network for early detection of oral cancer. *Oral Disease*, 1–8.
43. Ariji, Y., Sugita, Y., Nagao, T., et al. (2020). CT evaluation of extranodal extension of cervical lymph node metastases in patients with oral squamous cell carcinoma using deep learning classification. *Oral Radiology, 36*, 148–155.
44. Xia, J., Zhu, L., Yu, M., et al. (2020). Analysis and classification of oral tongue squamous cell carcinoma based on Raman spectroscopy and convolution neural networks. *Journal of Modern Optics, 67*, 481–489.
45. Fujima, N., Andreu-Arasa, V. C., Meibom, S. K., et al. (2020). Deep learning analysis using FDG-PET to predict treatment outcome in patients with oral cavity squamous cell carcinoma. *European Radiology, 30*, 6322–6330.
46. Fu, Q., Chen, Y., Li, Z., et al. (2020). A deep learning algorithm for detection of oral cavity squamous cell carcinoma from photographic images: A retrospective study. *EClinicalMedicine, 27*, 100558.
47. Ding, J., Yu, M., Zhu, L., et al. (2020). Diverse spectral band-based deep residual network for tongue squamous cell carcinoma classification using fiber optic Raman spectroscopy. *Photodiagnosis and Photodynmic Therapy, 32*, 102048.
48. Das, N., Hussain, E., Mahanta, L. B. Automated classification of cells into multiple classes in epithelial tissue of oral squamous cell carcinoma using transfer learning and convolutional neural network. *Neural Networks, 128*, 47–60.
49. Musulin, J., Štifanić, D., Zulijani, A., et al. (2021). An enhanced histopathology analysis: An ai-based system for multiclass grading of oral squamous cell carcinoma and segmenting of epithelial and stromal tissue. *Cancers, 13*, 1784.
50. Kirubabai, M. P., & Arumugam, G. (2021). View of deep learning classification method to detect and diagnose the cancer regions in oral MRI Images. *Medico Legal Update, 21*, 462–468.
51. Chu, C. S., Lee, N. P., Adeoye, J., et al. (2020). Machine learning and treatment outcome prediction for oral cancer. *Journal of Oral Pathology and Medicine, 49*, 977–985.
52. Welikala, R. A., Remagnino, P., Lim, J. H., et al. (2020). Automated detection and classification of oral lesions using deep learning for early detection of oral cancer. *IEEE Access, 8*, 132677–132693.
53. Paderno, A., Piazza, C., Del Bon, F., et al. (2021). Deep learning for automatic segmentation of oral and oropharyngeal cancer using narrow band imaging: Preliminary experience in a clinical perspective. *Frontier Oncology, 11*, 626602.
54. Tomita, H., Yamashiro, T., Heianna, J., et al. (2021). Deep learning for the preoperative diagnosis of metastatic cervical lymph nodes on contrast-enhanced computed tomography in patients with oral squamous cell carcinoma. *Cancers, 13*, 600.
55. Nanditha, B. R., Geetha Kiran, A., Chandrashekar, H. S., Dinesh, M. S., Murali, S. An ensemble deep neural network approach for oral cancer screening. *International Journal of Online Biomedical Engineering IJOE, 17*, 1–14.

56. Musulin, J., Štifanic, D., Zulijani, A., et al. (2021). An enhanced ´ histopathology analysis: An Ai-based system for multiclass grading of oral squamous cell carcinoma and segmenting of epithelial and stromal tissue. *Cancers, 13*, 1784.
57. Trajanovski, S., Shan, C., Weijtmans, P. J. C., et al. (2021). Tongue tumor detection in hyper-spectral images using deep learning semantic segmentation. *IEEE Transactions on Biomedical Engineering, 68*, 1330–1340.
58. Williams, A. M., Liu, Y., et al. (2018). Artificial intelligence, physiological genomics, and precision medicine. *Physiological Genomics, 50*, 237–243.
59. Xu, J., Yang, P., Xue, S., et al. (2019). Translating cancer genomics into precision medicine with artificial intelligence: applications, challenges and future perspectives. *Human Genetics, 138*, 109–124.
60. Jabeen, A., Ahmad, N., & Raza, K. (2018). Machine learning-based state-of-the-art methods for the classification of RNA-seq data. In N. Dey, A. Ashour & S. Borra (Eds.), *Classification in BioApps*. Lecture Notes in Computational Vision and Biomechanics (Vol. 26, pp. 133–172). Springer.
61. Wakai, T., Prasoon, P., Hirose, Y., et al. (2019). Next-generation sequencing-based clinical sequencing: Toward precision medicine in solid tumors. *International Journal of Clinical Oncology, 24*, 115–122.
62. Ang, M. Y., Low, T. Y., Lee, P. Y., et al. (2019). Proteogenomics: From next-generation sequencing (NGS) and mass spectrometry based proteomics to precision medicine *Clinica Chimica Acta, 498*, 38–46.
63. Mahmood, H., Shaban, M., Rajpoot, N., et al. (2021). Artificial intelligence-based methods in head and neck cancer diagnosis: An overview. *British Journal of Cancer., 124*, 1934–1940.
64. Kim, Y., Kang, J. W., Kang, J., et al. (2021). Novel deep learning-based survival prediction for oral cancer by analyzing tumor infiltrating lymphocyte profiles through CIBERSORT. *OncoImmunology, 10*, 1904573.
65. Epstein, B. J., Sciubba, J. J. (2010). Strategies for oral cancer detection. In *Early diagnosis and treatment of cancer series: Head and neck cancers* (pp. 45–58).
66. Kevin, B., Johnson, W.-Q. W., Weeraratne, D., Frisse, M. E., Misulis, K., Rhee, K., Zhao, J., Snowdon, J. L. (2020). Precision Medicine, AI, and the Future of Personalized Health Care 2020. https://doi.org/10.1111/cts.12884

Fuzzy Logic-Based Hybrid Models for Clinical Decision Support Systems in Cancer

Sahar Qazi, Naiyar Iqbal, and Khalid Raza

Abstract With the advent of *artificial intelligence in medicine* (AIM) many severe diseases are now being successfully diagnosed at the earliest with an efficient and accurate prognosis and treatment strategy. Expert intelligent systems such as—fuzzy logic systems, artificial neural networks, evolutionary algorithms, and their hybrid models have become essential for developing decision support systems. Clinical decision support systems (CDSS) are intelligent expert systems that are devised to aid consultants in taking crucial decisions. The deployment of the fuzzy logic systems and their hybrid models have proved to be highly influential in myriad global approximations of the disease progression and affected regions with greater applications in developing a person-centric treatment. There are several hybrid algorithms such as neuro-fuzzy systems, or adaptive genetic algorithms with fuzzy logic models that have been previously deployed for developing a clinical decision support system for oncology, psychiatric and cardiac-based diseases. This chapter highlights the potential of fuzzy logic systems and their hybrid intelligent models to develop CDSS in various cancers, including its limitations and future prospects.

Keywords Artificial intelligence in medicine · Artificial neural network · Clinical decision support system · Evolutionary algorithm · Fuzzy logic system · Hybrid system

Abbreviations

AGAF	Adaptive Genetic Algorithms with Fuzzy logic
AHP	Analytic Hierarchy Process
AIM	Artificial Intelligence in Medicine

S. Qazi · K. Raza (✉)
Department of Computer Science, Jamia Millia Islamia, New Delhi, India
e-mail: kraza@jmi.ac.in

N. Iqbal
Department of Computer Science and IT, Maulana Azad National Urdu University, Hyderabad, India

K. Raza (ed.), *Computational Intelligence in Oncology*, Studies in Computational Intelligence 1016, https://doi.org/10.1007/978-981-16-9221-5_12

ANFIS	Adaptive Neuro-Fuzzy Inference System
ANN	Artificial Neural Network
CDSS	Clinical Decision Support System
CIS	Computational Intelligent System
CNN	Convolutional Neural Network
DEMATE	Decision-Making Trial and Evaluation Laboratory
FCM	Fuzzy Cognitive Maps
FGA	Fuzzy Genetic Algorithms
FLS	Fuzzy Logic Systems
FMULTIMOORA	Fuzzy Multi-Objective Optimization on the basis of a Ratio Analysis
HNFS	Hybrid Neuro-Fuzzy Logic Systems
MCDM	Multi-Criteria Decision-Making
SWARA	Step-wise Weight Assessment Ratio Analysis
YOLO	You Only Look Once

1 Introduction

Clinical decision support systems (CDSS) are intelligent expert systems that are devised to aid consultants in taking crucial decisions. The main objective of CDSS is to provide better and robust healthcare decision-making, resulting in improved person-centric care [1]. Since the past decade, CDSS have been observed as an application of the advent of *artificial intelligence in medicine* (AIM) [2, 3]. For instance, the expert systems based on logical rules [4], learning theory-based models that can give more rational reasoning [5], fuzzy logic models, probabilistic methods-based networks like the Bayesian networks, artificial neural networks (ANNs), self-organizing maps (SOMs), etc. [6]. Fuzzy logic (FL) was first described by Zadeh in [7] and gave a concept of fuzzy logic sets [7]. This concept is used to make difficult, non-numerical, and imprecise (therefore the term—*Fuzzy*) information easy to understand, interpret, and representable.

The deployment of the fuzzy logic systems (FLS) and their hybrid models have proved to be highly influential in myriad global approximations of the disease progression and affected regions with greater applications in developing a person-centric treatment [8]. A fuzzy logic-based clinical decision support system (CDSS) was developed by Kunhimangalam et al. for early detection of peripheral neuropathy wherein the model used 24 input entries that combined the symptoms and pathological examination results. Their model had a 93% accuracy when compared to other existing expert systems [9]. A multi-layered Mamdani fuzzy inference system (ML-MFIS) has been deployed for diagnosing hepatitis B that categorizes the disease into three subtypes, namely normal, severe, and chronic [10]. The model was assessed using statistical methods based on system accuracy, specificity, and sensitivity and was recorded to be as 95.24%, 91.7%, and 96.17%, respectively. The research group discerned that an expert system like ML-MFIS could be deployed as an initial diagnosis approach in case of hepatitis. Another study executed by Hashmia and Khan discerns that a fuzzy control model (FCM) is suitable for diagnosing liver-based diseases in humans. Their research work was wrapped up by a 1.8% relative error in the simulated and calculated values [11]. A similar study carried out by Satarkar [12] was based on developing a fuzzy expert system for rectifying cirrhosis which was based on the sequential combination of the Bononcini score encapsulating aspartate transaminase (AST), alanine transaminase (ALT) ratio, platelet count, and international normalized ratio (INR). Their results showcased that the fuzzy-based system had provided an excellent performance in diagnosing the disease. Very similarly, there are several hybrid algorithms such as neuro-fuzzy systems, or adaptive genetic algorithms with fuzzy logic (AGAFL) models that have been previously deployed for developing a clinical decision support system for oncology, psychiatric and cardiac-based diseases [13]. Figure 1 highlights the potential of the amalgamation of fuzzy expert systems and their hybrids, consecutively termed as—computational intelligent systems and medical expertise and knowledge, that provides (a) holistic medic care to patients, (b) early screening, detection, and diagnosis of the disease, and (c) personalized treatment approaches for the patients.

This chapter highlights the potential of fuzzy logic systems and their hybrid intelligent models such as Decision-Making Trial and Evaluation Laboratory (DEMATEL), Fuzzy Cognitive Maps (FCM), Hybrid Neuro-Fuzzy Logic Systems (HNFS), Fuzzy Genetic Algorithms (FGA), etc. Since fuzzy logic systems have been tagged to simplify imprecise, non-numerical, and practically difficult problems to be represented, recognized, and interpret easily, along with the possibility of adaptive learning

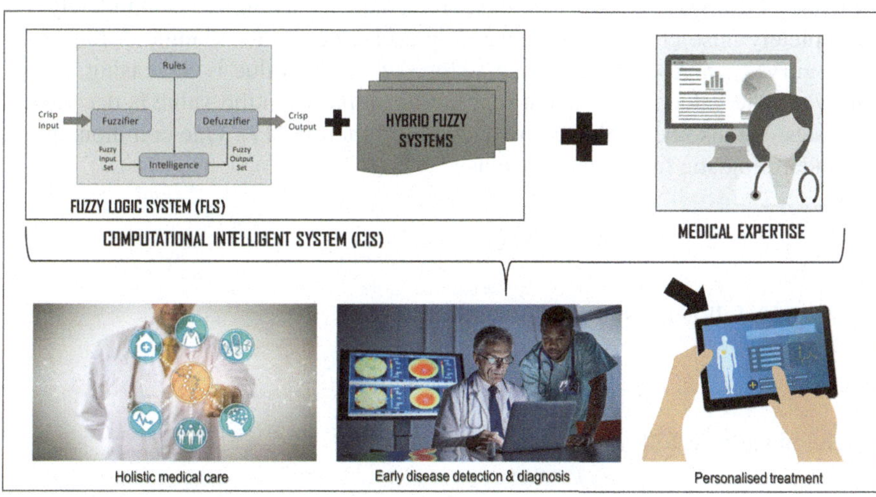

Fig. 1 The potential of fuzzy logic-based systems and medical expertise in providing a better and robust CDSS

properties, fuzzy logic systems, and hybrid models are the first choice of clinical practitioners in selecting them as clinical decision support systems (CDSS). They also allow depicting solutions in easy decision trees format too [8].

With the magnanimous amount of growing research evidence, drug development, prognostic marker identification, and discovery in cancers, the medical fraternity have opened their arms for computational intelligent expert systems so that they can help medical practitioners and staff in synthesizing the big medical data and also in guiding them regarding the final clinical decision. This chapter highlights the potential applications of fuzzy logic-based hybrid models that are being successfully adopted by the medical fraternity as a CDSS.

2 Background of Fuzzy Logic

The term "*fuzzy logic*" was first introduced by Lotfi Zadeh in 1965, however, the concept was studied back then in the early 1920s by Łukasiewicz and Tarski which was then referred to as—infinite valued logic [14]. Generally, fuzzy logic has been viewed differently by different people. Some researchers believe it is simply a way of disagreeing with the Western concept of having white and black thinking and highlighting the grey area too. While, for others, it is another way of lucidly describing our ordinary language not just as true or false, but in a more realistic manner [15]. Therefore, in terms of logic, fuzzy logic can be defined as a form of many-valued logic wherein the correct value of components may be any real number between 0 and 1. Since it deals with realistic values and not crisp values, it is deployed to tackle partial truth situations where the correct values may either be completely true or completely false [16]. Fuzzy sets are represented as either triangle or trapezoid-shaped curves where each value has a slope when the value is increasing, a peak point when the value is equivalent to 1, and a slope when the value is decreasing. Fuzzy sets can also be explained by a sigmoid function [17]. One common case is the standard logistic function defined as:

$$S(x) = \frac{1}{1 + e^{-x}}$$

having the following symmetry feature:

$$S(x) + S(-x) = 1$$

Here onwards, it follows the following rule:

$$(S(x) + S(-x)) \cdot (S(y) + S(-y)) \cdot (S(z) + S(-z)) = 1$$

Because of such aptness, the concept of fuzzy logic systems has been combined with existing artificial intelligent systems such as—neural networks, support vector machines (SVM), self-organizing maps (SOM), convolutional networks, and other deep learning models to support myriad medical and biological problems. One such rapidly growing sector is in clinical decision support systems. The common fuzzy logic-based hybrid models encapsulate—ANNs and fuzzy logic systems termed as *Neuro-Fuzzy* systems that have helped in enhanced pattern recognition efficiency [18], while another fusion of rule-based reasoning (RBR) and fuzzy logic has been deployed to predict the prioritization of patients as per consultant's views along with the emergency severity index (ESI) guidelines [19]. A fuzzy-based model named—*Intuitionistic fuzzy cognitive map* (iFCM) viz., an extension of a *fuzzy cognitive map* (FCM), helps in enhancing the manual screening of medical experts to predict the severity of disease [20]. Another hybrid model was developed by combining a *type-2 fuzzy logic* algorithm and the high-performance computing (HPC) cognitive aspects that can be easily deployed on medical big data to generate reliable prediction models along with accurate clinical decision systems for hospitals [21].

Evolutionary algorithms have also been combined with fuzzy logic systems, one of such fusions has resulted in an *Adaptive genetic algorithm with fuzzy logic* (AGAFL) model that has been proven to be effective in predicting the risk of cardiovascular diseases in their initial stages. This system has helped medical consultants in making a good and robust prognosis of the same [13].

3 Related Work

The application of fuzzy logic in CDSS is not new. Fuzzy logic along with its various hybrids has been extensively applied in CDSS, but poorly used in cancer. Kunhimangalam and collaborators [22] designed a novel CDSS with the integration of Electronic Medical Record (EMR) for Peripheral Neuropathy diagnosis. They applied the fuzzy experts' system that comes with a 93.7% accuracy rate. Nguyen and collaborator [23] proposed a fuzzy standard additive model (FSAM) based modified analytic hierarchy process (AHP). They used a gene microarray dataset for cancer classification using gene selection to diagnose diffuse large B-cell lymphoma (DLBCL), and leukemia and other diseases. They observed the dominance outcome of the proposed model over single ranking methods. Further, Uzoka and others [24] proposed a framework based on the fuzzy AHP (FAHP) for malaria disease prediction which showcases satisfactory outcomes. In their experiment, they found a better correlation between the Fuzzy system and the AHP method with 82.2%. El-Sappagh and collaborators [25] introduced a CDSS for the diagnosis of Hepatitis C for liver fibrosis. They applied hybridization of the fuzzy analytical hierarchy process (FAHP) and an adaptive neuro-fuzzy inference system (ANFIS) for the implementation of the CDSS. The system yields a good accuracy outcome with 93.3% for identification of Hepatitis C.

A hybrid of Rule-Based Reasoning (RBR) and Fuzzy Logic Classifier (FLC) for the prediction of triage level of patients have been proposed in [26]. From their analysis, this fuzzy-based hybrid system provides the highest rate of accuracy 99.44%.

Eghbali-Zarch et al. [27] presented a fuzzy Multi-Criteria Decision-Making (MCDM) system which combines a Step-wise Weight Assessment Ratio Analysis (SWARA) method with a modification of Fuzzy Multi-Objective Optimization Based on a Ratio Analysis and full multiplicative form (FMULTIMOORA) system for pharmacological therapy selection of Type 2 diabetes. Their results showcase close correspondence with other MCDM techniques fuzzy TOP-SIS, fuzzy VIKOR, and fuzzy SAW. An Adaptive Neuro-fuzzy Inference System (ANFIS) for the diagnosis of a social anxiety disorder (SAD), one of the critical mental disorders reported by WHO (World Health Organization), has been proposed in [28] that utilizes necessary preprocessing, normalization, feature selection, and anomaly identification based on SOM clustering technique. The outcome of their analysis found an accuracy of 98.67%, with sensitivity, and specificity of 97.14%, and 100%, respectively.

Colorectal Cancer (CRC), one of the most prevalent digestive system-related cancer, detection using computational intelligence-based approaches may significantly enhance the overall survival probability of patients. A fuzzy logic-based CDSS (FL-CDSS) was proposed by Nopour and collaborator [29] for the early detection of CRC where a C4.5 decision tree was applied to extract rules and FL-CDSS was implemented in MATLAB computing environment. It yielded an accuracy of 96%, with specificity and sensitivity of 97%, and 96%, respectively [29]. An FL-based method for the categorization of breast cancer was developed in [30], where a fuzzy inference system following the Fuzzy Omega algorithm for membership function generation was utilized. The method achieves a classification accuracy of 83.34%.

Melanoma, a kind of skin cancer, develops due to damage of melanocyte cells by excessive exposure to harmful UV radiation. Melanoma is more hazardous than other types of skin cancer because it quickly metastasizes if remained undetected and untreated at an early stage [31, 32]. The diagnosis of Melanoma could be perplexing and usually carried out based on histopathological and clinical features. A deep convolutional neural network (CNN)-based algorithm, called You Only Look Once (YOLO), was proposed to diagnose Melanoma from dermoscopic and digital images [33]. The YOLO algorithm, during the feature extraction process, infuses two-phase segmentation by using a blend of graph theory (minimal spanning tree), and L-type fuzzy-based approximations and extraction of the affected region of the lesion. YOLO reported achieving Jac scores of 79.84%, 86.99%, and 88.64% on ISIC 2019, ISBI 2017, and PH2 datasets, respectively [33].

The diagnosis of gastric cancer is difficult, as there is no systematic approach for its early diagnosis [34]. Safdari et al. [35] developed a fuzzy expert system to identify the risk levels of gastric cancer that utilizes the Mamdani inference technique and extracted a total of 67 fuzzy rules. The result achieves sensitivity and specificity of 92.1% and 83.1%, respectively. To estimate the risk of lung cancer and the effect of stress level on cancer, a neuro-fuzzy model has been proposed by Yilmaz et al. [36]. The model yields a prediction accuracy of 94.64%, while the accuracy of effects of stress was found to be 95.75%. The proposed system forms a pre-diagnosis tool for assessing the risk of getting cancer due to poor living styles, or working conditions, and also facilitates taking necessary precautions to avert the risk of cancer. To approximate the oxidation stress-related cancer risk of oral malignant disorders, a multi-criteria CDSS was developed based on serum malondialdehyde and proton donors' values using a fuzzy logic method [37]. It inferred 25 if–then rules and risk was estimated as numeric values on a 1 to 10 scale. The method may be integrated into a more complex computer-aided CDSS to aid in oral cancer- screening [37].

For the implementation of these systems, a database is one of the important resources for model development. Therefore, various prominent databases are available as an open accessed form such as NCBI-Sequence Read Archive (SRA), NCBI-Gene Expression Omnibus (GEO), ArrayExpress, and The Cancer Genome Atlas (TCGA).

A summary of FL-based hybrid approaches for CDSS in cancers has been presented in Table 1. Accuracy is one of the performance metrics of a machine learning-based confusion matrix that gives the percentage of correctly classified samples. Sensitivity calculates the proportion of predicted positive samples to the total actually positive samples. Specificity comes with predicted negative samples to the total actually negative samples.

4 Limitations of FL-Based CDSS

Since the past decade, computational biologists have employed and combined various FL-based systems with other existing machine learning algorithms and AI systems to improve CDSS. The accuracy, specificity, sensitivity, precision has been proved to be much better when compared to the traditional approaches i.e., manual checkup, screening, diagnosis, and prognosis of disease that is done by medical staff or consultant. Even with multitudinous applications in medical domains, practitioners with archaic or traditional approaches don't completely follow or adopt computational intelligent systems for clinical decisions for a particular disease or even for a second validation on their manual diagnosis. Lack of trust in computational intelligent systems and little or no awareness about their benefits is one of the apex limitations in medical settings.

Various other optimization and functionality problems are major problems in implementing fuzzy expert systems in CDSS. No expert intelligent system can provide exact solutions to complex medical problems, but they provide a direction to consultants and physicians in formulating a correct and plausible clinical decision to maladies.

Despite the above-mentioned limitations, there are other technical limitations of FL-based systems pointed out as follows [38]:

- The accuracy of fuzzy systems is sometimes compromised because it mostly works on imprecise inputs.
- FL-based systems are completely dependent on human knowledge and expertise.
- These systems need regular updation of rules.

Table 1 Application of fuzzy logic-based hybrid models in CDSS

Methods	Description	Disease	Evaluation (%)	References
Fuzzy expert system	A CDSS that integrates electronic medical records for peripheral neuropathy diagnosis	Peripheral neuropathy	Acc = 93.7	[22]
Fuzzy standard additive model-based modified analytic hierarchy process	Utilizes microarray dataset for gene selection to diagnose	Lymphoma, leukemia, and other diseases	Acc = 98 (Lymphoma) Acc = 97 (Leukemia)	[23]
Adaptive neuro-fuzzy inference system	A CDSS for the diagnosis of a social anxiety disorder	Social anxiety disorder	Acc = 98.67 Sn = 97.14 Sp = 100	[28]
Fuzzy logic-based CDSS (FL-CDSS)	A C4.5 decision tree was applied to extract rules, and FL-CDSS was implemented in MATLAB	Colorectal cancer	Acc = 96.0 Sn = 96.0 Sp = 97.0	[29]
Fuzzy inference system	Fuzzy inference system following Fuzzy Omega algorithm for membership function generation	Breast cancer	Acc = 83.34	[30]
YOLO	A deep CNN-based algorithm, called You Only Look Once (YOLO), that utilized two-phase segmentation and L-type fuzzy-based approximations during preprocessing and feature extraction	Skin cancer	Jac scores of 79.84%, 86.99%, and 88.64% on ISIC 2019, ISBI 2017, and PH2 datasets, respectively	[33]
Fuzzy expert system	Uses Mamdani inference technique, and extracted a total of 67 fuzzy rules	Gastric cancer	Sn = 92.1 Sp = 83.1	[35]
Neuro-fuzzy model	Model estimates estimate the risk of lung cancer and the effect of stress level on cancer	Lung cancer	Acc = 94.64 (prediction) Acc = 95.75 (effect of stress)	[36]

(continued)

Table 1 (continued)

Methods	Description	Disease	Evaluation (%)	References
Fuzzy logic	A multi-criteria CDSS based on serum malondialdehyde and proton donors' values	Oral cancer	Not available	[37]

Abbreviations Acc: Accuracy, Sn: Sensitivity, Sp: Specificity)

- It requires rigorous testing for the validation and verification of systems.
- Unlike neural systems, it can't perceive intelligence or recognize patterns.
- Lower speed and longer runtime for complex fuzzy systems.
- For designing a more accurate fuzzy system, more fuzzy grades are needed which would result in an exponential increase in the number of rules.
- Incapable to receive feedback for the implementation of the learning strategy.

5 Future Prospects of Fuzzy Logic Systems in CDSS

Recent growth and expansion in computational intelligent systems have paved a way for rich analytical expert systems that hold the potential to correctly detect cancers and other malignancies when compared to traditional statistical and manual diagnosis ones [30, 39, 40]. FL-based systems are highly deployed in clinical decisions because they can handle uncertainty, make approximate and precise decisions, and can tackle vague data easily. Moreover, this expert system is highly flexible and can be compiled in any computational language easily. In contrast to Boolean logic, fuzzy logic systems provide approximate reasoning to uncertain linguistic variables, therefore, making it a more human-like expert system [36, 41, 42]. There are multitudinous prospects for the future of FL-based systems for dealing with complex biomedical problems where there are doubts and where consultants cannot formulate a well medical decision. These intelligent expert systems give a variety of applications for best practices in medical infrastructure [43, 44].

Various fuzzy logic-based open and free software have been released in the past years that can perform simulations, predict outputs and help in giving an accurate clinical decision for a disease. In a recent study, the fuzzy logic system was used to classify and give a decision of diabetic retinopathy [45]. They used the MATLAB package named—Fuzzy-Calc which is the first package to compute fuzzy indicators with the aim to retrieve a synthetic performance value for the study variables of interest, while MATLAB fuzzy logic toolbox was deployed was used to compare the ultrasonography reports and decision outputs. Their study was able to give optimized medical classifications of diabetic retinopathy patients that were compared with ultrasonography reports that helped medical consultants to formulate an efficient prognosis.

6 Conclusion

The CDSS is intelligent expert system that is devised to aid consultants in taking crucial decisions. The main objective is to provide better and robust healthcare decision-making, resulting in improved person-centric care. Since the past decade, CDSS has been observed as an application of the advent of AIM. The deployment of the fuzzy logic systems and their hybrid models have proved to be highly influential in myriad global approximations of the disease progression and affected regions with greater applications in developing a person-centric treatment. FL-based systems are highly deployed in clinical decisions because they can handle uncertainty, make approximate and precise decisions, and can tackle vague data easily. Moreover, this expert system is highly flexible and can be compiled in any computational language easily.

Acknowledgements SQ is supported by the DST-INSPIRE fellowship provided by the Department of Science and Technology, Govt. of India. NI is supported by the UGC-NFOBC Fellowship provided by the University Grant Commission, Govt. of India.

Conflict of Interest None.

References

1. Osheroff, J. A., Teich, J., Levick, D., Saldana, L., Velasco, F., Sittig, D., Rogers, K., & Jenders, R. (2021). Improving outcomes with clinical decision support. https://doi.org/10.4324/9780367806125
2. Steels, L., & Lopez de Mantaras, R. (2018). The Barcelona declaration for the proper development and usage of artificial intelligence in Europe. *AI Communications, 31*(6), 485–494. https://doi.org/10.3233/aic-180607
3. Qazi, S., Raza, K., & Iqbal, N. (2021). 5 artificial intelligence in medicine (AIM): Machine learning in cancer diagnosis, prognosis and therapy. In D. Gupta, U. Kose, B. Le Nguyen & S. Bhattacharyya (Eds.), *Artificial intelligence for data-driven medical diagnosis* (pp. 103–126). De Gruyter. https://doi.org/10.1515/9783110668322-005
4. Kulikowski, C. A, Weiss, S. M., &Szolovits, P. (1982). Representation of expert knowledge for consultation: The CASNET and EXPERT projects chapter 2. In *Artificial intelligence in medicine*. Westview Press.
5. Hatzilygeroudis, I., & Prentzas, J. (2004). Integrating (rules, neural networks) and cases for knowledge representation and reasoning in expert systems. *Expert Systems with Applications, 27*(01), 63–75.
6. Montani, S., & Striani, M. (2019). Artificial intelligence in clinical decision support: A focused literature survey. *Yearbook of Medical Informatics, 28*(01), 120–127. https://doi.org/10.1055/s-0039-1677911
7. Zadeh, L. A. (1965). Fuzzy sets. *Information and Control [Internet], 8*(3), 338–353. Available from https://www.sciencedirect.com/science/article/pii/S001999586590241X?via%3Dihub
8. Cintula, P., Fermüller, C. G., & Noguera, C. (2016). Fuzzy logic (Stanford encyclopedia of philosophy) [Internet]. Stanford.edu. 2016. Available from https://plato.stanford.edu/entries/logic-fuzzy/

9. Kunhimangalam, R., Ovallath, S., & Joseph, P. K. (2014). A clinical decision support system with an integrated EMR for diagnosis of peripheral neuropathy. *Journal of Medical Systems, 38*(4), 1–4.
10. Ahmad, G., Khan, M. A., Abbas, S., Athar, A., Khan, B. S., & Aslam, M. S. (2019). Automated diagnosis of hepatitis B using multilayer mamdani fuzzy inference system. *Journal of Healthcare Engineering, 2019*, 1–11. https://doi.org/10.1155/2019/6361318
11. Hashmia, A., & Khan, M. S. (2015). Diagnosis blood test for liver disease using fuzzy logic. *International Journal of Sciences: Basic and Applied Research, 20*, 151–183.
12. Satarkar, S. (2014). Fuzzy expert system for the diagnosis of common liver disease. *International Engineering Journal for Research & Development, 1*.
13. Reddy, G. T., Reddy, M. P. K., Lakshmanna, K., Rajput, D. S., Kaluri, R., & Srivastava, G. (2019). Hybrid genetic algorithm and a fuzzy logic classifier for heart disease diagnosis. *Evolutionary Intelligence, 13*(2), 185–196. https://doi.org/10.1007/s12065-019-00327-1
14. Zadeh, L. A. (1965). Fuzzy sets. *Information and Control, 8*(3), 338–353. https://doi.org/10.1016/s0019-9958(65)90241-x
15. Pelletier, F. J. (2000). Petr Hájek. Metamathematics of fuzzy logic. Trends in logic, vol. 4. Kluwer Academic Publishers, Dordrecht, Boston, and London, 1998, viii + 297 pp. *Bulletin of Symbolic Logic, 6*(3), 342–346. https://doi.org/10.2307/421060
16. Zadeh, L. A., et al. (1996). *Fuzzy sets, fuzzy logic, fuzzy systems*. World Scientific Press. ISBN 978-981-02-2421-9.
17. Wierman, M. (2010). An introduction to the mathematics of uncertainty including set theory, logic, probability, fuzzy sets, rough sets, and evidence theory honors program [Internet]. 2010. Available from https://www.creighton.edu/fileadmin/user/CCAS/programs/fuzzy_math/docs/MOU.pdf
18. Vlamou, E., & Papadopoulos, B. (2019). Fuzzy logic systems and medical applications. *AIMS Neuroscience, 6*(4), 266–272. https://doi.org/10.3934/Neuroscience.2019.4.266
19. Dehghani Soufi, M., Samad-Soltani, T., Shams Vahdati, S., & Rezaei-Hachesu, P. (2018). Decision support system for triage management: A hybrid approach using rule-based reasoning and fuzzy logic. *International Journal of Medical Informatics, 114*, 35–44. https://doi.org/10.1016/j.ijmedinf.2018.03.008
20. Iakovidis, D. K., & Papageorgiou, E. (2011). Intuitionistic fuzzy cognitive maps for medical decision making. *IEEE Transactions on Information Technology in Biomedicine, 15*(1), 100–107. https://doi.org/10.1109/titb.2010.2093603
21. Benchara, F. Z., & Youssfi, M. (2020). A new distributed type-2 fuzzy logic method for efficient data science models of medical informatics. *Advances in Fuzzy Systems, 2020*, 1–10. https://doi.org/10.1155/2020/6539123
22. Kunhimangalam, R., Ovallath, S., & Joseph, P. K. (2014). A clinical decision support system with an integrated EMR for diagnosis of peripheral neuropathy. *Journal of Medical Systems, 38*(4), 1–14. https://doi.org/10.1007/s10916-014-0038-9
23. Nguyen, T., Khosravi, A., Creighton, D., & Nahavandi, S. (2015). Hierarchical gene selection and genetic fuzzy system for cancer microarray data classification. *PloS One, 10*(3), e0120364. https://doi.org/10.1371/journal.pone.0120364
24. Uzoka, F. M. E., Osuji, J., & Obot, O. (2011). Clinical decision support system (DSS) in the diagnosis of malaria: A case comparison of two soft computing methodologies. *Expert Systems with Applications, 38*(3), 1537–1553. https://doi.org/10.1016/j.eswa.2010.07.068
25. El-Sappagh, S., Ali, F., Ali, A., Hendawi, A., Badria, F. A., & Suh, D. Y. (2018). Clinical decision support system for liver fibrosis prediction in hepatitis patients: A case comparison of two soft computing techniques. *IEEE Access, 6*, 52911–52929. https://doi.org/10.1109/ACCESS.2018.2868802
26. Soufi, M. D., Samad-Soltani, T., Vahdati, S. S., & Rezaei-Hachesu, P. (2018). Decision support system for triage management: A hybrid approach using rule-based reasoning and fuzzy logic. *International Journal of Medical Informatics, 114*, 35–44. https://doi.org/10.1016/j.ijmedinf.2018.03.008

27. Eghbali-Zarch, M., Tavakkoli-Moghaddam, R., Esfahanian, F., Sepehri, M. M., & Azaron, A. (2018). Pharmacological therapy selection of type 2 diabetes based on the SWARA and modified MULTIMOORA methods under a fuzzy environment. *Artificial Intelligence in Medicine, 87*, 20–33. https://doi.org/10.1016/j.artmed.2018.03.003
28. Fathi, S., Ahmadi, M., Birashk, B., & Dehnad, A. (2020). Development and use of a clinical decision support system for the diagnosis of social anxiety disorder. *Computer Methods and Programs in Biomedicine, 190*, 105354. https://doi.org/10.1016/j.cmpb.2020.105354
29. Nopour, R., Shanbehzadeh, M., & Kazemi-Arpanahi, H. (2021). Developing a clinical decision support system based on the fuzzy logic and decision tree to predict colorectal cancer. *Medical Journal of the Islamic Republic of Iran (MJIRI), 35*(1), 341–348.
30. Miranda, G. H., & Felipe, J. C. (2015). Computer-aided diagnosis system based on fuzzy logic for breast cancer categorization. *Computers in Biology and Medicine, 1*(64), 334–346.
31. Schadendorf, D., Fisher, D. E., Garbe, C., Gershenwald, J. E., Grob, J. J., Halpern, A., Herlyn, M., Marchetti, M. A., McArthur, G., Ribas, A., & Roesch, A. (2015). Melanoma. *Nature Reviews Disease Primers, 1*(1), 1–20.
32. Schadendorf, D., van Akkooi, A. C., Berking, C., Griewank, K. G., Gutzmer, R., Hauschild, A., Stang, A., Roesch, A., & Ugurel, S. (2018). Melanoma. *The Lancet, 392*(10151), 971–984.
33. Banerjee, S., Singh, S. K., Chakraborty, A., Das, A., & Bag, R. (2020). Melanoma diagnosis using deep learning and fuzzy logic. *Diagnostics, 10*(8), 577.
34. Miyaoka, M., Yao, K., Tanabe, H., Kanemitsu, T., Otsu, K., Imamura, K., Ono, Y., Ishikawa, S., Yasaka, T., Ueki, T., Ota, A., Haraoka, S., & Iwashita, A. (2020). Diagnosis of early gastric cancer using image enhanced endoscopy: A systematic approach. *Translational Gastroenterology and Hepatology, 5*, 50.
35. Safdari, R., Arpanahi, H. K., Langarizadeh, M., Ghazisaiedi, M., Dargahi, H., & Zendehdel, K. (2018). Design a fuzzy rule-based expert system to aid earlier diagnosis of gastric cancer. *Acta Informatica Medica, 26*(1), 19.
36. Yılmaz, A., Arı, S., & Kocabıçak, Ü. (2016). Risk analysis of lung cancer and effects of stress level on cancer risk through neuro-fuzzy model. *Computer Methods and Programs in Biomedicine, 1*(137), 35–46.
37. Scrobotă, I., Băciuț, G., Filip, A. G., Todor, B., Blaga, F., & Băciuț, M. F. (2017). Application of fuzzy logic in oral cancer risk assessment. *Iranian Journal of Public Health, 46*(5), 612.
38. Behrooz, F., Mariun, N., Marhaban, M. H., Mohd Radzi, M. A., & Ramli, A. R. (2018). Review of control techniques for HVAC systems—Nonlinearity approaches based on fuzzy cognitive maps. *Energies, 11*(3), 495.
39. Baitharu, T. R., & Pani, S. K. (2016). Analysis of data mining techniques for healthcare decision support system using liver disorder dataset. *Procedia Computer Science, 85*, 862–870. https://doi.org/10.1016/j.procs.2016.05.276
40. Vijayarani, S., & Dhayanand, S. (2015). Data mining classification algorithms for kidney disease prediction. *International Journal on Cybernetics & Informatics, 4*(4), 13–25. https://doi.org/10.5121/ijci.2015.4402
41. Wang, C. Y., Lee, T. F., Fang, C. H., & Chou, J. H. (2012). Fuzzy logic-based prognostic score for outcome prediction in esophageal cancer. *IEEE Transactions on Information Technology in Biomedicine, 16*(6), 1224–1230.
42. Raza, K. (2019). Fuzzy logic based approaches for gene regulatory network inference. *Artificial Intelligence in Medicine, 1*(97), 189–203.

43. Lualdi, M., Cavalleri, A., Battaglia, L., Colombo, A., Garrone, G., Morelli, D., Pignoli, E., Sottotetti, E., & Leo, E. (2018). Early detection of colorectal adenocarcinoma: a clinical decision support tool based on plasma porphyrin accumulation and risk factors. *BMC Cancer, 18*(1). https://doi.org/10.1186/s12885-018-4754-2
44. Hernández-Julio, Y. F., Prieto-Guevara, M. J., Nieto-Bernal, W., Meriño-Fuentes, I., & Guerrero-Avendaño, A. (2019). Framework for the development of data-driven Mamdani-type fuzzy clinical decision support systems. *Diagnostics, 9*(2), 52. https://doi.org/10.3390/diagnostics9020052
45. de Oliveira Andrade, L. J., Franca, C. S., Andrade, R., Bittencourt, A. M., de Oliveira, G. C. (2020). Fuzzy logic use in classification of the severity of diabetic retinopathy. medRxiv, 2020 Jan 1.

Predicting Cancer Biomarkers, Therapeutic Targets, Drug Response, and Drug Design, Discovery, and Development

Predicting Biomarkers and Therapeutic Targets in Cancer

Rina Ningthoujam, Naorem BidyaLeima Chanu, Vivek Anumala, Punuri Jayasekhar Babu, Srimay Pradhan, Manasa Kumar Panda, Punabati Heisnam, and Yengkhom Disco Singh

Abstract The identification of specific patient therapeutic strategies, drug reactions, and efficacy of the management during the early period of cancer may help in guiding the medical oncologists in the selection of anti-cancer treatment for a person suffering from cancer. Also, it helps in calculating the improvable of the toxicity to benefit ratio. The success of this treatment is due to the emergence of predictive biomarkers. A predictive biomarker is a simple tool usually measured before treatment and provides information on the probability of response to a particular therapy. Several beneficial reports and appropriate evidence-based on the roles of prognostic and predictive biomarkers of known therapeutic targets in different cancer types including breast, colorectal, and non-small cell lung cancers in adults are also observed from different reviews. However, it is found that the utilization of predictive biomarkers incorporating with some drugs derived from natural sources such as trabectedin, cabazitaxel, and alvocidib is a bit slower than usual. Thus, this review paper covers the recent advances of cancer biomarkers which are used to

R. Ningthoujam · N. B. Chanu · V. Anumala
Department of Vegetable Science, College of Horticulture and Forestry, Central Agricultural University, Pasighat, Arunachal Pradesh 791102, India

P. J. Babu
Biomaterials and Bioengineering Research Laboratory, Department of Biotechnology, Pachhunga University College, Mizoram University (A Central University), Aizawl, Mizoram 796001, India

S. Pradhan
Department of Botany, School of Applied Sciences, Centurion University of Technology and Management, Bhubaneswar, Odisha, India

M. K. Panda
CSIR—Institute of Minerals and Materials Technology, Bhubaneswar 751013, India

P. Heisnam
Department of Natural Resource Management, College of Horticulture and Forestry, Central Agricultural University, Pasighat, Arunachal Pradesh 791102, India

Y. D. Singh (✉)
Biomaterials and Bioprocessing Research Laboratory, Department of Post-Harvest Technology, College of Horticulture and Forestry, Central Agricultural University, Pasighat, Arunachal Pradesh 791102, India

K. Raza (ed.), *Computational Intelligence in Oncology*, Studies in Computational Intelligence 1016, https://doi.org/10.1007/978-981-16-9221-5_13

forecast the effectiveness of selected natural compounds focusing on human clinical studies.

Keywords Predictive biomarkers · Oncology · Cancer therapies · Treatment · Diagnosis

1 Introduction

Biomarkers or biological markers are molecular in nature that show a usual or pathogenic procedure and can be applied to support disease diagnosis [1]. It also helps in explicating the susceptibility for a particular disease and finding out how well the body responds to a clinical and specific therapy. Furthermore, they help in regulating the development of rational drug interaction and monitoring the possible resistance mechanisms [2]. More than these, biomarkers provide detailed information about a particular drug as well as they can be implemented as a tool to choose a particular patient for a check-up in an early stage of clinical trials according to the molecular behavior of the tumor. Another superiority of this realization of targeted mutation shows the effect of a certain drug molecularly and describes the changes of a patient cohort in drug development programs of oncology as well as alter the attention from the enlargement of inexact cytotoxic chemotherapies to molecularly targeted therapeutics. Broadly, biomarkers are divided into four types. They are diagnostic, prognostic, predictive, and therapeutic [3].

Diagnostic biomarker helps in advance identification of cancer in a non-invasive way and consequently take action as secondary prevention of cancer whilst predictive biomarker permit the early prediction and reaction of the patient to a specific therapy [4]. It defines the advantage of the therapy over a patient. Likewise, a prognostic biomarker is a biological characteristic and helps in choosing patients who required the most intensive care or therapy [5] whereas a therapeutic biomarker uses a protein molecule and allows it to use for a specific therapy [6]. Among the four biomarkers, predicting biomarkers are considered to be symptomatic good, better survival, or an adverse outcome [7].

In the past years, predicting biomarkers is used in medical products and drew the attention of investigational therapy as it selects the patients who will show the positive and negative biomarkers. The concept of predicting biomarkers allows applying under diverse inventions such as medications, biologics, health devices, remedial procedures, and nutritional changes either for diagnosis or protection from infections. The application of predicting biomarkers does not have a boundary in the clinical trial setting. It is because these biomarkers support and assist information to the patient taking good decisions like observing the better treatment from various interventions. Simultaneously, the uses of predicting biomarkers on drugs depend upon the course of action of the nominated medicine and acknowledging of physiopathology. However, they possibly will also show the recognition experiment while following the previous studies. So, proper knowing the condition and consequence of mutually between the body as well as disease is necessary for effective growth along with ideal utilization of intercessions. Besides all these, predicting biomarkers are used as an agent in cancer therapy. They are used for future outcomes from the treatment of cancer. Some of the examples are squamous variation in non-small cell lung cancer could be the source of predicting biomarkers to detect the patients who should not be treated with pemetrexed. They show the result of the existence or advancement-free survival effect associated with management with further ordinary chemotherapies like docetaxel or cisplatin cooperating with gemcitabine [8]. Another good example is the use of mutation gene 1 and gene 2 of Breast CAncer (BRCA1/2) for predicting biomarkers. It is used for inspection of women through platinum-sensitive ovarian cancer, to screen out the sick person who is responsible similarly to suppressor of Poly (ADP-ribose) polymerase (PARP) [9]. In another study, it is reported that the presence of AASA haplotype in hormone receptors predicts the positive result on breast cancer patients while with lymph node says the negative and it is connected with low survival of premenopausal women. However, it does not affect the survival of postmenopausal women [10]. As a result, it is considered worthy to apply the different variants of predicting biomarkers in the therapy of various cancer types. Different databases can be referred to for predicting cancer diagnosis (Table 1).

2 MiRNA Databases

A microRNA (miRNA) might be taken as a diverse upshot taking place in cancer by acting mutually as a tumor inhibitor and an oncogene due to its ability to target numerous genes. MiRNAs can control gene appearance by modifying the epigenetic state of genes convoluted in cancer across the genome. The development of new anti-cancer treatments requires a thorough understanding of miRNA-epigenetic interactions in cancer [33]. The most researched short noncoding RNA is microRNA [34]. According to miRBase revision 22.1, this micro RNA was initially reported in 1993 [35] and presently has more than 38,589 sequences [36]. As a result, miRNA has a wide variety of databases and tools accessible[37]. Studies on miRNAs are more common than research on other ncRNAs, owing to their methods of regulation at the transcription and posttranscriptional levels of mRNAs [38]. Animals and plants have different miRNA biology, which influences biological assays and computational methods for these taxa [39–41]. Bioinformatics databanks and implements are a strong method meant for discovery, investigation of innovative ideas, and study of miRNA at numerous stages, for example, miRNA oneself, receptor functionality, web patterns) to astound tasks accompanied by means of organizing along with identifying miRNAs [42, 43]. The NRDR portal (Noncoding RNA Databases Resource), which catalogs above 200 records about noncoding RNAs, 50% of which are specific for the miRNA class, and Tools4miRs, a physically graded display place with over and above 170 procedures for miRNA study, are two of the foremost portals that possibly will support researchers hunt for miRNA databases and implements quickly (tools and databases) [44]. The NRDR source, which was initially

Table. 1. Data sources and selection

S. No.	Name of the database	Sub-data based and their description	References
1	UCI machine learning repository	Breast cancer data	[11]
		Original Wisconsin breast cancer database	
		Diagnostic Wisconsin breast cancer database	
		The data is formed to sort out difficulties connected to after-operative life suspense in lung cancer infected person: class 1—expiry of the patient within one-year afterward operation, class 2—survival	
		The dataset comprises circumstances from a study directed on the survival of sufferers who had experienced surgery for breast malignancy	
		Lung cancer data; no attribute definitions	
		Prognostic Wisconsin breast cancer database	
2	1000 genome project website	Data of cancer patient for tumor stage	[12]
3	Scopus biomedical database	Cancer risk assessment data	[13]
		Cancer recurrence data	
		Cancer survival data	
		Cancer prediction data	
4	COSMIC (catalogue of somatic mutations in cancer) database	COSMIC: the core of COSMIC, an expert-curated database of somatic mutations	[14]
		COSMIC-3D: an interactive view of cancer mutations in the context of 3D structures	
5	Sleeping beauty cancer driver database	Osteosarcoma—bone cancer	[15]
		Medulloblastoma—brain	
		Adenocarcinoma, adenoma, adenomyoepithelioma, adenosquamous carcinoma—breast	
		Intestine cancer (inferred)—Intestine	
		Hepatocellular adenoma, hepatocellular carcinoma (inferred)—liver	
		B-cell lymphoma, lymphoblastic lymphoma (non-T non-B), T-cell lymphoblastic lymphoma, T-cell lymphoma—lymph node and thymus	
		Rhabdomyosarcoma—muscle	
		Pancreatic ductal early carcinoma, Pancreatic ductal adenocarcinoma—pancreas	
		Adenocarcinoma—prostate	

(continued)

Table. 1. (continued)

S. No.	Name of the database	Sub-data based and their description		References
		Keratoacanthoma, melanoma, squamous cell carcinoma—skin		
		Undifferentiated myeloid leukemia—spleen		
		Gastric cancer (inferred)—stomach		
6	OncoVar: database	Inquiryboards for oncogenic driver variations in cancers		[16]
7	OGEE v2: database	Vital genes in human cancer cell lines		[17]
8	Drug–gene interaction database	GeneCards BioGPS CancerTracer Gene4Denovo SL-BioDP TargetDB OncoGemini	Predictive genomic biomarkers roles in oncology—a physically curated database that incorporates dissimilar coatings of annotations: cancer types, genes, variants, and sensitivity/resistance decorations to accepted and experimental agents under clinical examination	[18]
9	DriverDBv2: a database	Humanoid cancer driver gene data		[19]
10	SEER database	Cancer site, tumor pathology, stage, and cause of death data		[20]
11	ONCOMINE: a cancer microarray database and integrated data-mining platform	Database on a cancer microarray and web-based data-mining platform intended at enabling uncovering from genome-wide expression analyses		[21]
12	Tumor-associated gene (TAG) database	TAG database was calculated to exploit information from well-categorized oncogenes and tumor inhibitor genes to simplify cancer research. Whollymark genes were recognized through a text-mining method from the PubMed database		[22]
13	HLungDB: database	HLungDB is a database with the addition of the lung cancer-associated genes, proteins, and miRNAs organized with the agreeing clinical evidence. The chief determination of this platform is to start a setup of lung cancer-correlated molecules and to ease the mechanistic revision of lung carcinogenesis		[23]
14	TCGA (the cancer genome atlas)	A deprived prognostic issue in lung cancer and may assist as an in effect biomarker for expecting metastasis and prognosis of patients with lung cancer		[12]
15	OncoMX database	OncoMX will stand in a dynamic appointment among bioinformaticians and cancer biomarker scholars		[24]

(continued)

Table. 1. (continued)

S. No.	Name of the database	Sub-data based and their description	References
16	CBD—the Colorectal Cancer Biomarker Database	The CBD with the reliable fillings as an influential and time-saving implement offer extra inclusive and precise facts for additional Colorectal biomarker research	[25]
17	MarkerDB: an online database of molecular biomarkers	The chemical biomarkers in MarkerDB contain markers for a diversity of inborn-faults of metabolism or genetic conditions, cancers, metabolic sicknesses, transmissible illnesses, drug experiences, chemical/pollutant disclosures, and dietary consumption	[26]
18	CIViC (clinical interpretation of variants in cancer) database	Exploration of specific cancer models to comprehend the genes and paths elaborate on the expansion and progress of a cancer	[27]
19	Ovid database	MMP-9: invasion, metastasis	[28]
		SK1: cancer genesis, progression, metastasis	[29]
		NGAL: proliferation, survival, morphogenesis	[30]
		DcR3: tumorigenesis, progression	[31]
20	The GDSC database	It assists the documentation of molecular structures of cancers that foresee comeback to anti-cancer drugs	[32]

issued in 2012, has a comprehensive list and description of biological databases, as well as a user-friendly interface that allows for filtered searches. On NRDR, we discovered 110 miRNA-related libraries. The Tools4mirs repository is a carefully engineered library of miRNA tools and datasets [45]. MiRBase was the initial online repository for miRNA sequencing records and explanation, launched in 2006 [46]. It has been reorganized regularly since its first release, most recently in 2018. The database allows users to search for sequences by classes or miRNA and copy them in the FASTA layout. The different categories of miRNA databases can be categorized based on different approaches (Fig. 1).

MiRNAs are believed to play an important role in illness control, analysis, and progression, according to a variety of data. We mention dbDEMc [47], NCG [48], HNOCDB [49], and IGDB in the realm of cancer-related databases. NSCLC (Non-Small Cell Lung Cancer) [50]. The dbDEMc collection contains data on 14 different kinds of cancer in humans and these are nominated from 48 microarray datasets available in journals. The selected databanks utilize microarrays with importance analysis to find miRNAs with varying levels of expression in malignancies. In comparison to healthy tissues. The NCG database is primarily concerned with creating cancer gene networks by curating genes from the public domain literature. More than 1500 genes are stored in the database [51]. Among these genes, 518 of them are well-known to

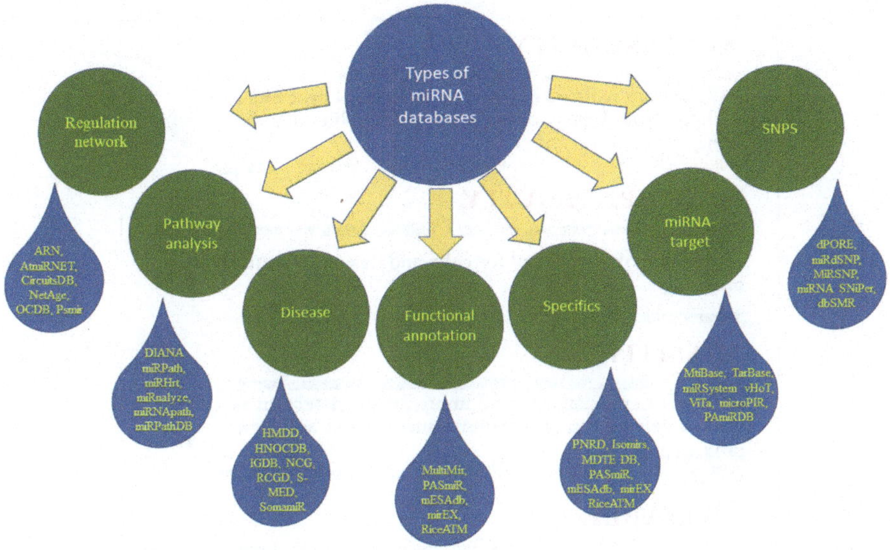

Fig. 1 Different categories of miRNA databases

cause cancer [52]. The HNOCDB is a database that focuses on Cancers of the upper part of the body such as the head, neck, and mouth. The set of data with several types of cancers are named further down via the subtype, as well as a chromosomal route of accompanying genes in addition to miRNAs. Last of all, we have IGDB in the cancer sector. NSCLC is a database that contains vetted and integrated data from many databases on cell lung cancer and allows for graphic display and tabular searches.

2.1 *MicroRNAs as* Predictive Biomarkers

MicroRNA (miRNA) is a minute (generally 21–25 nucleotide in length) RNA molecule, incapacitated of translation into protein but exhibit significant catalyst and gene regulator properties [53]. In the beginning, it was exposed in Caenorhabditis elegans later on, it existed identified to be eukaryotes including humans [42, 54, 55]. MicroRNAs are generally used as an indicator to detect any deviation in the regular biological activities, morbific processes, and pharmacologic effects as a response to medical treatment [56, 57] pioneered an experiment as a result of which miRNA was accepted as a biomarker for cancer diagnosis. Since then, it has been deployed in the detection and diagnosis of a variety of ailments. Some of the ideal characteristics possessed [53] by miRNAs as a potential biomarker are shown in Fig. 2.

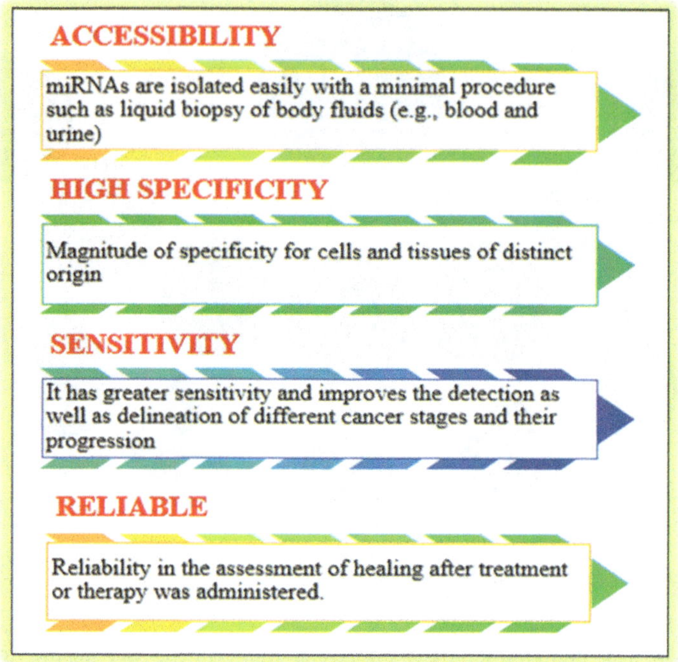

Fig. 2 Some important characteristics possessed by miRNAs

Due to the divergent nature of the cancer miRNAs have a significant role to play with a multi-marker approach in the early detection of carcinoma. This is supported by Xiong et al. [58] who reported the multi-marker signature comprising nine miRNA molecules for reliable diagnosis of breast cancer.

2.2 *Anomalous Expression of MiRNA in Cancer*

The anomalous appearance of miRNAs has been allied with cell sequences like cell multiplying, stress reaction, cell apoptosis, differentiation as well as inflammation. All these factors show a manifestation of a multitude kind of disorders and malignancies. Consequently, in the last few years miRNAs developed a course of biomarkers that give attention to research. Their class of biomarkers helps in the detection of diseases in an early stage. It also signifies a tough trial for analytical chemists who want to design not only the particular but also the greatly sensitive implements for their findings [59].

When the formation and development of cancer cells occurs, changes can be seen in miRNA levels. A different characteristic of abnormal behavior happens in the levels of mature miRNA and it is relevant with normal tissues. Various genome-wide studies found an association of anomalous (either upregulated or downregulated) behavior with the humans with vagaries of malignant carcinoma, which includes lymphoma [60] breast cancer [61], colorectal cancer [62], prostate cancer [63], and glioma [64].

The concept behind is certain genomic sites that are delicate in nature are coded for specific miRNA [65]. With the arousal of aberrations in cancer-associated genomic sites, alterations in the expression of miRNAs will be noticed. It might be due to chromosomal aberrations, genetic mutations, epigenetic changes, and changes in miRNA biogenesis at the affected sites. Based on the afore explained expressions, practical applicability may be possible for predictive use of biomarkers in cancer diagnosis [66]. MicroRNA (particularly of serum origin) a highly stable molecule, remains unaffected to different external factors like low or high pH (pH = 1–13), long storage, frequent thaw cycles, and have significant resistance against "RNase A" a cleavage enzyme [67].

Further, it is least affected to the degradation process during the formalin-fixed and paraffin-embedded (FFPE) procedure of sampling. Additionally, miRNAs can be encapsulated in delivery vehicles like exosomes [68], apoptotic bodies [69], and microparticles [70]. They are lipid-based derivatives of the cell. Exposure of miRNAs to nucleases that are found abundantly in extracellular spaces may lead to degradation. For self-protection, miRNAs are largely bound to RNA-linked proteins like argonaute (Ago1 or Ago2), nucleophosmin (NPM1), or ribosomal proteins [71]. They substantially the miRNAs possess significant advantages to be promoted as potential predictive biomarkers for cancer.

3 Generic Pipeline for Biomarkers Detection and Various State-of-the-Art Methods

Predictive and prognostic molecular biomarkers are usually applied in studies dealing with tumors [72]. Nevertheless, the utilization of these complex biomarkers is increasing enormously as well as their charge and time in decision making of practice. Moreover, biomarkers are highly necessary for clinical works and diagnosis. Nevertheless, normally accessible tumor tissue comprises copiousness clinically-related data which is not entirely subjugated. The hidden information can be unveiled with advanced technology like deep learning (DL), and artificial intelligence (AI). They provide histology images of cancer along with hypothetically clinical valuable information [73]. In addition to this, machine learning is a new practice model for biomarker detection in cancer investigation. Machine learning is a division of artificial intelligence (AI) that shows an unlimited prospective for shaping and acknowledgment in cryptic cancer datasets [74]. Meanwhile, the various form of data in velocity, volume, and diversity that are generated by means of health applications has produced enormous information. This information needs efficient space for storage and their management cannot reach the requirements of heterogeneous data. Hence, by the application of CI, the problem of insufficient space can be handled up to some extend and get better management [75]. It will also improve the performance and raise the level of accurateness in identification. Recently, many researchers are approaching to inspect the model of CI in medical data. This set of art help in the classification of CI techniques which are applied in medical fields in form of single and fusion. Some of the forms of CI are Support Vector Machine (SVM) and Artificial Immune Recognition System (AIRS). They come down in the category of single-based computational intelligence and are considered one of the finest systems in medical applications. Alternatively, the combination of Support Vector Machine (SVM) with additional ways like SVM Genetic Algorithm (SVM-GA), SVM-AIRS, SVM-Artificial Immune System (SVM-AIS), and fuzzy support vector machine (FSVM) obtained infinite performances. Also, it is more reliable and accomplished improved outcomes in relation to the accurateness, correctness, sensible, and results precisely. Furthermore, models like ANN and Fuzzy logic are applied in the evaluation of Huntington's disease symptoms [76].

4 Future Markers

Cancer is a condition marked by the uncontrollable growth of cells in the body due to a malfunctioning cell growth signaling system. It is a group of heterogeneous diseases with low predictability and a high rate of mortality [77]. Treatment of cancer is relatively easier if detected early upon removal of cancer-causing cells while it is near to impossibility at advanced stages. There are several means used by current medical researchers successfully one among which is widely exploited is biomarkers. 'Biomarkers' or 'Biological markers' are bio sources that can indicate information on cancer cells. Biomarkers are often exploited by samples drawn from blood, urine, and soft tissues [78]. Digital biomarkers and molecular digital biomarkers are novel futuristic markers that have a huge potential in indicating cancer cells with precise accuracy at very early stages. Biomarkers can be generally of several proteins released by the tumor cells in the blood or present themselves in the tumor cells. A recent addition to the definition of biomarkers includes the indication and measurements of biological process, pathological activity, and pharmacological reactions to therapeutic involvement. The concept of biological markers is quite simple as it detects the occurrence of diseases before the lethal period and generates enough time to undergo treatments during the latency period. Commonly exploited biomarkers are radioactive elements like 32P, 35S, 125I as radioactive marker, magnetic marker and optical marker are well-known types of presently used biomarkers in different medical fields.

For example in the treatment of Colorectal Cancer, the use and analysis of single markers for the diagnosis, identification, and prognosis of the disease are appropriate however it is frequently linked with little sensitivity and specificity in tedious medical practice. Therefore, another way to deal with this problem is the application of at least two or more markers at the same time. This application helps to upsurge their diagnostic utility. Moreover, circulating tumor cells analysis may also be a portion of an integrative medical method of the multimodal diagnostics, separate patient outlines as well as disease and person-specific biomarker patterns for treatment. Lately, technical and systematic developments have heightened scientific biomarker research [79]. In the upcoming future, we can say that the arrival of novel urinary assays will help in bringing high efficacy that would lessen CRC mortality [80]. Likewise, in recent reports, genetic biomarkers are used in differential expression analysis of ZIKV Infected Human RNA Sequence [81] and various approaches of genomics on differential expression analysis in Ovarian Cancer were also seen [82]. One of the ground-breaking recent discoveries of biomarkers by Abnova and Japan National Cancer Center Research Institute on pancreatic cancer early detection where proteins were used as the biomarker [83]. This identified pancreatic biomarker has outgrown all the limitations under previously exploited markers. Abnova the prime agent holds the exclusive right for commercialization of the resulting biomarkers while National Cancer Centre Research Institute will accept the royalty from sales of this particular product.

Futuristic markers are one of the most potent means to eradicate cancer from mankind. Advancements in the study area of proteomics have significantly boosted the study on tears as a high number of prostate cancer-related proteins are identified in tears for the detection of early prostate cancer in men. Thus tears can be used as a future biomarker for early detection of prostate cancer with further research refinement [84].

Though there are a number of means for the treatment of cancer are available but there is still a lack of high specificity and sensitivity towards an effective screening of cancer in the general population. Therefore, for efficient treatment of cancer, the focus must be made on early diagnosis using a variety of biomarkers upon its identification. There are several global institutes working on early cancer detection even prior to tumor formation. The clinical trials pose a high-cost demand with unpredictable and unreliable results. Therefore, the challenge is to search for a less cost involving, high accuracy with precision in detecting early cancer. It is high time to establish a cumulative approach by the public as well as private bodies to resolve the cancer biomarker problem worldwide.

5 Conclusions

Reviewing all the context, it is noticed that it gives a great significance for drug discovery and development [85] and also in the field of cancer therapy [86, 87]. Besides, different preclinical and clinical investigations illustrated that the achievement of using biomarkers to predict and effectiveness of cancer drug development and oncology practice. The usefulness of predictive cancer biomarkers has enlarged in recent years and brought successful goals in translational oncology. But still, caution should be taken while implementing predicting biomarkers in clinical trials. Additionally, reduction in cost and more studies are yet necessary before applying to cancer drug findings in the clinical setting. Discovered predictive biomarkers identification, clinical validation, and combination in everyday practice need considerable resources and working together with the international group. Thus, this helps in more invention of work and aims to go together with researchers from different fields and countries.

References

1. Chung, C., & Christianson, M. (2014). Predictive and prognostic biomarkers with therapeutic targets in breast, colorectal, and non-small cell lung cancers: A systemic review of current development, evidence, and recommendation. *Journal of Oncology Pharmacy Practice, 20*(1), 11–28.
2. Pezo, R. C., & Bedard, P. L. (2015) *Definition: Translational and personalised medicine, biomarkers, pharmacodynamics*. ESMO Handbook of Translational Research.
3. Carlomagno, N., Incollingo, P., Tammaro, V., Peluso, G., Rupealta, N., Chiacchio, G., Sandoval Sotelo, M. L., Minieri, G., Pisani, A., Riccio, E., & Sabbatini, M. (2017). Diagnostic, predictive, prognostic, and therapeutic molecular biomarkers in third millennium: A breakthrough in gastric cancer. *BioMed Research International*.
4. Animesh, S., Singh, Y. D. (2021). A comprehensive study on aptasensors for cancer diagnosis. *Current Pharmaceutical Biotechnology, 1;22*(8), 1069–1084.
5. Durães, C., Almeida, G. M., Seruca, R., Oliveira, C., & Carneiro, F. (2014). Biomarkers for gastric cancer: Prognostic, predictive or targets of therapy? *VirchowsArchiv, 464*(3), 367–378.
6. Lin, L. L., Huang, H. C., & Juan, H. F. (2012). Discovery of biomarkers for gastric cancer: A proteomics approach. *Journal of Proteomics, 75*(11), 3081–3097.
7. FDA-NIH Biomarker Working Group (2016). BEST (Biomarkers, Endpoints, and other Tools). https://www.ncbi.nlm.nih.gov/books/. Accessed December 22, 2016.
8. Scagliotti, G., Hanna, N., Fossella, F., Sugarman, K., Blatter, J., Peterson, P., Simms, L., & Shepherd, F. A. (2009). The differential efficacy of pemetrexed according to NSCLC histology: A review of two Phase III studies. *The Oncologist, 14*(3), 253–263.
9. Ledermann, J., Harter, P., Gourley, C., Friedlander, M., Vergote, I., Rustin, G., Scott, C., Meier, W., Shapira-Frommer, R., Safra, T., & Matei, D. (2012). Olaparib maintenance therapy in platinum-sensitive relapsed ovarian cancer. *New England Journal of Medicine, 366*(15), 1382–1392.
10. Buonaguro, F. M., Pauza, D., Tornesello, M. L., Hainaut, P., Franco, R., & Marincola, F. M. (2014). Cancer diagnostic and predictive biomarkers.
11. Wolberg, W. H., & Mangasarian, O. L. (1990). Multisurface method of pattern separation for medical diagnosis applied to breast cytology. *Proceedings of the National Academy of Sciences, 87*(23), 9193–9196.
12. Sun, Y., Zhu, S., Ma, K., Liu, W., Yue, Y., Hu, G., Lu, H., & Chen, W. (2019). Identification of 12 cancer types through genome deep learning. *Scientific Reports, 9*(1), 1–9.
13. Kourou, K., Exarchos, T. P., Exarchos, K. P., Karamouzis, M. V., & Fotiadis, D. I. (2015). Machine learning applications in cancer prognosis and prediction. *Computational and Structural Biotechnology Journal, 1*(13), 8–17.
14. Shan, L., Yu, J., He, Z., Chen, S., Liu, M., Ding, H., Xu, L., Zhao, J., Yang, A., & Jiang, H. (2020). Defining relative mutational difficulty to understand cancer formation. *Cell Discovery, 6*(1), 1–7.
15. Newberg, J. Y., Mann, K. M., Mann, M. B., Jenkins, N. A., & Copeland, N. G. (2018). SBCDDB: Sleeping beauty cancer driver database for gene discovery in mouse models of human cancers. *Nucleic Acids Research, 46*(D1), D1011–D1017.

16. Wang, T., Ruan, S., Zhao, X., Shi, X., Teng, H., Zhong, J., You, M., Xia, K., Sun, Z., & Mao, F. (2021). OncoVar: An integrated database and analysis platform for oncogenic driver variants in cancers. *Nucleic Acids Research, 49*(D1), D1289–D1301.
17. Chen, W. H., Lu, G., Chen, X., Zhao, X. M., Bork, P. (2016). OGEE v2: an update of the online gene essentiality database with special focus on differentially essential genes in human cancer cell lines. *Nucleic Acids Research, 45*(D1), D940–D944.
18. Freshour, S. L., Kiwala, S., Cotto, K. C., Coffman, A. C., McMichael, J. F., Song, J. J., Griffith, M., Griffith, O. L., Wagner, A. H. (2021). Integration of the drug–gene interaction database (DGIdb 4.0) with open crowdsource efforts. *Nucleic Acids Research, 49*(D1), D1144–1151.
19. Chung, I. F., Chen, C. Y., Su, S. C., Li, C. Y., Wu, K. J., Wang, H. W., & Cheng, W. C. (2016). DriverDBv2: A database for human cancer driver gene research. *Nucleic Acids Research, 44*(D1), D975–D979.
20. Huang, C. C., Chan, S. Y., Lee, W. C., Chiang, C. J., Lu, T. P., & Cheng, S. H. (2019). Development of a prediction model for breast cancer based on the national cancer registry in Taiwan. *Breast Cancer Research, 21*(1), 1–9.
21. Rhodes, D. R., Yu, J., Shanker, K., Deshpande, N., Varambally, R., Ghosh, D., Barrette, T., Pander, A., & Chinnaiyan, A. M. (2004). ONCOMINE: A cancer microarray database and integrated data-mining platform. *Neoplasia, 6*(1), 1–6.
22. Pradeepkiran, J. A., Sainath, S. B., Kumar, K. K., Balasubramanyam, L., Prabhakar, K. V., & Bhaskar, M. (2015). CGMD: An integrated database of cancer genes and markers. *Scientific Reports, 5*(1), 1–7.
23. Huang, C. H., Peng, H. S., & Ng, K. L. (2015). Prediction of cancer proteins by integrating protein interaction, domain frequency, and domain interaction data using machine learning algorithms. *BioMed Research International, 17*, 2015.
24. Dingerdissen, H. M., Bastian, F., Vijay-Shanker, K., Robinson-Rechavi, M., Bell, A., Gogate, N., Gupta, S., Holmes, E., Kahsay, R., Keeney, J., & Kincaid, H. (2020). OncoMX: A knowledgebase for exploring cancer biomarkers in the context of related cancer and healthy data. *JCO Clinical Cancer Informatics, 4*, 210–220.
25. Zhang, X., Sun, X. F., Cao, Y., Ye, B., Peng, Q., Liu, X., Shen, B., & Zhang, H. (2018). CBD: A biomarker database for colorectal cancer. *Database, 1*, 2018.
26. Wishart, D. S., Bartok, B., Oler, E., Liang, K. Y., Budinski, Z., Berjanskii, M., Guo, A., Cao, X., & Wilson, M. (2021). MarkerDB: An online database of molecular biomarkers. *Nucleic Acids Research, 49*(D1), D1259–D1267.
27. Lever, J., Jones, M. R., Danos, A. M., Krysiak, K., Bonakdar, M., Grewal, J. K., Culibrk, L., Griffith, O. L., Griffith, M., & Jones, S. J. (2019). Text-mining clinically relevant cancer biomarkers for curation into the CIViC database. *Genome Medicine, 11*(1), 1–6.
28. Song, J., Su, H., Zhou, Y. Y., & Guo, L. L. (2013). Prognostic value of matrix metalloproteinase 9 expression in breast cancer patients: A meta-analysis. *Asian Pacific Journal of Cancer Prevention, 14*(3), 1615–1621.
29. Zhang, Y., Wang, Y., Wan, Z., Liu, S., Cao, Y., & Zeng, Z. (2014). Sphingosine kinase 1 and cancer: A systematic review and meta-analysis. *PloS One, 9*(2), e90362.
30. Wang, Y. U., & Zeng, T. (2013). Neutrophil gelatinase-associated lipocalin protein as a biomarker in the diagnosis of breast cancer: A meta-analysis. *Biomedical Reports, 1*(3), 479–483.
31. Jiang, M., Lin, X., He, R., Lin, X., Liang, L., Tang, R., Xiong, D., Wei, K., Dang, Y., Feng, Z., & Chen, G. (2016). Decoy receptor 3 (DcR3) as a biomarker of tumor deterioration in female reproductive cancers: A meta-analysis. *Medical Science Monitor: International Medical Journal of Experimental and Clinical Research, 22*, 1850.
32. Ahmadi Moughari, F., & Eslahchi, C. (2021). A computational method for drug sensitivity prediction of cancer cell lines based on various molecular information. *PloS One, 16*(4), e0250620.
33. Arif, K. M., Elliott, E. K., Haupt, L. M., & Griffiths, L. R. (2020). Regulatory mechanisms of epigenetic miRNA relationships in human cancer and potential as therapeutic targets. *Cancers, 12*(10), 2922.

34. Paschoal, A. R., Maracaja-Coutinho, V., Setubal, J. C., Simões, Z. L., Verjovski-Almeida, S., & Durham, A. M. (2012). Non-coding transcription characterization and annotation: A guide and web resource for non-coding RNA databases. *RNA Biology, 9*(3), 274–282.
35. Kozomara, A., Birgaoanu, M., & Griffiths-Jones, S. (2019). miRBase: From microRNA sequences to function. *Nucleic Acids Research, 47*(D1), D155–D162.
36. Negri, T. D., Alves, W. A., Bugatti, P. H., Saito, P. T., Domingues, D. S., & Paschoal, A. R. (2019). Pattern recognition analysis on long noncoding RNAs: A tool for prediction in plants. *Briefings in Bioinformatics, 20*(2), 682–689.
37. Maracaja-Coutinho, V., Paschoal, A. R., Caris-Maldonado, J. C., Borges, P. V., Ferreira, A. J., Durham, A. M. (2019). Noncoding RNAs databases: Current status and trends. *Computational Biology of Non-Coding RNA, 2019*, 251–285.
38. Singh, N. K. (2017). microRNAs databases: Developmental methodologies, structural and functional annotations. *Interdisciplinary Sciences: Computational Life Sciences, 9*(3), 357–377.
39. Chen, L., Heikkinen, L., Wang, C., Yang, Y., Sun, H., & Wong, G. (2019). Trends in the development of miRNA bioinformatics tools. *Briefings in Bioinformatics, 20*(5), 1836–1852.
40. Szwacka, M., Pawełkowicz, M., Skarzyńska, A., Osipowski, P., Wojcieszek, M., Przybecki, Z., & Pląder, W. (2018). Biological significance, computational analysis, and applications of plant microRNAs. *Acta Physiologiae Plantarum, 40*(8), 1–30.
41. Bharadwaj, K. K., Srivastava, A., Panda, M. K., Singh, Y. D., Maharana, R., Mandal, K., Singh, M., Singh, D., Das, M., Murmu, D., Kabi, S. K. (2021) Computational intelligence in vaccine design against COVID-19. In *Computational intelligence methods in COVID-19: surveillance, prevention, prediction and diagnosis* (pp. 311–329). Singapore: Springer.
42. Lee, R. C., Feinbaum, R. L., Ambros, V. (1993). The C. elegans heterochronic gene lin-4 encodes small RNAs with antisense complementarity to lin-14. *Cell, 75*(5), 843–854.
43. Sarma, M. K., Ningthoujam, R., Panda, M. K., Babu, P. J., Srivastava, A., Das, M., & Singh, Y. D. (2021). Translational healthcare system through bioinformatics. In *Translational bioinformatics applications in healthcare*, 2021 Apr 19 (pp. 3–21). CRC Press.
44. Lukasik, A., Wójcikowski, M., & Zielenkiewicz, P. (2016). Tools4miRs–one place to gather all the tools for miRNA analysis. *Bioinformatics, 32*(17), 2722–2724.
45. Amorim, T. S., Pedro, D. L., & Paschoal, A. R. (2022). *MicroRNA databases and tools. InmiRNomics* (pp. 131–166). Humana.
46. Griffiths-Jones, S., Grocock, R. J., Van Dongen, S., Bateman, A., Enright, A. J. (2006). miRBase: microRNA sequences, targets and gene nomenclature. *Nucleic Acids Research, 34*(suppl_1), D140–D144.
47. Yang, Z., Ren, F., Liu, C., He, S., Sun, G., Gao, Q., Yao, L., Zhang, Y., Miao, R., Cao, Y., & Zhao, Y. (2010) *dbDEMC: a database of differentially expressed miRNAs in human cancers. InBMC genomics* (Vol. 11, No. 4, pp. 1–8). BioMed Central.
48. Repana, D., Nulsen, J., Dressler, L., Bortolomeazzi, M., Venkata, S. K., Tourna, A., Yakovleva, A., Palmieri, T., & Ciccarelli, F. D. (2019). The network of cancer genes (NCG): A comprehensive catalogue of known and candidate cancer genes from cancer sequencing screens. *Genome Biology, 20*(1), 1–2.
49. Mitra, S., Das, S., Das, S., Ghosal, S., & Chakrabarti, J. (2012). HNOCDB: A comprehensive database of genes and miRNAs relevant to head and neck and oral cancer. *Oral Oncology, 48*(2), 117–119.
50. Kao, S., Shiau, C. K., Gu, D. L., Ho, C. M., Su, W. H., Chen, C. F., Lin, C. H., & Jou, Y. S. I. G. D. B. (2012). NSCLC: Integrated genomic database of non-small cell lung cancer. *Nucleic Acids Research, 40*(D1), D972–D977.
51. Plon, S. E, Eccles, D. M., Easton, D., Foulkes, W. D., Genuardi, M., Greenblatt, M. S., Hogervorst, F. B., Hoogerbrugge, N., Spurdle, A. B., & Tavtigian, S. V. (2008). IARC unclassified genetic variants working group. Sequence variant classification and reporting: recommendations for improving the interpretation of cancer susceptibility genetic test results. *Human Mutation, 29*(11), 1282–1291.

52. Greenman, C., Stephens, P., Smith, R., Dalgliesh, G. L., Hunter, C., Bignell, G., Davies, H., Teague, J., Butler, A., Stevens, C., & Edkins, S. (2007). Patterns of somatic mutation in human cancer genomes. *Nature, 446*(7132), 153–158.
53. Lan, H., Lu, H., Wang, X., Jin, H. (2015). MicroRNAs as potential biomarkers in cancer: opportunities and challenges. *BioMed Research International.*
54. Perron, M. P., & Provost, P. (2008). Protein interactions and complexes in human microRNA biogenesis and function. *Frontiers in Bioscience: A Journal and Virtual Library, 1*(13), 2537.
55. Wightman, B., Ha, I., Ruvkun, G. (1993). Posttranscriptional regulation of the heterochronic gene lin-14 by lin-4 mediates temporal pattern formation in C. elegans. *Cell, 75*(5), 855–862.
56. Biomarkers Definitions Working Group, Atkinson, A. J., Colburn, W. A., DeGruttola, V. G., DeMets, D. L., Downing, G. J., Hoth, D. F., Oates, J. A., Peck, C. C., Schooley, R. T., & Spilker, B. A. (2001). Biomarkers and surrogate endpoints: Preferred definitions and conceptual framework. *Clinical Pharmacology & Therapeutics, 69*(3), 89–95.
57. Lawrie, C. H., Gal, S., Dunlop, H. M., Pushkaran, B., Liggins, A. P., Pulford, K., Banham, A. H., Pezzella, F., Boultwood, J., Wainscoat, J. S., & Hatton, C. S. (2008). Detection of elevated levels of tumour-associated microRNAs in serum of patients with diffuse large B-cell lymphoma. *British Journal of Haematology, 141*(5), 672–675.
58. Xiong, D. D., Lv, J., Wei, K. L., Feng, Z. B., Chen, J. T., Liu, K. C., Chen, G., & Luo, D. Z. (2017). A nine-miRNA signature as a potential diagnostic marker for breast carcinoma: An integrated study of 1110 cases. *Oncology Reports, 37*(6), 3297–3304.
59. Ciui, B., Jambrec, D., Sandulescu, R., & Cristea, C. (2017). Bioelectrochemistry for miRNA detection. *Current Opinion in Electrochemistry, 5*(1), 183–192.
60. Mazan-Mamczarz, K., & Gartenhaus, R. B. (2013). Role of microRNA deregulation in the pathogenesis of diffuse large B-cell lymphoma (DLBCL). *Leukemia Research, 37*(11), 1420–1428.
61. Ouyang, M., Li, Y., Ye, S., Ma, J., Lu, L., Lv, W., Chang, G., Li, X., Li, Q., Wang, S., & Wang, W. (2014). MicroRNA profiling implies new markers of chemoresistance of triple-negative breast cancer. *PloS One, 9*(5), e96228.
62. Dong, Y., Wu, W. K., Wu, C. W., Sung, J. J., Yu, J., & Ng, S. S. (2011). MicroRNA dysregulation in colorectal cancer: A clinical perspective. *British Journal of Cancer, 104*(6), 893–898.
63. Maugeri-Saccà, M., Coppola, V., Bonci, D., & De Maria, R. (2012). MicroRNAs and prostate cancer: From preclinical research to translational oncology. *The Cancer Journal, 18*(3), 253–261.
64. Tumilson, C. A., Lea, R. W., Alder, J. E., & Shaw, L. (2014). Circulating microRNA biomarkers for glioma and predicting response to therapy. *Molecular Neurobiology, 50*(2), 545–558.
65. Dash, R., Sahu, A., Panda, M. K., Das, M., & Singh, Y. D. (2021). Genomics in clinical care through precision medicine and personalized treatments. *Translational Bioinformatics in Healthcare and Medicine, 1*, 49–58.
66. Calin, G. A., & Croce, C. M. (2006). MicroRNA signatures in human cancers. *Nature Reviews Cancer, 6*(11), 857–866.
67. Chen, X., Ba, Y., Ma, L., Cai, X., Yin, Y., Wang, K., Guo, J., Zhang, Y., Chen, J., Guo, X., & Li, Q. (2008). Characterization of microRNAs in serum: A novel class of biomarkers for diagnosis of cancer and other diseases. *Cell Research, 18*(10), 997–1006.
68. Cheng, L., Sharples, R. A., Scicluna, B. J., & Hill, A. F. (2014). Exosomes provide a protective and enriched source of miRNA for biomarker profiling compared to intracellular and cell-free blood. *Journal of Extracellular Vesicles, 3*(1), 23743.
69. Zernecke, A., Bidzhekov, K., Noels, H., Shagdarsuren, E., Gan, L., Denecke, B., Hristov, M., Köppel, T., Jahantigh, M. N., Lutgens, E., & Wang, S. (2009). Delivery of microRNA-126 by apoptotic bodies induces CXCL12-dependent vascular protection. *Science Signalling, 2*(100), ra81.
70. Muralidharan-Chari, V., Clancy, J. W., Sedgwick, A., & D'Souza-Schorey, C. (2010). Microvesicles: Mediators of extracellular communication during cancer progression. *Journal of Cell Science, 123*(10), 1603–1611.

71. Turchinovich, A., Weiz, L., Langheinz, A., & Burwinkel, B. (2011). Characterization of extracellular circulating microRNA. *Nucleic Acids Research, 39*(16), 7223–7233.
72. Mehta, S., Shelling, A., Muthukaruppan, A., Lasham, A., Blenkiron, C., Laking, G., & Print, C. (2010). Predictive and prognostic molecular markers for cancer medicine. *Therapeutic Advances in Medical Oncology, 2*(2), 125–148.
73. Echle, A., Rindtorff, N. T., Brinker, T. J., Luedde, T., Pearson, A. T., & Kather, J. N. (2021). Deep learning in cancer pathology: A new generation of clinical biomarkers. *British Journal of Cancer, 124*(4), 686–696.
74. Jagga, Z., & Gupta, D. (2015). Machine learning for biomarker identification in cancer research—developments toward its clinical application. *Personalized Medicine, 12*(4), 371–387.
75. Sahu, A., Dash, R., Panda, M. K., & Singh, Y. D. (2021). Viroinformatics: A modern approach to counter viral diseases through computational informatics. In *Translational bioinformatics in healthcare and medicine*, 2021 Jan 1 (pp. 157–169). Academic Press.
76. Lauraitis, A., Maskeliūnas, R., & Damaševičius, R. (2018). ANN and fuzzy logic based model to evaluate Huntington disease symptoms. *Journal of Healthcare Engineering, 11*, 2018.
77. Martinkova, J., Gadher, S. J., Hajduch, M., & Kovarova, H. (2009). Challenges in cancer research and multifaceted approaches for cancer biomarker quest. *FEBS Letters, 583*(11), 1772–1784.
78. Hirsch, M. S., & Watkins, J. (2020). A comprehensive review of biomarker use in the gynecologic tract including differential diagnoses and diagnostic pitfalls. *Advances in Anatomic Pathology, 27*(3), 164–192.
79. Deschoolmeester, V., Baay, M., Specenier, P., Lardon, F., & Vermorken, J. B. (2010). A review of the most promising biomarkers in colorectal cancer: One step closer to targeted therapy. *The Oncologist, 15*(7), 699.
80. Jelski, W., & Mroczko, B. (2020). Biochemical markers of colorectal cancer-present and future. *Cancer Management and Research, 12*, 4789.
81. Jabeen, A., Ahmad, N., & Raza, K. (2019). Differential expression analysis of ZIKV infected human RNA sequence reveals potential genetic biomarkers. In *International work-conference on bioinformatics and biomedical engineering*, 2019 May 8 (pp. 283–294). Springer.
82. Zhang, Y., Qazi, S., & Raza, K. (2021). Differential expression analysis in ovarian cancer: A functional genomics and systems biology approach. *Saudi Journal of Biological Sciences, 28*(7), 4069–4081.
83. Kato, S., & Honda, K. (2020). Use of biomarkers and imaging for early detection of pancreatic cancer. *Cancers, 12*(7), 1965.
84. Li, Y. (2010). Detection of tear biomarkers for future prostate cancer diagnosis. *The Open Biomarkers Journal, 3*(1).
85. Atanasov, A. G., Yeung, A. W., & Banach, M. (2018). Natural products for targeted therapy in precision medicine, 1559–1562.
86. Moosavi, M. A., Haghi, A., Rahmati, M., Taniguchi, H., Mocan, A., Echeverría, J., Gupta, V. K., Tzvetkov, N. T., & Atanasov, A. G. (2018). Phytochemicals as potent modulators of autophagy for cancer therapy. *Cancer Letters, 28*(424), 46–69.
87. Singh, Y. D., Panda, M. K., Satapathy, K. B. (2020). Ethnomedicine for drug discovery. In *Advances in pharmaceutical biotechnology* (pp. 15–28). Singapore: Springer.

Computational Intelligence: A Step Forward in Cancer Biomarker Discovery and Therapeutic Target Prediction

Mohd Faizan Siddiqui, Azaroual Mouna, Gregory Nicolas, Syed Ali Abbas Rahat, Ainura Mitalipova, Nancy Emmanuel, and Nazgul Tashmatova

Abstract Computational intelligence (CI) is one of the most popular and advanced fields that mimics human intelligence and transforms numerous aspects of the healthcare industry. For the past two decades, CI has grown extensively and reached a new height in clinical research on cancer. The subfields of artificial intelligence, like deep learning and machine learning, are also applied to tackle various scientific problems. Cancer is one of the most aggressive and dreaded diseases, which every year costs more than 10 million lives globally, and it is expected that these tolls may reach 16.4 million by 2040. Hence, meticulous prognosis and early diagnosis of this disease are very significant to increase the chance of patient survival. In recent years, breakthroughs in various AI-based stratagems for precision oncology, digital pathology, and next-generation sequencing (NSG) are driving the need for new prognostic and predictive assays that facilitate the stratification and selection of patients for treatment. This chapter briefly includes the applications of CI and its subfields in cancer biomarkers and therapeutic target prediction. However, we explore how these applications have assisted in solving biomedical problems with unprecedented accuracy and deep learning. We also demonstrated how these data could be run on natural and mathematical algorithms to derive a classification of cancer genomes, identify potential biomarkers, therapeutic targets, drugs, and draw scientifically sound conclusions based on them. By providing a fresh viewpoint on how computational tools might aid enhance cancer detection, this chapter can help make significant advances in the medical disciplines and scientific community.

M. F. Siddiqui (✉) · S. A. A. Rahat · A. Mitalipova · N. Tashmatova
International Medical Faculty, Osh State University, Osh City 723510, Kyrgyzstan

A. Mouna
Tambov State Medical University, Tambov City 392000, Russia

G. Nicolas
Department of Plastic and Reconstructive Surgery, Hospital das Clinicas, Faculty of Medicine of the University of Sao Paulo, Sao Paulo, Brazil
e-mail: gregory.nicolas@hc.fm.usp.br

N. Emmanuel
Division of Research, Hospital das Clinicas, Faculty of Medicine of the University of Sao Paulo, Sao Paulo, Brazil
e-mail: Nancy.emmanuel@ijcrcentral.com

K. Raza (ed.), *Computational Intelligence in Oncology*, Studies in Computational Intelligence 1016, https://doi.org/10.1007/978-981-16-9221-5_14

Keywords Computational intelligence · Precision oncology · Cancer diagnosis · Machine learning · Image-based diagnosis · Prognosis prediction

1 Introduction

As one of the most dreaded illnesses of the twentieth century, cancer has become more prevalent. Its prevalence and incidence continue to rise in the twenty-first century; thus, it has become the world's second greatest cause of death, trailing only cardiovascular diseases. It is characterized by uncontrolled cell proliferation and a lack of cell death, resulting in an aberrant cell mass or tumor, except in hematological malignancies. Current cancer treatments include surgery, radiation, and chemotherapeutic medications, which frequently kill healthy cells with rapid growth rates and cause toxicity in patients, which is a severe side effect of chemotherapy. The indiscriminate destruction of normal cells, the toxicity of standard chemotherapeutic agents, and the emergence of multidrug resistance underscore the importance of developing new effective targeted treatments based on alterations in the tumor cells' molecular biology. As a result, experts are investigating techniques to destroy just malignant cells. The heterogeneity of cancer cells inside a tumor is the most significant obstacle to successful cancer therapy [1].

Big, multilayered, and highly interconnected datasets open the door to delivering new insights and speeding discoveries. Though the amount of available data has grown immensely, only a portion of it is being organized, analyzed, and interpreted. A result of modern systems that use high-speed, sophisticated image processing software, and ever-improving pattern recognition algorithms is the capacity to retrain machine learning to automate out difficult jobs in the fields of bioinformatics, medical imaging, and medical robotics [2].

Researchers have looked to imitate human intelligence by designing machines that can think and learn like humans. Machine learning is a kind of computational intelligence in which computers are programmed to become more efficient by using mathematics and statistics. Unlike other machine learning methods, deep learning uses multilayer artificial neural networks. The "deep learning" term denotes a collection of novel approaches, each of which is better than current industry-leading machine learning algorithms in numerous fields. Another key benefit of these techniques is their ability to improve accuracy in speech recognition and image categorization [3]. Thanks to these advances, deep learning has become a valuable tool for tackling diverse challenges in biomedicine. As we become more enlightened about the disease etiology and causes, we too are learning about the resources we already have at our access and which can be utilized in surprising ways. Deep learning has been shown to be a potent technique for detecting disease types based on the characterization of radiological or pathological pictures. A recent study concluded that deep learning is extremely accurate in diagnosing retinopathy based on fundus photos [4]. With the assumption that this technology would succeed, it is now being used in the drug discovery industry as well. Neural networks and variational autoencoders, among

Table 1 List of current and dynamic applications of computational intelligence (CI) in health care and medicine

Biomedical research (basic)	Translational research	Clinical practice
Experiments are automated [5]	Discovery of biomarkers	Diagnosis of disease
Data collection is automated [6]	Prioritization of drug target	Patient's genomes interpretation
Annotation of gene function [7]	Discovery of drugs	Selection of treatment
Transcription factor binding sites' prediction [8]	Repurposing of drugs	Automated surgery
Molecular dynamics stimulation [9]	Chemical toxicity prediction	Monitoring of patients
Mining of literature data [10]	Annotation of the genetic variant	Stratification of patient risk for primary prevention

other techniques, have played a major role in helping to advance the medical image analysis field and making it a much more dynamic area of study (Table 1).

We evaluate how these techniques could influence several parts of oncology, including their applications in assisting radiographic diagnosis, and highlight how these techniques are making significant progress in the field of oncology. We also discussed the challenges of clinical implementation and ways to improve the domain. We also outlined the existing solutions to these issues and constraints that are being implemented and how AI will affect future paths in the field of oncology in global health.

2 CI Impact of Precision Oncology in the Healthcare Industry

Healthcare will see significant changes in the future due to next-generation sequencing (NGS), data from large clinical trials, illness predictions, and image processing algorithms [11]. Cancer management has become a universal commitment in oncology, and AI is being pushed into the field to bring and introduce various advantages in this concern. It encompasses early detection and treatment that is customized or targeted depending on genetic information about the patient and forecasts the patient's future prognosis of the disease [12].

The capabilities of computational intelligence (CI) in complex algorithms and pattern recognition systems have the ability to improve patient care by increasing accuracy in early diagnosis and treatment. Precision medicine is more likely to succeed when ML is utilized as a tool in oncology. Complex neural networks can gather diagnostic imaging and genetic analysis data to forecast the probability of a disease and its associated treatment results. Radiomics, a machine vision field, usually uses deep learning to diagnose cancerous tumors that a human eye can't detect. And while in the case of tumor categorization and staging, tissue biopsy is still the major source of information. The biopsy is known to be vulnerable to sampling mistakes. Considering that tumors are often diverse, it may not be the ideal technique to investigate tumor biology [13].

However, imaging offers a technique to learn relevant tumor characteristics without the need to perform intrusive procedures. However, most derived images are of poor resolution, and some modalities expose patients to ionizing radiation. Diagnostic interpretations are often subjective, and it takes a long time to obtain and evaluate quantitative statistics. The results of the process also vary greatly depending on the imaging protocol, with low reproducibility (Fig. 1).

Quantitative imaging properties must be made more reproducible and diagnostically precise, as a result; these were the main drivers for radiomics developments, in which we aim to combine quantitative imagery characteristics with clinical outcomes and the classification of diseases [14]. The development, training, and validation of models that can help prevent disease and treatments, as well as patient stratification, which is key to precision medicine, are increasingly used in machine learning. Deep learning and radiomics are combined in order to give an accurate image analysis for diagnostic purposes. Medical care in health care is now being enhanced by the use of both AI and ML technologies. More progress in AI has led to a human-like approach to decision-making [15].

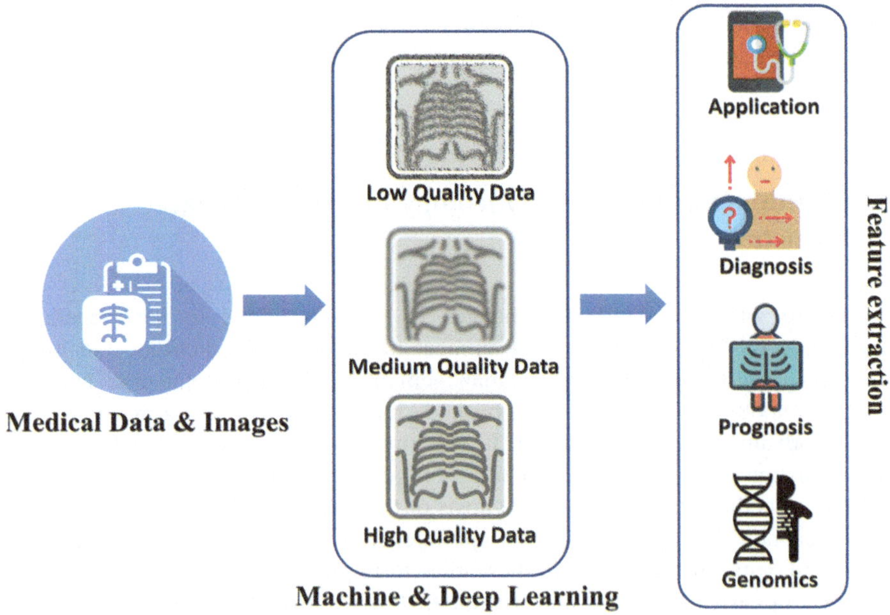

Fig. 1 Illustration of a deep learning and machine learning-based radiomics model for cancer prognosis

3 NGS-Aiding Molecular Profiling

Due to cancer's genetic complexity, precision medicine has been enhanced by increasing, understanding, and identifying major drivers of oncogenesis, along with progress in the testing of tumors by NGS and other profiling technology, and accessibility of novel treatment drugs. As the number of pharmacological aberrations and predictive biomarkers increases, NGS technology increasingly replaces conventional techniques like single-gene testing and tailored mutational platforms in molecular pathology. Conventional methods are very sensitive and specific in finding active mutations with demonstrated benefits from targeted treatments or in identifying mutations linked to drug resistance [16].

However, they must be pre-specified to identify biomarkers, and a specific test is required for each analyte. NGS can aid in analyzing a wide variety of gene mutations, copy number variations (CNV), translocations, and fusions, which is a lengthy procedure. Its high sensitivity in both tissue and cost savings offers more efficient tumor analysis than sequential single-biomarker studies [17]. Even considering the well-known genetic complexity inside malignancies, many studies have shown that using next-generation sequencing (NGS) for gene mutation scanning is comparable to traditional methods such as reverse-transcriptase (RT)-PCR and single-gene tests in everyday use. The compelling benefits of comprehensive genomic profiling by NGS, including a reduction in costs and turnaround time, and the ability to combine bioinformatics analysis and the harmonization of knowledge bases to assist clinical interpretation of genetic findings, are possible in the context of precision cancer treatment [18].

4 Biomarkers for Detecting the Onset of Disease, Its Diagnosis, and Forecasting the Prognosis

Cancer biomarkers, which include gene mutations, changes in gene transcription and translation, and protein modifications, are essential for identifying and monitoring the disease. Biomarkers are useful in determining the various phases of a disease, acting as a tool for diagnosis, prognosis, and prediction. Today, there are just a few biomarkers used in therapeutic settings. Carcinoembryonic antigen (CEA), prostate-specific antigen (PSA), and cancer antigen 125 (CA-125) are only a few examples of biomarkers in this category. But unfortunately, not enough specificity and sensitivity information is provided by any of these biomarkers for a precise diagnosis of the whole population [19, 20].

New biomarkers that can provide more accurate diagnostics are crucial. Diagnostic methods that use biomarkers for cancer detection are still primarily reliant on immunohistochemical, serological, or PCR testing. One of the significant drawbacks of immunohistochemistry is that it is invasive and requires tissue samples, and tumors may vary in biomarker content. Even with such serological methods as western blot, ELISA, and PCR, the major downside is the technical limits of each assay, which include limited detection capability and the usage of costly chemicals. Due to these factors, there has been a significant advance in the field of biosensors for initial cancer diagnosis, prognosis, and cancer therapy response prediction, as they have exhibited greater sensitivity. Consequently, the wait time for results may be shortened since the measurements can be completed in real time [21]. The most impacted CI methods and applications are listed in Table 2.

Table 2 List of CI methods and application in biomarkers and therapeutics target prediction

Application	Functioning and mechanism
Convolutional neural networks (CNNs)	CNNs are the most often used deep learning models for cancer prediction. The CNN approach is utilized to accurately and concurrently predict cancer/normal and cancer kinds based on gene expression patterns, and a novel model interpretation scheme is employed to highlight the biological significance of cancer marker genes once tissue-of-origin effects are eliminated [22]
Hybrid Taguchi-genetic algorithm (HTGA)	To detect high-order SNP barcodes, a Taguchi method is applied to a genetic algorithm. It is included to the GA just after crossover operations to improve the GA indexing [23]
Artificial neural network (ANN)	The most widely used analytical methods for biomarker identification in many cancer types [24]
Fuzzy logic selection	A novel technique to reliably detect gene signatures with higher classification capability. This approach uses computational intelligence algorithms to classify breast cancer molecular grade 2 into grade 1 and grade 2 to enhance patient prognosis. It paves the path for future research into novel biomarker combinations for applications like treatment response prediction [25]
Computer-aided detection (CADe) or computer-aided diagnosis (CADx)	The CI-based system structure lets professionals make choices quickly, improving radiologists' accuracy, and reducing time spent interpreting pictures and treating patients [26]
Support vector machine (SVM)	SVM outperforms other ML algorithms in detecting subtle patterns in large datasets. Oncology subtypes, outcome prognosis, therapeutic benefit forecasting, tumorigenesis drivers, or a tumor-specific biological system may all be classified or diagnosed using SVM algorithm [27]

5 Breakthrough of Deep Learning

The earliest deep learning methods were was derived from a model of artificial neurons originally published in 1943, which was designed to mimic the way that biological neurons process information. A neural network offers two types of layers: input, and output, with an optional set of hidden layers in between. A layer is made up of “units” or “features” that link the preceding and next levels. Each unit alters data by applying a nonlinear activation function [28].

Deep neural networks include many hidden layers (often over 100). The training process enables high-level characteristics from the previous layer to be combined with other high-level features and built on even more of them. This element can automatically be designed to solve the task. A range of different deep neural network designs exist. To analyze grid-like data such as images, a co-evolutionary neural network (CNN) may be utilized and configured to detect patterns in large datasets via many filters. Compared to a conventional CNN, a completely convolutional network (FCN) uses upsampling and deconvolution layers to replace fully connected layers, which are the reverse of convolution and pooling layers [29].

The RNN may also be used to analyze more complex data, such as genetic and linguistic sequences. In contrast to unsupervised learning, where data are trained without predefined responses, these neural networks are used in supervised learning techniques dependent on answers to train the network. Contrary to that, unsupervised learning doesn’t need labels. Unsupervised learning is used to generate outputs that are similar to the input data, and an autoencoder is a prime example of that [30]. There are two networks in a generative adversarial network (GAN): the generator and the discriminator. While the discriminator network identifies the fictitious data generated by the generator network, the generator produces bogus data to deceive the discriminator. This alternating training approach will help the generator eventually produce artificial data that seems indistinguishable from the genuine thing. Although we do not cover this in-depth, new architectures are being suggested and used in the medical field, like capsule ET and graphical convolution. Several existing frameworks or novel designs are expected to lead to a substantial rise in the use of neural networks to understand complicated events [31].

6 CI in Cancer Imaging and Diagnosis

Cancer research is progressively integrating quantitative, multiparametric, and functional imaging information. Radiomics, a rapidly expanding area of study, may allow for a more complex interpretation of imaging data, going well beyond the qualitative assessment of clearly apparent tissue changes [32]. Quantitative imaging data may be used in the future to provide more targeted and tumor-specific diagnostic workups and therapy strategies for oncology patients. This is especially in fields like radiology and radiation oncology, where the utilization of imaging data is currently high and only going to become more, this is especially critical [33]. A separate segmentation process may no longer be required for future analysis of cancer lesions due to significant increases in computer speed and improved efficiency of AI algorithms. Whole-body imaging data may instead be reviewed immediately by the AI algorithm. A holistic approach may also uncover organ structures that are not barely visible but might be exhibiting abnormal behavior [34].

For the resuscitation of affected individuals, the initial revealing of cancer is essential. Since spectacular success in the 2012 ImageNet Large Scale Visual Recognition Challenge (ILSVRC) image reconnaissance competition, many researchers and medical doctors have tried to exploit the influence of AI (or, more accurately, CNN) to be used in pathology and clinical radiology because of the elimination of the requirements for detailed feature generation. An example of a high-impact application is the successful categorization of dermoscopic pictures. AI was therefore demonstrated to be capable of annotating the lesions with the same accuracy as professional dermatologists with zone below the curve, including melanoma [35, 36].

AI has reached an accuracy level comparable to that of medical experts when interpreting mammograms for breast cancer screening. Furthermore, deep neural networks (DNNs) have been demonstrated to be efficient at detecting enlarging lymph nodes as well as colonic polyps in computed tomography images. Deep learning's many uses in radiology are discussed in more depth elsewhere. In industrialized countries, gathering digital images of diseased conditions and profound knowledge of pathological diagnosis has become a regular practice [37]. The ability of lymphocytes and the functions abstracted from that model (TIL maps) to identify tuberculosis infiltrators has been shown in 13 distinct cancer types, including breast, lung, and colorectal cancers. In addition, pathological slides from The Cancer Genome Atlas (TCGA) were subjected to a CNN analysis [38, 39].

6.1 Radiographic Imaging

One of the key elements of comprehensive cancer treatment is biomedical imaging, which offers many benefits, including real-time monitoring, the ability to do its job without the need to damage tissue, and little or no invasiveness [40]. For example, illnesses like cancer and their respective treatment times are spread throughout the spectrum, with milliseconds for things like protein binding and chemical processes and years for cancer. Molecules, cells, organs, and entire organisms all fall within the scale of size. Based on the radiology and non-radiology criteria, there are several AI-based clinical applications as well, including thoracic imaging, colonoscopy, abdominal and pelvic imaging, brain imaging, mammography, and radiation oncology come under radiology-based applications; moreover, pathology, dermatology, and DNA and RNA sequencing come under non-radiology-based applications (Fig. 2) [41].

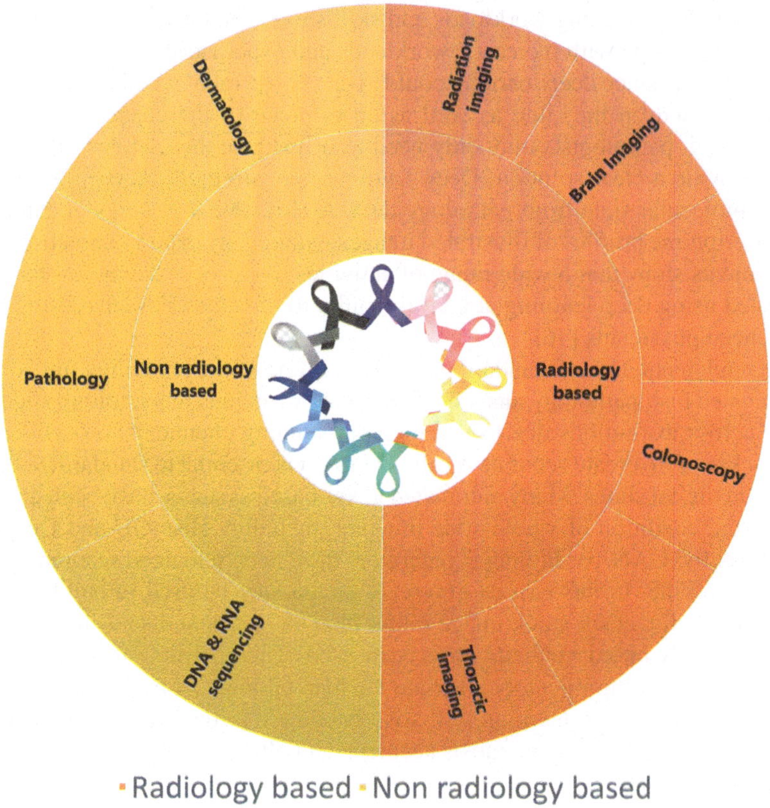

Fig. 2 Representation of clinical application areas of AI in oncology on radiological and non-radiological

6.2 Digital Pathology

Due to the fast development of technology for digitizing glass slides and the decrease in storage costs, there has been a significant rise in the usage of whole-slide images (WSIs), also known as virtual slides. WSIs allow us to view slides digitally on electronic screens at various magnifications. Numerous feasibility studies have been conducted, and regulatory authorities in major countries have authorized instruments for digital pathological imaging, primarily WSIs, for clinical use [42]. The College of American Pathologists (CAP) issued recommendations for the use of digital pathology as a first step. Shortly afterward, Philips' WSI scanner became the first to get CE certification in 2014. Increasing interest in digital pathology has led many laboratories worldwide to digitalize [43, 44]. This trend is comparable to the shift from films to DICOM in diagnostic imaging during the last two to three decades. The digitization of pathology practice enables the use of a variety of computer methods, including techniques of computational intelligence and machine learning. With increasing workloads and skill shortages, these strategies may help pathology labs cope with increased workloads and expertise shortages [45].

Furthermore, since deep learning could give a blueprint of where probable cancer cells are located on the slide as well as an estimate of the chance that the cells are malignant, pathologists may only need to investigate those slides for which AI cannot provide a clear solution. Deep learning may similarly be used to deduce a tumor's molecular state from pathology data. A HE2RNA CNN model can predict the transcriptome profiles of illustrated images without any expert annotation. These achievements show that a wide range of activities like cancer diagnosis have been performed using deep learning at a level similar to or sometimes surpassing that of experienced physicians [46].

The implementation of standard procedures is one of the remaining impediments to automated histopathology analysis. Color tone variations in pathology slides may appear across institutions due to variations in staining chemicals, procedures, and slice thickness. To create accurate AI algorithms, it is essential to standardize the tone of color in digital slides. Many automated CNN-based systems have been created to regulate the condition of whole-slide imaging, including HistoQC and DeepFocus [47]. Recently, GAN-based image generators have been remained recommended to resolve this issue. In this case, a grayscale image may be used to build a normalized hematoxylin–eosin-stuck image rather than inconsistent data as input. Beyond diagnosis, GAN-based methods have been used. These diverse instances demonstrate how AI may significantly alleviate the load on medical personnel engaged in tumor evaluation. Deep learning will soon become a critical tool for pathologists, enhancing histopathologic diagnosis accuracy and efficiency and informing therapy choices (Fig. 3) [48].

7 Computational Intelligence and Translational Oncology

Approaches based on computational intelligence (CI) have the possibility to impact many aspects of cancer treatment. These include medication research and development, and the clinical validation and eventual administration of these medicines at the point of care. At the moment, these procedures are prohibitively costly and time-consuming [49]. Additionally, treatments often result in a wide range of treatment results among individuals. The fusion of CI with cancer treatment has resulted in a plethora of answers to these problems. Computational intelligence systems ranging from machine learning to neural networks can help expedite drug development, correctly match patients to clinical trials, and fully customize cancer treatment using only the patient's data. These advancements suggest that CI-enabled cancer treatment may be on the horizon [50].

Using deep learning technology, oncologists can make better-informed treatment decisions. CI can determine the best treatment strategy for physicians by learning from clinical big data on cancer patients. Using deep learning technology, Printz et al. built a clinical decision support system (CDSS) that can collect and analyze

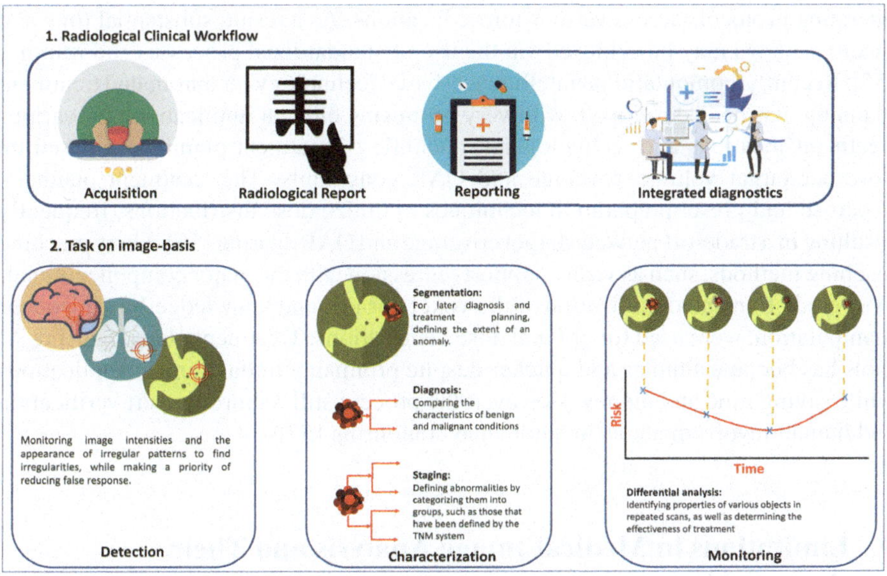

Fig. 3 Schematic outline of computational intelligence (CI) impression and workflow, i.e., clinical radiology workflow and image-based task within oncology imaging

a vast quantity of clinical data from medical records and provide treatment alternatives for cancer patients. According to the findings, AI technology may help doctors provide better cancer treatment recommendations for their patients [51, 52]. In order to minimize the overtreatment of patients, several algorithms have been developed that can assess digital pictures and diagnostic reports of patients and properly detect precancerous lesions that need to be treated. Reduce the overtreatment of lesions suspected of being cancerous using another machine learning method. As a result of the technology, clinicians may make better treatment choices and avoid performing unnecessary surgery on high-risk breast tumors [53].

8 Cancer Therapy: The Quantum Leap

Multidrug resistance is a key element that affects the outcome of illness treatment and poses a significant clinical risk. Treatment planning is based on dose per target volume coverage and OAR constraints. The treatment planner's expertise and preset preparation techniques are used to optimize dose distributions, frequently resulting in a trade-off between target coverage and OAR sparing [54].

This RT planning method is very intensive due to the many manual processes and many iterations required for dosimetric optimization. It is a collaborative effort of RTTs, dosimetrists, medical physicists, and doctors. There is a dearth of standard operating protocols across various tumor locations. As a result, substantial time and quality savings may be achieved via the use of standardized processes and routines [55]. Recently, computational intelligence-based technology for automated treatment planning has been developed, with very promising clinical implications for various treatment locations and technological modalities. Treatment planning is based on dose per target volume coverage and OAR constraints. The treatment planner's expertise and preset preparation techniques optimize dose distributions, frequently resulting in a trade-off between target coverage and OAR sparing [56]. Many machine teaching methods, such as vector support regression with the major components analysis, prediction and optimization of the voxel dosage, and knowledge-based isodose manipulation, were used for optimal dose distributions. Treatment planning using AI tools has become simpler and quicker despite promising initial clinical applications while saving time and money. However, the process still requires expert verification and human involvement, as in automated contouring [57].

9 Limitations in Medical Image Analysis and Their Proposed Solution

Generally, fewer than one million medical images are available for instruction, which vary in size from one order to another. Researchers have devised numerous methods to circumvent this constraint. Data augmentation, which involves randomly cropping, tilting, inverting, or reversing images to enhance their number, is one productive approach to deal with limited training sets. Another strategy includes dubbed transfer learning, which entails repurposing extracted features by machine learning from natural image datasets such as ImageNet for the latest idea of medical imaging [58]. A considerable number of deep learning researchers have been drawn after publishing a large, annotated dataset of fundus pictures as part of a master learning contest known as Kaggle in 2015. For example, researchers used the 48-layer CNN design known as the first CNN v3 which has been pre-trained using natural images in terms of specificity and sensitivity, and that managed to beat the present state-of-the-art model. These methods were also utilized for training AI for melanoma, the worst type of cancer of the skin. These findings provide an incentive for academics to share and open up image data to communities. Creating an increasing amount of AI available in medical images will lead to more robust and sophisticated algorithms being developed by researchers [59, 60].

10 Challenges and Future Aspects

The design concepts of various computer-based clinical equipment are already changing dramatically. The rate of adoption of newer deep learning algorithms in clinical radiography is hotly debated, with predictions ranging from a few years to decades. Autonomous deep learning solutions will start with the most common clinical concerns for which data is accessible [61]. These issues may arise when human knowledge is in short supply or when the data is much too complicated for human readers; examples include interpreting lung screening CTs, mammograms, and virtual colonoscopy images. A subsequent round of research is expected to focus on more difficult issues, such as multiparametric MRI. A frequent characteristic of contemporary AI technologies is their inability to do more than one job, as is true of any limited intellect [62].

10.1 A Unique Data Challenges

A complete computational intelligence (CI) system capable of detecting numerous disorders across the patients has expected to be created. Well, data remains a significant and fundamental component of developing AI systems. Substantial quantities of medical data are accessible and kept in a way that facilitates access and retrieval. However, such data are seldom vetted, posing a significant impediment to learning any AI model. Curation may relate to selecting appropriate patient cohorts for a particular AI job, but it can also apply to the segmentation of objects inside pictures [63]. Curation ensures that the classification model is devoid of potentially hazardous artifacts. Changes in data collection standards and imaging techniques, particularly in institutions, such as the time gap between contrast agent injection and imaging, may also be avoided. While non-experts may identify photographic pictures using methods such as crowdsourcing, medical images do need domain expertise. As a result, a qualified reader must do such curation to guarantee trustworthiness—a costly process. It is also very time-intensive, but new deep learning techniques promise to significantly decrease annotation time: Finding a seed point within the object that can be segmented into individual slices may potentially replace manual slice-by-slice segmentation [64].

10.2 Data Management, Annotation, and Storage

The amount of data that must be curated also varies depending on the AI approach, with deep learning being prone to overfitting and requiring more data. Unsupervised learning is one approach that allows automatic data curation. With generative adversarial networks and variational autoencoders, exclusionary traits may be learned without deliberate labeling. Recent research has examined unsupervised domain adaptation by segmenting brain MRI using adversarial networks, achieving unspecified and precise similarity to administered learning modules. To be sure, public archives like TCIA give unrivaled open access to labeled medical imaging data, allowing for rapid AI model creation and avoiding the need for long data curation processes. This paradigm shift away from algorithms with well-specified rules and those that learn directly from data reveals numerous previously hidden problems, despite the appearance that it increases intelligence [65].

As a result, understanding the implications of such continual learning of adaptive systems is crucial. Performing frequent evaluations at predetermined intervals may assist in ensuring learning, and the performance of its associated prediction is as expected. Moreover, such benchmarking tests must be adapted to account for AI-specific characteristics, including the sensitivity of CNN prediction probabilities. Additional ethical concerns may emerge as a result of the training of these AI systems using patient data. Data is stored inside medical institution networks, which often lack secure links to the AI system's state-of-the-art located somewhere. New developments in HIPAA-compliant storage have opened the door to even tighter privacy regulations in the future. Numerous research explores techniques for jointly training AI models without revealing the raw data sets—just the trained model is disclosed. Other projects approach learning in a decentralized, "federated" fashion. While local modifications are retained, a generalized prototype is developed by integrating them. Local inference of the shared model is then performed on live copies, obviating the requirement for privacy and data sharing concerns. The term "Cryptonets" refers to deep learning networks that are developed on encrypted data and then provide encrypted projections that can only be decrypted by the holder of a decryptor, so maintaining total secrecy across the workflow. Without sacrificing privacy or HIPAA compliance, these technologies have the ability to establish a viable "data to AI" ecosystem [66].

11 Conclusion

Health care digitalization transforms clinical procedures by making big data available including both patients as well as healthcare professionals. Experience-based medicine has given way to a data-driven, patient-centered approach. Computational intelligence (CI) will continue to have a significant influence on cancer research in the near future; hence, preparedness is required for both doctors and researchers. As a consequence, medical education should include not just biology and clinical care, but also statistics, computational, and bioinformatics skill. Many medical institutes, like the University of California, Irvine, California, United States; and Curie Institute France, started an initiative to offer short courses in collaboration with leading clinical experts on computational intelligence, cancer biology-related trending topics for free. Many open-source technologies and cloud computing companies are now making AI technology more user-friendly, which may enhance the quality of healthcare, advance medical research, and reshape the future of global healthcare.

While deep learning has gotten a lot of attention in recent years, there are still many issues that need to be worked out before it can be extensively utilized in health care and cancer research. In the next decade, AI will change oncology because of its fast development and several applications in cancer research. In the next few years, the combination of NGS with advanced bioinformatics will improve health care.

With the advent of precision oncology and the identification of novel biomarkers to assist in cancer diagnosis and therapy, the practical use of NGS is expanding. With recent technical advances, NGS systems are expected to become cheaper, quicker, and more sensitive, making them more widely available for research and clinical applications.

AI has had and will continue to have a significant impact on health care and precision oncology and will lead to a more accurate and quick diagnosis, which not only improvise and upgrade the current clinical-decision-making process of the healthcare providers but will ultimately lead to better and effective health outcomes for cancer patients and those at risk around the globe. Despite the fact that most research examining the use of AI in oncology has not been rigorously tested for repeatability and generalizability, the findings clearly point to increased concentrated attempts to bring AI technology into clinical usage and to influence future paths in cancer treatment.

References

1. Goldenberg, S. L., Nir, G., & Salcudean, S. E. (2019). A new era: Artificial intelligence and machine learning in prostate cancer. *Nature Reviews. Urology, 16*(7), 391–403. https://doi.org/10.1038/s41585-019-0193-3
2. Nguyen, V. T., Benchoufi, M., Young, B., Ghosn, L., Ravaud, P., & Boutron, I. (2019). A scoping review provided a framework for new ways of doing research through mobilizing collective intelligence. *Journal of Clinical Epidemiology, 110*, 1–11. https://doi.org/10.1016/j.jclinepi.2019.02.007
3. Bi, W. L., et al. (2019). Artificial intelligence in cancer imaging: Clinical challenges and applications. *CA: A Cancer Journal for Clinicians, 69*(2), 127–157. https://doi.org/10.3322/caac.21552
4. Callaway, N. F., & Mruthyunjaya, P. (2019). Widefield imaging of retinal and choroidal tumors. *International Journal of Retina Vitreous, 5*(S1), 49. https://doi.org/10.1186/s40942-019-0196-5
5. Yang, Y., Li, Y.-X., Yao, R.-Q., Du, X.-H., & Ren, C. (2021). Artificial intelligence in small intestinal diseases: Application and prospects. *World Journal of Gastroenterology, 27*(25), 3734–3747. https://doi.org/10.3748/wjg.v27.i25.3734
6. Hirasawa, T., et al. (2021). Current status and future perspective of artificial intelligence applications in endoscopic diagnosis and management of gastric cancer. *Digestive Endoscopy, 33*(2), 263–272. https://doi.org/10.1111/den.13890
7. Nagarajan, N., Yapp, E. K. Y., Le, N. Q. K., Kamaraj, B., Al-Subaie, A. M., & Yeh, H.-Y. (2019). Application of computational biology and artificial intelligence technologies in cancer precision drug discovery. *BioMed Research International, 2019*, 8427042. https://doi.org/10.1155/2019/8427042
8. Koromina, M., Pandi, M.-T., & Patrinos, G. P. (2019). Rethinking drug repositioning and development with artificial intelligence, machine learning, and omics. *OMICS: A Journal of Integrative Biology, 23*(11), 539–548. https://doi.org/10.1089/omi.2019.0151
9. Liang, G., Fan, W., Luo, H., & Zhu, X. (2020). The emerging roles of artificial intelligence in cancer drug development and precision therapy. *Biomedicine & Pharmacotherapy, 128*, 110255. https://doi.org/10.1016/j.biopha.2020.110255
10. Pinsky, P. (2020). Artificial intelligence and data mining to assess lung cancer risk: Challenges and opportunities. *Annals of Internal Medicine, 173*(9), 760–761. https://doi.org/10.7326/M20-5673

11. Siddiqui, M. F. (2021). IoMT Potential Impact in COVID-19: Combating a Pandemic with Innovation. In K. Raza (Ed.), *Computational intelligence methods in COVID-19: Surveillance, prevention, prediction and diagnosis* (Vol. 923, pp. 349–361). Springer. https://doi.org/10.1007/978-981-15-8534-0_18
12. Chua, I. S., et al. (2021). Artificial intelligence in oncology: Path to implementation. *Cancer Medicine, 10*(12), 4138–4149. https://doi.org/10.1002/cam4.3935
13. Summers, R. M. (2019). Are we at a crossroads or a plateau? Radiomics and machine learning in abdominal oncology imaging. *AbdomRadiol (NY), 44*(6), 1985–1989. https://doi.org/10.1007/s00261-018-1613-1
14. Huang, S., Yang, J., Fong, S., & Zhao, Q. (2020). Artificial intelligence in cancer diagnosis and prognosis: Opportunities and challenges. *Cancer Letters, 471*, 61–71. https://doi.org/10.1016/j.canlet.2019.12.007
15. Niu, P.-H., Zhao, L.-L., Wu, H.-L., Zhao, D.-B., & Chen, Y.-T. (2020). Artificial intelligence in gastric cancer: Application and future perspectives. *World Journal of Gastroenterology, 26*(36), 5408–5419. https://doi.org/10.3748/wjg.v26.i36.5408
16. Shimizu, H., & Nakayama, K. I. (2020). Artificial intelligence in oncology. *Cancer Science, 111*(5), 1452–1460. https://doi.org/10.1111/cas.14377
17. Guan, Y.-F., et al. (2012). Application of next-generation sequencing in clinical oncology to advance personalized treatment of cancer. *Chinese Journal of Cancer, 31*(10), 463–470. https://doi.org/10.5732/cjc.012.10216
18. Hosny, A., Parmar, C., Quackenbush, J., Schwartz, L. H., & Aerts, H. J. W. L. (2018). Artificial intelligence in radiology. *Nature Reviews Cancer, 18*(8), 500–510. https://doi.org/10.1038/s41568-018-0016-5
19. Sheth, D., & Giger, M. L. (2020). Artificial intelligence in the interpretation of breast cancer on MRI. *Journal of MagnReson Imaging, 51*(5), 1310–1324. https://doi.org/10.1002/jmri.26878
20. Hoshino, A., et al. (2020). Extracellular vesicle and particle biomarkers define multiple human cancers. *Cell, 182*(4), 1044-1061.e18. https://doi.org/10.1016/j.cell.2020.07.009
21. Coon, J., Kingsley, K., & Howard, K. M. (2020). miR-365 (microRNA): Potential biomarker in oral squamous cell carcinoma exosomes and extracellular vesicles. *International Journal of Molecular Sciences, 21*(15), E5317. https://doi.org/10.3390/ijms21155317
22. Munir, K., Elahi, H., Ayub, A., Frezza, F., & Rizzi, A. (2019). Cancer diagnosis using deep learning: A bibliographic review. *Cancers (Basel), 11*(9), E1235. https://doi.org/10.3390/cancers11091235
23. Chuang, L.-Y., Yang, C.-S., Yang, H.-S., & Yang, C.-H. (2020). Identification of high-order single-nucleotide polymorphism barcodes in breast cancer using a hybrid Taguchi-genetic algorithm: Case-control study. *JMIR Medical Informatics, 8*(6), e16886. https://doi.org/10.2196/16886
24. Checcucci, E., et al. (2020). Artificial intelligence and neural networks in urology: Current clinical applications. *Minerva UrolNefrol, 72*(1), 49–57. https://doi.org/10.23736/S0393-2249.19.03613-0
25. Kempowsky-Hamon, T., et al. (2015). Fuzzy logic selection as a new reliable tool to identify molecular grade signatures in breast cancer–the INNODIAG study. *BMC Medical Genomics, 8*, 3. https://doi.org/10.1186/s12920-015-0077-1
26. Firmino, M., Angelo, G., Morais, H., Dantas, M. R., & Valentim, R. (2016). Computer-aided detection (CADe) and diagnosis (CADx) system for lung cancer with likelihood of malignancy. *Biomedical Engineering Online, 15*, 2. https://doi.org/10.1186/s12938-015-0120-7
27. Huang, S., Cai, N., Pacheco, P. P., Narrandes, S., Wang, Y., & Xu, W. (2018). Applications of support vector machine (SVM) learning in cancer genomics. *Cancer Genomics & Proteomics, 15*(1), 41–51. https://doi.org/10.21873/cgp.20063
28. Suh, H. B., et al. (2018). Primary central nervous system lymphoma and atypical glioblastoma: Differentiation using radiomics approach. *European Radiology, 28*(9), 3832–3839. https://doi.org/10.1007/s00330-018-5368-4
29. Kniep, H. C., et al. (2019). Radiomics of brain MRI: Utility in prediction of metastatic tumor type. *Radiology, 290*(2), 479–487. https://doi.org/10.1148/radiol.2018180946

30. Shin, H., et al. (2020). Early-stage lung cancer diagnosis by deep learning-based spectroscopic analysis of circulating exosomes. *ACS Nano, 14*(5), 5435–5444. https://doi.org/10.1021/acsnano.9b09119
31. Wang, C., et al. (2020). Crowdsourcing in health and medical research: A systematic review. *Infectious Diseases of Poverty, 9*(1), 8. https://doi.org/10.1186/s40249-020-0622-9
32. Raza, K., & Singh, N. K. (2021). A tour of unsupervised deep learning for medical image analysis. *Current Medical Imaging, 17*(9), 1059–1077. https://doi.org/10.2174/1573405617666210127154257
33. Singh, N. K., & Raza, K. (2021). Medical image generation using generative adversarial networks: A review. In R. Patgiri, A. Biswas & P. Roy (Eds.), *Health informatics: A computational perspective in healthcare* (Vol. 932, pp. 77–96). Singapore. https://doi.org/10.1007/978-981-15-9735-0_5
34. Eychenne, R., Bouvry, C., Bourgeois, M., Loyer, P., Benoist, E., & Lepareur, N. (2020). Overview of radiolabeled somatostatin analogs for cancer imaging and therapy. *Molecules, 25*(17), E4012. https://doi.org/10.3390/molecules25174012
35. Chan, H.-P., Samala, R. K., & Hadjiiski, L. M. (2020). CAD and AI for breast cancer-recent development and challenges. *British Journal of Radiology, 93*(1108), 20190580. https://doi.org/10.1259/bjr.20190580
36. Wani, N., & Raza, K. (2018). Multiple Kernel-learning approach for medical image analysis. In *Soft computing based medical image analysis* (pp. 31–47). Elsevier. https://doi.org/10.1016/B978-0-12-813087-2.00002-6
37. Hachey, S. J., et al. (2021). An *in vitro* vascularized micro-tumor model of human colorectal cancer recapitulates *in vivo* responses to standard-of-care therapy. *Lab on a Chip, 21*(7), 1333–1351. https://doi.org/10.1039/D0LC01216E
38. Afshar-Oromieh, A., et al. (2016). The rise of PSMA ligands for diagnosis and therapy of prostate cancer. *Journal of Nuclear Medicine, 57*(Suppl 3), 79S-89S. https://doi.org/10.2967/jnumed.115.170720
39. Trebeschi, S., et al. (2019). Predicting response to cancer immunotherapy using noninvasive radiomic biomarkers. *Annals of Oncology, 30*(6), 998–1004. https://doi.org/10.1093/annonc/mdz108
40. Papanikolaou, N., Matos, C., & Koh, D. M. (2020). How to develop a meaningful radiomic signature for clinical use in oncologic patients. *Cancer Imaging, 20*(1), 33. https://doi.org/10.1186/s40644-020-00311-4
41. Geras, K. J., Mann, R. M., & Moy, L. (2019). Artificial intelligence for mammography and digital breast tomosynthesis: Current concepts and future perspectives. *Radiology, 293*(2), 246–259. https://doi.org/10.1148/radiol.2019182627
42. Vuong, L. M., et al. (2015). Differential effects of hepatocyte nuclear factor 4α isoforms on tumor growth and T-cell factor 4/AP-1 interactions in human colorectal cancer cells. *Molecular and Cellular Biology, 35*(20), 3471–3490. https://doi.org/10.1128/MCB.00030-15
43. Bera, K., Schalper, K. A., Rimm, D. L., Velcheti, V., & Madabhushi, A. (2019). Artificial intelligence in digital pathology—New tools for diagnosis and precision oncology. *Nature Reviews. Clinical Oncology, 16*(11), 703–715. https://doi.org/10.1038/s41571-019-0252-y
44. Zhang, Y., Qazi, S., & Raza, K. (2021). Differential expression analysis in ovarian cancer: A functional genomics and systems biology approach. *Saudi Journal of Biological Sciences, 28*(7), 4069–4081. https://doi.org/10.1016/j.sjbs.2021.04.022
45. Cuocolo, R., Caruso, M., Perillo, T., Ugga, L., & Petretta, M. (2020). Machine Learning in oncology: A clinical appraisal. *Cancer Letters, 481*, 55–62. https://doi.org/10.1016/j.canlet.2020.03.032
46. Kumar, M., Salem, K., Tevaarwerk, A. J., Strigel, R. M., & Fowler, A. M. (2020). Recent advances in imaging steroid hormone receptors in breast cancer. *Journal of Nuclear Medicine, 61*(2), 172–176. https://doi.org/10.2967/jnumed.119.228858
47. Yang, S. J., et al. (2020). Establishment and clinical testing of pancreatic cancer faster R-CNN AI system based on fast regional convolutional neural network. *Zhonghua Wai Ke Za Zhi, 58*(7), 520–524. https://doi.org/10.3760/cma.j.cn112139-20191017-00515

48. Ardila, D., et al. (2019). End-to-end lung cancer screening with three-dimensional deep learning on low-dose chest computed tomography. *Nature Medicine, 25*(6), 954–961. https://doi.org/10.1038/s41591-019-0447-x
49. Alam, A., Imam, N., Siddiqui, M. F., Ali, Md. K., Ahmed, M. M., & Ishrat, R. (2021). Human gene expression profiling identifies key therapeutic targets in tuberculosis infection: A systematic network meta-analysis. *Infection, Genetics and Evolution, 87*, 104649. https://doi.org/10.1016/j.meegid.2020.104649
50. He, Z.-Y., et al. (2020). Corrigendum to 'up-regulation of RFC3 promotes triple negative breast cancer metastasis and is associated with poor prognosis via EMT' [translational oncology 10 (2017); 1–9]. *Translation Oncology, 13*(6), 100803. https://doi.org/10.1016/j.tranon.2020.100803
51. Printz, C. (2017). Artificial intelligence platform for oncology could assist in treatment decisions. *Cancer, 123*(6), 905–905. https://doi.org/10.1002/cncr.30655
52. Meyer, P., Noblet, V., Mazzara, C., & Lallement, A. (2018). Survey on deep learning for radiotherapy. *Computers in Biology and Medicine, 98*, 126–146. https://doi.org/10.1016/j.compbiomed.2018.05.018
53. Hu, L., et al. (2019). An observational study of deep learning and automated evaluation of cervical images for cancer screening. *JNCI: Journal of the National Cancer Institute, 111*(9), 923–932. https://doi.org/10.1093/jnci/djy225
54. Ibrahim, A., et al. (2020). Artificial intelligence in digital breast pathology: Techniques and applications. *Breast, 49*, 267–273. https://doi.org/10.1016/j.breast.2019.12.007
55. Le Berre, C., et al. (2020). Application of artificial intelligence to gastroenterology and hepatology. *Gastroenterology, 158*(1), 76-94.e2. https://doi.org/10.1053/j.gastro.2019.08.058
56. Habowski, A. N., Habowski, T. J., & Waterman, M. L. (2021). GECO: Gene expression clustering optimization app for non-linear data visualization of patterns. *BMC Bioinformatics, 22*(1), 29. https://doi.org/10.1186/s12859-020-03951-2
57. Huynh, E., et al. (2020). Artificial intelligence in radiation oncology. *Nature Reviews. Clinical Oncology, 17*(12), 771–781. https://doi.org/10.1038/s41571-020-0417-8
58. Liu, S.-L., et al. (2019). Establishment and application of an artificial intelligence diagnosis system for pancreatic cancer with a faster region-based convolutional neural network. *Chinese Medical Journal (English), 132*(23), 2795–2803. https://doi.org/10.1097/CM9.0000000000000544
59. Niazi, M. K. K., Parwani, A. V., & Gurcan, M. N. (2019). Digital pathology and artificial intelligence. *The Lancet Oncology, 20*(5), e253–e261. https://doi.org/10.1016/S1470-2045(19)30154-8
60. Gao, Y., et al. (2019). Deep neural network-assisted computed tomography diagnosis of metastatic lymph nodes from gastric cancer. *Chinese Medical Journal (English), 132*(23), 2804–2811. https://doi.org/10.1097/CM9.0000000000000532
61. Wang, C., Zhu, X., Hong, J. C., & Zheng, D. (2019). Artificial intelligence in radiotherapy treatment planning: present and future. *Technology in Cancer Research & Treatment, 18*, 1533033819873922. https://doi.org/10.1177/1533033819873922
62. Wei, J., et al. (2020). Radiomics in liver diseases: Current progress and future opportunities. *Liver International, 40*(9), 2050–2063. https://doi.org/10.1111/liv.14555
63. El Naqa, I., Haider, M. A., Giger, M. L., & Ten Haken, R. K. (2020). Artificial intelligence: Reshaping the practice of radiological sciences in the 21st century. *British Journal of Radiology, 93*(1106), 20190855. https://doi.org/10.1259/bjr.20190855
64. Hamidinekoo, A., Denton, E., Rampun, A., Honnor, K., & Zwiggelaar, R. (2018). Deep learning in mammography and breast histology, an overview and future trends. *Medical Image Analysis, 47*, 45–67. https://doi.org/10.1016/j.media.2018.03.006
65. Aneja, S., Chang, E., & Omuro, A. (2019). Applications of artificial intelligence in neurooncology. *CurrOpin Neurol, 32*(6), 850–856. https://doi.org/10.1097/WCO.0000000000000761
66. Jiang, Y., Yang, M., Wang, S., Li, X., & Sun, Y. (2020). Emerging role of deep learning-based artificial intelligence in tumor pathology. *Cancer Communication (London), 40*(4), 154–166. https://doi.org/10.1002/cac2.12012

Computational Intelligence-Based Cheminformatics Model as Cancer Therapeutics

Ritushree Biswas, Abira Dey, Ria Puri, Sarra Akermi, Sagarika Sahoo, Rishabh Panesar, Chandramohan Jana, Sunil Jayant, Anshul Nigam, Jean Bernard, Subrata Sinha, and Surabhi Johari

Abstract A cancer is used to describe disorders in which abberant cells divide uncontrollably and infect neighboring tissues. The development of novel and more effective anti-cancer chemotherapies is a rapidly expanding field of research. The structural characteristics and chemical properties of chemical structures are used in recent cheminformatics-inspired techniques to provide essential information regarding lead molecule associations. This strategy could help scientists to better comprehend biology and boost research, especially when it comes to finding new biomarkers. Cheminformatics has been proved effective in anti-cancer drug designing and investigating the pathway of drug delivery. In recent years artificial intelligence (AI) is progressing in the field of cancer prognosis and cancer diagnosis. The studies reveal that AI predicts the cancer prognosis more accurately utilizing deep learning

---

Ritushree Biswas, Abira Dey and Ria Puri are equal contribution.

R. Biswas · S. Akermi · S. Sahoo · R. Panesar
Annotation Analytics Pvt. Ltd., 36, Ward No. -14, Biswa, Amarpura, Gurgaon, Haryana 122001, India

A. Dey · S. Jayant
Indian Science and Technology Foundation (ISTF), C-1/131, Yamuna Vihar, New Delhi 110053, India

R. Puri · S. Johari (✉)
Institute of Management Studies University Courses Campus, Ghaziabad, Uttar Pradesh 201002, India
e-mail: surabhi.johari@imsuc.ac.in

A. Nigam
Amity University Mumbai, Bhatan Post—Somathne, Panvel, Mumbai, Maharashtra 410206, India

C. Jana
Department of Chemistry, Michael Madhusudan Memorial College, Durgapur, West Bengal 713216, India

J. Bernard
Insight Biosolutions, 35000 Rennes, France

S. Sinha
Centre for Biotechnology and Bioinformatics, Dibrugarh University, Dibrugarh, Assam 786001, India

K. Raza (ed.), *Computational Intelligence in Oncology*, Studies in Computational Intelligence 1016, https://doi.org/10.1007/978-981-16-9221-5_15

(DL), artificial neural networks (ANN). Also, It is proved that convolutional neural networks (CNN), are an evolving approach in many cases of cancer diagnosis particularly classifying cancer lesions. With the use of these bioinformatics models, the development of novel disease-curing treatments is possible these days. Cheminformatics has a bright future ahead with improved solutions to drug therapeutics in cancer studies.

Keywords Artificial intelligence · Cancer · Cheminformatics · Therapeutics

1 Introduction

Cheminformatics is a branch of computer science that deals with learning from chemical data and modeling problems that chemists face. In the last few years, the field has evolved significantly, influencing how chemical research is conducted by allowing access to chemical data on a scale not possible with previous approaches. Structure data has been used to predict a variety of physical, chemical, and biological facts. Methods have been created for the early stages of drug design that are employed by all major pharmaceutical corporations. Cheminformatics approaches, on the other hand, can assist all fields of chemistry; many areas that are not yet well established but could profit significantly from the use of cheminformatics methods [1].

Chemical sciences are critical to the development of clinically effective anti-cancer medicines, utilizing a variety of cheminformatics models. The number of therapeutic targets available has expanded as our understanding of the cellular, molecular, and genetic foundation of cancer has improved. The chemical techniques employed in the development of drugs that target specific properties of cancer cells improve the efficacy of novel therapeutics. Over the decades, chemical synthesis and understanding of drug uptake have played important roles in drug development, as well as chemical insights of drug molecules interactions [2]. The main issue with drug design and development is the amount of time it takes and the expense of production. In addition, the distribution and development of pharmaceuticals are hindered by inefficiency, imprecise target delivery, and insufficient dosage. With advancements in technology, computer-assisted drug development using artificial intelligence algorithms can reduce competition and save effort. Machine learning approaches that include supervised learning, unsupervised learning, and reinforcement learning, and artificial are providing a great help in the designing of drugs [3]. Furthermore, deep learning, a subset of machine learning, has been widely used in medication development and design. Artificial neural networks (ANNs), deep neural networks (DNNs), support vector machines (SVMs), and classification are all examples of artificial neural networks. Computational intelligence principles have been applied to active and inactive drug classification, drug release monitoring, pre-clinical and clinical development, primary and secondary drug screening, biomarker development, pharmaceutical manufacturing, bioactivity identification, and physiochemical properties, toxicity prediction, and mode of action identification [4]. The AI models that are described in this chapter will provide a guide for in silico drug design processes.

2 Structure-Based Cheminformatics Model for Cancer

Structure-based machine learning predominantly focuses on categorizing the small molecules which can indubitably target the protein site under study thereby resulting in the minimization of the trial–and–error cost and multiplication of fruitful results [5]. It mainly predicts the binding affinity or score between the target site or molecule under study and the small molecules [2]. Then the binding affinity or score is utilized to list the small molecules in descending order according to their affinity of binding with the target site or molecule under study. It is generally considered that greater binding affinity or score betwixt the target site or molecule understudy better is the target–molecule interaction.

The technique of using physical chemistry along with computer science and information technology is popularly known as the "in silico" technique. This in silico technique is used by different chemical and pharmaceutical companies and researchers to find the mechanistic pathways of drug delivery and also in well-defined drug designs [1]. Ever since the in-silico molecular modeling was initiated, structure-based machine learning has expanded the procedure of drug discovery to a greater extent. There are many structure-based machine learning models that are used for identifying the target-drug interactions. Some of them are listed below.

2.1 Molecular Docking and Molecular Dynamics Simulation

Molecular modeling girdles every theoretical and computational technique to replicate or mimic the response of molecules [6]. Molecular docking is a method belonging to the domain of molecular modeling that previses the favorable interaction of two molecules (target site or molecule under study and the small or drug molecules), when they are bound with each other, for the formation of a stable complex [7]. The target-molecule interaction is studied by calculating the free energy of binding (ΔG) and is considered that the complex having the least (or most negative) ΔG value has more binding affinity which implies the most stable complex formed [8].

Pattanayak et al. performed the interaction study of 23 furanocoumarins compounds (Marmesin, Xanthotoxol, Khellin, Psoralen, Bergapten, Angelicin, Methoxsalen, Visnagin, Isobergapten, Sphondin, Lanatin, Xanthotoxin, Apterin, 6,7-dihydroxy bergamottin, Imperatonin, Isopimpinellin, Trioxsalen, Bergamottin, Isoimperatonin, and Phellopterin) regarded to have anti-cancer properties with target receptors namely, Estrogen receptor (Erα), Progesterone receptor (PR), Epidermal growth factor receptor (EGFR) and mammalian target of rapamycin (mTOR) for the breast cancer treatment. They used FlexX docking tool for the study and the best docking score was found for Xanthotoxol and therefore it can be regarded as a powerful anti-cancer drug [17]. Kumar et al. performed a docking study with different cancer macromolecules (VEGFR-2, CDK-2, Bcl-2, CDK-6, G-Quadruplexes, and IGF-1R kinase) and pyridoacridines that contains natural anti-cancer pigments. They used the Glide docking tool for the study and the best docking score found for CDK-6 and therefore it is regarded as the most acceptable anti-cancer target [18]. Few of the tools utilized to carry out these experiments are highlighted in Table 1.

The molecular dynamic simulation was first put forward by Wainwright and Alder in the late 1950s. Molecular dynamics is the technique of computer simulation that is involved in examining the physical motions of the molecules and atoms, therefore, the modus operandi involves the modeling of microscopic particles on a molecular scale [19]. In Fig. 1, we have depicted different types of tools used for molecular dynamics simulation [20].

Table 1 Tools used for molecular docking

S. No.	Tools	Links	References
1	ParDOCK	http://www.scfbio-iitd.res.in/dock/pardock.jsp	[9]
2	PatchDock	https://bioinfo3d.cs.tau.ac.il/PatchDock/	[10]
3	HADDOCK	https://wenmr.science.uu.nl/haddock2.4/submit/1	[11]
4	DockThor	https://dockthor.lncc.br/v2/	[12]
5	AutoDock	https://autodock.scripps.edu/	[13]
6	Discovery Studio	https://www.3ds.com/products-services/biovia/products/molecular-modeling-simulation/biovia-discovery-studio/	[14]
7	FlexX	https://www.biosolveit.de/products/	[14]
8	UCSF Dock	http://dock.compbio.ucsf.edu/	[15]
9	GOLD	https://www.ch.cam.ac.uk/computing/software/gold-suite	[16]

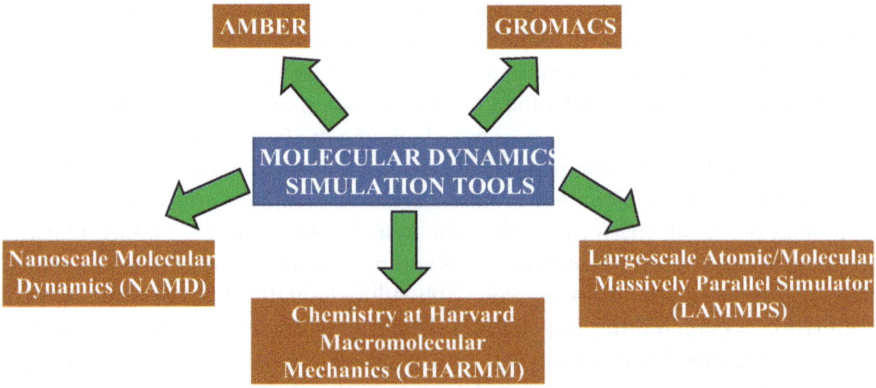

Fig. 1 Different molecular dynamics tools used for simulation

Yasuda et al. introduced a molecular dynamic simulation-based model that has the potency of studying mutations in complex cancer and suggested that their model is a potent tool for precision medicine to non-small cell lung carcinoma victims bearing unusual epidermal growth factor receptor gene (EGFR) mutations [21]. Gurung et al. used AMBER16 program which is available on the Ligand and Receptor Molecular Dynamics (LARMD) server for carrying out the molecular dynamic simulation of *Ficus carica* L. plant extracts in order to investigate the mechanistic pathway of its anti-cancer property and concluded that the *Ficus carica* L. plant extracts can be valuable in anti-cancer treatments [22].

2.2 Cheminformatics

The process in which the concepts of physical chemistry, mainly quantum chemistry and force-field molecular modeling, is combined with the methodology of the information technology and computer science in order to describe and prescribe different issues related to chemistry, biology, and other related molecular fields is known as cheminformatics or chemoinformatics [19]. According to Frank K. Brown, "Cheminformatics is the mixing of those information resources to transform data into information and information into knowledge for the intended purpose of making better decisions faster in the arena of drug lead identification and optimization" [20]. In contrast to bioinformatics, cheminformatics mainly deals with small molecules. Although, the cooperation of bioinformatics and cheminformatics is required to predict various biomolecular processes like finding the interaction of receptor molecules with ligands, the effect of a catalyst in enzyme catalysis reactions, and so on [21]. Cheminformatics has been regarded as a time-effective technology since a number of analyses can be done at a time with the least possibility of intercepting errors. Thus, a person practically analyzing one or two compounds for days or weeks can analyze hundreds or thousands of compounds at the same interval of time using cheminformatics [22]. Tools used for cheminformatics can support and examine an endless amount of chemical data using proper databases and act as a novel technique to extract those data whenever required in order to model the structural relationships and biological activities between chemical compounds (Fig. 2) [23, 24].

Sardari et al. used three cheminformatics tools (ChemDraw Ultra-[0.8, 2004] for drawing structure of the compounds, PubChem and NCI/CADD group server for similarity search) to study five novel herbal extracts that were combined with cisplatin and doxorubicin which were used to stimulate human renal adenocarcinoma (ACHN) and human ovarian carcinoma, resistant to cisplatin (A2780/cp) cells and overpower multidrug resistance (MDR) phenomenon which acts as a crucial obstruction to anti-cancer treatment [25].

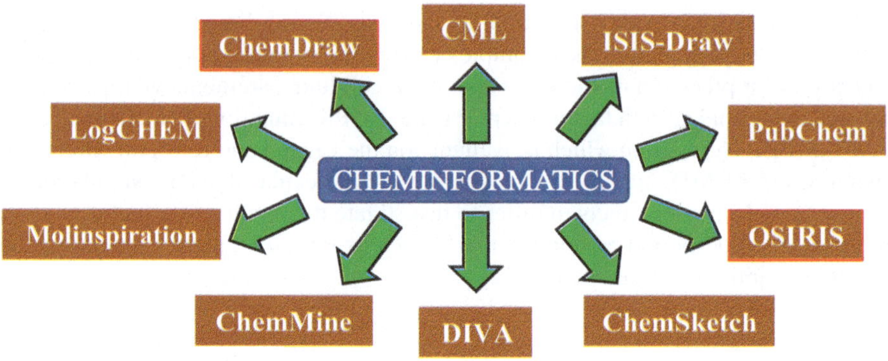

Fig. 2 Different tools used in cheminformatics

2.3 *Proteo-chemometrics*

The combined extraction of features from both target protein and drugs is advantageous to establish prognostic models of drug activity. This combinative perspective is known as proteo-chemometrics [26]. Albanese et al. coordinated DrugGenEx-Net, a proteo-chemometrics system, with normal and prostate cancer cells and they concluded that their procedure is broadly capable of recognizing and examining the approved drugs that can possibly avert or at least retard the reappearance of the primary prostate cancer in patients [27]. Estrogen-dependent breast cancer is found in many women all over the world and one of the main reasons for such cancer is aromatase, an enzyme that acts as a catalyst to convert androgen to estrogen. Nantasenamat et al. developed a proteo-chemometrics model in order to formulate some powerful aromatase inhibitors and studied their interaction with the aromatase enzyme and suggested that their findings provide the significant perception that can pave the way in designing dynamic aromatase inhibitors for the treatment of breast cancer [28].

2.4 *Molecular Dynamics Simulation*

This method was first put forward by Wainwright and Alder in the late 1950s. Molecular dynamics is the technique of computer simulation that is involved in examining the physical motions of the molecules and atoms, therefore, the modus operandi involves the modeling of microscopic particles on a molecular scale [29].

Yasuda et al. introduced a molecular dynamic simulation-based model that has the potency of studying mutations in complex cancer and suggested that their model is a potent tool for precision medicine to non-small cell lung carcinoma victims bearing unusual epidermal growth factor receptor gene (EGFR) mutations [30]. Gurung et al. used AMBER16 program which is available on the Ligand and Receptor Molecular

Dynamics (LARMD) server for carrying out the molecular dynamic simulation of *Ficus carica* L. plant extracts in order to investigate the mechanistic pathway of its anti-cancer property and concluded that the *Ficus carica* L. plant extracts can be valuable in anti-cancer treatments [31].

3 Ligand-Based Cheminformatics Cancer Models

Ligand-based drug design is a technique that uses information of molecules that bind to the desired biological target [32]. This approach is devoid of any knowledge of the receptor molecule. It is dependent on the basic principle that molecules having similar structures are likely to have similar properties [3, 33–35]. Ligand-based drug design technique uses various computational algorithms for describing the features of small molecules [36–38]. These features or properties are termed as descriptors. These properties are basically derived from the structure of the molecules. Ligand-based drug design includes three methods, namely: molecular fingerprint and similarity searches; pharmacophore modeling, and QSAR.

The molecular fingerprint method collects a cluster of molecules based on structural similarity. This technique is less computationally expensive in comparison to pharmacophore mapping and QSAR models. One of the important features of this method lies in the fact that this technique equally consider all parts of the molecule and avoids focussing only on parts of a molecule that are thought to be the most important for activity [39–43].

The idea of pharmacophore was first brought forward by Ehrlich in 1909. The basis behind the pharmacophore model is that their mode of binding the inhibitors against a specific target may possess a set of common physicochemical properties. There are three processes involved in pharmacophore modeling:

- Finding the features required for particular biological activity.
- Determining molecular conformation necessary (i.e., bioactive conformation).
- Developing an alignment rule for the series of compounds.

Developing molecular alignment is a challenge in pharmacophore modeling. There are two approaches for molecular alignment: (a) property-based approach and (b) point-based approach. In the case of the property-based approach, the superimposition is generated using molecular descriptors. Such molecular descriptors constitute Gaussian functions. Grid-based interaction energies, atomic property fields, fuzzy pattern recognition are some recently developed alignment methods. In a point-based approach, superimposition is done using least-squares fitting. The points such as fragments or pairs of atoms are aligned using this method. In this approach, the anchor points need to be predefined which can be considered as one of its major limitations [44–46].

QSAR is a procedure for creating a mathematical or computational model which finds a correlation between the structure and property of a compound. These properties are well known as descriptors. Some molecular descriptors in QSAR are partition coefficient (log P), Hansch's substitution constant, solubility parameter, Hammett constant, ionization constant, molar volume, Van der Waals radius, etc. On the basis of dimensionality of molecular representation, molecular descriptors are 0D, 1D, 2D, 3D. Molecular weight, rotatable bonds, double bonds, aromatic bonds are some examples of 0D descriptors. The number of primary carbon, tertiary carbon, number of H-bond acceptor atoms come under 1D descriptors. 2D descriptors are all topological descriptors. 3D descriptors include the radius of gyration, 3D Wiener index, surface area, polar surface area, etc. The goal of QSAR is to correlate the change taking place in the biological activity on altering the structure. There are several software tools that calculate such descriptors for any given structure [47–50].

Ligand-based machine learning approaches is of huge importance in recent years. The essence of machine learning lies in the fact that it is able to train a model when numerous data is available. For an instance, Allen et al. have designed a neural network model to assess the kinase activity across the human kinome. With the advancement of cases in cancer, there has also been an unprecedented development in machine learning in cancer prognosis and diagnosis. Deep learning models are able to screen databases containing a large number of compounds for a kinase that is important for multiple types of cancer.

One of the most prominent issues identified in the research reviewed in this evaluation was a failure to pay attention to data size and learner validation. A sufficiently big data collection that can be partitioned into disjoint training and test sets or subjected to some reasonable kind of n-fold cross-validation for smaller data sets is a minimum need for any machine learning project.

4 Random Forest-Based Cancer Model

Random forest or random decision forest is a method of conglomeration learning for categorization, regression, and other missions that work by establishing a large number of decision trees at the time of trial. Tim Kam Ho had established the first algorithm for a random forest. However, different types of algorithms for random forests are found nowadays (Fig. 3). When categorization is the work to be done, the result of random forest is the category that is chosen by most trees. When regression is the task to be done, the result is the midway prediction of discrete trees [51, 52]. Further, we have depicted the different algorithms for the random forest in Fig. 3 [53–56].

Predicting and designing a drug to treat a disease have always been a complicated process and when it comes to cancer therapy it becomes even more difficult. Pathologically some cancers might look similar but their response to the same drug may vary to a great extent [57]. The random forest machine learning model has found its importance to deal with such difficulties with a high accuracy rate. Moreover, the random forests method has also ranked among the best executing algorithms as suggested by the NCI-DREAM drug sensitivity prediction challenge [58]. Few of the algorithms used in the experimental studies are described in Fig. 3.

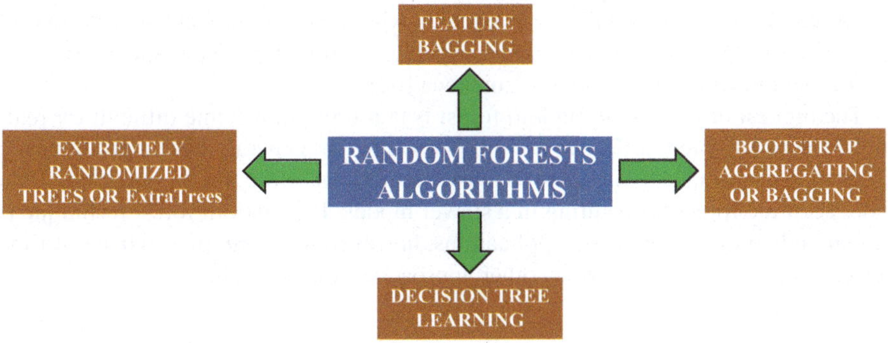

Fig. 3 Different types of algorithms for random forests

Anderson et al. studied 145 oncogene mutations and rejected 95 avoiding any change in the classification accuracy using a fivefold cross-validation random forest model and suggested that their analysis might find its importance in drug discovery applications and aid drug reprocessing which is extremely helpful for productive drug treatments for different cancer patients [59]. Rajini et al. proposed a model to predict lung cancer using K-fold cross-validation random forest classification machine learning model and found that their studied model has a very high accuracy rate thereby concluding that their studied model can assist medical experts in diagnosing lung cancer at an early stage [60]. Chen et al. employed a random forest algorithm for the diagnostic case studies of breast cancer and the results obtained had a high accuracy rate. Thus, they suggest that their model has experimental significance for additional medical diagnosis [61]. Hepatocellular carcinoma patients are not frequently treated by liver transplantation due to a shortage of liver organ donors, therefore they are given secondary curative treatment like liver resection [62]. Guba et al. proposed a clinical parameter-based random forest model, whose workflow included preprocessing, recursive feature elimination, reconstructing, training, and cross-validation, which was highly capable of predicting cancer-free survival for patients who undergo liver resection [63]. Women suffering from cervical cancer are treated by surgical resection, for early stage cancer, and concurrent chemoradiotherapy, for middle and advanced-stage cancer, but the treatment efficacy in chemoradiotherapy is still poor [64]. Liu et al. constructed and enhanced a random forest model using open-source toolkit scikit-learn and suggested that their proposed model has the capability to predict the potency of neoadjuvant chemotherapy–radiation therapy on advanced-stage cervical cancer patients [65]. Now—a—days, many people are diagnosed which acute myeloid leukemia, a deadly blood cancer, but the manual diagnostic techniques are not up to the mark because they are time-consuming, labor concerted, and also face variation among observers [66]. Dasariraju et al. designed a random forest algorithm to detect and classify immature leukocytes and suggested that their studied model can be utilized as sustainable equipment to diagnose acute myeloid leukemia with a high accuracy rate of detecting and classifying immature leukocytes [67]. Lui et al. constructed a random forest model for the prediction of bone metastasis in patients who are freshly detected with thyroid cancer and suggest that their model is capable of providing medic specialists with more customized decision-making guidance [68].

The biggest drawback of random forest is that it might become difficult for real-time forecasts to predict if there are too many trees. In general, these algorithms are quick to learn yet take a long time to make predictions. More trees are required for a more accurate forecast, resulting in a slower model. The random forest technique is fast enough in most real-world applications, however, there are times when run-time performance is critical, and thus, other approaches are preferable.

5 Deep Learning Cancer Models

Deep learning (DL), a branch of machine learning has recently shown a huge advancement in health care areas, drug design, cancer prognosis, and many other fields. Deep learning may also be addressed as a deep neural network [69]. It consists of many layers of artificial neurons that imitate neurons present in human brains. The major breakthrough in deep learning techniques is because of the growth in computation power and exponential rise in data capture by devices. Neural networks can be both supervised and unsupervised. A supervised learning algorithm requires training data containing inputs and outputs. Some of the examples of such supervised learning algorithms are linear and logistic regression, naïve Bayes, classification trees, gradient boosting, and many more. On the contrary unsupervised learning finds out the pattern depending on the inputs, it does not require pre-existing output. Word2vec and Latent Dirichlet Allocation are some popular unsupervised learning algorithms. Like machine learning, deep learning inherently uses statistics and basic probability. However deep learning has a better predictive ability and more flexibility. With a view to making more advancement in deep learning, deep belief networks (DBNs) have been applied in image recognition, speech recognition, and natural language processing [70–74]. The performance of a DL-based method is assessed by measuring the area under the receiver-operating curve (AUROC). In most of the cases, it shows accordance with the results from pathologists [75].

In recent years, the application of deep learning in cancer prognosis is mentionworthy. A multivariate regression named as Cox proportional hazards model (Cox-PH) plays a great role in cancer studies [69]. It has the ability to compare the survival features between two or more treatment groups. Because of the wide range of approval of the Cox regression model in the prediction of survival, it was utilized as the output layer to construct a neural network to anticipate cancer survival. DeepSurv, a neural network model built by Katzman et al. that performs survival analysis. RankDeepSurvival has been adapted by using the basic infrastructure of DeepSurv but has 3–4 hidden layers for performing survival analysis in cancer datasets. However, RankDeepSurivival model surpassed the DeepSurv model in breast cancer datasets from the German Breast Cancer Study Group (GBSG) and Molecular Taxonomy of Breast Cancer International Consortium (METABRIC). A lung cancer screening trial was performed in 2019, which was a deep learning-based analysis. The method was a huge success and widely acceptable. The DL method has also shown powerful results in the detection of skin cancer. In recent advancements, it has been found that the DL system is capable to predict cancer from Hematoxylin and eosin stain (H and E) histology images [76–80].

Caffe, Theano, Torch, DMTK, MXNet, TensorFlow are some deep learning frameworks. Despite the wide range of applications of DL, challenges are still there in its application. However deep learning is gradually approaching artificial intelligence (AI). The data size of the genomic sequencing model is one of the restrictions, which may limit the model's training process. Another drawback is that one can only have restricted access to the datasets and can only deal with publicly accessible samples with a limited quantity of data.

6 Cancer-Based Phenotypic Models

Cancer is a disease that resulted from the disturbance of the cell cycle, especially proliferation and cell death. By understanding and identifying the disturbance of the cell cycle can lead to better and improved cancer therapy, drug, and data regarding such.

The systematic cellular functions are carefully arranged in the molecular system that reacts to the stimuli both external and internal. The disturbance of such a system is due to the mutation in the molecular system leading to avoiding of cell apoptosis of a healthy cell. Such disturbance happens due to factors that hinder and alter the system functioning leading to mutation driving the initiation of cancer cell proliferation. Conventional therapies of cancer treatment make use of cancer's deficiencies in DNA repair. In traditional chemotherapy, the drugs induce DNA damage to the cancer cell leading to a halt to the growth of cancer. Another conventional treatment uses drugs or ionizing radiation to target them, however, they are not narrow in cell selection, hence leading to damaging of the normal, healthy cells which also can cause other severe side effects.

With the modern treatment of cancer that is, targeting a specific malfunction of the cell using specific drugs for the same can be more effective and less severe on side effects than the traditional treatment, however, the resistance shown by the cells for the drugs poses a challenge to face. Finding the mechanism of the cancer functioning can aid in facing the resistance problem. Hence, the use of systematic modeling of the cellular signaling of the cancer cell can impart knowledge regarding the confrontation of drug resistance. A positive aspect of modeling is that they can be tested in various aspects in silico with drugs and novel treatment methods.

The cancer models give the area of experiment with the cellular interactions with each other and the microenvironment and also with the study of the regulation of genetic and protein levels [72]. The use of computational models for drug development has a great effect on faster development. However, in cancer research there are a few limitations to it, the models created have been limited due to the chemically small space or molecule clubbed together to create the model, another limitation includes the use of a single cancer cell line, as different cancer cell line exhibit a different response to the same chemical or drug-associated, and lastly the models published up till now will not have the same responses and results [4].

Pancreatic cancer is one of the world's most aggressive out of the many neoplasms. The early diagnosis is quite difficult and the majority are diagnosed in incurable states of it. The chemotherapeutic treatment has gotten reduced due to the growing resistance to the known drugs. Hence, the emphasis on using the multitarget model for quantitative structure–activity relationship (mt-QSAR) to resolve the said drawback of the existing models. Several models based on this technique predicted simultaneously the multiple biomolecule activities interacting with non-biomolecule targets. The mt-QSAR is a grouped in silico advance technique that combines the perturbating theory ideas and machine learning (PTML) modeling [66]. Some of the challenges of the phenotypic model method for cancer treatment are as follows:

- The models to be created must be chemically small spaced or molecularly clubbed together.
- Model creation focuses mostly on single cancer cell lines to record the drugs or treatments effect, however, the response is not always the same with other cancer cell lines.
- The models published so to date will be outdated, as the same cancer cell lines may not respond like the model.

7 Electronic Health Records-Based ML Methods

Electronic health records (EHRs) are the digital collection of the patient's medical information that includes past treatments, drugs administrated, diagnosis, tests, and so on. Such gathered information has the relevant information of the medical events of the patients [81].

The use of EHR, aids in the analysis of the particular disease diagnosed in a patient, methodologies have been fabricated for such, using the major characteristics of EHR:

- *Heterogeneity*: The data collected here are large amounts of the patients' medical information like diagnosis, treatments, and laboratory tests, these are distinct from each other.
- *Incomplete information*: Here the values observed are outnumbered by the missing values. The use of the real-world medical database brings upon the characteristics of the missing values of the EHR's data.

The use of the above two characteristics features of EHR's can lead to the making of the methodology needed to diagnose and treat a particular disease in patients, with lack of value of all medical information and comorbidity that leads to the uncertainty of medical actions truly associated to the particular disease or not.

The method fabricated for the same uncertainty constitutes the identification of (i) actions for the particular disease in a health care system, (ii) information of patients with complete treatment of the disease, and (iii) common treatment pathway followed by the patients with a specific diagnosis.

EHR's are used for mining the knowledge of the clinical patterns and treatment patterns in the health database, however, they are not always well structured and extremely diverse leading to complex models that are difficult to study. Machine learning techniques aids in the analysis of such models by homogeneous subgrouping. These are done by hierarchical clustering with similarities followed by multiple scans and data mining to narrow it down even further. The models known so far are incompetent in dealing with the challenges of clinical data such as inaccuracy, incompleteness, comorbidities, and treatment which gives a partial perspective of the medical history of a patient. Some approaches after the clustering techniques show the most frequent medical activities instead of the whole set of medical activities implied that gives a partial knowledge of the medical treatment rather than the complete one.

The new methodology tackles the complete treatment pathway with accuracy in the analysis of the disease [82]. Cancer patients often suffer from the symptoms that are either because of the disease or treatment or sometimes both. Obtaining the overview of a patient's symptom information is quite a challenge due to the patients' information gathered and compiled into huge numbers of clinical notes tends to cause errors. These errors often get led to ignorance to adding to the symptoms one displays in a disease. If the symptom's knowledge and its creation are strengthened, easy access to the outcomes of the health care research will become patient-centric. The use of EHRs makes information mining much easier and precise but as its limit, most of them should be categorized in subgroups which are more effective than large variable data scattered in the system. For such large variable data, machine learning models come as an asset in identifying those similar symptoms of the current patients from records of clinical records [83].

By using the EHRs as the inputs of one of the major human cancer, cervical cancer dominating in women. With the prevention through the organized screening of this, cancer has become rarer in Sweden, but still, some cases do emerge every year. The age range of women that are diagnosed for this is 46 years, hence given the fact, it strikes at an early stage of age. The prevention of its growth can happen with the improved prediction of it, leading to the intervening of the precancerous lesion through surgical removal at an early stage. The early detection can also improve the quality of the treatment's outcome and life as well, along with the high rates of survival, such improvement for cancer, such as cervical cancer, which has a high mortality rate at the higher stages of the cancer development [84]. The machine learning model, developed from the EHRs with high accuracy can lead to improved diagnostics and treatment at early stages. The use of the model has been applied for predicting a number of different outcomes for both the disease and also for the risks like mortality, etc. with the increase in risk prediction models.

The use of EHR is difficult due to the diverse and unstructured data leading to increase complexity in the study of the same. The partial information stored by patients can make the model study incompetent.

8 Conclusion

Every year, the practice of medicine evolves, with more automated technologies that aid and enhance the healthcare professional's ability to be more efficient with treatments and accurate in their evaluations. Machine learning boosts the value of data and redefines diagnostic approaches. Cancer research has progressed and diversified into several sectors over time, including deep learning approaches such as image screening and genomic sequencing. Furthermore, new therapies and diagnostic methodologies have improved the accuracy of cancer predicting methods.

There is no doubt that in the near future AI will bring revolutionary improvements to the drug design and development process in cancer therapeutics. There is a certain inevitable challenge that still needs to be overcome to include AI tools in the drug discovery cycle. Apart from all challenges faced in the development of AI-based models, this approach has undoubtedly reduced the time consumption spent in the trial-and-error approach used in traditional drug design studies. With the advent of next-generation computational infrastructure and tools, Computational Intelligence-based cheminformatics models will be a breakthrough in the field of cancer therapeutics.

References

1. Ekins, S., Mestres, J., & Testa, B. (2007). In silicopharmacology for drug discovery: Methods for virtual ligand screening and profiling. *British Journal of Pharmacology, 152*(1), 9–20. https://doi.org/10.1038/sj.bjp.0707305
2. Leach, A. R., Shoichet, B. K., & Peishoff, C. E. (2006). Prediction of protein–ligand interactions. Docking and scoring: Successes and gaps. *Journal of Medicinal Chemistry,* 49(20), 5851–5855. https://doi.org/10.1021/jm060999m
3. Ekins, S., Puhl, A. C., Zorn, K. M., Lane, T. R., Russo, D. P., Klein, J. J., Hickey, A. J., & Clark, A. M. (2019). Exploiting machine learning for end-to-end drug discovery and development. *Nature Materials, 18*, 435–441.
4. Raza et al. (2020). *An introduction to computational intelligence for COVID-19: Surveillance, prevention, prediction, and diagnosis. Computational intelligence methods in COVID-19: Surveillance, prevention, prediction and diagnosis, studies in computational intelligence (SCI)* (vol 923, pp 3–18). Springer.
5. Issa, N. T., Stathias, V., Schürer, S., & Dakshanamurthy, S. (2021). Machine and deep learning approaches for cancer drug repurposing. *Seminars in Cancer Biology, 68*, 132–142. https://doi.org/10.1016/j.semcancer.2019.12.011
6. Leach, A. R. (2009). *Molecular modelling: Principles and applications*. Pearson Prentice Hall.
7. Lengauer, T., & Rarey, M. (1996). Computational methods for biomolecular docking. *Current Opinion in Structural Biology, 6*(3), 402–406. https://doi.org/10.1016/s0959-440x(96)80061-3
8. Bronowska, A. K. (2011). Thermodynamics of ligand-protein interactions: Implications for molecular design. In J. C. M. Piraján (Ed.), *Thermodynamics—Interaction studies—Solids, liquids and gases* (pp. 1–49). IntechOpen. https://doi.org/10.5772/19447
9. Gupta, A., Gandhimathi, A., Sharma, P., & Jayaram, B. (2007). ParDOCK: An all atom energy based monte carlo docking protocol for protein-ligand complexes. *Protein and Peptide Letters, 14*(7), 632–646.

10. Schneidman-Duhovny, D., Inbar, Y., Nussinov, R., & Wolfson, H. (2005). PatchDock and SymmDock: Servers for rigid and symmetric docking. *Nucleic Acids Research, 33*(Web Server), W363–W367.
11. van Zundert, G. C. P., Rodrigues, J. P. G. L. M., Trellet, M., Schmitz, C., Kastritis, P. L., Karaca, E., Melquiond, A. S. J., van Dijk, M., de Vries, S. J., & Bonvin, A. M. J. J. (2016). The HADDOCK2.2 webserver: User-friendly integrative modeling of biomolecular complexes. *Journal of Molecular Biology, 428*, 720–725.
12. dos Santos, K. B., Guedes, I. A., Karl, A. L. M., & Dardenne, L. (2020). Highly flexible ligand docking: Benchmarking of the DockThorProgram on the LEADS-PEP protein-peptide dataset. *Journal of Chemical Information and Modeling*. https://doi.org/10.1021/acs.jcim.9b00905
13. Morris, G. M., Huey, R., Lindstrom, W., Sanner, M. F., Belew, R. K., Goodsell, D. S., & Olson, A.J. (2009). AutoDock4 and AutoDockTools4: Automated docking with selective receptor flexibility. *Journal of Computational Chemistry, 30*(16), 2785–91. PubMed Central PMCID: PMC2760638.
14. BIOVIA Discovery Studio - BIOVIA - Dassault Systèmes®. (2021). From https://www.3ds.com/products-services/biovia/products/molecular-modeling-simulation/biovia-discovery-studio
15. Allen, W. J., Balius, T. E., Mukherjee, S., Brozell, S. R., Moustakas, D. T., Lang, P. T., Case, D. A., Kuntz, I. D., & Rizzo, R. C. (2015). DOCK 6: Impact of new features and current docking performance. *Journal of Computational Chemistry, 36*, 1132–1156.
16. Jones, G., Willett, P., Glen, R. C., Leach, A. R., & Taylor, R. (1997). *Journal of Molecular Biology, 267*, 727–748. https://doi.org/10.1006/jmbi.1996.0897
17. Acharya, R., Chacko, S., Bose, P., Lapenna, A., & Pattanayak, S. P. (2019). Structure based multitargeted molecular docking analysis of selected furanocoumarins against breast cancer. *Scientific Reports, 9*(1), 15743. https://doi.org/10.1038/s41598-019-52162-0
18. Sharma, V., Sharma, P. C., & Kumar, V. (2016). In Silico molecular docking analysis of natural pyridoacridines as anticancer agents. *Advances in Chemistry, 2016*(5409387), 1–9. https://doi.org/10.1155/2016/5409387
19. Varnek, A., & Baskin, I. I. (2011). Chemoinformatics as a theoretical chemistry discipline. *Molecular Informatics, 30*(1), 20–32. https://doi.org/10.1002/minf.201000100
20. Brown, F. (1998). Chapter 35 – chemoinformatics: What is it and how does it impact drug discovery. In J. A. Bristol (Ed.), *Annual reports in medicinal chemistry, 33* (pp. 375–384). Academic Press.
21. Martinez-Mayorga, K., Madariaga-Mazon, A., Medina-Franco, J. L., & Maggiora, G. (2020). The impact of chemoinformatics on drug discovery in the pharmaceutical industry. *Expert Opinion on Drug Discovery, 15*, 1–14. https://doi.org/10.1080/17460441.2020.1696307
22. Brown, N. (2009). Chemoinformatics—An introduction for computer scientists. *ACM Computing Surveys, 41*(2), 1–38. https://doi.org/10.1145/1459352.1459353
23. Begam, B. F., & Kumar, J. S. (2012). A study on cheminformatics and its applications on modern drug discovery. *Procedia Engineering, 38*, 1264–1275. https://doi.org/10.1016/j.proeng.2012.06.156
24. Guha, R., Gilbert, K., Fox, G., Pierce, M., Wild, D., & Yuan, H. (2010). Advances in cheminformatics methodologies and infrastructure to support the data mining of large, heterogeneous chemical datasets. *Current Computer Aided-Drug Design, 6*(1), 50–67. https://doi.org/10.2174/157340910790980115
25. Ghavami, G., Sardari, S., & Ali Shokrgozar, M. (2011). Cheminformatics-based selection and synergism of herbal extracts with anticancer agents on drug resistance tumor cells—ACHN and A2780/CP cell lines. *Computers in Biology and Medicine, 41*(8), 665–674. https://doi.org/10.1016/j.compbiomed.2011.06.002
26. Cortes-Ciriano, I., van Westen, G. J., Lenselink, E. B., Murrell, D. S., Bender, A., & Malliavin, T. (2014). Proteochemometricmodeling in a Bayesian framework. *Journal of Cheminformatics, 6*(1), 35, 1–16. https://doi.org/10.1186/1758-2946-6-35

27. Naeem, A., Dakshanamurthy, S., Walthieu, H., Parasido, E., Avantaggiati, M., Tricoli, L., Kumar, D., Lee, R. J., Feldman, A., Noon, M. S., Byers, S., Rodriguez, O., & Albanese, C. (2020). Predicting new drug indications for prostate cancer: The integration of an in silico proteochemometric network pharmacology platform with patient-derived primary prostate cells. *The Prostate, 80*(14), 1233–1243. https://doi.org/10.1002/pros.24050
28. Simeon, S., Spjuth, O., Lapins, M., Nabu, S., Anuwongcharoen, N., Prachayasittikul, V., Wikberg, J. E. S., & Nantasenamat, C. (2016). Origin of aromatase inhibitory activity via proteochemometricmodeling. *PeerJ, 4*, e1979. https://doi.org/10.7717/peerj.1979
29. Wainweight, T., & Alder, B. (1958). Molecular dynamics computations for the hard sphere system. *Il Nuovo Cimento, 1955–1965*(9), 116–132. https://doi.org/10.1007/bf02824238
30. Ikemura, S., Yasuda, H., Matsumoto, S., Kamada, M., Hamamoto, J., Masuzawa, K., Kobayashi, K., Manabe, T., Arai, D., Nakachi, I., Kawada, I., Ishioka, K., Nakamura, M., Namkoong, H., Naoki, K., Ono, F., Araki, M., Kanada, R., Ma, B., ... Soejima, K. (2019). Molecular dynamics simulation-guided drug sensitivity prediction for lung cancer with rare EGFR mutations. *Proceedings of the National Academy of Sciences, 116*(20), 10025–10030. https://doi.org/10.1073/pnas.1819430116
31. Gurung, A. B., Ali, M. A., Lee, J., Farah, M. A., & Al-Anazi, K. M. (2021). Molecular docking and dynamics simulation study of bioactive compounds from *Ficus carica* L. with important anticancer drug targets. *PLoS ONE, 16*(7), e0254035. https://doi.org/10.1371/journal.pone.0254035
32. Issa, N. T., Stathias, V., Schürer, S., & Dakshanamurthy, S. (2020). Machine and deep learning approaches for cancer drug repurposing. *Seminars in Cancer Biology, 68*, 132–142. https://doi.org/10.1016/j.semcancer.2019.12.011
33. Nosengo, N. (2016). Can you teach old drugs new tricks? *Nature, 534*(7607), 314–316.
34. Kitchen, D. B., Decornez, H., Furr, J. R., & Bajorath, J. (2004). Docking and scoring in virtual screening for drug discovery: Methods and applications. *Nature Reviews. Drug Discovery, 3*(11), 935–949.
35. Friesner, R. A., Banks, J. L., Murphy, R. B., Halgren, T. A., Klicic, J. J., Mainz, D. T., Repasky, M. P., Knoll, E. H., Shelley, M., Perry, J. K., Shaw, D. E., Francis, P., & Shenkin, P. S. (2004). Glide: A new approach for rapid, accurate docking and scoring. 1. Method and assessment of docking accuracy. *Journal of medicinal chemistry, 47*(7), 1739–1749. https://doi.org/10.1021/jm0306430
36. Mirza, S. B., Salmas, R. E., Fatmi, M. Q., & Durdagi, S. (2016). Virtual screening of eighteen million compounds against dengue virus: Combined molecular docking and molecular dynamics simulations study. *Journal of Molecular Graphics & Modelling, 66*, 99–107. https://doi.org/10.1016/j.jmgm.2016.03.008
37. Kumar, V., Krishna, S., & Siddiqi, M. I. (2015). Virtual screening strategies: Recent advances in the identification and design of anti-cancer agents. *Methods (San Diego, Calif.), 71*, 64–70. https://doi.org/10.1016/j.ymeth.2014.08.010
38. Hafeez, B. B., Ganju, A., Sikander, M., Kashyap, V. K., Hafeez, Z. B., Chauhan, N., Malik, S., Massey, A. E., Tripathi, M. K., Halaweish, F. T., Zafar, N., Singh, M. M., Yallapu, M. M., Chauhan, S. C., & Jaggi, M. (2017). Ormeloxifene suppresses prostate tumor growth and metastatic phenotypes via inhibition of oncogenic β-catenin signaling and EMT progression. *Molecular Cancer Therapeutics, 16*(10), 2267–2280. https://doi.org/10.1158/1535-7163.MCT-17-0157
39. Cereto-Massagué, A., Ojeda, M. J., Valls, C., Mulero, M., Garcia-Vallvé, S., & Pujadas, G. (2015). Molecular fingerprint similarity search in virtual screening. *Methods, 71*, 58–63. https://doi.org/10.1016/j.ymeth.2014.08.005
40. Kirchmair, J., Distinto, S., Markt, P., Schuster, D., Spitzer, G. M., Liedl, K. R., & Wolber, G. (2009). How to optimize shape-based virtual screening: Choosing the right query and including chemical information. *Journal of Chemical Information and Modeling, 49*(3), 678–692. https://doi.org/10.1021/ci8004226
41. Grant, J. A., Gallardo, M. A., & Pickup, B. T. (1996). A fast method of molecular shape comparison: A simple application of a Gaussian description of molecular shape. *Journal of Computational Chemistry, 17*(14), 1653–1666.

42. Singh, J., Chuaqui, C. E., Boriack-Sjodin, P. A., Lee, W. C., Pontz, T., Corbley, M. J., Cheung, H. K., Arduini, R. M., Mead, J. N., Newman, M. N., Papadatos, J. L., Bowes, S., Josiah, S., & Ling, L. E. (2003). Successful shape-based virtual screening: The discovery of a potent inhibitor of the type I TGFbeta receptor kinase (TbetaRI). *Bioorganic & Medicinal Chemistry Letters, 13*(24), 4355–4359. https://doi.org/10.1016/j.bmcl.2003.09.028
43. Yang, S. Y. (2010). Pharmacophore modeling and applications in drug discovery: Challenges and recent advances. *Drug Discovery Today, 15*(11–12), 444–450. https://doi.org/10.1016/j.drudis.2010.03.013
44. Wermuth, C. G. (2006). Pharmacophores: Historical perspective and viewpoint from a medicinal chemist. In T. Langer & R. D. Hoffmann (Eds.), *Pharmacophores and pharmacophore searches* (pp. 3–13). Wiley–VCH.
45. Dror, O., Shulman-Peleg, A., Nussinov, R., & Wolfson, H. J. (2004). Predicting molecular interactions in silico: I. A guide to pharmacophore identification and its applications to drug design. *Current Medicinal Chemistry*, 11(1), 71–90. https://doi.org/10.2174/0929867043456287
46. Verma, J., Khedkar, V. M., & Coutinho, E. C. (2010). 3D-QSAR in drug design—A review. *Current Topics in Medicinal Chemistry, 10*(1), 95–115. https://doi.org/10.2174/156802610790232260
47. Labute, P. (1999). Binary QSAR: A new method for the determination of quantitative structure activity relationships. In *Pacific Symposium on Biocomputing. Pacific Symposium on Biocomputing* (pp. 444–455). https://doi.org/10.1142/9789814447300_0044
48. Kubinyi, H. (2004). 2D QSAR models: Hansch and Free-Wilson analyses. In P. Bultinck, H. D. Winter, W. Langenaeker & J. P. Tollenaere (Eds.), *Computational chemistry for drug discovery* (pp. 539–570). Marcel Dekker.
49. Martin, Y. C. (1998). 3D QSAR: Current state, scope, and limitations. In H. Kubinyi, G. Folkers, & Y. C. Martin (Eds.), *3D QSAR in drug design—Recent advances* (pp. 3–23). Kluwer Academic Publishers.
50. Wise, M., Cramer, R. D., Smith, D., & Exman, I. (1983). Progress in three dimensional drug design: The use of real time colour graphics and computer postulation of bioactive molecules in DYLOMMS. In J. Dearden (Ed.), *Quantitative approaches to drug design* (pp. 145–146). Elsevier.
51. Ho, T. K. (1995) Random decision forests. In *Proceedings of 3rd International Conference on Document Analysis and Recognition* (pp. 278–282). IEEE. https://doi.org/10.1109/icdar.1995.598994
52. Ho, T. K. (1998). The random subspace method for constructing decision forests. *IEEE Transactions on Pattern Analysis and Machine Intelligence, 20*(8), 832–844. https://doi.org/10.1109/34.709601
53. Suthaharan, S. (2016). Decision tree learning. *Integrated Series in Information Systems, 36*, 237–269. https://doi.org/10.1007/978-1-4899-7641-3_10
54. Grandvalet, Y. (2004). Bagging equalizes influence. *Machine Learning, 55*(3), 251–270. https://doi.org/10.1023/b:mach.0000027783.34431.42
55. Geurts, P., Ernst, D., & Wehenkel, L. (2006). Extremely randomized trees. *Machine Learning, 63*(1), 3–42. https://doi.org/10.1007/s10994-006-6226-1
56. Lazarevic, A., & Kumar, V. (2005, January). Feature bagging for outlier detection. In *Proceeding of the Eleventh ACM SIGKDD International Conference on Knowledge Discovery in Data Mining* (pp. 157–166). ACM. https://doi.org/10.1145/1081870.1081891
57. Haibe-Kains, B., El-Hachem, N., Birkbak, N. J., Jin, A. C., Beck, A. H., Aerts, H. J. W. L., & Quackenbush, J. (2013). Inconsistency in large pharmacogenomic studies. *Nature, 504*(7480), 389–393. https://doi.org/10.1038/nature12831
58. Wan, Q., & Pal, R. (2014). An ensemble based top performing approach for NCI-DREAM drug sensitivity prediction challenge. *PLoS ONE, 9*(6), e101183. https://doi.org/10.1371/journal.pone.0101183
59. Lind, A. P., & Anderson, P. C. (2019). Predicting drug activity against cancer cells by random forest models based on minimal genomic information and chemical properties. *PLoS ONE, 14*(7), e0219774. https://doi.org/10.1371/journal.pone.0219774

60. Rajini, A., & Jabbar, M. A. (2021). Lung cancer prediction using random forest. *Recent Advances in Computer Science and Communications, 14*(5), 1652–1659. https://doi.org/10.2174/2213275912666191026124214
61. Dai, B., Chen, R.-C., Zhu, S.-Z., & Zhang, W.-W. (2018). Using random forest algorithm for breast cancer diagnosis. In *2018 International Symposium on Computer, Consumer and Control (IS3C)* (pp. 449–452). IEEE. https://doi.org/10.1109/is3c.2018.00119
62. Schoenberg, M. B., Bucher, J. N., Vater, A., Bazhin, A. V., Hao, J., Guba, M. O., Angele, M. K., Werner, J., & Rentsch, M. (2017). Resection or transplant in early hepatocellular carcinoma. *DeutschesArzteblatt International, 114*(31–32), 519–526. https://doi.org/10.3238/arztebl.2017.0519
63. Schoenberg, M. B., Bucher, J. N., Koch, D., Börner, N., Hesse, S., De Toni, E. N., Seidensticker, M., Angele, M. K., Klein, C., Bazhin, A. V., Werner, J., & Guba, M. O. (2020). A novel machine learning algorithm to predict disease free survival after resection of hepatocellular carcinoma. *Annals of Translational Medicine, 8*(7), 434–434. https://doi.org/10.21037/atm.2020.04.16
64. Bhatla, N., Berek, J. S., CuelloFredes, M., Denny, L. A., Grenman, S., Karunaratne, K., Kehoe, S. T., Konishi, I., Olawaiye, A. B., Prat, J., Sankaranarayanan, R., Brierley, J., Mutch, D., Querleu, D., Cibula, D., Quinn, M., Botha, H., Sigurd, L. et al. (2019). Revised FIGO staging for carcinoma of the cervix uteri. *International Journal of Gynaecology and Obstetrics: The Official Organ of the International Federation of Gynaecology and Obstetrics, 145*(1), 129–135.https://doi.org/10.1002/ijgo.12749
65. Liu, D., Zhang, X., Zheng, T., Shi, Q., Cui, Y., Wang, Y., & Lui, L. (2021). Optimisation and evaluation of the random forest model in the efficacy prediction of chemoradiotherapy for advanced cervical cancer based on radiomics signature from high-resolution T2 weighted images. *Arch GynecolObstet, 303*(3), 811–820. https://doi.org/10.1007/s00404-020-05908-5
66. Prinyakupt, J., & Pluempitiwiriyawej, C. (2015). Segmentation of white blood cells and comparison of cell morphology by linear and naïve Bayes classifiers. *BioMedical Engineering OnLine, 14*(1), 63. https://doi.org/10.1186/s12938-015-0037-1
67. Dasariraju, S., Huo, M., & McCalla, S. (2020). Detection and classification of immature leukocytes for diagnosis of acute myeloid leukemia using random forest algorithm. *Bioengineering, 7*(4), 120. https://doi.org/10.3390/bioengineering7040120
68. Liu, W. C., Li, Z. Q., Luo, Z. W., Liao, W. J., Liu, Z. L., & Liu, J. M. (2021). Machine learning for the prediction of bone metastasis in patients with newly diagnosed thyroid cancer. *Cancer Medicine, 10*(8), 2802–2811. https://doi.org/10.1002/cam4.3776
69. Zhu, W., Xie, L., Han, J., & Guo, X. (2020). The application of deep learning in cancer prognosis prediction. *Cancers, 12*(3), 603. https://doi.org/10.3390/cancers12030603
70. Siegel, R. L., Miller, K. D., & Jemal, A. (2019). Cancer statistics, 2019. *CA: A Cancer Journal for Clinicians,* 69(1), 7–34. https://doi.org/10.3322/caac.21551
71. Yu, M. K., Ma, J., Fisher, J., Kreisberg, J. F., Raphael, B. J., & Ideker, T. (2018). Visible machine learning for biomedicine. *Cell, 173*(7), 1562–1565. https://doi.org/10.1016/j.cell.2018.05.056
72. van IJzendoorn, D., Szuhai, K., Briaire-de Bruijn, I. H., Kostine, M., Kuijjer, M. L., & Bovée, J. (2019). Machine learning analysis of gene expression data reveals novel diagnostic and prognostic biomarkers and identifies therapeutic targets for soft tissue sarcomas. *PLoS Computational Biology, 15*(2), e1006826.https://doi.org/10.1371/journal.pcbi.1006826
73. AlQuraishi, M. (2019). AlphaFold at CASP13. *Bioinformatics (Oxford, England), 35*(22), 4862–4865. https://doi.org/10.1093/bioinformatics/btz422
74. Katzman, J. L., Shaham, U., Cloninger, A., Bates, J., Jiang, T., & Kluger, Y. (2018). DeepSurv: Personalized treatment recommender system using a Cox proportional hazards deep neural network. *BMC Medical Research Methodology, 18*(24), 1–12. https://doi.org/10.1186/s12874-018-0482-1
75. Echle, A., Rindtorff, N. T., Brinker, T. J., Luedde, T., Pearson, A. T., & Kather, J. N. (2021). Deep learning in cancer pathology: A new generation of clinical biomarkers. *British Journal of Cancer, 124*, 686–696. https://doi.org/10.1038/s41416-020-01122-x
76. Yu, D., & Deng, L. (2011). Deep learning and its applications to signal and information processing. *IEEE Signal Processing Magazine, 28*, 145–154. https://doi.org/10.1109/MSP.2010.939038

77. Hinton, G. E., Osindero, S., & Teh, Y. W. (2006). A fast learning algorithm for deep belief nets. *Neural Computation, 18*(7), 1527–1554. https://doi.org/10.1162/neco.2006.18.7.1527
78. Hinton, G. E., & Salakhutdinov, R. R. (2006). Reducing the dimensionality of data with neural networks. *Science (New York, N.Y.), 313*(5786), 504–507. https://doi.org/10.1126/science.1127647
79. Gautam, P., Jaiswal, A., Aittokallio, T., Al-Ali, H., & Wennerberg, K. (2019). Phenotypic screening combined with machine learning for efficient identification of breast cancer-selective therapeutic targets. *Cell Chem Biology, 26*(7), 970–979. https://doi.org/10.1016/j.chembiol.2019.03.011
80. Sirinukunwattana, K., Ahmed Raza, S. E., Tsang, Y.-W., Snead, D. R., Cree, I. A., & Rajpoot, N. M. (2016). Locality sensitive deep learning for detection and classification of nuclei in routine colon cancer histology images. *IEEE Transactions on Medical Imaging, 35*(5), 1196–1206. https://doi.org/10.1109/TMI.2016.2525803
81. Qazi, S., & Raza, K. (2021). Translational bioinformatics in healthcare: past, present, and future. *Translational Bioinformatics in Healthcare and Medicine*, 1–12.https://doi.org/10.1016/B978-0-323-89824-9.00001-X
82. Zaballa, O., Pérez, A., Gómez Inhiesto, E., AcaiturriAyesta, T., & Lozano, J. A. (2020). Identifying common treatments from electronic health records with missing information. An application to breast cancer. *PloS one, 15*(12), e0244004. https://doi.org/10.1371/journal.pone.0244004
83. Forsyth, A. W., Barzilay, R., Hughes, K. S., Lui, D., Lorenz, K. A., Enzinger, A., Tulsky, J. A., & Lindvall, C. (2018). Machine learning methods to extract documentation of breast cancer symptoms from electronic health records. *Journal of Pain and Symptom Management, 55*(6), 1492–1499. https://doi.org/10.1016/j.jpainsymman.2018.02.016
84. Weegar, R., & Sundström, K. (2020). Using machine learning for predicting cervical cancer from Swedish electronic health records by mining hierarchical representations. *PLoS ONE, 15*(8), e0237911. https://doi.org/10.1371/journal.pone.0237911
85. Friedman, R., Boye, K., & Flatmark, K. (2013). Molecular modelling and simulations in cancer research. *Biochimica et Biophysica Acta (BBA) - Reviews on Cancer, 1836*(1), 1–14. https://doi.org/10.1016/j.bbcan.2013.02.001

Gene Expression Signature: An Influential Access to Drug Discovery in Ovarian Cancer

Anam Beg and Rafat Parveen

Abstract Ovarian cancer is the worst gynecological malignancy around the globe because of its asymptomatic existence. Due to the lack of diagnostic strategies in ovarian cancer, it is being detected at an advanced stage. It will continue to rise in the future as well because of the rapidly aging population and lifestyle. At the individual level, the financial burden is relatively high. Currently, there is no remedy for disease treatment and the perfect way to reduce its morbidity and incidence is to detect it early. In clinical trials, the advancement in molecular biology, bioinformatics, and laboratory technology have broadened the use and feasibility of applying biomarkers in disease treatment. Amidst all these, the applications of Gene expression signatures (GES) have shown to be a powerful tool. GES are dominant tools that can unfold a spectrum of biologically and clinically relevant aspects of biological samples. Over the past few years differentiation has been made in different subtypes of tumors with the help of gene expression signatures. It also helps in predicting clinical outcomes in cancer and model the signaling pathways activation. During the past two decades, gene signatures detection from genomic data has always been an important topic of discussion in the medical field. This chapter deals with gene expression signature and its role in complex diseases. Further, we also describe the prognostic relevance of gene expression signature in ovarian cancer.

Keywords Ovarian cancer · Biomarkers · Gene expression signatures · Drug discovery · High throughput screening

1 Introduction

Ovarian cancer is the most lethal gynecologic malignancy having a survival rate of only 30%. The heterogeneous nature and high mortality make it difficult for the early detection and primary prevention in ovarian cancer, but still, little improvement

A. Beg (✉) · R. Parveen
Department of Computer Science, Jamia Millia Islamia, New Delhi 110025, India

R. Parveen
e-mail: rparveen@jmi.ac.in

K. Raza (ed.), *Computational Intelligence in Oncology*, Studies in Computational Intelligence 1016, https://doi.org/10.1007/978-981-16-9221-5_16

is being made over the past many decades. Currently, 295,414 cases of OC are being estimated by GLOBOCAN [1, 2]. It also gives the estimate that 184,799 cases of ovarian cancer are related to mortality in 2018. The late-stage diagnosis is the cause of high mortality rates in OC. Around 75% of patients with extensive metastasis are being detected at stages III and IV [1]. Pathological studies suggested that ovarian tumors are distinguished into three subtypes, i.e., stromal, epithelial sex cord, and germ cells tumors. Out of which EOC constitutes 80–85% of OC [3, 4]. Further EOC is being categorized into low grade serous, high grade serous, mucinous, endometrioid, and clear cell carcinoma. Among all EOC 75% of mortalities are due to HGSOC and are most lethal [4]. Although it originates from surface epithelium, recent studies indicate that majorities of HGSOC arise from fallopian tube fimbriae [5]. In 90% of HGSOC patients, TP53 is mutated. With the advancement of next-generation sequencing (NGS) it is revealed that BRCA1 and BRCA2 mutations including DNA repair pathways are common in 50% HGSOC; which has contributed to the development of PARP inhibitors; a targeted therapy [3].

At present, the diagnostic methods for monitoring and detection include transvaginal ultrasound, pelvic examination, and measurement of CA125 [6], (HE4) [7], p53 [8], and Wnt/beta-catenin [9]; all these methods lack adequate sensitivity and specificity and it is, therefore, OC is detected at late stages. Around 75% of patients in ovarian cancer die due to late-stage detection however early-stage detection is curable but the majority of women are being diagnosed at stage III/IV [10]. For decades combinations of chemotherapies (platinum-taxane) along with Cytoreductive surgery have remained the mainstay of therapy. The main aim of cytoreductive surgeries is the complete removal of all macroscopic diseases. It's a surgical procedure where the tumor/cancer tissues are removed in order to reduce the disease load of the patient and also to relieve symptomatic problems. Lowering the number of tissues/tumors more effectively will be the treatment with cytotoxic chemotherapy. However, the efficacy of a particular treatment in a particular patient is not determined by a clinicopathological assessment that results in ineffective treatment outcomes due to excessive therapy in a lot of patients. There are a few drawbacks of clinicopathological assessments which include limited morphological data from patients at intermediate, advanced, and terminal disease stages, according to current clinical guidelines biopsies are not recommended for diagnosis, also, there is little consensus on the evaluation of key histopathological features, notably histological grading (degree of differentiation) but with the advancement of—omics technologies new era have emerged for the gene identification that can differentiate between different types of Ovarian Cancer into molecular subtypes, find the genes that are frequently mutated in Ovarian Cancer or linked with hereditary Ovarian Cancer, leading to a massive amount of data exploring resistance, metastasis, OC development, and disease progression, and opening the extremities for precision medicine and personalized treatment case for patient. For the early detection and therapeutic option, many approaches have emerged with a gene signature for different Ovarian Cancer subtypes. With the help of Gene-expression profiling, genomic tests have been developed that provide a better estimation of clinical outcomes in comparison to traditional and pathological standards.

Thousands of mRNA transcripts can be measured in a single experiment with the help of Gene-expression profiling using DNA microarrays. Results from such studies confirmed that cancers are not a single disease instead it's a group of molecularly distinct neoplastic disorders. Besides these GES are also used in the de novo generation of hit-like molecules using artificial intelligence; recently a research article from neuroscience has concluded that a dopamine-induced gene expression signature regulates neuronal function and cocaine response. Furthermoregene expression analyses are used in the identification of potential gene signatures that serve as potential biomarkers in ovarian cancer and are responsible for the vulnerability to develop complicated diseases. Apart from all these continuous progress has been made in the field of deep learning, machine learning, and numerous bioinformatics tools and techniques are developed to hasten the gene expression, identification of gene biomarkers, finding prognostic genes, etc. in various other diseases. For instance, a machine learning model called GVES is used for the identification of prognostic genes with small data sets. Similarly, HE2RNA, a model based on the integration of multiple data modes is used to predict RNA-seq expression of tumors from whole slide images. In the case of ovarian cancer, Cox Proportional Hazard regression models are employed to identify gene expression patterns associated with disease mortality and progression. For the interpretation of genomic signatures GATHER tool is used and for the simplification of gene expression signature analysis a web-based resource called SIGNATURE, has been developed which provides software, data, and protocols to perform the analysis successfully. Hence efforts are being made to understand the mechanism behind molecular signatures which could help us anticipate the potency of ovarian cancer. Many biomarkers have already been studied and many are underway to know the onset of Ovarian Cancer: for example the deregulation in tumor suppressor genes, miRNAs, and epigenetics. The list is beyond our expectations, and it would not be an easy job to analyze those genes one by one in each individual. Here in this chapter, we are going to elaborate on the development and progression of ovarian cancer and the prognostic relevance of GES in OC. We will also highlight a few gene signatures that have been found to have an association with ovarian cancer. Further, we will add how the gene expression signatures are helpful in drug discovery in OC.

2 Progression and Development in Ovarian Cancer

Ovarian cancer is characterized by peritoneal disseminated metastasis having a survival rate of only thirty percent. The metastasizing tumor differs from cancer cells because it first disperses within the peritoneal cavity and is superficially invasive. Metastasis is a complex stepwise growth involving critical interactions between stromal components and cancer cells in the tumor microenvironment, which thoroughly influence the contrasting aspects of the metastatic cascade. Many genetic and epigenetic changes also lead to cell transformation in ovarian cancer. As mentioned above the site of origin in ovarian cancer, i.e., fallopian tube, ovary surfaces, or the peritoneal cavity lined by mesothelium which plays crucial roles in tumorigenesis and invasion. Disease progression is a multistep process where the carcinoma advances to a well-defined type 1 carcinoma from a borderline tumor or it involves a genetically unstable type of carcinoma involving epithelial cells. This subtype of ovarian cancer also metastasizes rapidly. The cell's ovarian carcinoma go-through transition of epithelial-to-mesenchymal which occurs during initial tumorigenesis. It affects and alters the proteolytic pathways upregulation and expression of integrin and cadherin. The first steps of metastasis are carried out by composing interaction between proteases and adhesion receptors, whereas the late metastasis is oncogene-driven, i.e., Rapid growth of tumor outgrowth on the covered surfaces of mesothelium thereby obstructing bowel movement, ascites, and tumor cachexia.

Due to non-specific symptoms like back pain, abdominal bloating, early satiety, nausea, abdominal distension, fatigue, loss of weight, and change in bowel function, (which usually appear when cancer progresses in advanced stage), lack of screening strategies to detect ovarian cancer in an advanced stage; the mortality rate is high [11, 12]. Pelvic ultrasound and CA125 are the initial investigations but further investigations like abdomen or pelvis CTs and a pelvic MRI are needed to accurately predict the extension of ovarian cancer. Initial staging requires surgical treatment and involves total abdominal hysterectomy and analysis of peritoneal surfaces via biopsy or removal of different infected areas [12]. The staging process helps decide the surgical stage of the disease, organizations like FIGO (International Federation of Gynecology and Obstetrics) and the Joint American committee on cancer have defined the process of staging [13, 14]. Pathological diagnosis of tumors is important as ovarian cancer has pathological subtypes and the treatment and disease progression vary greatly from one another. Despite many ongoing screening programs, development of many high throughput technologies, only a limited number of women are being able to diagnose at an early stage of OC. Studies on Microarray-based gene expression states that ovarian cancer is a heterogeneous disease in nature and clinically diverse with distinct gene expression patterns in each subtype that are correlated with different subtypes and are statistically significant [12]. Numerous challenges are being faced by GES due to the heterogeneous nature of ovarian cancer which includes the use of different platforms for gene expression, different methods for analysis, overfitting the data, restriction to mostly high grade serous ovarian cancer histology, and most importantly, all studies to date were retrospective in nature. Most studies which all intended to define an independent prognostic gene signature were not able to define a common gene signature that would be robustly reproducible across different studies. But still, further assessments are required to predict which signature subtype is exclusively selected in therapy for a particular patient. Figure 1 represents the brief intervention in ovarian cancer and its ongoing treatment options available.

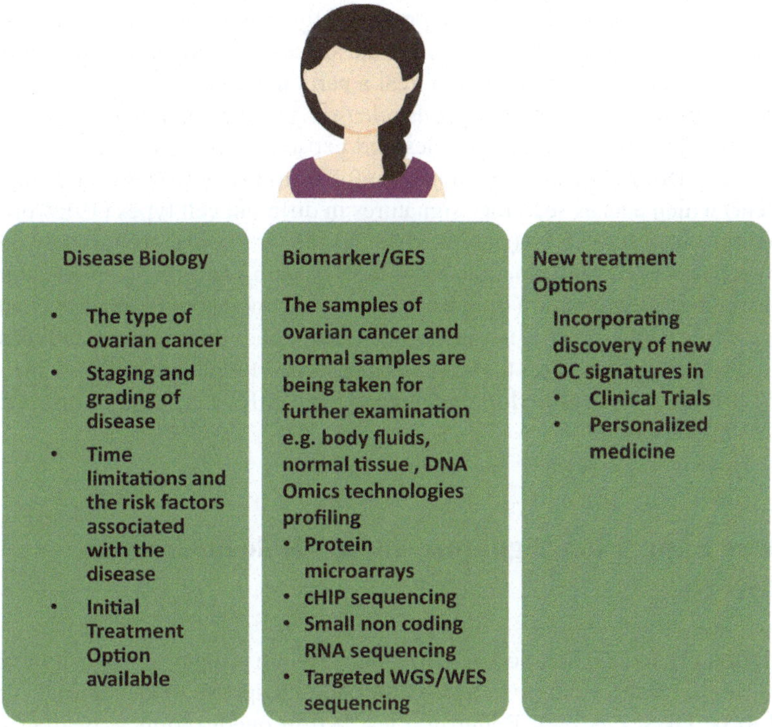

Fig. 1 Understanding the etiology and biology in ovarian cancer and novel application in omics-based technologies in research and clinical trials

3 Cancer Biomarkers

Biomarkers are proteomic and genetic signatures that are used to differentiate between diseased and healthy persons. These biomarkers are used to determine the patient's prognosis and diagnosis thereby helping in regulating the possible outcome in targeted therapy. Therefore, it is crucial to interpret the emerging panorama in cancer genetics and to associate biomarker-based targeted therapy (Bevacizumab or Avastin) as the known targeted therapy being given to patients with ovarian cancer and it belongs to a class of drugs called angiogenesis inhibitors. This particular drug attaches to a protein VEGF (that is responsible for the formation of blood vessels) and slows or stops cancer growth) with tumor aberrations [15]. These signatures include protein (peptides and antibodies); DNA (dsDNA, ssDNA, and retrotransposons), RNA (mRNA, miRNA, circRNA, and lncRNA). On the basis of the site of isolation and secretion, these biomarkers are classified [15]. Cancer biomarkers are classified into three types that are based on particular signatures associated with and these are: diagnostic, predictive, and prognostic biomarkers [15, 16]. Disease outcomes are predicted by diagnostics biomarkers that are linked with a particular malignancy; the risk of disease and its recurrence are predicted by prognostic biomarkers followed by predictive biomarkers which speculate the successful outcome of an appropriate therapeutic approach being applied to treat a particular disease.

Researchers revealed that tumor cells release EVs (at a much higher amount than the normal cells) such as microvesicles and exosomes into the extracellular environment [17, 18]. EVs carry the Genetic information (RNA, DNA, and fragments of protein) which acts as secretory signatures in different cell types [19]. Collection and recognition of these EVs (stream, serum, urine, or plasma) from cancer patients could reveal important information about their genetic constituents, molecular variants, etc. Hence Identification of these EVs serves as potential biomarkers that have enabled advanced therapeutic targets for the treatment of different cancer types. Few identified secretory signatures that serve as therapeutic targets are miRNAs in ovarian cancer [20], HGF is identified in melanoma called MET [21], and in breast cancer HER2/neu [22], etc.

4 Gene Expression Signature and Its Role in Complex Diseases

A small synchronized collection of genes that have the prognostic capacity to distinguish the entire transcriptome in a tissue or cell in response to an external stimulus is said to be GES; [23, 24]. Being in a test bed in oncogenomics; ovarian cancer studies uncovered many mRNA markers of disease recurrence, which cater suitable information in guiding the particular treatment. These clinically inspired multi-genes markers are known as signatures; these signatures are obtained from tumoral profiles of whole-genome mRNA by choosing only those genes whose expressions are correlated with the outcome, or with known offensive markers such as grade of particular cancer and its proliferation [25]. Many signatures are also derived from biological states or the markers of specific mechanisms and these include stem cells signatures, aneuploidy, wound healing, ALK5; loss of PTEN; perturbations of E2F1 [26]. Meta-analysis of different signatures is highly correlated with disease proliferation and it also shows that they have high prognostic performance. Multiple statistical methods are used to get GES in diseased and normal states; differentially expressed genes usually <100 are used in a set that can differentiate between both the states. The high-throughput method is used after profiling gene expression changes in diseased and normal states [27, 28]. Further, NGS, real-time PCR, or multiplex techniques are used to measure GES in interested samples [23, 25]. The signature Genes can be cross-checked through a literature survey that has already been reported and through in silico studies-based databases where a number of Genes with their annotation are submitted like TCGA and ahead of all validation experimental validation will reveal their exact function. The GES is a dynamic tool in the treatment and diagnosis of heterogeneous diseases like cancer in the breast, ovaries, hepatocellular carcinoma, diabetes, etc. Figure 2 represents the role of gene expression signature in complex

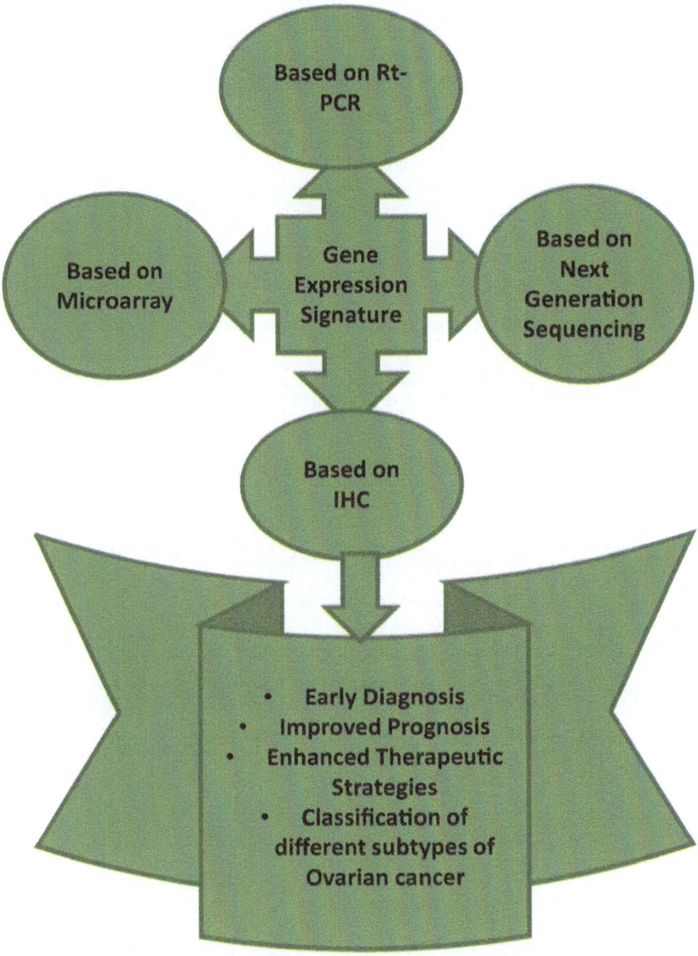

Fig. 2 Role of GES based on various omics technologies in complex diseases

diseases and Fig. 3 represents a summary about how GES analysis is being used to predict cancer biomarkers.

5 Prognostic Relevance of GES in Ovarian Cancer

The future of OC basically depends upon prognostic and predictive value, i.e., whether an ovarian cancer patient needs therapy or a patient will benefit from the ongoing therapy. After an organized Medline search we found literature in ovarian cancer that describes gene expression studies. Among that literature, the

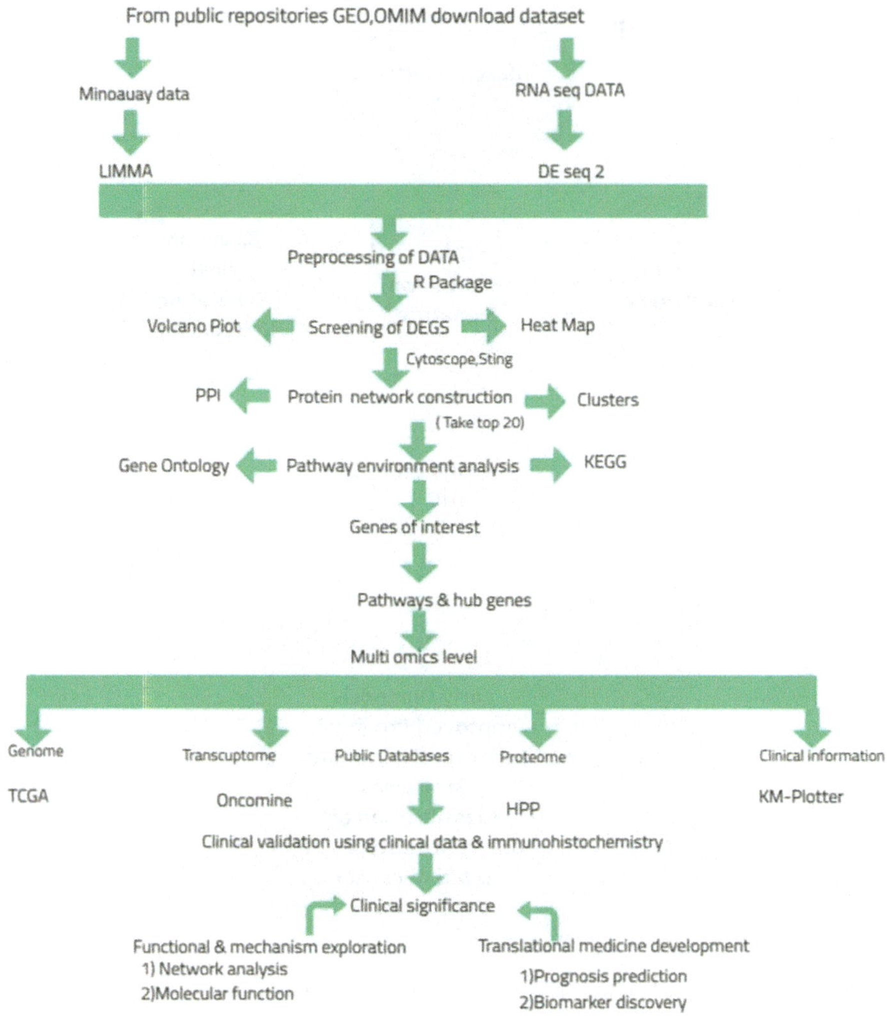

Fig. 3 A summary to predict cancer biomarkers using GES analysis

early data/studies of GES profiling mainly focus on the prognostic value of GES in ovarian cancer. However, there were several limitations in many of these studies which include different platforms of gene expression, overfitting the data, different analysis methods, restriction in the histology of HGSOC, etc. The majority of prognostic genes that were identified in different studies were not able to identify familiar gene signatures [29]. Table 1 represents the studies based on gene expression analysis in OC and its prognostic relevance of gene signature. All these prognostic models being published before 2012 still need accuracy in defining the accurate clinical value. To improve the metastatic potential in ovarian cancer we need master genes

Table 1 Studies based on gene expression analysis on ovarian cancer and its prognostic relevance of gene signature

S. No	Figo staging	Gene expression assay (array)	Number of genes associated with OC signatures	Prognostic significances		References
				Training set	Validation set	
1	I–IV	Affymetrix	26	NA	0.007	[33]
2	I–IV	Affymetrix	300	0.009	0.007	[34]
3	I–IV	Affymetrix	14	<0.001	<0.001	[35]
4	I–IV	Affymetrix	60 (BRCA signature)	NA	0.006	[36]
5	III/IV	Affymetrix	115	0.004	0.01	[37]
6	III/IV	Agilent	TCGA subtype signature	0.004	0.04	[38]
7	I/IV	Agilent	200 (POSTN/TGFBI)	0/009	0.001	[39]
8	III/IV	Agilent	126	<0.001	0.003	[40]
9	III/IV	Agilent	88 (PFS)	<0.001	<0.001	[41]
10	I/IV	cDNA	85	<0.001	NA	[42]
11	III/IV	cDNA	14 (P)FS	<0.001	<0.05	[43]
12	III/IV	Affymetrix Agilent	14 DNA repair genes	<0.001	<0.05	[44]
13	III/IV	Affymetrix Agilent	100 (CLOVAR survival signature)	<0.001	0.004	[45]
14	III/IV	Affymetrix Agilent	193 genes (TCGA prognostic signature)	NA	NA	[46]
15	I/IV	cDNA	C1-C6 subtype signature	<0.001	0.354	[47]

that can improve the reproducibility of prognostic gene signature. Hence in this regard construction of prognostic and predictive tools will benefit validation studies. For example, Bernards et al. in 2002 first developed and approved the 70-gene signature in 295 patients with breast cancer. Mamma Print test is the first 'prognostic gene signature', which has been given approval by FDA and is being used in various studies. Microarray-based gene expression profiling in breast cancer sets an example for ovarian cancer and every other gynecological malignancy.

Therefore, we urgently need novel therapies to improve the outcomes of ovarian cancer. Hence the development of prominent biomarkers will lead to the success of new drug development in OC with the help of which patients will be benefitted from the new therapy. The development of gene expression profiling based on microarray leads to major advancement in OC prediction, classification, and prognostication.

Although in the past 10 years many prognostic and predictive molecular classifications have emerged in OC, the clinical implication of OC is not clear and studies are still underway for the successful clinical findings of gene expression profiling in OC [15]. The patients suffering from Ovarian cancer (BRCA1/2 wild-type) are categorized into high survival rates and low survival rates having prominent signatures based on different non-coding RNAs which include lncRNAs (LINC01234 and CCDC144NL-AS1) and two miRNAs (miR-637 and miR-129-5p) signatures based on genome-wide lncRNA and miRNA expression profiles [30]. Wang et al. identified 7 lncRNAs (NR_073113, NR_036503, NR_103801, XR_948297, XR_947831, XR_938728, and XR_938392) that are mostly deregulated in samples of ovarian tumor and found to have shown a symbolic correlation in an epithelial ovarian cancer patient with a poor chemotherapeutic response [31]. Numerous lncRNAs like CTD-2555A7.3, LINC01514, ZFAS1, RP11-16E12.1, RP11-136I14.5, RP5-1061H20.5, RP11-489O18.1, and TUG1 are the identified signature lncRNA by Rong Liu et al. that act as diagnostic markers and they play important role in chemotherapeutic resistance of HGS-OvCa [32].

6 Gene Expression as a Drug Discovery Tool

The biggest milestone that was achieved in 1995, was the development of microarray, i.e., when microarrays have led to the development in DNA chip technology and genetics research [48]. The first gene expression signature was presented in 1999 by Golub [49]. Monitoring of gene expression in case of acute leukemia was being done by T. R. Golub using DNA microarray for the production of a classifier that could distinguish AML (acute myeloid leukemia) and ALL (acute lymphoblastic leukemia) [49]. Thenceforth numerous gene expression signatures have been developed and used to classify different tumor types, recognize different stages of tumors as well as predict the prognosis of the diseases. Due to limitations in clinicopathologic parameters, there are still many challenges in predicting the disease prognosis which is crucial for cancer malignancies and their management. Prognostic GES can help in improving the patient's therapy by allocating tumors into different groups, thereby providing directions for a personalized treatment decision. Bernards et al. in 2002 first developed and validated the 70-gene signature in 295 patients with breast cancer. MammaPrint test is the first 'prognostic gene signature', which has been given approval by FDA and is being used in various studies [50, 51]. MammaPrint test is commercially promoted as AGENDIA and is used in clinical diagnostics on the use of adjuvant chemotherapy for early breast cancer [51]. Following its approval, numerous prognostic gene expression signatures were discovered for different organs and tissues [52–55]. The post-treatment in case of leukemia cells the gene expression can be used to screen candidate compounds to induce the target phenotype. The mechanisms of phenotypic differentiation are usually complex and involve multiple signaling pathways. Although many improvements have been made to detect a particular phenotype, the primary screen still lagged behind to measure the function of single molecular targets [56, 57].

Drug discovery in homogenous diseases is accomplished by screening various libraries that bind to a particular drug target. However, in complex diseases, multiple signaling pathways are involved. Hence the prevalent drug discovery approach fails to inflict the origin of heterogeneous diseases. High throughput screening based on GES is adopted; it does not require prior learning about the target; instead, compounds are identified based on overall cellular structure. The method used by GES in a cellular model has its own defined set of conditions; where two states of interest are created, from which transcriptome is modeled and measured to generate GES. Further, this model is screened with a drug library to measure the expression level of GES using the qPCR technique; to analyze those drugs which have a decisive influence on GES genes. In addition, to make qPCR more throughputs the readout measurement can be performed at 97-384-well format. Various drug libraries can be screened for efficacy, as the GES approach is high throughput and unbiased (Evans & Guy, 2004). The majority of medications that are being used to treat cancer are non-specific cytotoxic agents which are simultaneously affecting both tumors as well as normal cells [57]. To improve the curing rates in all human malignancies selective agents are required to reduce the host toxicity. Advancement in the field of human genetics, cancer biology, bioinformatics, and disease pathogenesis promises the discovery of new approaches for targeted drugs [58]. Sequencing in human genome projects and advancement in recent technologies have paved the way for a broad analysis of cancer cells and it also facilitates synthesis and screening of huge libraries to define particular drug targets [59]. The computational and cost-effective methods of virtual screening are used to identify potential drug targets which helped a lot in cancer treatment. These days along with these potential drug targets in combination with radiotherapy small molecule drugs and monoclonal antibodies are also effectively used in treating ovarian cancer [58, 59].

7 Conclusion

Improved therapies are needed, with the increasing mortality rate for ovarian cancer that is affecting women worldwide. At the initial stages Classical anticancer drug interference are usually profitable but as the progression of disease starts these drugs sooner or later miscarry the treatment outcomes. This inadequacy is associated not only with these drugs but also with the incompetency to understand the complicated pathways being associated with the disease. The advancement in understanding the complete genome has provided a better understanding of the complex diseases and pathways involved with it but still, we have to go a long way to sufficiently identify appropriate targets. The drug discovery method based on GES is a completely different approach where the selection of drugs is based on an entire measurement as of how a cell responds to them (Schadt et al., 2009) moreover this approach has proven to be more fruitful in various complex diseases. Due to disease heterogeneity and different omics datasets, various milestones are present in finding gene signatures for OC development or progression. Therefore it is important first to address the entire question before extrapolating genetic targets in ovarian cancer.

Acknowledgements The authors are thankful for the high computing infrastructure in the Department of Computer Science, Jamia Millia Islamia, New Delhi. Anam Beg is also thankful for the award of Senior Research Fellowship from the Indian Council of Medical Research (ICMR). This work is supported by the Indian Council of Medical Research.

Fundings This work was supported by the Indian Council of Medical Research (ICMR); PROJECT ID: 2019-4178.

References

1. Ghafouri-Fard, S., Shoorei, H., & Taheri, M. (2020). miRNA profile in ovarian cancer. *Experimental and Molecular Pathology, 113*, 104381.
2. Biamonte, F., et al. (2019). MicroRNA let-7g acts as tumor suppressor and predictive biomarker for chemoresistance in human epithelial ovarian cancer. *Scientific Reports, 9*(1), 1–12.
3. Dwivedi, S. K. D., et al. (2021). Small non-coding-RNA in gynecological malignancies. *Cancers, 13*(5), 1085.
4. Devouassoux-Shisheboran, M., & Genestie, C. (2015). Pathobiology of ovarian carcinomas. *Chinese Journal of Cancer, 34*(1), 50–55.
5. Labidi-Galy, S. I., et al. (2017). High grade serous ovarian carcinomas originate in the fallopian tube. *Nature Communications, 8*(1), 1–11.
6. Dochez, V., et al. (2019). Biomarkers and algorithms for diagnosis of ovarian cancer: CA125, HE4, RMI and ROMA, a review. *Journal of Ovarian Research, 12*(1), 1–9.
7. Hellström, I., et al. (2003). The HE4 (WFDC2) protein is a biomarker for ovarian carcinoma. *Cancer Research, 63*(13), 3695–3700.
8. Brachova, P., et al. (2015). TP53 oncomorphic mutations predict resistance to platinum- and taxane-based standard chemotherapy in patients diagnosed with advanced serous ovarian carcinoma. *International Journal of Oncology, 46*(2), 607–618.
9. Bodnar, L., et al. (2014). Wnt/β-catenin pathway as a potential prognostic and predictive marker in patients with advanced ovarian cancer. *Journal of Ovarian Research, 7*(1), 1–10.
10. Steinberga, I., Jansson, K., Sorbe, B. (2019). Quality indicators and survival outcome in stage IIIB-IVB epithelial ovarian Cancer treated at a single institution. *In vivo, 33*(5), 1521–1530.
11. Goff, B. A., et al. (2004). Frequency of symptoms of ovarian cancer in women presenting to primary care clinics. *JAMA, 291*(22), 2705–2712.
12. Lheureux, S., et al. (2019). Epithelial ovarian cancer. *The Lancet, 393*(10177), 1240–1253.
13. Edge, S., et al. (2010). American Joint Committee on Cancer cancer staging manual. *Annals of Surgical Oncology, 17*, 1471–1474.
14. Prat, J., & F. C. o. G. (2014). Oncology, staging classification for cancer of the ovary, fallopian tube, and peritoneum. *International Journal of Gynecology & Obstetrics, 124*(1), 1–5.
15. Hora, S., Pandey, A. K., Jha, S. (2018). Biomarker-based targeted therapeutics. *Neoplasm*, 159.
16. Goossens, N., et al. (2015). Cancer biomarker discovery and validation. *Translational Cancer Research, 4*(3), 256.
17. Raposo, G., & Stoorvogel, W. (2013). Extracellular vesicles: Exosomes, microvesicles, and friends. *Journal of Cell Biology, 200*(4), 373–383.

18. Van Doormaal, F., et al. (2009). Cell-derived microvesicles and cancer. *The Netherlands Journal of Medicine, 67*(7), 266–273.
19. Valadi, H., et al. (2007). Exosome-mediated transfer of mRNAs and microRNAs is a novel mechanism of genetic exchange between cells. *Nature Cell Biology, 9*(6), 654–659.
20. Taylor, D. D., & Gercel-Taylor, C. (2008). MicroRNA signatures of tumor-derived exosomes as diagnostic biomarkers of ovarian cancer. *Gynecologic Oncology, 110*(1), 13–21.
21. Peinado, H., et al. (2012). Melanoma exosomes educate bone marrow progenitor cells toward a pro-metastatic phenotype through MET. *Nature Medicine, 18*(6), 883–891.
22. Ciravolo, V., et al. (2012). Potential role of HER2-overexpressing exosomes in countering trastuzumab-based therapy. *Journal of Cellular Physiology, 227*(2), 658–667.
23. Sithara, S., et al. (2017). Gene expression signature: A powerful approach for drug discovery in diabetes. *Journal of Endocrinology, 232*(2), R131–R139.
24. Bevilacqua, J. L. B., et al. (2007). Doctor, what are my chances of having a positive sentinel node? A validated nomogram for risk estimation. *Journal of Clinical Oncology, 25*(24), 3670–3679.
25. Venet, D., Dumont, J. E., & Detours, V. (2011). Most random gene expression signatures are significantly associated with breast cancer outcome. *PLoS Computational Biology, 7*(10), e1002240.
26. Kalia, M. (2013). Personalized oncology: Recent advances and future challenges. *Metabolism, 62*, S11–S14.
27. Jabeen, A., Ahmad, N., & Raza, K. (2019). Differential expression analysis of ZIKV infected human RNA sequence reveals potential genetic biomarkers. In *Lecture notes in bioinformatics 2019* (Vol. 11465, pp. 1–12). Springer.
28. Zhang, Y., Qazi, S., & Raza, K. (2021). Differential expression analysis in Ovarian Cancer: A functional genomics and systems biology approach. *Saudi Journal of Biological Sciences, 28*(7), 4069–4081.
29. Konecny, G. E., Winterhoff, B., & Wang, C. (2016). Gene-expression signatures in ovarian cancer: Promise and challenges for patient stratification. *Gynecologic Oncology, 141*(2), 379–385.
30. Guo, L., et al. (2017). Expression profiles analysis reveals an integrated miRNA-lncRNA signature to predict survival in ovarian cancer patients with wild-type BRCA1/2. *Oncotarget, 8*(40), 68483.
31. Wang, L., et al. (2017). Identification of long non-coding RNA signature for paclitaxel-resistant patients with advanced ovarian cancer. *Oncotarget, 8*(38), 64191.
32. Liu, R., et al. (2017). Long noncoding RNA expression signature to predict platinum-based chemotherapeutic sensitivity of ovarian cancer patients. *Scientific Reports, 7*(1), 1–10.
33. Berchuck, A., et al. (2005). Patterns of gene expression that characterize long-term survival in advanced stage serous ovarian cancers. *Clinical Cancer Research, 11*(10), 3686–3696.
34. Denkert, C., et al. (2009). A prognostic gene expression index in ovarian cancer—Validation across different independent data sets. *The Journal of Pathology: A Journal of the Pathological Society of Great Britain and Ireland, 218*(2), 273–280.
35. Jochumsen, K. M., et al. (2009). Gene expression profiles as prognostic markers in women with ovarian cancer. *International Journal of Gynecologic Cancer, 19*(7).
36. Konstantinopoulos, P. A., et al. (2010). Gene expression profile of BRCAness that correlates with responsiveness to chemotherapy and with outcome in patients with epithelial ovarian cancer. *Journal of Clinical Oncology, 28*(22), 3555.
37. Spentzos, D., et al. (2004). Gene expression signature with independent prognostic significance in epithelial ovarian cancer. *Journal of Clinical Oncology, 22*(23), 4700–4710.
38. Konecny, G. E., et al. (2014). Prognostic and therapeutic relevance of molecular subtypes in high-grade serous ovarian cancer. *JNCI: Journal of the National Cancer Institute, 106*(10).
39. Karlan, B. Y., et al. (2014). POSTN/TGFBI-associated stromal signature predicts poor prognosis in serous epithelial ovarian cancer. *Gynecologic Oncology, 132*(2), 334–342.
40. Yoshihara, K., et al. (2012). High-risk ovarian cancer based on 126-gene expression signature is uniquely characterized by downregulation of the antigen presentation pathway. *Clinical Cancer Research, 18*(5), 1374–1385.

41. Yoshihara, K., et al. (2010). Gene expression profile for predicting survival in advanced-stage serous ovarian cancer across two independent datasets. *PloS One, 5*(3), e9615.
42. Jazaeri, A. A., et al. (2005). Gene expression profiles associated with response to chemotherapy in epithelial ovarian cancers. *Clinical Cancer Research, 11*(17), 6300–6310.
43. Hartmann, L. C., et al. (2005). Gene expression profiles predict early relapse in ovarian cancer after platinum-paclitaxel chemotherapy. *Clinical Cancer Research, 11*(6), 2149–2155.
44. Kang, J., D'Andrea, A. D., & Kozono, D. (2012). A DNA repair pathway–focused score for prediction of outcomes in ovarian cancer treated with platinum-based chemotherapy. *Journal of the National Cancer Institute, 104*(9), 670–681.
45. Verhaak, R.G., et al. (2012). Prognostically relevant gene signatures of high-grade serous ovarian carcinoma. *The Journal of clinical investigation, 123*(1).
46. Network, C. G. A. R. (2011). Integrated genomic analyses of ovarian carcinoma. *Nature, 474*(7353), 609.
47. Tothill, R. W., et al. (2008). Novel molecular subtypes of serous and endometrioid ovarian cancer linked to clinical outcome. *Clinical Cancer Research, 14*(16), 5198–5208.
48. Schena, M., et al. (1995). Quantitative monitoring of gene expression patterns with a complementary DNA microarray. *Science, 270*(5235), 467–470.
49. Golub, T. R., et al. (1999). Molecular classification of cancer: Class discovery and class prediction by gene expression monitoring. *Science, 286*(5439), 531–537.
50. Van De Vijver, M. J., et al. (2002). A gene-expression signature as a predictor of survival in breast cancer. *New England Journal of Medicine, 347*(25), 1999–2009.
51. Qian, Y., et al. (2021). Prognostic cancer gene expression signatures: Current status and challenges. *Cells, 10*(3), 648.
52. Cardoso, F., et al. (2016). 70-gene signature as an aid to treatment decisions in early-stage breast cancer. *New England Journal of Medicine, 375*(8), 717–729.
53. Ye, Q.-H., et al. (2003). Predicting hepatitis B virus–positive metastatic hepatocellular carcinomas using gene expression profiling and supervised machine learning. *Nature medicine, 9*(4), 416–423.
54. Bullinger, L., et al. (2004). Use of gene-expression profiling to identify prognostic subclasses in adult acute myeloid leukemia. *New England Journal of Medicine, 350*(16), 1605–1616.
55. Lossos, I. S., et al. (2004). Prediction of survival in diffuse large-B-cell lymphoma based on the expression of six genes. *New England Journal of Medicine, 350*(18), 1828–1837.
56. Bleicher, K. H., et al. (2003). Hit and lead generation: Beyond high-throughput screening. *Nature reviews Drug discovery, 2*(5), 369–378.
57. Evans, W. E., & Guy, R. K. (2004). Gene expression as a drug discovery tool. *Nature Genetics, 36*(3), 214–215.
58. Beg, A., & Parveen, R. (2021). Role of bioinformatics in cancer research and drug development. *Translational bioinformatics in healthcare and medicine* (pp. 141–148). Elsevier.
59. Beg, A., et al. (2019). High throughput screening, docking, and molecular dynamics studies to identify potential inhibitors of human calcium/calmodulin-dependent protein kinase IV. *Journal of Biomolecular Structure and Dynamics, 37*(8), 2179–2192.

Machine Learning-Based Approach for Early Diagnosis of Breast Cancer Using Biomarkers and Gene Expression Profiles

Ankita Sahu, Sahar Qazi, Khalid Raza, Astha Singh, and Saurabh Verma

Abstract Breast cancer is a heterogeneous disease and the most frequent malignancy in women globally each year. Emerging applications of gene expression profiles are important to determine the clinical outcomes for breast cancer. Biomarker dataset from Gene Expression Omnibus (GEO), The Cancer Genome Atlas (TCGA), and Oncomine databases are used to analyze the potential therapeutic target for the expression level of hub gene based on their microarray technology. Several computational intelligent techniques, such as—Naïve Bayes, Support vector machines (SVM), K-nearest neighbor, and decision trees, are mostly used to classify different types of breast cancers. These also have been appreciated in the field for identifying new gene biomarkers for breast cancer. Out of these major algorithms, SVM has been proved to have higher accuracy and specificity while detecting breast cancers during initial diagnosis. The benchmark of these algorithms can be attributed to the development of new computational biology strategies, characterization performance for gene expression profile data, and the ability to predict biomedical outcomes. This chapter focuses on an array of successful computational intelligent systems that are deployed for identifying potential biomarkers, strongly related to breast cancer survivability. Furthermore, we will also address the recent advancement in techniques, their challenges, possible opportunities, and clinical implementation in their assessment.

Keywords Breast cancer · Machine learning · Microarray · Gene Expression Omnibus · The Cancer Genome Atlas · Oncomine databases

A. Sahu · A. Singh · S. Verma (✉)
Tumor Biology, ICMR-National Institute of Pathology, New Delhi 110029, India

S. Qazi · K. Raza
Department of Computer Science, Jamia Millia Islamia, New Delhi 110025, India

K. Raza (ed.), *Computational Intelligence in Oncology*, Studies in Computational Intelligence 1016, https://doi.org/10.1007/978-981-16-9221-5_17

1 Introduction

Breast cancer is the most frequent malignancy in the female population, and its treatment process is long, expensive due to its heterogeneity, high recurrence, and poor survival [1]. Owing to the current advancement in high-throughput techniques for measuring the expression level of genes across various samples, such as microarrays and RNA-seq, these have emerged as important tools for gene expression profiling and detection of clinical outcomes for several diseases including breast cancer. In fact, gene expression profiling is done in order to identify specific signatures (gene biomarkers) associated with disease diagnosis, prediction, and prognosis [2, 3]. By utilizing the power of computational intelligent systems, early screening, diagnosis, the prognosis that use gene expression profiling data can continue to improve the current scenario of person-centric treatment approach for oncology. Machine learning algorithms are widely utilized for developing robust prognostic models for analyzing the gene expression profile data better classification.

This chapter provides an array of successful computational intelligence systems used to identify a potential set of biomarkers, strongly associated with the survivability of breast cancer and addresses the recent advancement in techniques, their challenges, possible opportunities, and clinical implementation in their assessment.

1.1 Biomarkers and Their Role in Breast Cancer Diagnosis

Biomarkers are molecules that have been identified for various diseases such as cancer, cardiovascular disease, nephropathy, and retinopathy [4]. It is used to describe potential markers of cancer development and progression, produced by tumor cells, or other cells of the body. The most promising use of biomarkers is particularly important in cancer that can enhance the rational development, approval of new innovative drugs and therapeutic biomedical products [5]. Numerous types of biomolecules including genetic material (DNA, methylated DNA, RNA), proteins, or hormones, assist as biomarkers, all express something about the body [6, 7].

Breast cancer biomarkers have been discovered and are still in their discovery stage. The evidence of biomarkers requires to provide an earlier stage diagnosis of breast cancer [8]. There are a tremendous variety of biomarkers that are found in different types of cancer, and levels of the same tumor marker may be associated with more than one cancer. The established biomarkers (ER, PR, and human epidermal growth factor eceptor-2 also named ER-2) and emerging biomarkers (Ki67, cyclin D1, cyclin E, and Erβ) are applied for breast cancer diagnosis and treatment [9]. These markers are verified to facilitate breast cancer diagnosis and management, especially for early detection, accurately predict metastatic cell behaviors, selection, and clinical trial of appropriate therapy. These biomarkers predict response to chemotherapy in breast cancer.

Protein biomarkers in biological fluid have been associated with breast cancer to improve breast cancer diagnosis. CA 15.3, CEA, and HER2 are useful as tumor protein biomarkers for early diagnosis of metastases for prognosis, recurrence, and monitoring of breast cancer [10, 11]. These biomarkers are periodically linked with the predisposition of breast cancer and predict patient response to treatment. The specificity and sensitivity of these markers are imperative in establishing their potential clinical settings for a precise type of neoplasm. It can be detected by blood, saliva, or urine. Working with biomarkers allows a better understanding of disease processes that are elucidated by the graphical Figure 1. Biomarkers that detect disease earlier are more valuable and help us to provide treatment for the disease; if it can't be detected, it becomes incurable in advanced stages. Hence, the biomarker is enormously important for the early detection and treatment of cancer [5].

Clinical biomarkers can be applied to describe the measurable biological indicators for the diagnosis and monitoring of a certain disease. It determines the optimal treatments based on their phenotypes and genotypes in medical settings [12]. These biomarkers are the process in the field of computational intelligence systems with the help of gene expression profiles in breast cancer.

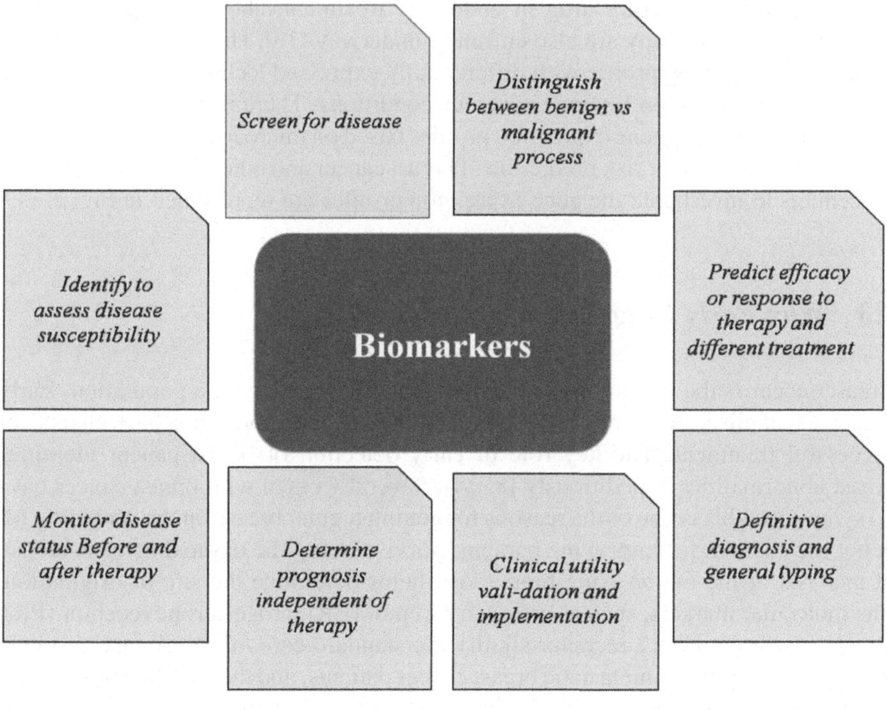

Fig. 1 Different aspects of cancer biomarkers

1.2 Gene Expression Profiles

Cancer can also be called a disease of altered gene expression. Numerous proteins act as on/off switches such as on (gene activation) or off (gene silencing), deeply altering the cell's overall activity. A key goal of biology is to relate gene expression profiling, determine the particular pattern of expressed genes by several cell types at the level of transcription and measure mRNA levels [13]. To understand the differential expression behavior and its involvement in various biological pathways in breast cancer are processed by genes expression patterns data such as The Cancer Genome Atlas (TCGA), Gene expression Omnibus (GEO), Oncomine databases, Surveillance, Epidemiology, and End Results (SEER), and Sequence Read Archive (SRA). These expression studies in breast cancer usually investigate at early time-points after uncontrolled growth of the abnormal cell. The analysis of gene expression is the process by which the genes are transcribed and converted to synthesize functional gene products such as protein products or functional RNA. The regulation of gene expression is engaged in many normal cellular processes, such as differentiation, and abnormal or pathological processes. For evidence in drug targeting in breast cancer, several new gene expression analyses are carried out at gaining the capability to determine the selecting drug in endocrine treatment, chemotherapy, and neo-adjuvant medical therapy are also currently underway [13]. High-throughput large-scale gene expression profile with differentially expressed technology has aided the breast cancer prediction like precancerous conditions. There is currently immersed interest in identifying gene expression profiles based on microarrays for breast cancer diagnosis, as well as for risk prediction of breast cancer and other diseases. The entire procedures to investigate the gene expression profiles are represented in Fig. 2.

1.3 Why Early Diagnosis of Breast Cancer?

Breast cancer is the second most diagnosed cancer in the female population. Early diagnosis of disease opens the door to the future and holds the best chance of successful treatment. The key role of early detection of breast cancer identifies breast abnormalities expeditiously [8, 14]. Several women with breast cancer have no symptoms; this is one of the reasons for getting regular breast cancer screening for better the chances for improving patients' survival rate. The tissue diagnosis biopsy of analysis of the tumor using biomarkers helps determine the site of origination. The molecular markers, such as estrogen receptor (ER), progesterone receptor (PR), together with the HER2 receptor signify the standard care of all primary systemic therapy, recurrent, and metastatic breast cancer patients, and the ER/PR/HER2 status is the standardized assessment of every newly diagnosed breast cancer [6]. Therefore, more specific biomarkers are an urgent need for identifying breast cancer. In earlier studies, several biomarkers have been developed related to early detection and diagnosis for breast cancer such as uPA [15], Rs/DJ-1 [16], and recently, circulating

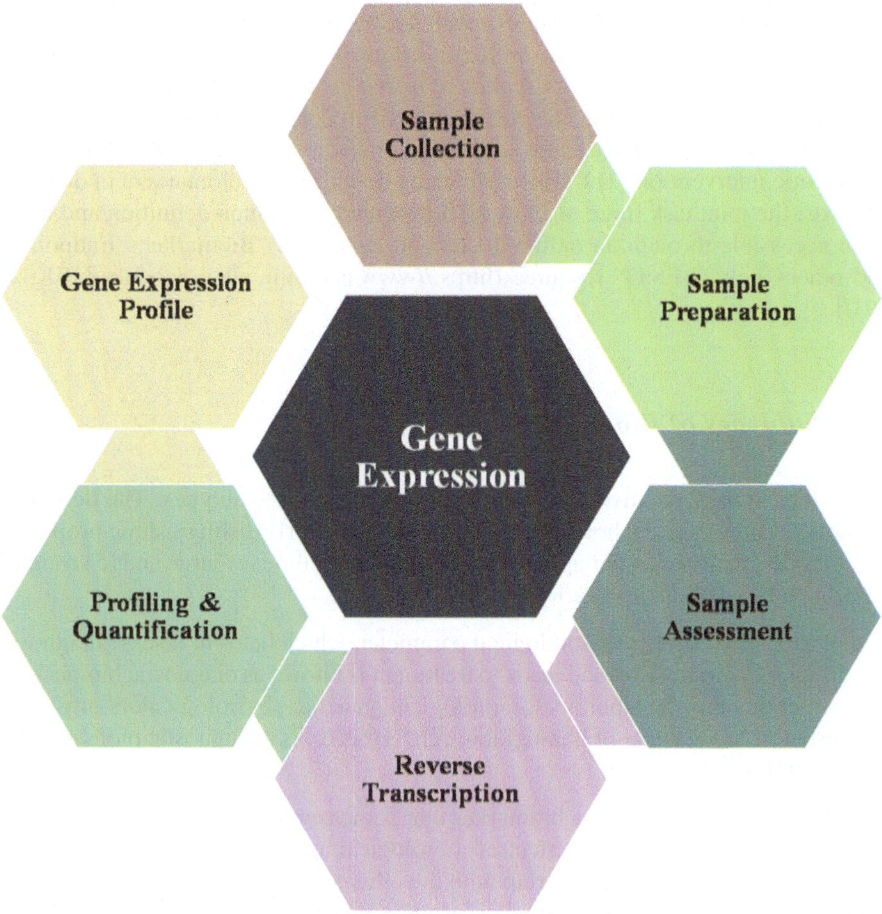

Fig. 2 Schematic flowchart of entire procedures to investigate the gene expression profiles of breast cancer

miRNAs [17], serum uPAR Hao and Friedman [18], KiSS1 [19], CD24 [20], etc. are more strongly associated with breast cancer development. These biomarkers provide information on the specific therapeutic target and also offer the overall information of the particular cancer maker.

2 Biomarkers and Gene Expression Databases for Breast Cancer

According to National Cancer Institute (NCI), National Institute of Health (NIH), the term biomarker (also called molecular marker or signature) is defined as "*A biological molecule found in blood, other body fluids, or tissues that is a sign of a normal or abnormal process, or a condition or disease. A biomarker may be used to see how well the body responds to a treatment for a disease or condition.*" In simple terms, biomarkers are measures used to carry out a clinical assessment and monitor and predict the states of health in patients in order to plan appropriate therapeutic intervention [21]. Due to differing definitions of biomarkers in different contexts, the joint task force of FDA-NIH provided a common definition and made them accessible through an online document, called the "Biomarkers, EndpointS, and other Tools (BEST)" resource (https://www.ncbi.nlm.nih.gov/books/NBK326791/).

2.1 Subtypes of Biomarkers

According to their putative applications, biomarkers have subtypes. The definition of subtypes may overlap; however, they would have clearly distinguishing properties that describe their particular application. The BEST online resource and [5] roughly categorize biomarkers into various subtypes (Fig. 3).

Diagnostic biomarkers: Any biological parameter, which helps in disease diagnosis, determines its progression and leads to treatment is known as diagnostic biomarkers. These markers may be laboratory, radiological, genetic, physiological, or any other. For instance, blood sugar or hemoglobin A1c (HbA1c) is a diagnostic biomarker for type-2 diabetes.

Monitoring Biomarker: It is a biomarker that is measured sequentially to assess the disease status or to detect an effect of a biological agent on the disease condition. Monitoring biomarkers may overlap with the other subtypes of biomarkers and have pivotal applications in clinical care. For instance, when blood pressure (BP) is treated, or low-density lipoprotein (LDL) also known as "bad" cholesterol-lowering drugs is used, the level of BP or LDL cholesterol is monitored [5].

Predictive biomarkers: If presence or change in the biological marker predicts an individual or group that is expected to experience the effect from the exposure to a medical product or an environmental agent, it is known as a predictive biomarker. It is usually measured before treatment in order to assess the probability of response to a particular therapy. For instance, a predictive biomarker in breast cancer is the expression of the human epidermal growth factor receptor 2 (HER2 sometimes referred to as HER2/neu) protein [22].

Prognostic Biomarker : A biomarker that is used to detect the probability of a clinical event, disease recurrence, and progression, or death in patients independent of treatment received, is known as a prognostic biomarker. For instance, prostate-specific antigen (PSA) level is a prognostic biomarker in prostate cancer and PIK3CA mutation with HER2 in breast cancer [23].

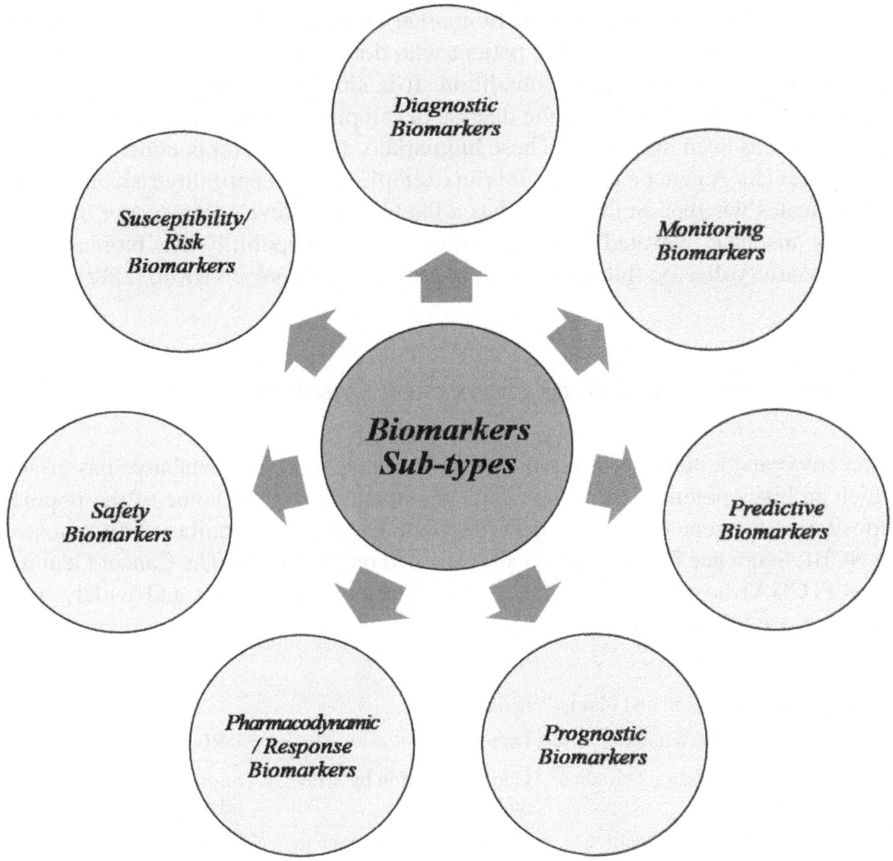

Fig. 3 Subtypes of the biomarkers

Pharmacodynamic/Response Biomarker: When the level of biomarker changes due to exposure to a biological agent, or a medical product, it is known as a *pharmacodynamic/response biomarker*. It is useful in clinical practice and the early stages of therapeutic development. For instance, if blood pressure or glucose level is not reduced while treating hypertension or diabetes, there is a need to avoid that intervention and try another. These biomarkers are also used to determine the drug-dosing response by measuring changes in *pharmacodynamic/response biomarkers* [5].

Safety Biomarker: It is a biomarker indicative of the likelihood, presence, or extend of toxicity as an adverse effect of a medical product or an environmental agent. Safety biomarkers help identify adverse effects of treatment in patients. Further, safety biomarkers can be utilized to balance the safety and benefits of therapies in the patients.

Susceptibility/Risk Biomarker: This biomarker designates the prospects to develop a disease or health condition in a patient who does not currently have a clinically apparent illness or other health condition. It is similar to prognostic biomarkers, except that it is associated with the disease development rather than prognosis after the disease has been diagnosed. These biomarkers are useful for conducting disease risk studies [5]. A genetic biomarker is an example of a susceptibility/risk biomarker that indicates whether an individual has a likelihood of developing cancer in future life. For instance, elevated LDL cholesterol is a susceptibility/risk biomarker of coronary artery disease (https://www.ncbi.nlm.nih.gov/books/NBK402288/).

2.2 Biomarkers and Gene Expression Databases

In recent years, a plethora of biomarkers and gene expression databases has grown which archives potential information for therapeutics targets. Some of the popular repositories for gene expression data are Gene Expression Omnibus (GEO) hosted on NCBI, Sequence Read Archive (SRA) hosted on NCBI, and The Cancer Genome Atlas (TCGA) hosted on the GDC portal. The most prominent and widely used databases are listed in Table 1.

Table 1 Gene expression and biomarkers databases

S. No.	Name of the database	Data types	URL
1	Gene Expression Omnibus (GEO)	Gene expression by array and sequence	https://www.ncbi.nlm.nih.gov/geo/
2	Sequence Read Archive (SRA)	High-throughput sequence	https://www.ncbi.nlm.nih.gov/sra
3	The Cancer Genome Atlas (TCGA)	Harmonized cancer datasets	https://portal.gdc.cancer.gov
4	Oncomine	Cancer microarray database and data mining platform	https://www.oncomine.org/
5	MarkerDB	General biomarkers	https://markerdb.ca/
6	BiomarkersDB	General biomarkers	https://wwwapps.criver.com/BiomarkersDB/
7	OncoMX	Cancer biomarker	https://www.oncomx.org/
8	DisGeNET	Gene-disease and variant-disease association	https://www.disgenet.org/
9	GoBIOM	General biomarkers	https://www.gobiomdbplus.com/
10	BIONDA	General biomarkers	https://bionda.mpc.ruhr-uni-bochum.de/
11	BmDR	Safety biomarker	https://c-path.org/programs/bmdr/

2.3 Digital Biomarkers: The Future

The term "biomarker" is already defined in the previous section. The digital refers to the method of collecting data. Instead of blood tests and medical imaging, digital biomarkers are identified/measured using connected sensors and algorithms across a plethora of reachable linked hardware and software tools [24]. The term "digital biomarker" is defined as quantifiable physiological and behavioral data that are collected and measured through portable, wearable, implantable, or digestible digital devices that aim to explain, influence, or health-related predicted outcomes. The rapid advancement in wearable digital technologies for healthcare applications is generating a vast amount of data (e.g., big healthcare data) in order to produce actionable insights related to the biological state of individuals, acts as biomarkers, but are measured and collected using digital tools [25]. These portable and wearable devices enable digital biomarker discovery that would help the detection and monitoring of various chronic diseases. Its algorithms provide important aggregation of high-resolution, intra-individual data to summary metrics that are interpretable and actionable [26].

Owing to the advancement in smart biosensors and Internet of Things (IoT) technologies, a variety of biosensors are available in the consumer market that is capable to monitor an individual's various biological activities and dynamic signs, such as an electrocardiogram (ECG), heart rate, pulse rate, sweat, pedometer, sleeping profiles, and other parameters are increasingly available [25]. Research into the digital biomarkers discovery algorithm has been carried out to screen various diseases including atrial fibrillation using photoplethysmographic rhythm analysis [27], digital biomarkers in sweat, saliva and exhaled breath for tuberculosis and antibiotic stewardship [25], Alzheimer's disease [28], and so on.

As far as the challenging role of digital biomarkers in cancer research is concerned, it has a great impact on various clinical decision support. The digital biomarkers facilitate the oncologist to track their patients' treatment journey in a real-world setting. Gresham et al. [29] predicted performance status scores in patients with advanced stage of cancer. Ingestible sensors can be used to transmit time medication and collect data on physiological changes of the digestive system, which in turn can be potentially used to control therapy adherence. Rodríguez-Ruiz et al. [30] attempt to screen breast cancer using mammography images. In pathology, new biomarkers are being tested to determine the PD-L1 expression in cancer tissue [31]. In skin cancer, diagnosis relies mostly on the chromatic and morphological features of lesions detected by dermatologists. The information flow in a newly developed artificial neural network (ANN) may predict the malignancy potential of skin lesions more efficiently than trained dermatologists [32].

In a nutshell, digital biomarkers have tremendous application and are currently changing cancer research and gradually improving the health outcome in the clinical decision-making process. They can derive from various sources like body sensors, health platforms, image processing, and electronic medical records or and will have a significant impact on clinical research and patient care [33].

3 Computational Intelligence System for Early Diagnosis of Cancer

At present, computer-aided diagnosis has become a common feature in clinical diagnosis procedures for disease detection using medical images like histopathological, mammography and become a most major topic in the imaging and diagnosis process. The computational intelligence system (CIS) is a substantial requirement for early diagnostic of breast cancer to reduce human errors and deliver significant growth in histopathology imagery and medical health applications. Various surveys have been reported in current years reviewing the computer-aided diagnosis that covers the history and detailed information of general computational intelligence techniques. The process of the system is carried out in five steps (Fig. 4):

(a) *Preprocessing of breast profiling*: Preprocessing is a basic and more suitable step for machine learning to transform raw data into meaningful patterns for further subsequent analysis [34]. The preprocessing is used in mammography films to enhance the visibility of peripheral areas and improve the intensity distribution [35, 36]. The standardized dataset is used by the following Equation (1):

$$Z = \frac{\chi - \mu}{\sigma}. \tag{1}$$

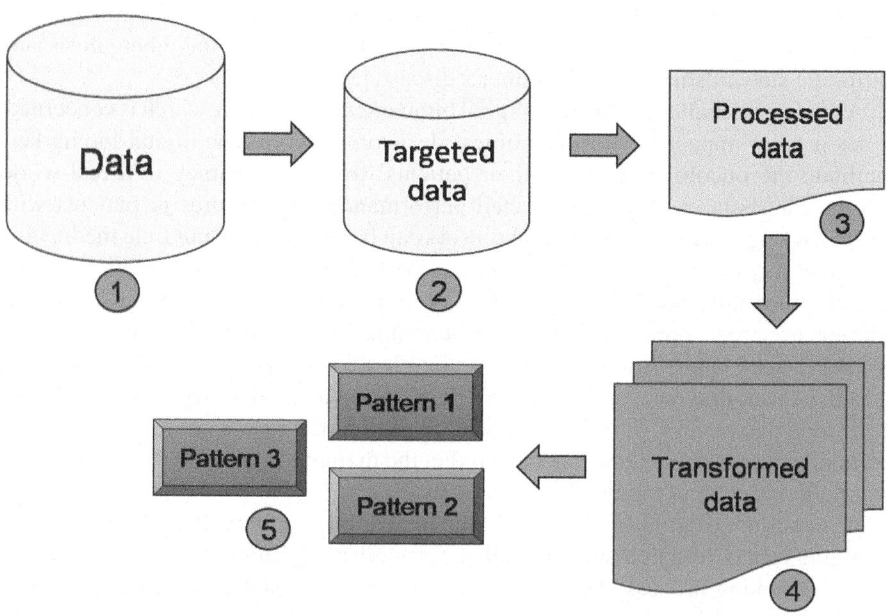

Fig. 4 Workflow of the computational intelligence system for breast cancer diagnosis

where χ represent a standardized feature, μ denotes mean, and σ is a standard deviation (SD). The Python script is used for data standardization [37].

(b) *Features Selection*: After the preprocessing step, creating an effective predictive feature selection model is being used. Feature selection methods have been reported to assist in this process to serve the improved current problem domain, in terms of classes **(supervised)** and clusters **(unsupervised)** methods [35]. This step helps distinguish benign tumors from malignant tumor [38]. The key benefits to performing the feature selection methods: (a) reduce the complexity (b) reduce overfitting (c) effective and reduce the training time (d) improve accuracy. Filter, wrapper, and embedded methods are the three main approaches in supervised feature selection methods [39]. Filter selection is a faster and better approach when the number of features is enormous [40]. Correlation, chi-square test, information gain are generally used as filter methods. The correlation-based feature (CFS) rank attribute calculates those features which are highly correlated with class labels. Gain ratio memory-based feature evaluation measures the information gain of a feature based on the mathematical formula for entropy. The second method wrapper exits around the predictive model algorithm. Forward selection, backward elimination, and stepwise selection are widely used as wrapper methods. The embedded method is a mixed feature of filter and wrapper method; this method addressed their own in-build feature selection with less computationally expensive and less likely to overfitting [34, 35].

(c) *Training a Machine Learning model:* A machine learning algorithm is a winning solution for early detection and diagnosis of breast cancer. Numerous methods have been developed for predicting cancer such as Naïve Bayes, decision trees (DT) [41], k-nearest neighbor (KNN), artificial neural network (ANN) [42], support vector machine (SVM) [43], convolutional neural network (CNN), random forest (RF), logistic regression (LR), and the radiant boosting classifier(GB) [35]. These models have been discussed in the following section.

(d) *Parameter Optimization:* The best feature searching in the subset is a complex and challenging processing task for assuring the model's parameter optimization. It basically depends on large population size, numbers of generations, crossover rate (CR), and so forth. In the previous studies, several metaheuristic biostatistical approaches have been used for the optimization of models parameters that help in the medical disease detection, diagnosis, prognosis, and therapeutic targets [35, 40, 44].

(e) *Testing, evaluation, and deployment:* The approach of selecting datasets for training and test samples plays a major key role in obtaining better performance and result validation. Several evolutionary algorithms are accessible in the previous literature to improve the accuracy of the classification techniques and solve several problems and conquer the desired results.

We have understood that computational intelligence (CI) is different from artificial intelligence in terms of the theory, design, application, and development of nature-motivated computational paradigms. Conventionally, there are five main pillars of

CI, namely—ANNs, FLS, evolutionary algorithms (EA), learning theory, and probabilistic methods and are represented in Fig. 5 [45] and described in the following section.

Fuzzy Logic Systems (FLS): It was first described by Zadeh in 1964 to resolve the issue of uncertainty that is omnipresent in engineering problems. A fuzzy logic system was first deployed for solving power system problems in 1979. Fuzzy set theory is simply a generalization of the classical set theory, wherein a component of the system falls into one category or doesn't fall at all. Therefore, the association degree of the component is crisp. However, in the case of fuzzy set theory, the association of a component is variable. In terms of mathematics, a fuzzy set is a membership function from the system as in values of the closed interval [0, 1]. The main advantage of fuzzy logic systems (FLS) is that they can endure incompleteness and ignore the data in a process model referring to the fact that it doesn't require exact knowledge as in the case of artificial intelligence systems [46]. It has been widely used for control, image processing, and clinical decision-making purposes [47].

Artificial Neural Networks (ANN): One of the natures-inspired computational algorithms is ANN that works similar to the human nervous systems and brain by processing information that encapsulates a processing system consisting of humongous interconnected processing units called—*neurons*. These neurons work in unity to solve complex problems and adapt to situations by learning from examples. Initially demonstrated by Hebb in 1949, wherein, he postulated that a network of neurons could showcase adaptive learning behavior just like human beings. The neurons are exposed to some initial training sets, and then, they accordingly adjust their weights to a specific learning rule during their training tenure. Unlike the majority of AI systems, ANNs are not programmed, but they adapt themselves according to examples and situations to solve the problem via interconnections with

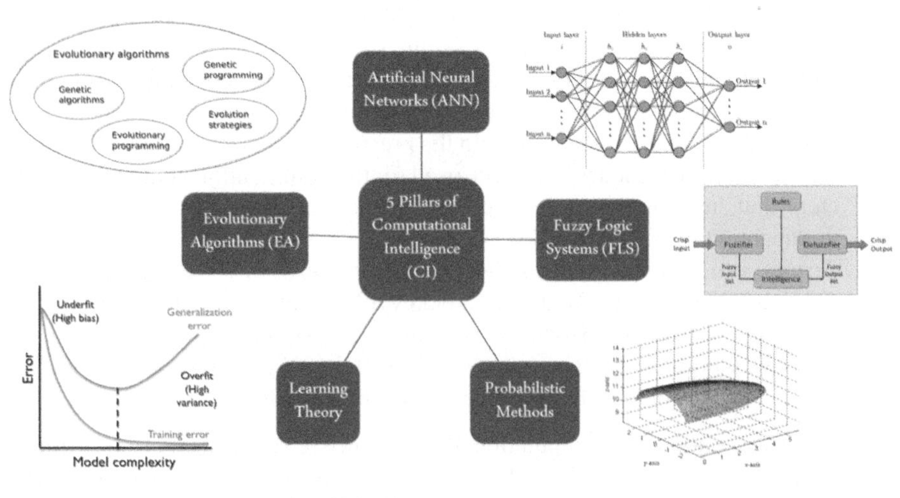

Fig. 5 Five pillars of computational intelligence

the surrounding. Only, a short computation takes place at every individual neuron, and there is no explicit memory in the neural network but is implicit in the connections between every neuron [46]. Moreover, ANNs share the advantage of data clustering with their counterpart FLS [48].

Evolutionary Algorithms (EAs): As the name suggests, evolutionary algorithms (EAs) are based on the biological concept of evolution that was lucidly described by Charles Darwin with his concept of "natural selection" and "survival of the fittest." This computational paradigm allows us to check the strength of natural evolution to develop artificial evolutionary methods and also to solve optimization-based problems [49]. This class of algorithms also falls into the category of *nature-inspired* algorithms just like ANNs. The main operators on which these algorithms work are as follows—*reproduction, mutation, recombination*, and *selection*. Probable solutions in the optimization problem constitute individuals in a population, wherein the fitness function provides the optimal number of solutions to that optimization problem. The evolution of the population gets repeated on the abovementioned operators until the best non-redundant solution is achieved with the least error and bias [50]. Some of the algorithms that are included in EAs are genetic algorithm (GA), genetic programming (GP), evolutionary programming (EP), gene expression programming (GEP), swarm optimization, metaheuristic algorithms, evolutionary strategy (ES), differential evolution (DE), neuroevolution (NE), etc. [51].

Learning Theory: The main objective of computational intelligent systems is to achieve human-like reasoning and rationality. That is why, learning theory is one main concept to bring together the human-like *cognitive, emotional,* and *adaptive* skills and expertise to enrich and enhance knowledge that can be further used for real-life problem-solving [52]. Learning theories aid computational researchers in predicting how these experiences are processed in algorithms and further help in making the right decisions in different real-life problems [53]. There are myriad approaches to computational learning theory on making different assumptions based on inferencing that can allow in generalizing limited data. They include—*exact learning, probability approximately correct learning* (PAC), *VC theory, Bayesian inference*, and *algorithmic learning theory* (ALT) [52].

Probabilistic Methods: First introduced by Paul Erdos and Joel Spencer in 1974, probabilistic methods compute the results of a computational intelligent system by using the randomness factor. These methods share the main core with fuzzy logic systems. Henceforth, probabilistic methods provide solutions to the problems using pre-existing knowledge [54].

4 Emerging Machine Learning Methods for Breast Cancer Diagnosis

There are several CIS methods that have allowed to help medical consultants, physicians, and researchers in decoding myriad aspects of various diseases including cancers. The CIS including Naïve Byes, decision tree, SVM, ANNs, SOM, FS, and hybrid models have helped in developing appropriate diagnosis and prognosis of breast cancer.

Naïve Bayes is supervised, an intuitive probabilistic generative model of machine learning algorithm used to solve classification problems based on Bayesian theorem [38, 55], considering the stimulating task within machine imaging processing in a large sample size. This implicitly assumes that the high sensitivity to the expression form of an independent predictor of each input variable is the main limitation of Naive Bayes [55, 56]. Among decision tree-based algorithms, Iterative Dichotomiser 3 (ID3) that was first introduced by Quinlan [57] is known to be the best in identifying the optimal solution to a problem that tends to over fit. There are many decision tree algorithms that are accessible to data classification, including ID3, C4.5, C5, CHAID, and J48 [58, 59] which are effectively applied in the biomedical area to diagnose and predict the numerous diseases. It can deal with many factors in prediction resolving, classification, pattern recognition, and completion [58]. Using the ID3 algorithm on the Wisconsin breast dataset by using 35 features, Pritom et al. [60], when ranked the features, obtained an accuracy of 76.30% with a false-positive rate (FPR) of 75.10% and a ROC score of 0.745. They obtained an accuracy of 73.70% with an FPR of 50.70% and a ROC score of 52.80 when they did not rank the features. Similarly, another group of researchers deployed the C4.5 decision tree algorithm for the Wisconsin breast cancer (WBC) database classification where they used only 11 features and retrieved an accuracy of 91.13% [61–63].

As far as the application of ANN in breast cancer is concerned, it has been used to quantify the risk of breast cancer by using a dataset that contains mammographic features, ultrasonography, IR imaging, and demographic data [42, 64]. Researchers recently proposed a soft computing-based cloud computational intelligent system named—BCP-T1F-SVM with two different models' type-1 fuzzy logic (T1F) and type-1 support vector machine (T1-SVM). The T1F-SVM model describes the stage and the type of cancer, while T1-SVM provides the higher precision of breast cancer detection. After analysis and computations, researchers suggest that T1-SVM is better than T1F. The T1F had an accuracy percentage of 96.56, while the T1-SVM had an accuracy of 97.06%, and thus, T1-SVM must be deployed as the initial breast cancer diagnosis system [65]. Usually, image screening becomes a problem in deploying CIS systems for breast cancer detection. Blurry mammograms or erroneous scans tend to decrease the specificity of CIS systems. For this problem, researchers have come up with *convolutional neural networks* (CNN). By deploying the *traditional convolutional neural network* (TCNN) and *supported convolutional neural network* (SCNN) approaches, the image detection problem can be overcome easily. Also, by using the flipped rotation-based approach (FRbA), it is possible to enrich the accuracy of breast cancer prediction as it considers different directions of the tumor mass to retrieve suitable features to form the exact image of the tumor [66]. The deep belief network (DBN) technique was first used for supervised image classification by Liu et al. [67]. Although this is still a novel field in breast cancer image classification, Zhang et al. have deployed both the RBM and Point-wise Gated RBM (pgRBM) for shear-wave electrography image classification of 227 images. Their hybrid model showed an accuracy of 93.40% with a sensitivity of 88.60% and specificity of 97.10%, respectively [68].

A hybrid computational intelligence model is proposed based on both supervised and unsupervised learning that combines ANNs and SOM for the accurate identification of breast cancer. The research group proposed this hybrid model, wherein they categorized it in two stages. In the first stage, the input features were subjected to the SOM algorithm to club patients with similar characteristics. In the second stage, for each club that was formed from SOM, the features of the patient were applied to a complex-valued neural network (CVNN) and were further classified for breast cancer rectification based on tumor severity. The retrieved results were then compared to the traditional diagnosis results with the help of receiver operating characteristic (ROC) analyses and a confusion matrix. The group discerned that in the testing phase, the disease detection ratio was 95%, while healthy patient detection came out to be 94%, respectively. With the results in hand, the researchers proposed that their hybrid CIS model (SOM + CVNN) was reliable for deploying it as an early detection system in the case of breast cancer in females [69].

5 Discussion and Future Perspectives

The development of biomarkers covers multiple processes, namely (i) connectivity preliminary discovery in basic studies design, (ii) validation, and (iii) clinical implementation [70]. The ultimate goal of the processes of establishing the biomarker is early diagnosis, disease recurrence, drug-target identification, and evaluating the patient's response to the treatment and recurrence of the disease [9]. Established biomarkers and numerous emerging biomarkers have been discovered which are clinically applicable to improve understanding of the multifaceted nature of the tumor microenvironment process in breast cancer [9]. Several predictive biomarkers based on a single protein or single gene are currently underway in the clinical trial phase II/III (depends on numerous factor) evaluation along with their therapeutic agents [71]. These biomarkers may be used and monitor the progression of breast cancer.

In previous studies, ML has been used to learn gene expression patterns in disease biology [72]. *Gene expression* profiling has the potential to predict the biological behavior of *breast cancer in terms of which genes are expressed.* The potential biomarkers support detection of the finest therapy for the patients based on their testing of gene expression [73]. It can be used to generate the profiling data and analyzed using different machine learning algorithms to better identify the several pathways and provide strong links to cancer progression. Large-scale gene expression profiling with distinguish expressed technology such as GEO, SRA, Oncomine databases, SEER, and TCGA is used for the early detection of breast cancer disease diagnostic and treatments [74, 75].

Numerous methods have been developed for the ensuing stages of processing and analysis of the breast cancer dataset. Informative and discriminative features can make the applicable selections to keep the notable features and reduce the dataset size. The preprocessing supports the region of interest (ROI) localization for abnormality search that improves the accuracy and reduces the access time complexity of an algorithm [36, 39]. All the selection features are based on the number of criteria to extract the top features. In the machine learning (ML) algorithm, optimization methods face tremendous challenges due to increased practical demand and significantly increase the complexity of models [44, 76].

Several studies have verified that ML algorithms have the potential to effectively aid in mammography interpretation and diagnosis of breast cancer. The historical data/input data are used to provide the new predictive output values in this algorithm. We have discussed the six ML methods that provide intense accurate information of the disease. The breast diagnosis methods illustrate that ML has aided to improve the diagnostic performance of the breast computer-aided diagnostic system, but still challenges remain, and expanded research is required [36, 37].

The learning algorithm may be weak due to the bad selection of the learning parameter value. There is a growing curiosity in developing effective models for breast cancer detection and diagnosis, due to the high computational power and practical use of ML algorithms. The future perspective on biomarker development is a major issue for effective clinical validation and implementation in the oncology field. ML technique for the diagnosis of breast cancer should focus on enlightening the performance. Feature selection and different algorithms may play key steps in developing a computational intelligence system. A wide variety of features selection methods for the classification of breast cancer have been developed over the last few years. Hence, more research is needed to produce a high accuracy rate.

6 Conclusion

This chapter addresses and summarizes the most useful methods for early detection and diagnosis of breast cancer from the outlook of biomarkers and gene expression profiles and their applications in machine learning. Promisingly, breast cancer biomarkers are definitely well known in standard care in breast cancer treatment and could also be applied to other meaningful diagnoses. The significant result of ML methods might reduce the diagnosis error in the diagnosis process and reduce cancer financial impacts. These techniques proceed to emerge every year, not only is mammography limited with the intention of improving the accuracy of interpretation but also endeavor to help the researcher to detect and comprehend the vital sign of the machine learning approach.

Acknowledgements AS is grateful to the Indian Council of Medical Research (Grant No. 45/17/2019-PHA/BMS), Govt. of India for financial assistance as ICMR-Research Associate fellowship. SQ is supported by the DST-Inspire Fellowship, provided by the Department of Science and Technology (DST), Govt. of India.

References

1. Harbeck, N., Penault-Llorca, F., Cortes, J., Gnant, M., Houssami, N., Poortmans, P., Ruddy, K., Tsang, J., & Cardoso, F. (2019). Breast cancer. *Nature Reviews Disease Primers*, *5*(1), 1–31. https://doi.org/10.1038/s41572-019-0111-2.
2. Raza, K., & Hasan, A. N. (2015). A Comprehensive evaluation of machine learning techniques for cancer class prediction based on microarray data. *International Journal of Bioinformatics Research and Applications, Inderscience, 11*(5), 397–416. https://doi.org/10.1504/IJBRA.2015.071940
3. Raza, K. (2016). Reconstruction, topological and gene ontology enrichment analysis of cancerous gene regulatory network modules. *Current Bioinformatics, 11*(2), 243–258. https://doi.org/10.2174/1574893611666160115212806
4. Duffy, M. J., Walsh, S., McDermott, E. W., & Crown, J. (2015). Biomarkers in breast cancer: Where are we and where are we going? *Advances in Clinical Chemistry*, *71*, 1–23. https://doi.org/10.1016/bs.acc.2015.05.001.
5. Califf, R. M. (2018). Biomarker definitions and their applications. *Experimental Biology and Medicine (Maywood, N.J.), 243*(3), 213–221. https://doi.org/10.1177/1535370217750088
6. Bertozzi, S., Londero, A. P., Seriau, L., Vora, R. D., Cedolini, C., & Mariuzzi, L. (2018). Biomarkers in breast cancer. In *Biomarker—Indicator of abnormal physiological process*. IntechOpen. https://doi.org/10.5772/intechopen.77320
7. Henry, N. L., & Hayes, D. F. (2012). Cancer biomarkers. *Molecular Oncology, 6*(2), 140–146. https://doi.org/10.1016/j.molonc.2012.01.010
8. Wang, L. (2017). Early diagnosis of breast cancer. *Sensors (Basel, Switzerland), 17*(7), 1572. https://doi.org/10.3390/s17071572
9. Weigel, M. T., & Dowsett, M. (2010). Current and emerging biomarkers in breast cancer: Prognosis and prediction. *Endocrine-Related Cancer, 17*(4), R245–R262. https://doi.org/10.1677/ERC-10-0136
10. Pedersen, A. C., Sørensen, P. D., Jacobsen, E. H., Madsen, J. S., & Brandslund, I. (2013). Sensitivity of CA 15–3, CEA and serum HER2 in the early detection of recurrence of breast cancer. *Clinical Chemistry and Laboratory Medicine, 51*(7), 1511–1519. https://doi.org/10.1515/cclm-2012-0488
11. Stieber, P., Nagel, D., Blankenburg, I., Heinemann, V., Untch, M., Bauerfeind, I., & Di Gioia, D. (2015). Diagnostic efficacy of CA 15-3 and CEA in the early detection of metastatic breast cancer-A retrospective analysis of kinetics on 743 breast cancer patients. *ClinicaChimica Acta; International Journal of Clinical Chemistry, 448*, 228–231. https://doi.org/10.1016/j.cca.2015.06.022
12. Li, C.-J., Chen, H.-M., & Lai, J.-C. (2020). Diagnostic, prognostic, and predictive biomarkers in breast cancer. *Journal of Oncology, 2020*, e1835691. https://doi.org/10.1155/2020/1835691
13. Güler, E. N. (2017). Gene expression profiling in breast cancer and its effect on therapy selection in early-stage breast cancer. *European Journal of Breast Health, 13*(4), 168–174. https://doi.org/10.5152/ejbh.2017.3636
14. Milosevic, M., Jankovic, D., Milenkovic, A., & Stojanov, D. (2018). Early diagnosis and detection of breast cancer. *Technology and Health Care: Official Journal of the European Society for Engineering and Medicine, 26*(4), 729–759. https://doi.org/10.3233/THC-181277

15. Jänicke, F., Schmitt, M., Pache, L., Ulm, K., Harbeck, N., Höfler, H., & Graeff, H. (1993). Urokinase (uPA) and its inhibitor PAI-1 are strong and independent prognostic factors in node-negative breast cancer. *Breast Cancer Research and Treatment, 24*(3), 195–208. https://doi.org/10.1007/BF01833260
16. Naour, F. L., Misek, D. E., Krause, M. C., Deneux, L., Giordano, T. J., Scholl, S., & Hanash, S. M. (2001). Proteomics-based Identification of RS/DJ-1 as a novel circulating tumor antigen in breast cancer. *Clinical Cancer Research, 7*(11), 3328–3335.
17. Zhao, H., Shen, J., Medico, L., Wang, D., Ambrosone, C. B., & Liu, S. (2010). A Pilot Study Of Circulating miRNAs as potential biomarkers of early stage breast cancer. *PLoS ONE, 5*(10), e13735. https://doi.org/10.1371/journal.pone.0013735
18. Hao, W., & Friedman, A. (2016). Serum uPAR as biomarker in breast cancer recurrence: A mathematical model. *PLoS ONE, 11*(4), e0153508. https://doi.org/10.1371/journal.pone.0153508
19. Singh, R., Bhatt, M. L. B., Singh, S. P., Kumar, V., Goel, M. M., Mishra, D. P., & Kumar, R. (2016). Evaluation of KiSS1 as a prognostic biomarker in North Indian breast cancer cases. *Asian Pacific Journal of Cancer Prevention, 17*(4), 1789–1795. https://doi.org/10.7314/APJCP.2016.17.4.1789
20. Jing, X., Cui, X., Liang, H., Hao, C., Yang, Z., Li, X., Yang, X., & Han, C. (2018). CD24 is a potential biomarker for prognosis in human breast carcinoma. *Cellular Physiology and Biochemistry, 48*(1), 111–119. https://doi.org/10.1159/000491667
21. Strimbu, K., & Tavel, J. A. (2010). What are biomarkers? *Current Opinion in HIV and AIDS, 5*(6), 463–466. https://doi.org/10.1097/COH.0b013e32833ed177
22. Pezo, R. C., & Bedard, P. L. (2015). 11 definition: Translational and personalised medicine, biomarkers, pharmacodynamics. In *ESMO handbook of translational research.*
23. Ballman, K. V. (2015). Biomarker: Predictive or Prognostic? *Journal of Clinical Oncology: Official Journal of the American Society of Clinical Oncology, 33*(33), 3968–3971. https://doi.org/10.1200/JCO.2015.63.3651.
24. McCarthy, A. (2020). The biomarker future is digital. *Clinical OMICs, 7*(1), 24–28. https://doi.org/10.1089/clinomi.07.01.19.
25. Brasier, N., Osthoff, M., De Ieso, F., & Eckstein, J. (2021). Next-generation digital biomarkers for tuberculosis and antibiotic stewardship: Perspective on novel molecular digital biomarkers in sweat, saliva, and exhaled breath. *Journal of Medical Internet Research, 23*(8), e25907. https://doi.org/10.2196/25907.
26. Bent, B., Cho, P. J., Henriquez, M., Wittmann, A., Thacker, C., Feinglos, M., Crowley, M. J., & Dunn, J. P. (2021). Engineering digital biomarkers of interstitial glucose from noninvasive smartwatches. *NPJ Digital Medicine, 4*(1), 1–11. https://doi.org/10.1038/s41746-021-00465-w.
27. Brasier, N., & Eckstein, J. (2019). Sweat as a source of next-generation digital biomarkers. *Digital Biomarkers, 3*(3), 155–165. https://doi.org/10.1159/000504387.
28. Kourtis, L. C., Regele, O. B., Wright, J. M., & Jones, G. B. (2019). Digital biomarkers for Alzheimer's disease: The mobile/wearable devices opportunity. *NPJ Digital Medicine, 2*, 9. https://doi.org/10.1038/s41746-019-0084-2.
29. Gresham, G., Schrack, J., Gresham, L. M., Shinde, A. M., Hendifar, A. E., Tuli, R., Rimel, B. J., Figlin, R., Meinert, C. L., & Piantadosi, S. (2018). Wearable activity monitors in oncology trials: Current use of an emerging technology. *Contemporary Clinical Trials, 64*, 13–21. https://doi.org/10.1016/j.cct.2017.11.002.
30. Rodríguez-Ruiz, A., Krupinski, E., Mordang, J. -J., Schilling, K., Heywang-Köbrunner, S. H., Sechopoulos, I., & Mann, R. M. (2019). Detection of breast cancer with mammography: Effect of an artificial intelligence support system. *Radiology, 290*(2), 305–314. https://doi.org/10.1148/radiol.2018181371.
31. Kapil, A., Meier, A., Zuraw, A., Steele, K. E., Rebelatto, M. C., Schmidt, G., & Brieu, N. (2018). Deep semi supervised generative learning for automated tumor proportion scoring on NSCLC tissue needle biopsies. *Scientific Reports, 8*(1), 17343. https://doi.org/10.1038/s41598-018-35501-5.

32. Esteva, A., Kuprel, B., Novoa, R. A., Ko, J., Swetter, S. M., Blau, H. M., & Thrun, S. (2017). Dermatologist-level classification of skin cancer with deep neural networks. *Nature, 542*(7639), 115–118. https://doi.org/10.1038/nature21056.
33. Rodler, S., Schulz, G., Buchner, A., Stief, C., Staehler, M., & Casuscelli, J. (2019). The role of digital biomarkers in cancer research and patient care. *Biomedical Journal of Scientific & Technical Research, 17*(3), 12870–12872. https://doi.org/10.26717/BJSTR.2019.17.003009.
34. Kourou, K., Exarchos, T. P., Exarchos, K. P., Karamouzis, M. V., & Fotiadis, D. I. (2015). Machine learning applications in cancer prognosis and prediction. *Computational and Structural Biotechnology Journal, 13*, 8–17. https://doi.org/10.1016/j.csbj.2014.11.005
35. Dhahri, H., Al Maghayreh, E., Mahmood, A., Elkilani, W., & Faisal Nagi, M. (2019). Automated breast cancer diagnosis based on machine learning algorithms. *Journal of Healthcare Engineering, 2019*, e4253641. https://doi.org/10.1155/2019/4253641
36. Gardezi, S. J. S., Elazab, A., Lei, B., & Wang, T. (2019). Breast cancer detection and diagnosis using mammographic data: Systematic review. *Journal of Medical Internet Research, 21*(7), e14464. https://doi.org/10.2196/14464
37. Gupta, P., & Garg, S. (2020). Breast cancer prediction using varying parameters of machine learning models. *Procedia Computer Science, 171*, 593–601. https://doi.org/10.1016/j.procs.2020.04.064
38. Dhahri, H., Rahmany, I., Mahmood, A., Al Maghayreh, E., & Elkilani, W. (2020). Tabu search and machine-learning classification of benign and malignant proliferative breast lesions. *BioMed Research International, 2020*, e4671349. https://doi.org/10.1155/2020/4671349
39. Sajjadnia, Z., Khayami, R., & Moosavi, M. R. (2020). Preprocessing breast cancer data to improve the data quality, diagnosis procedure, and medical care services. *Cancer Informatics, 19*, 1176935120917955. https://doi.org/10.1177/1176935120917955
40. Hambali, M. A., Oladele, T. O., & Adewole, K. S. (2020). Microarray cancer feature selection: Review, challenges and research directions. *International Journal of Cognitive Computing in Engineering, 1*, 78–97. https://doi.org/10.1016/j.ijcce.2020.11.001
41. Ayer, T., Chen, Q., & Burnside, E. S. (2013). Artificial neural networks in mammography interpretation and diagnostic decision making. *Computational and Mathematical Methods in Medicine, 2013*, e832509. https://doi.org/10.1155/2013/832509
42. Mehdy, M. M., Ng, P. Y., Shair, E. F., Saleh, N. I. M., & Gomes, C. (2017). Artificial neural networks in image processing for early detection of breast cancer. *Computational and Mathematical Methods in Medicine, 2017*, e2610628. https://doi.org/10.1155/2017/2610628
43. Zafiropoulos, E., Maglogiannis, I., & Anagnostopoulos, I. (2006). A support vector machine approach to breast cancer diagnosis and prognosis. In I. Maglogiannis, K. Karpouzis, & M. Bramer (Eds.), *Artificial intelligence applications and innovations* (pp. 500–507). Springer US. https://doi.org/10.1007/0-387-34224-9_58
44. Daelemans, W., Hoste, V., De Meulder, F., & Naudts, B. (2003). Combined optimization of feature selection and algorithm parameters in machine learning of language. In N. Lavrač, D. Gamberger, H. Blockeel, & L. Todorovski (Eds.), *Machine learning: ECML 2003* (pp. 84–95). Springer. https://doi.org/10.1007/978-3-540-39857-8_10
45. Sharma, R., Agarwal, M., Gupta, M., Somendra, S., & Saxena, S. K. (2020). Clinical characteristics and differential clinical diagnosis of novel coronavirus disease 2019 (COVID-19). *Coronavirus Disease 2019 (COVID-19)*, 55–70. https://doi.org/10.1007/978-981-15-4814-7_6
46. Saxena, D., Singh, S. N., & Verma, K. S. (2010). Application of computational intelligence in emerging power systems. *International Journal of Engineering, Science and Technology, 2*(3), 1–7. https://doi.org/10.4314/ijest.v2i3.59166
47. Muhammad, L. J., & Algehyne, E. A. (2021). Fuzzy based expert system for diagnosis of coronary artery disease in Nigeria. *Health and Technology, 11*(2), 319–329. https://doi.org/10.1007/s12553-021-00531-z
48. Somers, M. J., & Casal, J. C. (2009). Using artificial neural networks to model nonlinearity: The case of the job satisfaction—Job performance relationship. *Organizational Research Methods, 12*(3), 403–417. https://doi.org/10.1177/1094428107309326

49. Vikhar, P. A. (2016). Evolutionary algorithms: A critical review and its future prospects. In *2016 International Conference on Global Trends in Signal Processing, Information Computing and Communication (ICGTSPICC)* (pp. 261–265). https://doi.org/10.1109/ICGTSPICC.2016.7955308
50. Maier, H. R., Razavi, S., Kapelan, Z., Matott, L. S., Kasprzyk, J., & Tolson, B. A. (2019). Introductory overview: Optimization using evolutionary algorithms and other metaheuristics. *Environmental Modelling & Software, 114*, 195–213. https://doi.org/10.1016/j.envsoft.2018.11.018
51. Cohoon, J., Kairo, J., & Lienig, J. (2003). Evolutionary algorithms for the physical design of VLSI circuits. In A. Ghosh & S. Tsutsui (Eds.), *Advances in evolutionary computing: Theory and applications* (pp. 683–711). Springer. https://doi.org/10.1007/978-3-642-18965-4_27
52. Siddique, & Adeli. (2013). Introduction to computational intelligence. In *Computational intelligence* (pp. 1–17). John Wiley & Sons, Ltd. https://doi.org/10.1002/9781118534823.ch1.
53. Angluin, D. (1992). Computational learning theory: Survey and selected bibliography. In *Proceedings of the Twenty-Fourth Annual ACM Symposium on Theory of Computing* (pp. 351–369). https://doi.org/10.1145/129712.129746.
54. Palit, A. K., & Popovic, D. (Eds.). (2005). Computational intelligence: An introduction. In *Computational intelligence in time series forecasting: Theory and engineering applications* (pp. 1–15). Springer. https://doi.org/10.1007/1-84628-184-9_1.
55. Karabatak, M. (2015). A new classifier for breast cancer detection based on Naïve Bayesian. *Measurement, 72*, 32–36. https://doi.org/10.1016/j.measurement.2015.04.028.
56. Xiong, Y., Ye, M., & Wu, C. (2021). Cancer classification with a cost-sensitive Naive Bayes stacking ensemble. *Computational and Mathematical Methods in Medicine, 2021*, e5556992. https://doi.org/10.1155/2021/5556992.

57. Quinlan, J. R. (1986). Induction of decision trees. *Machine Learning, 1*(1), 81–106. https://doi.org/10.1007/BF00116251.
58. Shankar, J. S. R., Nithish, S., Babu, M. N., Karthik, R., & Afridi, A. S. (2021). Breast cancer prediction using decision tree. *Journal of Physics: Conference Series, 1916*(1), 012069. https://doi.org/10.1088/1742-6596/1916/1/012069.
59. Verma, A. K., Chakraborty, M., & Biswas, S. K. (2021). Breast cancer management system using decision tree and neural network. *SN Computer Science, 2*(3), 234. https://doi.org/10.1007/s42979-021-00644-2.
60. Pritom, A. I., Munshi, Md. A. R., Sabab, S. A., & Shihab, S. (2016). Predicting breast cancer recurrence using effective classification and feature selection technique. In *2016 19th International Conference on Computer and Information Technology (ICCIT)* (pp. 310–314). https://doi.org/10.1109/ICCITECHN.2016.7860215.
61. Asri, H., Mousannif, H., Moatassime, H. A., & Noel, T. (2016). Using machine learning algorithms for breast cancer risk prediction and diagnosis. *Procedia Computer Science, 83*, 1064–1069. https://doi.org/10.1016/j.procs.2016.04.224.
62. Muhammad, L. J., Abba Haruna, A., Mohammed, I. A., Abubakar, M., Badamasi, B. G., & Musa Amshi, J. (2019). Performance evaluation of classification data mining algorithms on coronary artery disease dataset. In *2019 9th International Conference on Computer and Knowledge Engineering (ICCKE)* (pp. 1–5). https://doi.org/10.1109/ICCKE48569.2019.8964703.
63. Muhammad, L. J., BesiruJibrin, M., Yahaya, B. Z., Mohammed BesiruJibrin, I. A., Ahmad, A., & Amshi, J. M. (2020). An improved C4.5 algorithm using principle of equivalent of infinitesimal and arithmetic mean best selection attribute for large dataset. In *2020 10th International Conference on Computer and Knowledge Engineering (ICCKE)* (pp. 006–010). https://doi.org/10.1109/ICCKE50421.2020.9303622.
64. Sepandi, M., Taghdir, M., Rezaianzadeh, A., & Rahimikazerooni, S. (2018). Assessing breast cancer risk with an artificial neural network. *Asian Pacific Journal of Cancer Prevention: APJCP, 19*(4), 1017–1019. https://doi.org/10.22034/APJCP.2018.19.4.1017.
65. Khan, F., Khan, M. A., Abbas, S., Athar, A., Siddiqui, S. Y., Khan, A. H., Saeed, M. A., & Hussain, M. (2020). Cloud-based breast cancer prediction empowered with soft computing approaches. *Journal of Healthcare Engineering, 2020*, e8017496. https://doi.org/10.1155/2020/8017496.
66. Alfifi, M., Alrahhal, M. S., Bataineh, S., & Mezher, M. (2020). Enhanced artificial intelligence system for diagnosing and predicting breast cancer using deep learning. *International Journal of Advanced Computer Science and Applications (IJACSA), 11*(7), Article 7. https://doi.org/10.14569/IJACSA.2020.0110763.
67. Liu, Y., Zhou, S., & Chen, Q. (2011). Discriminative deep belief networks for visual data classification. *Pattern Recognition, 44*(10–11), 2287–2296. https://doi.org/10.1016/j.patcog.2010.12.012.
68. Zhang, J., Silber, J. I., & Mazurowski, M. A. (2015). Modeling false positive error making patterns in radiology trainees for improved mammography education. *Journal of Biomedical Informatics, 54*, 50–57. https://doi.org/10.1016/j.jbi.2015.01.007.
69. Zadeh Shirazi, A., Seyyed Mahdavi Chabok, S. J., & Mohammadi, Z. (2018). A novel and reliable computational intelligence system for breast cancer detection. *Medical & Biological Engineering & Computing, 56*(5), 721–732. https://doi.org/10.1007/s11517-017-1721-z.
70. Parkinson, D. R., McCormack, R. T., Keating, S. M., Gutman, S. I., Hamilton, S. R., Mansfield, E. A., Piper, M. A., Deverka, P., Frueh, F. W., Jessup, J. M., McShane, L. M., Tunis, S. R., Sigman, C. C., & Kelloff, G. J. (2014). Evidence of clinical utility: An unmet need in molecular diagnostics for patients with cancer. *Clinical Cancer Research: An Official Journal of the American Association for Cancer Research, 20*(6), 1428–1444. https://doi.org/10.1158/1078-0432.CCR-13-2961.
71. Goossens, N., Nakagawa, S., Sun, X., & Hoshida, Y. (2015). Cancer biomarker discovery and validation. *Translational Cancer Research, 4*(3), 256–269. https://doi.org/10.3978/j.issn.2218-676X.2015.06.04.

72. van IJzendoorn, D. G. P., Szuhai, K., Bruijn, I. H. B., Kostine, M., Kuijjer, M. L., & Bovée, J. V. M. G. (2019). Machine learning analysis of gene expression data reveals novel diagnostic and prognostic biomarkers and identifies therapeutic targets for soft tissue sarcomas. *PLOS Computational Biology*, *15*(2), e1006826.https://doi.org/10.1371/journal.pcbi.1006826.
73. Tabl, A. A., Alkhateeb, A., ElMaraghy, W., Rueda, L., & Ngom, A. (2019). A machine learning approach for identifying gene biomarkers guiding the treatment of breast cancer. *Frontiers in Genetics, 10*, 256. https://doi.org/10.3389/fgene.2019.00256.
74. Kim, S. Y., Kawaguchi, T., Yan, L., Young, J., Qi, Q., & Takabe, K. (2017). Clinical relevance of microRNA expressions in breast cancer validated using the cancer genome Atlas (TCGA). *Annals of Surgical Oncology, 24*(10), 2943–2949. https://doi.org/10.1245/s10434-017-5984-2.
75. Marchetti, M. A., Coit, D. G., Dusza, S. W., Yu, A., McLean, L., Hu, Y., Nanda, J. K., Matsoukas, K., Mancebo, S. E., & Bartlett, E. K. (2020). Performance of gene expression profile tests for prognosis in patients with localized cutaneous melanoma. *JAMA Dermatology, 156*(9), 1–10. https://doi.org/10.1001/jamadermatol.2020.1731.
76. Rama Krishna, S., & Sirajuddin, M. (2022). A role of emerging technologies in the design of novel framework for COVID-19 data analysis and decision support system. In J. Nayak, B. Naik, & A. Abraham (Eds.), *Understanding COVID-19: The role of computational intelligence* (pp. 313–337). Springer International Publishing. https://doi.org/10.1007/978-3-030-74761-9_14.

Exosomes: Supramolecular Biomarker Conduit in Cancer

Manmeet Kaur and H. S. Sodhi

Abstract Cancer is a complex disease attributed to genetic distortions and cellular and non-cellular host responses. Tumors contain a variety of cell types that interact in a dynamic manner to maintain cancer-specific signaling networks. Extrinsic vesicles (EVs) are formed and retrieved as part of cell communication. Even tumor cells release exosomes, which are "30–100 nm" membrane vesicles that come from endosomes. Parental cells proteins and nucleic acids enrich their repertoire, and intercellular signals are thought to be transmitted by them. DNA and RNA are released into all body fluids as well as protein biomarkers that can be used to identify tumors and therapeutic targets. Patients with cancer may be screened for tumors based on the presence of exosomes secreted by tumor cells. Biomarkers for clinical diagnoses, such as exosomal proteins and microRNAs, are attracting considerable interest. The unique biogenesis of exosomes, their pervasive production by all cell types, and their biological features in liquid biopsy samples have all contributed to a growing interest in exosomes as cancer biomarkers. Cancer 'prognosis', 'diagnosis' and 'progression' may be more comprehensively assessed using these biomarkers, which reflect the heterogeneous biological changes associated with tumor growth. This chapter provides a brief overview of exosomal initiation, function, isolation, and the current roles of computation in oncology in the context of multi-omic technologies.

Keywords Cancer · Exosomes · Extracellular vesicles · Biomarkers · miRNAs · Body fluids · Computational oncology · Machine learning · Artificial intelligence

1 Introduction

There were approximately eighteen million new cases and nearly 10 million deaths per year in 2017, making cancer the second leading cause of death in the world [1]. Well over a quarter of the global total will be assessed with metastatic carcinoma at a certain point in their lives. For a high success rate, swift cancer treatment is

M. Kaur (✉) · H. S. Sodhi
Department of Microbiology, Punjab Agricultural University, Ludhiana 141004, India
e-mail: manmeet1-mb@pau.edu

K. Raza (ed.), *Computational Intelligence in Oncology*, Studies in Computational Intelligence 1016, https://doi.org/10.1007/978-981-16-9221-5_18

crucial [2]. 'Radiation-based computer tomography', 'ultrasound', 'endoscopy', and 'tissue biopsy' can detect cancer up to 20 years after its onset. These liquid biopsies are gaining popularity due to 'smaller sample volume', 'ease-of-use', 'minimal invasiveness', and 'cost saving' as well as greater accuracy and high throughput for personalized cancer treatment [3]. The vast bulk of cancer cases can be viewed more adequately in the formative development. Angiogenesis and metastasis require tumor cells to converse and transmogrify among each other and non-tumor host cells [4]. A central role is presumed to be completed by tumor cell exosomes in this process by transferring biomolecules such as 'proteins', 'fatty acids', 'RNA', and 'DNA' [5]. However, cells are far less stable and more susceptible to degradation enzymes, such as 'RNAses', than tissues. Small non-coding RNA (sncr) is a family of molecules that includes microRNAs (miRNAs). Because they alter the expression of oncogenes and tumor suppressor genes, these cancer-specific miRNAs play a crucial role in cancer development. To promote tumor formation or growth, onco-miRNAs are abnormally expressed in cancer cells and target the degradation of key tumor suppressor messenger RNAs (mRNAs). By inhibiting the expression of oncogenes, cancer cell growth is generally slowed down when tumor-suppressive miRNAs are expressed at a high level [6].

2 Exosomes

Most eukaryotic cells secrete exosomes, which range in size from 40 to 160 mm in diameter. In the late 1980s, exosomes were identified as cellular waste products [7]. Although exosomes represent an innovative mode of intercellular communication, individuals are now realizing that they play a role in a wide range of biological processes, including cancer. Lipids, metabolites, proteins, and nucleic acids are some of the bioactive cargos that exosomes hold, and these cargos can be delivered to target cells [8]. Exosomes (TEXs) derived from tumors are thought to play a pivotal role in cancer. Because of their pleiotropic biological activity, "exosomes" have attracted attention. As defined by the International Organization for Standardization (ISO), exosomes are vesicles formed by "inward/reverse budding" of the multivesicular bodies (MVB) limiting membrane in the late endocytic compartment [9]. There are three different classes of membrane-derived extracellular vehicles, based on their 'size', 'content', 'dimensions', 'cellular origin', 'mode of release', and 'function'.

"Exosomes (30–100 nm)", "microvesicles (100–1000 nm)", and "apoptotic bodies (500–3000 nm)" are three of the most common. Pan and Johnstone were the first to discover exosomes in 1983. [10]. When viewed under electron microscopy, exosomes have a "cup-shaped" or "saucer-like" morphology. Cancer cells secrete more exosomes after receiving radiation treatment, a process that may involve activation of the "tumor suppressor-activated pathway 6 (TsAP6)" and subsequent up-regulation of the transmembrane protein [11]. Based on cellular origin, exososmes are classified as (Fig. 1).

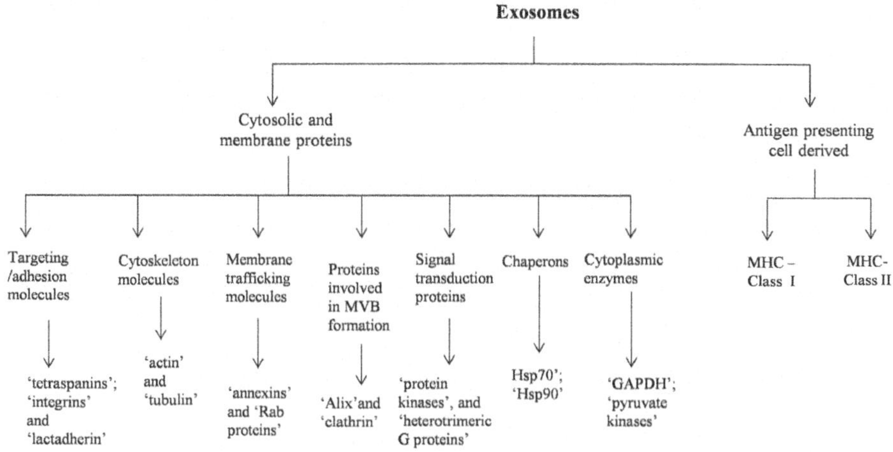

Fig. 1 Membrane-derived vesicles based on the cellular origin

These exosomes are now known to be important mediators of cell communication. How these particles interact with and influence the feature of target cells is not yet clear. Massive amounts of interactions are developed based on observational evidence and in vitro assays, including:

(1) Attachment of vesicles to the surface of a recipient cell via exosomal adhesion molecules.
(2) After adhesion direct fusion of vesicles with the recipient plasma membrane.
(3) Internalization of vesicles through phagocytosis.

Their absorption, but not their fusion with target cells such as 'dendritic cells,' may be aided by "phatidyl-ethanolamine" membrane repartitioning. Through the interaction between exosomes and 'target cells', 'bioactive lipids', 'growth factors', 'membrane receptor transfer', and 'protein delivery' can be delivered directly to the target cell surface. Also, exosomes could facilitate the transfer of genetic material between cells [8].

3 Formation and Composition of Exosomes

Many "intraluminal endosomal vesicles" are carried by MVBs, which are late endosomes. Some integrate with the 'cell membrane' and release the intracellular vesicles into the interstitial spaces, while others are degraded in lysosomes. Exosomes, which have a diameter of 30–120 nm, and microvesicles, which have a diameter of 120–1000 nm, are the smaller vehicles released [12]. The endosomal sorting complex required for transport (ESCRT) is mandated for exosome formation because it recognizes ubiquitylated proteins. Exosomes with certain biochemical compositions are produced by mechanisms other than ESCRT. The 'tetraspanins', 'CD63',

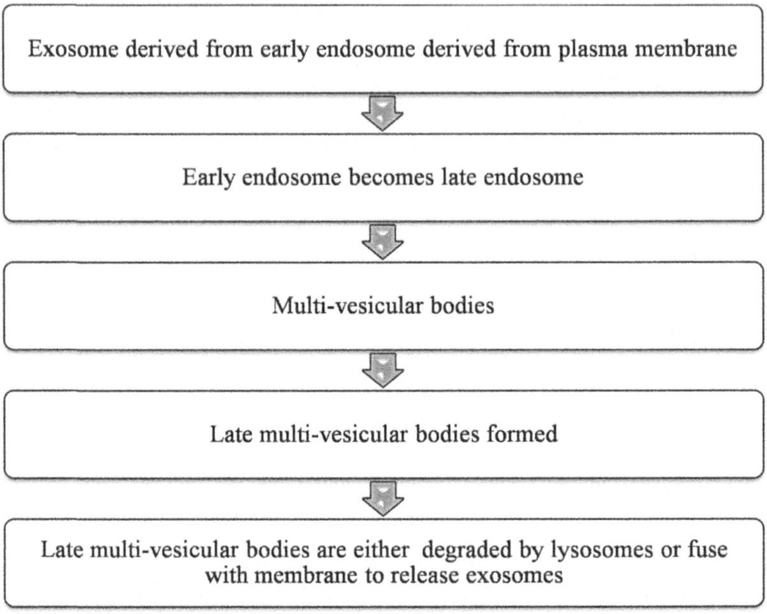

Fig. 2 Formation and release of exosomes

and 'CD81' are the most commonly used exosomal markers. Lipids make up the majority of the exosomes' composition [13]. Early endosomes are formed from the plasma membrane, followed by inward budding of the endosomal vesicle membrane, resulting in MVBs that are composed of ILVs, and finally, the fusion of these MVBs with either the lysosome or plasma membrane, which releases the vesicular contents known as exosomes (late endosomes) (Fig. 2). The limiting membrane of the late endosome undergoes invagination and budding to form ILVs, which results in the sorting of transmembrane proteins.

4 Signalings in the Regulation of Early Endosome

Both 'clathrin-dependent and independent' endocytic vesicles deliver cargo to early endosomes. Early endosomes are frequently found along the microtubules near the cytoplasm's periphery, close to the plasma membrane. Early endosomes have a vacuolar and tubular domain made up of vacuoles morphologically. 'Rab5' is thought to have a role in the transition of early endosomes to late endosomes. Rab5 and its effector proteins coupled to internalized ubiquitinated proteins. As a result, Rab5 can form a complex on the early endosome's cytosolic side. The Rab5 complex then acts as a catalyst for the early endosome to move through the microtubules [14].

'Phosphatidylinositol-3 phosphate' is produced by PI3K, which facilitates the recruitment of numerous effector proteins, resulting in the selectivity of the endosome through cargo binding. The fact that Hrs is associated with PI (3) P suggests that protein sorting may occur at the earliest endosomal stage. As a consequence, 'clathrin' and members of 'ESCRT' are found on the cytosolic side of early endosomes, where they begin to sort mono-ubiquitinated membrane proteins into ILVs. As the early endosome matures, subdomains harboring different 'Rab proteins' (such as "Rab4" and "Rab11") are found along the membrane. 'Rab4' and 'Rab11' sort the receptors that need to be recycled into tubular domains and transport them to the plasma membrane. 'Rab5' to 'Rab7' conversion governs the transition of early endosomes to late endosomes. The most widely accepted explanation for this switch currently involves the recruitment of 'Rab7' to convert "Rab5-GTP to Rab5-GDP". It's also been suggested that the quantity of 'Rab5' decreases with time as 'Rab7' levels rise, resulting in Rab7's conquest [15].

5 Signaling in the Regulation of Exosome Cargo Loading to Late Exosomes

Late endosomes, unlike early endosomes, have a spherical shape, indicating that they have matured from the vacuole domain of early endosomes. The late endosome's limiting membrane comprises 'cholesterol' and 'sphingolipid rafts', 'clathrin', and 'ESCRT' components. The ESCRT machinery recognizes and sorts transmembrane proteins after they have been mono-ubiquitinated. As shown in Table 1, the ESCRT machinery consists of four complexes that lead to the formation of MVBs [16].

Ceramide enhanced the inward budding of the limiting membrane of late endosomes in oligodendroglial cells without the help of the ESCRT machinery. 'Hrs' and 'STAM' help ESCRT-0 detect mono-ubiquitinated cargo. The cargo transfer from ESCRT-0 to ESCRT-I is started by the contact between 'Hrs' and 'Tsg101'. Through the interaction of 'Vps28' and 'Vps36', cargo is transported from ESCRT-I to ESCRT-II. 'Vps20' is recruited by ESCRT-II component 'Vps25', which in turn recruits ESCRTIII components 'CHMP4', 'Vps24', 'Vps2' and 'Vps4' in that sequence. The development of ESCRT-III results in the removal of ubiquitin from the limiting membrane of MVB, as well as invagination and scission of sorted cargo into ILVs in the lumen. Ceramide can also start freight sorting without the help of ESCRT technology. Ceramide is generated when sphingomyelin is converted to neutral sphingomyelinase, which induces invaginations in MVBs' limiting membrane and ultimately budding into ILVs [17].

Table 1 ESCRT machinery complex [16]

S. No.	ESCRT machinery complex	Components	Activity
1	ESCRT Complex 0	• Hepatocyte growth factor-regulated kinase • The signal transducing adapter molecule • Clathrin • Eps15	Recognizes mono-ubiquitinated proteins on limiting membrane of late endosomes through the ubiquitin-binding domains
2	ESCRT Complex I	• Tgs 101 • Vps 28 • Vps37 • Mvb12	Initiates binding of ESCRT-I to ESCRT-II
3	ESCRT Complex II	• Vps36 • Vps22 • Vps25	Ubiquitin-binding domains that transfer and sort mono-ubiquitinated proteins on limiting membrane
4	ESCRT Complex III	• Vps20 • Vps24 • Vps2	Removes ubiquitin tags, and inward bud sorted proteins

6 Signaling in the Regulation of Exosome Release

The intracellular trafficking of MVBs to the cell periphery and the fusion of MVBs with the cell membrane are both required for exosome release. Several Rab GTPases, including 'Rab11', 'Rab27a/b'; and 'Rab35', have been demonstrated to regulate MVB trafficking to the plasma membrane. Savina et al. discovered that 'GFPRab11' was localized to MVBs and activated MVB fusion and docking using time-lapse confocal imaging. In comparison to cells expressing the mutant 'Q70L GFP-Rab11', they discovered that 'K562' cells infected with 'GFP-Rab11' WT produced larger MVBs and released more exosomes [18]. 'Rab27a' and 'Rab27b' role in regulating exosome release was recently discovered in the "HeLa B6H4" tumor cell line, where silencing of 'Rab27a' and 'Rab27b' reduced exosome docking at the plasma membrane. Rab27a silencing, on the other hand, increased the size of MVBs, whilst Rab27b silencing caused MVBs to be localized to the cell's perinuclear area [19].

7 Exosomes: Specific Purpose

Exosomes can meld with recipient cells and release their contents. Exosomes play an essential part in cell-to-cell communication by 'transferring proteins', 'RNAs', and 'lipids' from one cell to another [20]. According to the cell or tissue they originate from, exosomes have a wide variety of functions. Some immune cells, such as 'Dendritic cells' and 'B cells' produce exosomes that may arbitrate adaptive immune responses to pathogens and tumors Oncogenes and onco-miRNAs are transferred between cancer cells and the tumor stroma via tumor cell-derived exosomes [21]. The use of exosomes by viruses and other pathogens to transfer pathogenic molecules between host cells has been demonstrated in recent studies, implicating them in the viral spread and immune evasion [22]. Biomarkers such as exosomes and en outre have a great deal of potential for molecular diagnostics.

8 Biological Functions of Exosomes in Cancer

A fundamental biological function of the exosome is to facilitate intercellular communication, induce physiological changes in recipient cells, and have been implicated in a wide range of disease states such as 'cancer', 'cardiovascular disease', and 'autoimmune syndromes'[23]. Consequently, tumor cell-released exosomes play a crucial role in:

- Preferment of foremost tumor evolvement
- Incitement of angiogenesis
- Reactivation of stromal fibroblasts
- Chiseling the cancer extracellular matrix adherence
- Creation of a premetastatic habitat
- Refrainment of the host immune response
- Counteracting cell death
- Evolving drug resistance.

Selecting, binding, and uptaking of exosomes to the surface of recipient cells is mediated by different proteins such as *Tetraspanins, Immunoglobulins, Proteoglycans,* and *Intercellular adhesion molecules* (e.g., integrins).

The transmission of exosome cargo molecules into the recipient cell at new sites can result from these connections, potentially changing their biology (Table 2) [24].

At a distance from the donor cell, exosomes can transport oncogenic proteins and nucleic acids. In order for cancer cells to colonize a site in the future, new

Table 2 Extracellular vesicles: their biological properties [24]

S. No.	Extracellular vesicles	Exosomes	Apoptotic bodies	Microvesicles
1	Size	30–100 nm	500–3000 nm	100–1000 nm
2	Sedimentation	100,000 × g	1200–100,00 × g	1200–100,000 × g
3	Shape	Cup-shaped	Heterogenous	Irregular
4	Mode of release	Multivesicular endosomes	Condensed apoptotic fragments	Exocytosis
5	Biomarkers	CD24, Rab 27, HSP 90	Histones, chemokines	Selectins, integrins

blood vessels (angiogenesis) must be formed. Oncogenic cells produce exosomes, which have a variety of functions, including promoting neoangiogenesis in their premetastatic niche and cancerous cell migration. Several tumor cell-released miRNAs and cytokines have been shown to promote neovascularization and metastasis, including *miR-9*, *miR-23a,* and *IL-6,* and *IL-8, miR-105, miR-126, miR-135b,* and *miR-210,* and *miR-221. MiR-105* induces vascular leakiness and promotes metastasis [25]. It is estimated that more than 90% of cancer-related deaths are the result of metastasis. Cancerous tumor cells stretched and reconquer organ systems, resulting in secondary tumors. "Tumor-derived exosomes" play a pivotal role in the pathology of 'tumor metastasis' through tumor-signaling pathways such as HIF-1a, miR-21, miR-105, miR-210, and oncogenic kinases [26].

9 Isolation of Exosomes

Because of their small size and low density, exosomes are usually separated from bodily fluids and cell culture media using differential ultracentrifugation. It is centrifuged at 10,000 × g to eliminate extra cells and cell debris from the biofluid. At 100,000 × g for 1 h or more, the supernatant is accumulated and ultra-centrifuged. The phosphate buffer solution is used to wash the pellet containing crude exosomes, removing any remaining proteins or contaminants. After an ultracentrifugation at 100,000 × g, the sample is purified. As a result of recent technological advances, exosome isolation has become easier, faster, and more cost-effective. By using antibodies or lectins against exosomal markers such as "CD63", "CD81", "EpCAM" and "Rab5", exosomes have also been isolated by immunoaffinity capture. Another method for rapid exosome isolation has been explored: precipitation followed by centrifugation. Modern exosome isolation methods, such as ExoQuick, require only a single precipitation step [27]. In order to 'isolate', 'detect' and 'quantify exosomemiRNA' from body fluids for research, there is a need for a "delicate," "sudden," and "outlay" global standard method. Only 0.1 percent of exo-miRNA is found in body fluids [28].

10 Physical Characterization and Molecular Analysis Techniques for Exosomes

The small size of exosomes (30–100 nm) makes accurate quantification and characterization difficult. As a result of these challenges, numerous tools have been introduced and applied in recent years described in Table 3 [29].

Table 3 Techniques used for the characterization and analysis of exosomes [29]

S. No.	Techniques	Application
1	Nanoparticle tracking analysis	Exosome size and quantity determined
2	Cryoelectron microscopy	Physical characterization
3	Scanning electron microscopy	
4	Atomic force microscopy	
5	Transmission electron microscopy	
6	Dynamic light scattering	
7	Tunable resistive pulse sensing	
8	Western blotting	Molecular methods used to analyze the concentration, quantitative, and profile of exosomes
9	Whole-genome sequencing	
10	Microarray profile	
11	Exome-targeted sequencing	
12	Quantitative real-time PCR	
13	ELISA	

11 Exosome-Derived MiRNAs: Cancer Biomarkers

A sensitive miRNA-based biomarker assay should be used to detect tumors at the earliest possible stage (0–1). Because circulating miRNA possess all of the characteristics of tissue biopsy biomarkers, they can be detected in liquid biopsy, moreover wholesome and cancer biopsies from patients are not required. Circulating miRNA research is a new and expanding field in biomarker research. Physicians and researchers can detect cancer at an early stage using body fluids, such as blood samples. Momen-Heravi et al., [30] found that exosomes provide an enriched and protective stable source of miRNA in body fluids, preventing the decadence of their biological molecules under non-physiological conditions such as 'freeze drying', 'extensive storage' and 'pH' [30]. According to research, exosomally derived miRNA can withstand freezing and thawing cycles for up to five years [4]. As a result, it could be used as a biomarker to detect cancer and other diseases. miRNAs are known to regulate gene expression in a fundamental way. They have important roles in 'tumorigenesis', 'metastasis', and resistance to various treatments.

MiRNAs can be transferred to target cells using exosomes. Exosomes defend miRNAs from degeneration so they are extra reliable than free miRNAs and could be accurately engrained by precise recipient cells. MiRNAs can therefore provide relevant data about the cell type from which they are derived, the target, and the cellular state, including resistance to therapy, within the exosome cargo. Tumor cell exosomes are increasingly being implicated in tumor cell proliferation, invasion, angiogenesis, and distant metastasis by transmitting onco-miRNA. A malignant tumor's growth and metastasis are dependent on angiogenesis even though new blood vessels provide extra oxygen, nutrients, and waste removal [31]. Scientists have found evidence that "exosomal miRNAs 21, 23, 29, 103, and 210", which are released by cancer cells, promote 'tumor proliferation', 'angiogenesis', and 'tumor migration'. A growing body of evidence suggests that "exo-miR-21" is an enticing biomarker for a wide variety of cancer types. The miRNA cargoes, in particular, contribute to the manipulation of the transcriptome pool of target cells. The discovery of exosomalmiRNAs in biology may provide insight into the mechanisms that promote tumor aggressiveness. The role of exosomal miRNAs as biomarkers in carcinogenesis and 'cancer progression, however, still requires further study [32].

12 Relationship Between Exosome and Tumor Microenvironment

It consists of an extracellular matrix, stromal cells ('fibroblasts' and 'adipocytes'), and immune cells ('T and B lymphocytes', 'tumor-associated macrophages', and 'natural killer cells'). As a key player in tumor biology, TME plays an important role in the tumor's genesis, progression, and treatment response. In the TME, exosomes play a key role. These chemicals serve as effective 'signaling molecules' between cancer cells and the TME cells that surround them (Fig. 3). As will be explained in the next sections, exosomes play a key function in the TME [33].

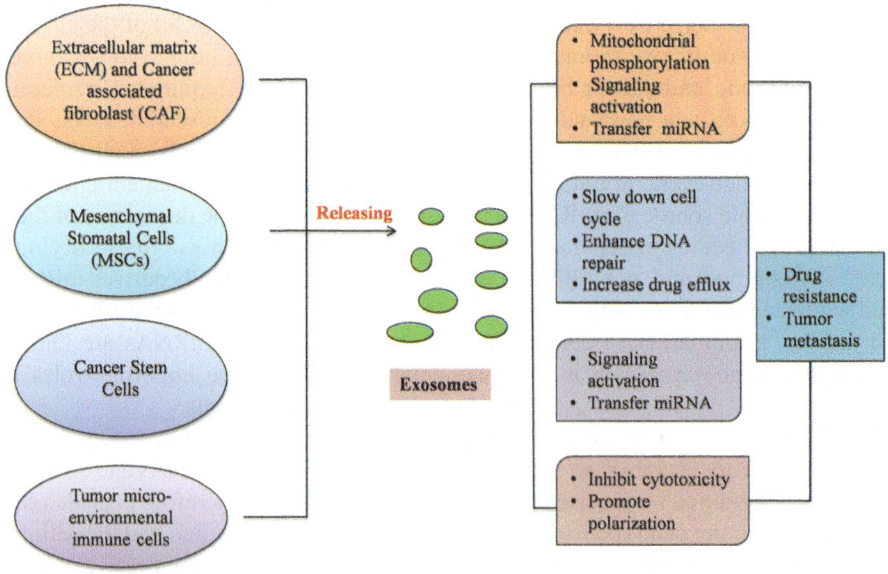

Fig. 3 Signal transduction pathway of exosomes in the tumor microenvironment

12.1 Exosome and Cancer-Associated Fibroblasts

In most solid tumors, the TME is predominantly made up of cancer-associated fibroblasts (CAF) [34]. "CAF-derived exosomes (CDEs)" are one of the most critical contributors in oncogenic transformation [35]. CDEs inhibit mitochondrial oxidative phosphorylation, which promotes cancer cell proliferation by increasing glycolysis and glutamine-dependent reduction carboxylation. CDEs enhance drug resistance and tumor metastasis in addition to promoting cancer growth and dissemination. When cancer cells are exposed to CDEs, they may become dedifferentiated via the 'Wnt pathway'. Chemical resistance in CRC would increase as a result of this. TGF-1 regulates lncRNA expression in CAF exosomes [36].

12.2 Exosomes and Cancer Stem Cells (CSCs)

They are a small subset of tumor tissue's diverse cells. CSCs, which have an infinite ability such as:

(a) Influence tumor initiation
(b) Self-renewal and diversification
(c) Recurrence
(d) Metastasis
(e) Therapeutic resistance.

CSC resistance is caused by a number of factors, including increased 'anti-apoptotic capabilities' & 'DNA repair efficiency' as well as slower 'drug efflux', 'cell cycle progression', and the production of detoxification enzymes [37].

12.3 Exosome and Mesenchymal Stem Cells (MSCs)

Because of their accessible availability and pluripotency qualities of 'osteoblasts'; 'adipocytes'; 'neurons' & 'cardiomyocytes', and, MSCs are considered one of the most promising seed cells in tissue engineering. Exosomes generated from MSCs influence tumor markers and help tumor growth by delivering unique miRNA to surrounding cells. Exosomes secreted by MSCs from bone marrow after "CaMKII" silencing protected CSCs from oxidative stress [38]. "MiR-16" and "miR-100", which suppress angiogenesis in breast cancer cells by targeting vascular endothelial growth factors in the TME. MSC-derived exosomes play a key role in tissue healing and inflammation [39].

12.4 Exosome and Tumor Microenvironmental Immune Cells

T- and B-cells are the most common immune cells in the tumor microenvironment [40]. Tumor cell-derived exosomes (TEXs) are a good source of immune-stimulating cellular components, such as 'alarmins' [41]. TEXs also have antigen-presenting and immune-stimulatory capabilities, allowing them to activate anticancer responses and aid in the recruitment and reconstruction of tumor microenvironmental components. By communicating through the "CD95 (Fas) receptor" and "FasL^{+}exosomes", exosomes produced by oral squamous cell carcinoma and histiocytic lymphoma could decrease immunological responses [42]. In the tumor microenvironment, immune cells also create exosomes. "CTLA-4" expression on 'Treg cells' and 'adenosine antitumor immunity' play a role in tumor genesis and progression. The primary immune cells that govern inflammation in the TME are macrophages, which come in two phenotypes: 'M1' and 'M2'. 'M1 macrophages' have the ability to destroy viruses and bacteria by secreting "IL-2" and "IL-3" [43].

13 Exosomal Diagnostics

Exosomes are ejected by cells in both healthy and diseased states. They transport 'nucleic acids' and 'proteins' from their host cells that are symptomatic of pathophysiological conditions, and they are widely regarded as critical in the development of biomarkers for clinical diagnosis. Exosomes with tumor-specific RNAs are released by tumor cells and could be exploited for cancer diagnosis. Exosomes include nucleic acids and proteins linked in cancer, as well as 'neurological', 'metabolic', 'viral', and other disorders, according to multiple research published in the last few years. Exosomes may also be extracted from readily available biofluids including blood and urine, making them an appealing target for diagnostic use.

13.1 Exosomal Proteins

Exosomes contain membrane-related proteins as well as proteins that are particular to the cell's functions and circumstances. A number of exosomal proteins have recently been identified as possible biomarkers for a variety of illnesses. 'Tetraspanins' which are abundant in exosomes are among the scaffolding membrane proteins. "CD63" is a tetraspanin that is present on exosomes and belongs to the tetraspanin family. Malignant cancer cells have been discovered to have higher levels of exosomal 'CD63' than non-cancer cells [44]. The exosomal marker 'CD81' (tetraspanin family) is important for the Hepatitis C virus's attachment and/or cell entrance (HCV). This shows that exosomal 'CD81' could be a helpful diagnostic and therapy response

Table 4 Exosomal proteins for clinical diagnostic applications

S. No.	Biofluid	Disease	Associated proteins	References
1	Plasma	Melanoma	HSP90, CD63, HSP70	[46]
		Prostate cancer	Survivin	[47]
		Glioblastoma	Epidermal growth factor receptor VIII	[48]
2	Cell culture medium	Human ovarian cancer	CD24, Claudin	[49]
3	Urine	Liver injury	CD10, CD26	[50]
		Bladder cancer	Resistin, retinoic acid-induced protein 3	[51]
		Prostate cancer	PSA, PCA3	[52]
		Acute kidney injury	ATF3	[53]

marker for hepatitis C [45]. These exosomal proteins should be investigated further. The putative exosomal protein biomarkers for diagnostic applications that have been revealed so far are included in Table 4.

13.2 *Exosomal Nucleic Acids*

Valadi's revelation in 2007 that exosomes contain RNAs, particularly miRNAs, as diagnostic biomarkers sparked a lot of interest [54]. Exosomal miRNAs are shielded from RNase destruction, making these biomarkers appropriate for clinical diagnostic applications [55]. ExosomalmiRNAs are the most commonly used cancer biomarkers. This test has a limited 'specificity' and a high 'false-positive rate', which can result in indolent prostate tumors being overtreated. As a result, new prostate cancer markers with improved diagnostic accuracy are required immediately. For prostate cancer, 'miR-14′1 is a reliable diagnostic marker [56]. ExosomalmiRNAs could be used as biomarkers for the detection of esophageal squamous cell carcinoma (ESCC). Exosomal 'miR21' levels are higher in ESCC patients than in those with benign tumors who do not have systemic inflammation. Furthermore, tumor development and aggressiveness are linked to exosomal miR-21. The only reservoir of miRNA-21 in circulation is exosome-derived miRNA-21 [57]. In addition, a few studies have shown that exosomal mRNAs, like miRNAs, could be used as biomarkers in clinical diagnosis. To date, putative exosomal RNA biomarkers for diagnostic applications have been reported, as shown in Table 5.

Table 5 Exosomal RNAs for clinical diagnostic applications

S. No.	Biofluid	Disease	Associated proteins	References
1	Plasma	Ovarian cancer	miR-21,-203	[58]
		Breast cancer	miR-21	[59]
		Lung cancer	miR-17, let-7f	[60]
2	Cell culture medium	Gastric cancer	Let-7 family miRNA	[61]
		Colorectal cancer	mRNA	[62]
3	Urine	Renal fibriosis	miR-29c	[63]

13.3 Exosomes from Other Biofluids

According to current research, exosomes can be found in physiological fluids other than serum and urine. Exosomal markers in amniotic fluid were also looked into as a possible source. Human saliva includes hundreds of stable mRNA core transcripts, which could be exploited for disease diagnosis [64]. Saliva exosomes could be used as a biomarker for pancreatic cancer diagnosis [65].

14 Role of Computation in the Age of Cancer Multi-omics

The four major roles that computation performs in high-throughput data analysis. These include obtaining raw data from high-throughput equipment, converting raw data to quantitative data, storing and managing enormous omics data, such as in remote repositories, and lastly deploying data analysis models.

14.1 Data Acquisition and Processing

Because of the usage of specialized bioinformatics pipelines, the acquisition, processing, and manipulation of omic data generated in high throughput studies is required. As the complexity of these datasets grows as a result of the natural expansion of such technologies, the problems that are associated with it expand as well [66]. Bioinformatics workflow management systems can be used to create, maintain, and encourage the reproducibility of a pipeline or workflow.

14.1.1 Genomics

Genomic analyses are the earliest omic technologies, focusing on the genomic sequence and its variants, such as 'INDELs', 'single nucleotide variations (SNVs)', 'copy number variations (CNVs)' and so on. The link between genetic changes and cancer is well-established. Microarrays have been utilized for genotyping for a long time. Despite the fact that microarray technology varies by manufacturer, most current DNA microarrays can be studied with well-established tools found in the Arrays database [67]. While DNA microarrays are still in use, next-generation sequencing (NGS) is soon becoming the norm. The procedure for analyzing NGS data includes sequencing capture and alignment to a reference genome. For instance, a variant discovery workflow might include 'variant calling', 'filtering', 'annotation', and 'prioritization' [68].

14.1.2 Epigenomics

With the contemporary introduction of high-throughput omic technologies to examine chemical alterations in tumor genomes, it has become increasingly clear that such epigenomic modifications are prevalent and likely play a role in a variety of malignancies. DNA methylation and histone modifications, both in oncogenes and other cancer-related genes, are examples of these alterations. Several tumor forms have also been identified to have mutations in genes involved in epigenetic control. The computational study of epigenomic data may reveal new information on the onset and course of cancer. Perhaps more importantly, such research will open the door for more rapid discovery of genetic and epigenetic biomarkers for diagnosis, prognosis, and therapeutic response. As a result, the development of novel therapeutic techniques may be accelerated. The epigenome is a combination of chemical changes to DNA and histone proteins that can influence gene expression activity and are possibly inheritable [69]. The epigenomics idea encompasses a number of mechanisms, each of which necessitates the use of a distinct high-throughput molecular approach for assessment. Each of these methods, in turn, necessitates the employment of a certain set of computational tools, as seen in Table 6.

14.1.3 Transcriptomics

The presence and quantity of RNA in a specific physiological setting are measured using transcriptomic studies [73]. The measurement of gene expression is perhaps the most prevalent application of transcriptomic technologies. A phenotype's gene expression profile can be utilized as a barcode for its biological state. Through differential expression analysis, such barcodes may be compared to pinpoint cellular alterations in malignancies [74]. The gene regulatory program encoded in the genome and the epigenome combine to create the expression profile. Cancer-related omic investigations frequently rely on customized analytics. AFMs are particularly well-suited to investigating the role and quantity of fusion transcripts that may give rise to chimeric proteins in cancer transcriptomics [75]. Another rationale for using AFMs is that different RNASeq pipelines are known to have differences that could be crucial for evaluating cancer genomes and transcriptomes [76].

Table 6 Computational tools required in the epigenomics

S. No.	Inheritable modifications	Activity	Technique	References
1	DNA methylation	Alter its transcriptional activity	Data array-based methods such as methylation array analysis, sequence-based methods such as *bsseq*	[70]
2	Chromatin remodeling	Nucleosomes are sparse, physical access to DNA is enabled	Nucleotide genome sequencing techniques such as *ATAC*-seq	[71]
3	Chromosome confirmation	Capture techniques that are able to quantify interactions between genomic loci; able to quantify interactions between a single pair of loci	*GenomicInteraction* tool	[72]

14.1.4 Metabolomics and Lipidomics

Changes in metabolism have a significant role in the development of cancer [77]. Cancer metabolomics has emerged as a hot area in oncology research, with the promise of new insights into cancer formation and therapeutic alternatives. Lipidomics is a subcategory of metabolomics [78]. Cancer lipidomics research could lead to the discovery of biomedically significant findings, such as novel biomarkers. There are currently frameworks for analyzing metabolomic and lipidomic data. Metabolomics data produced from gas chromatography–mass spectrometry data can be analyzed using the metab tool. The metaRbolomics software is a multi-purpose toolkit that may be used for everything from data processing to functional analysis. Similarly, the lipid package is a comparable framework that focuses on data from lipidomics [79].

14.1.5 Proteomics

Proteomic analyses are used to determine the number of proteins present in a biological system of interest and to quantify them. The study of cancer proteomes has the potential to uncover biomarkers and therapeutic targets [80]. The use of surface-enhanced laser desorption/ionization time-of-flight (SELDI-TOF) mass spectrometry has been one of the most promising approaches to the proteomic identification of marker genes. The use of serum proteomic patterns to diagnose ovarian cancer has been shown to have high sensitivity and specificity. More research is needed to confirm these findings, but the strategy appears to be quite promising. The SELDI-TOF approach, on the other hand, has significant drawbacks, and the methodology needs to be refined further. Nevertheless, it does show that the proteomics approach, when combined with computational tools, has the potential to uncover clinically important tumor markers. SELDI found three peaks in the 17–23 kDa mass range from tumor cells in a study of lung tumor tissue, which was significantly higher than normal tissues. The discovery of this protein profile in malignant lung tissue, which is highly repeatable, could lead to a screening technique that could be used to research people at risk for lung cancer and track their response to chemopreventive medicines [81].

14.2 Data Management

Since the commencement of the Human Genome Project, there has been a push for open data in the field of biomedical genomics, resulting in the creation of a thriving Genomic Commons [82]. Making data available in public repositories speeds up scientific discovery, but there are ethical and legal as well as technological difficulties to solve [83]. Determining the sort of data to be stored and how to store it, as well as policies for data access, sharing, and re-use, and long-term archiving policies, are all challenges in data management. NIH's Genome Data Commons is arguably the most successful archive of cancer multi-omics (GDC). The information is arranged as a directed graph (Fig. 4) of interconnected entities, each with its own set of properties and links. The systematic re-analysis of data available in huge public datasets can yield a wealth of information [84].

15 AI in Cancer Medical Imaging

Deep learning algorithms have proven to be an effective tool in medical imaging for illness monitoring, diagnosis, surgical operations, and disease management. The use of AI in radiology for multiple modalities with increased quality, such as X-rays, ultrasounds, computed tomography (CT/CAT), magnetic resonance imaging (MRI), positron emission tomography (PET), and digital pathology is critical in most oncology-related diagnostics [85]. With enhanced speed and precision, images are analyzed using highly sophisticated algorithms. The ability to distinguish between normal and abnormal medical images is critical for correct diagnosis. This is especially important for early cancer detection since it ensures a better prognosis. AI has improved the quality of images, computer-aided image interpretation, and radiomics in medical imaging, and the future of AI in medical imaging will focus on speed and cost reduction [86].

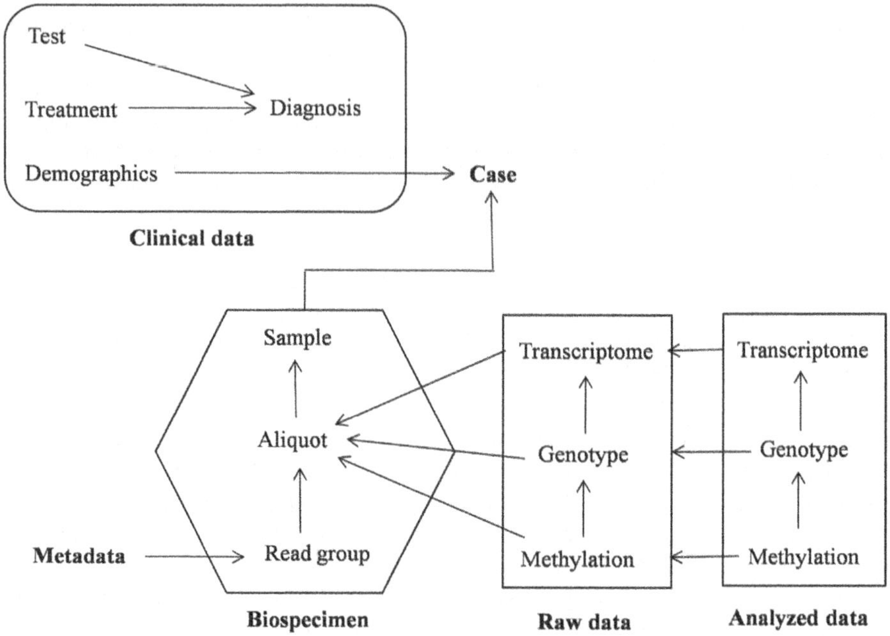

Fig. 4 Representation of data structure used to store the cancer genome atlas

15.1 Radiographic Imaging

Medical imaging is an important and effective tool for detecting cancer, tracking its course, and predicting illness prognosis (s). Mammography, for example, is the first-line imaging screening for breast cancer. Ultrasound is the best method for younger women with thick breasts. The use of medical imaging to diagnose the disease early is critical in lowering mortality rates. Medical imaging is not always possible in low and middle-income nations due to a scarcity of well-trained radiologists. Computer-assisted automated technologies would revolutionize the healthcare sector in such circumstances. The influence of AI on breast imaging was established by [87]. Recently, an AI-based breast cancer detection system was hailed as a game-changing breakthrough in cancer diagnosis. The Food and Drug Administration (FDA) has authorized Quant X as the first computer-aided system for breast cancer diagnosis. When compared to previous imaging systems, Quant X improves accuracy by 20% and provides radiologists with additional clinical patient-related information for diagnosis [88].

15.2 Digital Pathology

For many years, pathology has relied on microscopic examination of pigmented cells and tissues. Pathology will alter as a result of technological and AI advancements, which will reduce labor-intensive microscopic tasks, increase efficiency, and preserve quality for better clinical care. AI in digital pathology improves workflow by allowing clinicians to access images for accurate analysis and by standardizing methods, it decreases subjectivity. Digital pathology also allows for larger-scale image viewing and more consistent color information. This allows for the successful identification of unique indicators linked to disease-specific biomarkers for diagnosis, prognosis, and treatment [89]. A computer algorithm to predict patient prognosis using anatomic glass pathology slides of breast cancer. The computer algorithm was developed by taking measurements on digital images of 700 breast cancer patients in order to create a predictive model. They created a computer program that generated a predicted measure/score that was proportionate to the patient survival rate. This study proved that digital images created from glass slides can be utilized to train computer algorithms that can estimate patient prognosis [90].

Deep learning systems have also lately been intended to facilitate pathologists in distinguishing between benign and malignant prostate tumors, as well as morphological patterns used to grade this cancer. Scientists have created a deep learning method to score and quantify prostatectomy specimens using Gleason grading. The findings of this deep learning system, which trained over 900 pathology glass slides, were consistent with those supplied by certified pathologists [91] (Fig. 5).

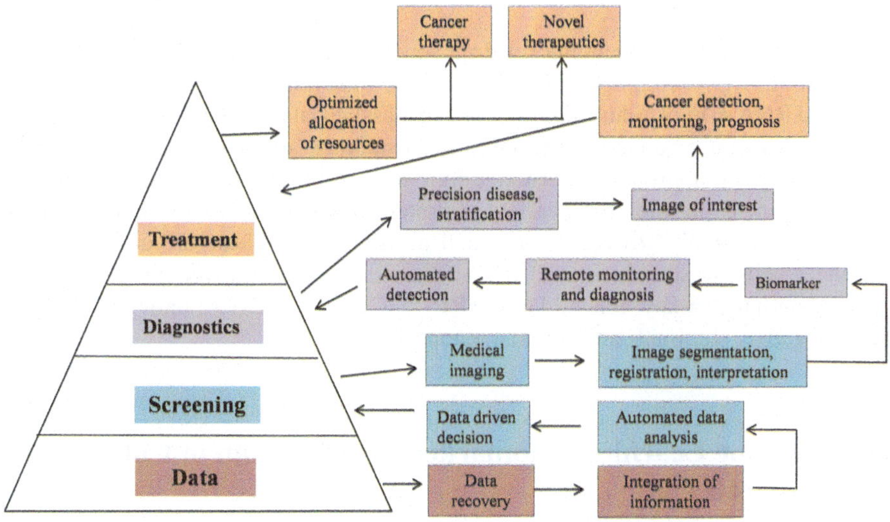

Fig. 5 Artificial intelligence in medical imaging

16 AI and Translational Oncology

16.1 Cancer Therapy

Multidrug resistance is an important element in the outcome of disease therapy and poses a significant clinical issue. This can be resolved by identifying novel drug resistance-inducing genes and biological mechanisms. These genes and pathways are frequently used as possibilities for new medication development and discovery. Additionally, medication resistance could be caused by a variety of epigenetic changes. For instance, drug resistance has been observed in estrogen receptor-positive breast tumors and ovarian malignancies. An estimated 30–55 percent of metastatic receptor-positive subtypes in breast cancer develop secondary resistance to therapy after receiving neoadjuvant aromatase inhibitor treatment. The existence of mutant ESR1 is blamed for drug resistance [92]. Several biological mechanisms contribute to drug resistance, including 'apoptosis' to avoid drug-induced 'cytotoxicity', 'tumor migration', 'drug metabolism', 'enhanced DNA repair', and 'activation of molecular' pathways that promote tumor angiogenesis. The mismatched DNA repair mechanism, the "p53 pathway"; the 'P-glycoprotein', and multidrug resistance-associated protein have all been proposed as biological routes for treatment resistance in ovarian cancer [93].

16.2 Drug Discovery

The high throughput sequencing for drug screening is a major benefit of NGS as a clinical tool. High-throughput screening enables for simultaneous sequencing of both DNA and RNA in high quantities, resulting in massive datasets. Pathogenic mutations and cancer-specific transcriptome alterations, such as 'alternative splicing', can be discovered in this approach. Alternative splicing is a complex biological process that regulates gene expression for a variety of proteins involved in 'DNA repair', 'angiogenesis', 'adhesion', 'invasion', and 'cell proliferation'. These are characteristics of cancer cells. Researchers used RNA sequencing to find novel subtype-specific splicing variants in key genes like 'LARP1', 'CDK4', 'ADD3', and 'PHLPP2' in triple-negative, 'luminal' and 'human' cancers [94].

17 Machine Learning: Biomarker Identification in Cancer Research

The panacea for finding patterns in opaque datasets from various domains is machine learning (ML), a subfield of artificial intelligence. Machine learning has proved

Table 7 Machine learning methods used for cancer biomarker studies

S. No.	Cancer	Data source	Machine learning algorithm	Reference
1	Breast cancer	Microarray	Linear-discriminant analysis	[96]
2	B-cell lymphoma	SELDI–TOF MS	Decision tree classification	[97]
3	Colorectal cancer	Microarray	Correlation-based feature selection	[98]
4	Lung cancer	Multiplexed immunoassay	Rule learning approach	[99]
5	Multiple cancer dataset	Meta-analysis	Clustering	[100]
6	Pancreatic cancer	Electronic health record via text mining	Vector machine	[101]

promise to address mining cancer-specific patterns in 'cancer prediction' and 'prognosis'; in 'cancer diagnosis', 'management' and customized treatment since a diversified and enormous number of cancer datasets are already in the public domain [95]. Table 7 lists the machine learning approaches employed in cancer biomarker research.

18 Exosome Simplification in Metastatic Cancer Therapy

Tumor cells have biological vulnerabilities at various phases of metastasis, and these vulnerabilities can be exploited to stop the spread of cancer. Exosomes are implicated in metastatic cascades and have features that make them appealing for therapeutic administration. The following are some exosome-based treatment methods with promising clinical applications:

(a) **Decreasing production and uptake of exosomes**: Exosome secretion and absorption can be blocked, which could help to prevent metastasis. Targeting the 'heparanase/syndecan-1 axis' which is involved in the creation of exosomes and tumor cell dispersion, has been suggested in preclinical and clinical research as a way to at least partially alleviate metastatic malignancies [102]. For example, discovered that heparin can effectively prevent oral squamous carcinoma spread by reducing the uptake of tumor-derived exosomes [103]. These findings suggest that therapeutic antibodies that target metastasis-related exosomes could be a viable treatment option. Targeted antibodies have also been shown to inhibit cancer spread by encouraging macrophages to eliminate tumor-derived exosomes [104]. A new gadget has also been developed to stop or divert the spread of malignant cells. The trapping of ovarian tumor cells within the peritoneum and redirection of the tumor cells away from their initial target areas was achieved by implanting tumor exosomes in a 3D scaffold and then transplanting the scaffold into the peritoneal cavity of mice. At a distance, this method effectively reduced tumor metastasis [105].

(b) **ExosomalmiRNAs**: Exosomes include a number of miRNAs that can be used to prevent exosome-mediated cancer spread [106]. ExosomalmiRNAs produced from colorectal cancer (CRC) have been demonstrated to increase tumor cell proliferation, allowing for the use of gene therapy to suppress tumor metastasis by designing exosomalmiRNAs [62]. Furthermore, it was discovered that 'miR-379' in CRC-derived exosomes inhibits CRC cell migration and that transferring these engineered miR-379-overexpressing exosomes to recipient cells inhibited their migration [107]. Similarly, Zaharie et al. found that exosomal 'microRNA-375' reduces tumor cell spread in colon cancer by blocking 'Bcl-2', implying that exosomal 'microRNA-375' could be a therapeutic target [108].

(c) **Exosomes as promising delivery systems**: Exosomes can be chemically or biologically manipulated to produce delivery systems that can improve the treatment outcomes of chemotherapeutic medicines while also reducing drug toxicity, thanks to their excellent physicochemical stability and biocompatibility [109]. Exosomes can be utilized to deliver doxorubicin selectively to tumor tissues by intravenous injection, reducing tumor development without causing overt damage [110]. Exosomes that have been genetically modified have also been found to slow the progression of schwannoma tumors by releasing suicide mRNAs and proteins [111].

19 Conclusion

Exosome-mediated cell-to-cell and cell-to-distant communication are gaining traction as a novel mode of communication and a delivery mechanism for their contents. Because of their 'small size', 'natural origin', and 'innocuous qualities' they are a great delivery mechanism for anticancer miRNAs and antitumor medicines in therapeutic interventions. The study of tumor-derived exosomal miRNAs is a rapidly developing topic that aims to develop new cancer prevention, early detection, diagnostic, and individualized therapy strategies. The expression patterns of miRNA in tumor cells are very different from those in healthy cells. Variations in expression profiles have been found to be linked to tumor angiogenesis, invasion, and metastasis. Scientists are exploring the possibility of using engineered exosomes to deliver therapeutic chemicals, such as cancer medicines and functional antitumor miRNAs, to cancer cells or tissues that are being treated individually. Preventing the progression of mature onco-miRNA seems to be another envisaged therapeutic intervention. Exosome depletion could be accelerated as well. As a result, exosomes are completely 'biocompatible'; have little 'toxicity' and 'immunogenicity' are extremely stable in physiological fluids, and can be loaded with specific chemicals to kill cancer cells. Finally, exosomes are microscopic particles that play an important function in the development of cancer. Additional efforts are needed to create more sensitive, quick, and cost-effective approaches to better describe and understand the roles of exosomal miRNAs in body fluids, as well as to build a plan for cancer prevention, early diagnosis, and therapy.

The availability of greater resolution molecular data from inexpensive technology has supplied an incentive to translate the potential of a customized medicine approach. Molecular characterization of tumor cells leads to molecular stratification of the illness with probable clinical applicability. A tailored molecular characterization is the way of the future, allowing for suitable therapy combinations for each patient and at each stage of disease progression. Given the heterogeneity of most malignancies, it is necessary to categorize them at the molecular level rather than using broad phenotypes. Personalized medicine will become a part of regular clinical practices due to the availability of lower and more affordable sequencing technology, as well as breakthroughs in systems biology. Nonetheless, this subject is developing, and AI and machine learning have a lot to offer in terms of cancer detection and prognosis.

References

1. Bray, F., Ferlay, J., Soerjomataram, I., Siegel, R. L., Torre, L. A., & Jemal, A. (2018). Global cancer statistics 2018: GLOBOCAN estimates of incidence and mortality worldwide for 36 cancers in 185 countries. *CA: A Cancer Journal for Clinicians, 68*(6), 394–424.
2. Li, W., Li, C., Zhou, T., et al. (2017). Role of exosomal proteins in cancer diagnosis. *Molecular Cancer, 16*(1), 145.
3. Bu, H., He, D., He, X., & Wang, K. (2019). Exosomes: Isolation, analysis, and applications in cancer detection and therapy. *ChemBioChem, 20*(4), 451–461.
4. Thind, A., & Wilson, C. (2016). ExosomalmiRNAs as cancer biomarkers and therapeutic targets. *Journal of Extracellular Vesicles, 5*, 31292.
5. Mathieu, M., Martin-Jaular, L., Lavieu, G., & Thery, C. (2019). Specificities of secretion and uptake of exosomes and other extracellular vesicles for cell-to-cell communication. *Nature Cell Biology, 21*(1), 9.
6. Dakubo, G. D. (2016). Advanced technologies for body fluid biomarker analyses. In G. D. Dakubo (Ed.), *Cancer biomarkers in body fluids: Principles* (pp. 55–74). Springer Nature.
7. Ruivo, C. F., Adem, B., Silva, M., & Melo, S. A. (2017). The biology of cancer exosomes: Insights and new perspectives. *Cancer Research, 77*, 6480–6488.
8. SkotlandT, S. K., & Llorente, A. (2017). Lipids in exosomes: Current knowledge and the way forward. *Progress in Lipid Research, 66*, 30–41.
9. Denzer, K., Kleijmeer, M. J., Heijnen, H. F. G., Stoorvogel, W., & Geuze, H. J. (2000). Exosome: From internal vesicle of the multivesicular body to intercellular signaling device. *Journal of Cell Science, 113*(19), 3365–3374.
10. Clayton, A., TurkesA, N. H., Mason, M. D., & Tabi, Z. (2005). Induction of heat shock proteins in B-cell exosomes. *Journal of Cell Science, 118*(16), 3631–3638.
11. LespagnolA, D. D., Beekman, C., et al. (2008). Exosome secretion, including the DNA damage-induced p53-dependent secretory pathway, is severely compromised in TSAP6/Steap3-null mice. *Cell Death and Differentiation, 15*(11), 1723–1733.
12. Sun, D., Zhuang, X., Zhang, S., et al. (2013). Exosomes are endogenous nanoparticles that can deliver biological information between cells. *Advanced Drug Delivery Reviews, 65*(3), 342–347.
13. Olver, C., & Vidal, M. (2007). Proteomic analysis of secreted exosomes. *Sub Cell Biochemistry, 43*, 99–131.

14. Huotari, J., & Helenius, A. (2011). Endosome maturation. *EMBO Journal, 30*(17), 3481–3500.
15. Del Conte-Zerial, P., Brusch, L., Rink, J. C., Collinet, C., Kalaidzidis, Y., Zerial, M., et al. (2008). Membrane identity and GTPase cascades regulated by toggle and cut-out switches. *Molecular Systems Biology, 4*, 206.
16. Mukherjee, S., & Maxfield, F. R. (2004). Membrane domains. *Annual Review Cell Development Biology, 20*, 839–866.
17. Trajkovic, K., Hsu, C., Chiantia, S., Rajendran, L., Wenzel, D., Wieland, F., et al. (2008). Ceramide triggers budding of exosome vesicles into multivesicular endosomes. *Science, 319*(5867), 1244–1247.
18. Savina, A., Fader, C. M., Damiani, M. T., & Colombo, M. I. (2005). Rab11 promotes docking and fusion of multivesicular bodies in a calcium-dependent manner. *Traffic, 6*, 131–143.
19. Ostrowski, M., Carmo, N. B., Krumeich, S., Fanget, I., Raposo, G., Savina, A., et al. (2010). Rab27a and Rab27b control different steps of the exosome secretion pathway. *Nature Cell Biology, 12*, 19–30.
20. Schorey, J. S., & Bhatnagar, S. (2008). Exosome function: From tumor immunology to pathogen biology. *Traffic, 9*(6), 871–881.
21. Kharaziha, P., Ceder, S., Li, Q., & Panaretakis, T. (2012). Tumor cell-derived exosomes: A message in a bottle. *Biochimica et BiophysicaActa: Reviews on Cancer, 1826*(1), 103–111.
22. Pegtel, D. M., van de Garde, M. D. B., & Middeldorp, J. M. (2011). Viral miRNAs exploiting the endosomal-exosomal pathway for intercellular cross-talk and immune evasion. *Biochimica et Biophysica Acta, 1809*(11–12), 715–721.
23. Markopoulos, G. S., Roupakia, E., Tokamani, M., et al. (2017). A step-by-step microRNA guide to cancer development and metastasis. *Cellular Oncology, 40*(4), 303–339.
24. van Niel, G., D'angelo, G., & Raposo, G. (2018). Shedding light on the cell biology of extracellular vesicles. *Nature Reviews Molecular Cell Biology, 19*, 213.
25. Zhou, W., Fong, M. Y., Min, Y., et al. (2014). Cancer-secreted miR-105 destroys vascular endothelial barriers to promote metastasis. *Cancer Cell, 25*, 501–515.
26. Wang, N., & Xie, L. (2017). Diagnostic and therapeutic applications of tumor-associated exosomes. *Precision Radiation Oncology, 1*, 34–39.
27. RekkerK, S. M., Roost, A. M., et al. (2014). Comparison of serum exosome isolation methods for microRNA profiling. *Clinical Biochemistry, 47*(1–2), 135–138.
28. Chen, J. F., Mandel, E. M., Thomson, J. M., et al. (2006). The role of microRNA-1 and microRNA-133 in skeletal muscle proliferation and differentiation. *Nature Genetics, 38*(2), 228–233.
29. Lee, K., Fraser, K., Ghaddar, B., et al. (2018). Multiplexed profiling of single extracellular vesicles. *ACS Nano, 12*(1), 494–503.
30. Momen-Heravi, F., Getting, S. J., & Moschos, S. A. (2018). Extracellular vesicles and their nucleic acids for biomarker discovery. *Pharmacology and Therapeutics, 192*, 170–187.
31. Martial, S. (2016). Involvement of ion channels and transporters in carcinoma angiogenesis and metastasis. *American Journal of Physiology Cell Physiology, 310*, C710–C727.
32. Rahbarghazi, R., Jabbari, N., Sani, N. A., et al. (2019). Tumor-derived extracellular vesicles: Reliable tools for cancer diagnosis and clinical applications. *Cell Communication and Signaling: CCS, 17*(1), 73.
33. Roma-Rodrigues, C., Mendes, R., Baptista, P. V., & Fernandes, A. R. (2019). Targeting tumor microenvironment for cancer therapy. *International Journal of Molecular Science, 20*, 840.
34. Zhao, H., et al. (2016). Tumor microenvironment derived exosomespleiotropically modulate cancer cell metabolism. *eLife, 5*, e10250.
35. Whiteside, T. L. (2016). Tumor-derived exosomes and their role in cancer progression. *Advances in Clinical Chemistry, 74*, 103–141.
36. HaoY, B. D., & Ten Dijke, P. (2019). TGF-beta-mediated epithelial-mesenchymal transition and cancer metastasis. *International Journal of Molecular Science, 20*, 27–67.
37. Wang, J., Zheng, Y., & Zhao, M. (2016). Exosome-based cancer therapy: Implication for cancer. *Stem Cells Front Pharmacology, 7*, 533.

38. Sharma, A. (2018). Role of stem cell derived exosomes in tumor biology. *International Journal of Cancer, 142*, 1086–1092.
39. Ti, D., HaoH, Fu. X., & Han, W. (2016). Mesenchymal stem cells-derived exosomal microRNAs contribute to wound inflammation. *Science China Life Science, 59*, 1305–1312.
40. Yong, S. B., et al. (2019). Non-viral nano-immunotherapeutics targeting tumor microenvironmental immune cells. *Biomaterials, 219*, 119401.
41. Ramos-Zayas, Y., et al. (2019). Immunotherapy for the treatment of canine transmissible venereal tumor based in dendritic cells pulsed with tumoralexosomes. *Immunopharmacology and Immunotoxicology, 41*, 48–54.
42. Muller, L., et al. (2017). Human tumor-derived exosomes (TEX) regulate Treg functions via cell surface signaling rather than uptake mechanisms. *Oncoimmunology, 6*, e1261243.
43. Sakai, C., & Nishikawa, H. (2018). Immunosuppressive environment in tumors. *Gan Kagaku Ryoho, 45*, 222–226.
44. Yoshioka, Y., Konishi, Y., Kosaka, N., Katsuda, T., Kato, T., & Ochiya, T. (2013). Comparative marker analysis of extracellular vesicles in different human cancer types. *Journal of Extracellar Vesicles, 2*, 14–23.
45. Welker, M. W., Reichert, D., Susser, S., et al. (2012). Soluble serum CD81 is elevated in patients with chronic hepatitis c and correlates with alanine aminotransferase serum activity. *PLoS ONE, 7*, e30796.
46. Peinado, H., Aleckovic, M., Lavotshkin, S., et al. (2012). Melanoma exosomes educate bone marrow progenitor cells toward a prometastatic phenotype through MET. *Nature Medicine, 18*, 883–891.
47. Khan, S., Jutzy, J. M. S., Valenzuela, M. M. A., et al. (2012). Plasma-derived exosomal survivin, a plausible biomarker for early detection of prostate cancer. *PLoS ONE, 7*, e46737.
48. Skog, J., Wurdinger, T., van Rijn, S., et al. (2008). Glioblastomamicrovesicles transport RNA and proteins that promote tumour growth and provide diagnostic biomarkers. *Nature Cell Biology, 10*, 1470–1476.
49. Li, J., Sherman-Baust, C. A., Tsai-Turton, M., Bristow, R. E., Roden, R. B., & Morin, P. J. (2009). Claudin-containing exosomes in the peripheral circulation of women with ovarian cancer. *BMC Cancer, 9*, 244.
50. Conde-Vancells, J., Rodriguez-Suarez, E., & Gonzalez, E., et al. (2010). Candidate biomarkers in exosome-like vesicles purified from rat and mouse urine samples. *PROTEOMICS—ClinAppl, 4*, 416–425.
51. Smalley, D. M., Sheman, N. E., Nelson, K., & Theodorescu, D. (2008). Isolation and identification of potential urinary microparticle biomarkers of bladder cancer. *Journal of Proteome Research, 7*, 2088–2096.
52. Nilsson, J., Skog, J., Nordstrand, A., et al. (2009). Prostate cancer-derived urine exosomes: A novel approach to biomarkers for prostate cancer. *British Journal of Cancer, 100*, 1603–1607.
53. Zhou, H., Cheruvanky, A., Hu, X., et al. (2008). Urinary exosomal transcription factors, a new class of biomarkers for renal disease. *Kidney International, 74*, 613–621.
54. ValadiH, E. K., Bossios, A., Sjostrand, M., Lee, J. J., & Lotvall, J. O. (2007). Exosome-mediated transfer of mRNAs and microRNAs is a novel mechanism of genetic exchange between cell. *Nature Cell Biology, 9*(6), 654–659.
55. Hunter, M. P., Ismail, N., Zhang, X., et al. (2008). Detection of microRNA expression in human peripheral blood microvesicles. *PLoS ONE, 3*(11), e3694.
56. Mitchell, P. S., Parkin, R. K., Kroh, E. M., et al. (2008). Circulating microRNAs as stable blood-based markers for cancer detection. *Proceedings of the National Academy of Sciences of the United States of America, 105*, 10513–10518.
57. Tanaka, Y., Kamohara, H., Kinoshita, K., et al. (2013). Clinical impact of serum exosomal microRNA-21 as a clinical biomarker in human esophageal squamous cell carcinoma. *Cancer, 119*, 1159–1167.
58. Taylor, D. D., & Gercel-Taylor, C. (2008). MicroRNA signatures of tumor-derived exosomes as diagnostic biomarkers of ovarian cancer. *Gynecologic Oncology, 110*, 13–21.

59. Corcoran, C., Friel, A. M., Duffy, M. J., Crown, J., & O'Driscoll, L. (2011). Intracellular and extracellular microRNAs in breast cancer. *Clinical Chemistry, 57*, 18–32.
60. Silva, J., Garcıa, V., Zaballos, A., et al. (2011). Vesicle-related microRNAs in plasma of non-small cell lung cancer patients and correlation with survival. *European Respiratory Journal, 37*, 617–623.
61. Ohshima, K., Inoue, K., Fujiwara, A., et al. (2010). Let-7 microRNA family is selectively secreted into the extracellular environment via exosomes in a metastatic gastric cancer cell line. *PLoS ONE, 5*, e13247.
62. Hong, B. S., Cho, J. H., Kim, H., Choi, E. J., Rho, S., Kim, J., Kim, J. H., Choi, D. S., Kim, Y. K., Hwang, D., & Gho, Y. S. (2009). Colorectal cancer cell-derived microvesicles are enriched in cell cycle-related mRNAs that promote proliferation of endothelial cells. *BMC Genomics, 10*, 556.
63. Lv, L. L., Cao, Y. H., Pan, M. M., et al. (2014). CD2AP mRNA in urinary exosome as biomarker of kidney disease. *Clinica Chimica Acta, 428*, 26–31.
64. Palanisamy, V., Sharma, S., Deshpande, A., Zhou, H., Gimzewski, J., & Wong, D. T. (2010). Nanostructural and transcriptomic analyses of human saliva derived exosomes. *PLoS ONE, 5*, e8577.
65. Lau, C., Kim, Y., Chia, D., et al. (2013). Role of pancreatic cancer-derived exosomes in salivary biomarker development. *Journal of Biological Chemistry, 288*, 26888–26897.
66. Davis-Turak, J., Courtney, S. M., Hazard, E. S., Glen, W. B., da Silveira, W. A., Wesselman, T., et al. (2017). Genomics pipelines and data integration: Challenges and opportunities in the research setting. *Expert Review of Molecular Diagnostics, 17*, 225–237.
67. Maintainer, B. P. (2019). *Arrays: Using bioconductor for microarray analysis.*
68. Roy, S., Coldren, C., Karunamurthy, A., Kip, N. S., Klee, E. W., Lincoln, S. E., et al. (2018). Standards and guidelines for validating next-generation sequencing bioinformatics pipelines. *Journal of Molecular Diagnostics, 20*, 4–27.
69. Bernstein, B. E., Meissner, A., & Lander, E. S. (2007). The mammalian epigenome. *Cell, 128*, 669–681.
70. Hansen, K. D., Langmead, B., & Irizarry, R. A. (2012). BSmooth: From whole genome bisulfite sequencing reads to differentially methylated regions. *Genome Biology, 13*, R83.
71. Buenrostro, J. D., Wu, B., Chang, H. Y., & Greenleaf, W. J. (2015). ATAC-seq: A method for assaying chromatin accessibility genome-wide. *Current Protocols in Molecular Biology, 109*, 21–29.
72. Harmston, N., Ing-Simmons, E., Perry, M., Barešic, A., & Lenhard, B. (2015). Genomic interactions: An R/bioconductor package for manipulating and investigating chromatin interaction data. *BMC Genomics, 16*, 963.
73. Zhang, H., He, L., & Cai, L. (2018). Transcriptome sequencing: RNA-seq. In T. Huang (Ed.), *Computational systems biology* (pp. 15–27). Humana Press.
74. Jeong, E., Moon, S. U., Song, M., & Yoon, S. (2017). Transcriptome modeling and phenotypic assays for cancer precision medicine. *Archives of Pharmacal Research, 40*, 906–914.
75. Yang, X., Saito, Y., Rao, A., Kim, H. J., Singh, P., Scott, E., et al. (2019). Alignment free filtering for cfNA fusion fragments. *Bioinformatics, 35*, i225–i232.
76. Babarinde, I. A., Li, Y., & Hutchins, A. P. (2019). Computational methods for mapping, assembly and quantification for coding and non-coding transcripts. *Computer Structure Biotechnology of Journal, 17*, 628–637.
77. Vazquez, A., Kamphorst, J. J., Markert, E. K., Schug, Z. T., Tardito, S., & Gottlieb, E. (2016). Cancer metabolism at a glance. *Journal of Cell Science, 129*, 3367–3373.
78. Yang, K., & Han, X. (2016). Lipidomics: Techniques, applications, and outcomes related to biomedical sciences. *Trends in Biochemical Sciences, 41*, 954–969.
79. Mohamed, A., Molendijk, J. (2019). *Lipidr: Data mining and analysis of lipidomics datasets.* R package version 200.
80. Yakkioui, Y., Temel, Y., Chevet, E., & Negroni, L. (2017). Integrated and quantitative proteomics of human tumors. *Methods in Enzymology, 586*, 229–246.

81. Cho, W. C. (2017). Mass spectrometry-based proteomics in cancer research. *Expert Review of Proteomics, 14*, 725–727.
82. Cook-Deegan, R., & McGuire, A. L. (2017). Moving beyond Bermuda: Sharing data to build a medical information commons. *Genome Research, 27*, 897–901.
83. Jansen, P., van den Berg, L., van Overveld, P., & Boiten, J. W. (2018). Research data stewardship for healthcare professionals. In P. Kubben, M. Dumontier, & A. Dekker (Eds.), *Fundamentals of clinical data science* (pp. 37–53). Springer.
84. Grossman, R. L., Heath, A. P., Ferretti, V., Varmus, H. E., Lowy, D. R., Kibbe, W. A., et al. (2016). Toward a shared vision for cancer genomic data. *New England Journal of Medicine, 375*, 1109–1112.
85. Wani, N., & Raza, K. (2018). Multiple kernel learning approach for medical image analysis. In: Dey, N., Ashour, A., Shi, F., Balas, E. (Eds.), *Soft computing based medical image analysis*, (pp. 31–47). Elsevier. https://doi.org/10.1016/B978-0-12-813087-2.00002-6
86. Gore, J. C. (2020). Artificial intelligence in medical imaging. *Magnetic Resonance Imaging, 68*, A1-4.
87. Rodriguez-Ruiz, A., et al. (2019). Detection of breast cancer with mammography: Effect of an artificial intelligence support system. *Radiology, 290*, 305–314.
88. Newswire, P. (2020). QuantX artificial intelligence (AI) breast cancer diagnosis system receives 2020 gold edison award. Available: https://www.prnewswire.com/news-releases/quantx-artificial-intelligenceai-breast-cancer-diagnosis-system-receives-2020-gold-edison-award301027112.html
89. Bera, K., Schalper, K. A., Rimm, D. L., Velcheti, V., & Madabhushi, A. (2019). Artificial intelligence in digital pathology—New tools for diagnosis and precision oncology. *Nature Reviews Clinical Oncology, 16*, 703–715.
90. Beck, A. H., et al. (2011). Systematic analysis of breast cancer morphology uncovers stromal features associated with survival. *Science Translational of Medicine, 108*, ra113
91. Nagpal, K., et al. (2019). Development and validation of a deep learning algorithm for improving gleason scoring of prostate cancer. *NPJ Digital Medicine, 2*, 48.
92. Harbeck, N., et al. (2019). Breast cancer. *Nature Reviews Disease Primers, 5*, 66.
93. Pokhriyal, R., Hariprasad, R., Kumar, L., & Hariprasad, H. (2019). Chemotherapy resistance in advanced ovarian cancer patient. *Biomark Cancer, 11*, 1179299X19860815.
94. Eswaran, J., et al. (2013). RNA sequencing of cancer reveals novel splicing alterations. *Science and Reports, 3*, 1689.
95. Vellido, A., Biganzoli, E., Lisboa, P. J. (23–25 April 2008). *Machine learning in cancer research: implications for personalised medicine.* At: The 16th European symposium on artificial neural networks ESANN.
96. Sun, Y., Goodison, S., Li, J., Liu, L., & Farmerie, W. (2007). Improved breast cancer prognosis through the combination of clinical and genetic markers. *Bioinformatics, 23*, 30–37.
97. Zhang, X., Wang, B., Zhang, X. S., Li, Z. M., Guan, Z. Z., & Jiang, W. Q. (2007). Serum diagnosis of diffuse large B-cell lymphomas and further identification of response to therapy using SELDITOF-MS and tree analysis patterning. *BMC Cancer, 7*, 235.
98. Garcia-Bilbao, A., Armananzas, R., Ispizua, Z., et al. (2012). Identification of a biomarker panel for colorectal cancer diagnosis. *BMC Cancer, 12*, 43.
99. Bigbee, W. L., Gopalakrishnan, V., Weissfeld, J. L., et al. (2012). A multiplexed serum biomarker immunoassay panel discriminates clinical lung cancer patients from highrisk individuals found to be cancer-free by CT screening. *Journal of Thoracic Oncology, 7*, 698–708.
100. Lanara, Z., Giannopoulou, E., & Fullen, M. et al. (2013). *Comparative study and meta-analysis of meta-analysis studies for the correlation of genomic markers with early cancer detection*, (pp. 7–14). Hum. Genomics.
101. Zhao, D., & Weng, C. (201). Combining PubMed knowledge and EHR data to develop a weighted bayesian network for pancreatic cancer prediction. Journal Biomedicine Informatics 44, 859–868.

102. Thompson, C. A., Purushothaman, A., Ramani, V. C., Vlodavsky, I., & Sanderson, R. D. (2013). Heparanase regulates secretion, composition, and function of tumor cell-derived exosomes. *Journal of Biological Chemistry, 288*, 10093–10099.
103. Sento, S., Sasabe, E., & Yamamoto, T. (2016). Application of a persistent heparin treatment inhibits the malignant potential of oral squamous carcinoma cells induced by tumor cell-derived exosomes. *PLoS ONE, 11*, e0148454.
104. Nishida-Aoki, N., Tominaga, N., Takeshita, F., Sonoda, H., Yoshioka, Y., & Ochiya, T. (2017). Disruption of circulating extracellular vesicles as a novel therapeutic strategy against cancer metastasis. *Molecular Theraphy, 25*, 181–191.
105. de la Fuente, A., Alonso-Alconada, L., Costa, C., Cueva, J., Garcia-Caballero, T., LopezLopez, R., & Abal, M. (2015). M-trap: Exosome-based capture of tumor cells as a new technology in peritoneal metastasis. *Journal of National Cancer Institute, 107*, djv184.
106. Zhang, Y., Yang, P., & Wang, X. F. (2014). Microenvironmental regulation of cancer metastasis by miRNAs. *Trends in Cell Biology, 24*, 153–160.
107. Clancy, C., Khan, S., Glynn, C. L., Holian, E., Dockery, P., Lalor, P., Brown, J. A., Joyce, M. R., Kerin, M. J., & Dwyer, R. M. (2016). Screening of exosomal microRNAs from colorectal cancer cells. *Cancer Biomarkers, 17*, 427–435.
108. Zaharie, F., Muresan, M. S., Petrushev, B., Berce, C., Gafencu, G. A., Selicean, S., Jurj, A., Cojocneanu-Petric, R., Lisencu, C. I., Pop, L. A., et al. (2015). Exosome-carried microRNA375 inhibits cell progression and dissemination via Bcl-2 blocking in colon cancer. *Journal of Gastrointestinal and Liver Diseases, 24*, 435–443.
109. Dos Anjos, P. B., da Luz Andres Cordero, F., Socorro Faria, S., Peixoto Ferreira de Souza, L., Cristina Brigido Tavares, P., Alonso Goulart, V., Fontes, W., Ricardo Goulart, L., & Jose Barbosa Silva, M. (2017). The multifaceted role of extracellular vesicles in metastasis: Priming the soil for seeding. *International Journal of Cancer, 140*, 2397–407.
110. Tian, Y., Li, S., Song, J., Ji, T., Zhu, M., Anderson, G. J., Wei, J., & Nie, G. (2014). A doxorubicin delivery platform using engineered natural membrane vesicle exosomes for targeted tumor therapy. *Biomaterials, 35*, 2383–2390.
111. Mizrak, A., Bolukbasi, M. F., Ozdener, G. B., Brenner, G. J., Madlener, S., Erkan, E. P., Strobel, T., Breakefield, X. O., & Saydam, O. (2013). Genetically engineered microvesicles carrying suicide mRNA/protein inhibit schwannoma tumor growth. *Molecular Theraphy, 21*, 101–108.

The Revelation and Therapeutic Role of Medicinal Phytochemicals in the Treatment of Cancer: A Brief Review

Muhammad Mazhar Fareed and Muhammad Mohsin Ali

Abstract Medicinal phytochemical-based plants have been used initially in human cultivation, including mostly evident from in the ancient era as well as herbal-based phytochemicals in traditional ways. The use of plants as therapeutics, clinical treatment, and pharmaceuticals-based interest not on phyto herbal plants studies as compared to the artificial, celluloid drugs. Most of the time, the lack of information related to herbal medicine in the clinical therapeutics uses is responsible to draw the research-oriented observation of scientists to contemplate throughout the herbal hits for the acts like potential drugs for various diseases, such as cancers and tumors. In this review, we will cover all about the terms related to a scientific perspective based on successful clinically approach phytochemical like anti-tumors, anticancer drugs. Furthermore, to enhance this research-oriented data space between botanists, oncological researchers, and clinical biologists, we also add the synthetic chemistry analysis to spot the target of the genome, proteome-based study, and efficient drug conveyance framework has made it simpler for the researcher to build up phytochemicals as an efficient anticancer medication in future purposes.

Keywords Phytochemicals · Medicinal plants · Therapeutics uses · Anticancer

1 Introduction

In this modern era cancer is the most prevalent disorder causing great and irreparable damage resulting in the death of millions of people every year. As the presence of advanced techniques in the modern area still these techniques are not providing a helping hand that's why becoming a challenge for the medical world of this era. According to research by the UK research center conducted in 2019 which shows

M. M. Fareed (✉)
Faculty of Life Sciences, Department of Bioinformatics and Biotechnology, Government College University, Faisalabad, Pakistan
e-mail: mmazharfareed22@gcuf.edu.pk

M. M. Ali
Faisal Institute of Health Sciences Faisalabad, Affiliated with Government College University Faisalabad, Faisalabad, Pakistan

K. Raza (ed.), *Computational Intelligence in Oncology*, Studies in Computational Intelligence 1016, https://doi.org/10.1007/978-981-16-9221-5_19

a mortality rate of more than 5000 people as they were diagnosed with cervical cancer, furthermore, other cancer ratios are higher than this one. As in 2018 patients diagnosed with cancer died resulting in a mortality rate of about 9.1 million people and still, cases are reported day by day. According to this ratio, just after 30 years later in 2050 mortality rate will be increased up to 28.5 billion people diagnosed with cancer approximately [1, 2]. It is predicted that there will be 27.5 million new cancer diagnosed cases worldwide each year by 2040 if the recent trend keeps in the incidence of major cancers with respect to population growth seen globally by Cancer Research UK [3, 4].

The major factor in initiating cancer, as reported was uncontrolled symmetric cell division which induces tumor genesis (cancer cells formation) well known as carcinogenesis. The purpose is to produce anticancer drugs/antineoplastic drugs that help to cure cancer by stopping symmetric/asymmetric cell division resulting in increased uptake of body phosphorus causing tumor genesis. As a traditional approach for the production of anticancer drugs is time-consuming and expensive. Thus, we aim to search for non-expensive and time-saving drugs like the production of drug compounds from the medicinal plant; they are low cost as compared to conventional synthetic compounds. Thus, we use phytochemicals for anticancer drugs which are of two types; primary phytochemicals and secondary phytochemicals include polyphenols, terpenoids, thiols, and other nitrogen-containing compounds [5, 6]. Mainly phytochemicals act as antioxidants because they have the ability to provide cell protection that can cause cancer thus used in anticancer activities. There is a wide variety of phytochemicals that plays a therapeutic role against different type of tumor-causing cells like *organosulphur compounds, nitrogen-containing compounds, polyphenols, lignin, chlorophyllin, furyl compounds, proteins-peptides, and thiophenes*, etc. Plants synthesize different types of secondary metabolites against biotic and abiotic stress [7]. Thus, these metabolites are derived from plants and used to prepare anticancer drugs like we derive *atropine taxol, vinblastine, and topotecan* were in clinical studies via in-vivo, in-silico, and in-vitro aspects [8, 9].

In this chapter, all phytochemicals are screened through in-silico approaches by using various natural product-based compounds, natural phytochemicals compound like; PubChem-database, ZINC database, MPD3 database, Chinese medicinal compounds phytochemicals, and different drug-ligand databases using Molecular Operating Environment (MOE) software for docked [10]. Also, we will be investigating the effective and successful plant-based phytochemical anti-tumor and anticancer drugs and the future perspective in the emerging era via drug-screened therapies in the form of screening phytochemicals and advancement of the drug system such as; drug design (computer-aided drug design CADD) in various phytochemicals like alkaloids, flavonoids, and others are already mentioned in this chapter, specific cell type function against different types of cancer, production of anti-tumor phytochemical drugs will be discussed and mentioned in Fig. 1.

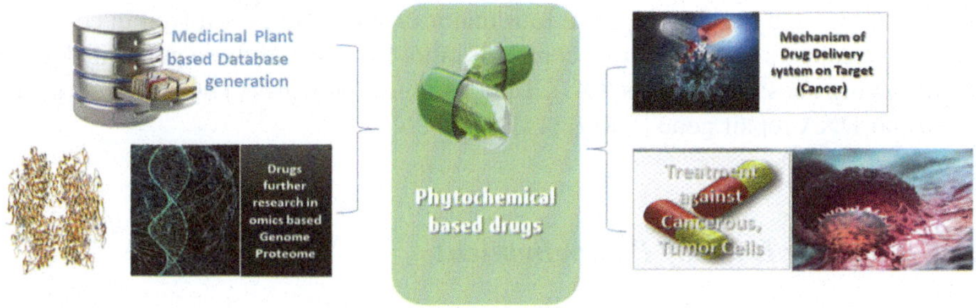

Fig. 1 The systematic diagram related to drug conveyance framework in different anticancer medication

2 Phytochemical-Based Treatment of Tumor and Cancer

2.1 Cancer, Tumor Cell Processing

Cell division can be measured as cell growth and proliferation. For the proper functioning of cells, tissues, and organs, this process must be controlled very wisely. When cells begin to multiply, their high speed and uncontrolled outcomes may be devastating. In advance of a cell division process to begin through semiconservative replication of DNA molecules, a copy of one strand is made and then each strand, in turn, is transferred to daughter cells that are genetically comparable to each other. In cell division, hundreds of various proteins are involved and some of them give information regarding cell division. Some of them show exquisite care for the replication of DNA. So that DNA can be replicated properly [10]. But most of them are involved in the process of cell division and are responsible for the separation of chromosomes toward the poles and the number of cells was doubled. Currently, cancer is considered a human catastrophe. Deaths caused by cancer are increasing gradually day by day. As cancer is the uncontrolled development of eccentric cells in the body. New methods seem to be designed to cure and stop cancer [11]. Control and survival of the cell are essential in cancer organization and treatment. Apoptosis is the programmed death of unauthorized and non-functional cells in the body. As for cancerous cells, they do not undergo apoptosis resulting in the administration of anticancer agents to put an end to cancerous cells while producing side effects on healthy cells and to reduce those side effects alternative therapeutic approaches were recommended side by side with the anticancer drug administration. Apoptosis is a series of morphological changes in the cell and organs that involve cell condensation and rapid budding that have undergone apoptosis are also well-maintained cell organelles. Induction of apoptosis is a marker for anti-toxic and anticancer drugs. Some common substances such as plant-mined metabolites use various mechanisms to produce apoptosis in cancerous cells that are blocked. Mixtures of plant extracts such as podophyllotoxin, vinca alkaloid compounds have been used in cancer treatment [12, 13]. But usually due to uncontrolled cell division, it is associated with one or several mutated genes. There are four major types of genes involved in cell division; most cancers have defective copies of more than one of these genes including the following ones: Oncogenes (OG), Tumor suppressor genes (TSG), Suicide genes (SG), and DNA repair gene (DRG) [14].

2.2 Looking Back of Phytochemical

Approximately 5000 years ago, the most ancient text embedded in the Sumerian clay slab was found from the Asian part (i.e., India and Nagpur). It states the practice of medicinal plants, as it comprises therapeutics detail about the usage of poppy, henbane, and mandrake. Subsequently, embedded in ancient Chinese literature older evidence of medicinal plants was demonstrated by "*Shen-Nung*" (the father of Chinese medicine) 2695 BCE. Furthermore, a Greek botanist "*Pedanius Dioscorides*" wrote a book on the uses of medicinal plants *"De Materia Medica"* which comprises a total of five-volume [8, 11]. His work was immensely successful and was employed as a physician in the Roman army. During the Islamic golden age, the legacy of the Roman Empire was carried by "Ibn al Baitar". He (Islamic scholar) mentioned more than a thousand medicinal plants in his book, *"Liber Magnae Collectionis Simplicum Alimentorum Et Medicamentorum*". The emergence of advanced synthetic chemistry in the early nineteenth century enables us to interpret the mechanism, isolation, and synthesis of active compounds from medicinal plants. While in the twentieth century, research on medicinal plants did not go forward. The pharmaceutical industry's reluctance about plant-based components has prompted a major change in focus on drug development from plant to synthetic chemistry [8].

2.3 Phytochemical-Based Anticancer Drugs

Till now, many thousands of plant species with distinguished anticancer potential have been reported. *Catharanthus roseus G* and *Madagascar periwinkle*-like plants are isolated for different chemo drugs like; vinca alkaloids and vinblastine, which are being used to treat cancer. Another big accomplishment via natural ingredients drug discovery is *Taxaceae*, obtained from the bark of Pacific Yew, also known as *Taxus brevifolia Nutt* from which scientists discover paclitaxel (Taxol) "*a type of chemotherapy drug used to treat cancer*" [12]. The usage of many parts of this plant and its other species (e.g., *Taxus baccata* L.) were identified by several Native American Tribes. They ignite the concept of indigenous knowledge-based medicinal plants. A derivative of ellipticine is isolated from a Fijian medicinal plant that is *Elliptinium. Bleekeria-vitensis* used for treating cancer [13]. Therapeutic plants have been utilized from the start of human development, which is generally apparent from the old content and conventional homegrown medication formula. In spite of the generally enhanced exhibit about the utilization of plants as therapeutics, the drug enterprises need an interest in phytochemical research contrasted and engineered drugs. For the most part, the shortfall of data about plant-based restorative therapeutics is mindful to draw the consideration of analysts to consider normal items expected medication for impeding sicknesses, like malignant growth [8].

2.4 Leading Role of the Phytochemicals

To find drug targets and unparallel changes in the drug delivery system cutting edge, drug design technique is used to accelerate with the recent advancement of numerous medicinal plant databases from local and global researchers. Due to advancements in the recent years of genomics, proteomics, transcriptomics, and metabolomics; it is simpler than ever to find out the target of potential phytochemicals. The final frontier of the use of natural products as cancer treatment relies on an effective drug delivery system [14, 15]. Luckily, the emergence of nanotechnology and its usage in the drug delivery system made rapid progress in all biological terminology of this area over the last few years.

2.5 Phytochemicals as a Source of Anticancer Agents

2.5.1 Phenolics

In fruits, secondary phenolic metabolites are widely present. As more than one aromatic ring is observed along with one or more hydroxyl groups in these compounds. The key phenolic compounds found in foods are divided into three categories: simple phenols, hydroxycinnamic acid derivatives, and flavonoids. In addition to defense mechanisms against pathogens, parasites, and natural enemies they also play an important role in plant growth and reproduction. The main attribute to their antioxidant capacity and ability to prevent certain diseases is the increased activity of these compounds [16]. Interestingly, health benefits can be achieved by daily consumption and bioavailability of phytochemicals. Simple phenols are the pioneers of the fusion of other compounds such as flavonoids and tannins. They act as a natural defensive system for the plants in order to avoid infectious diseases and thus decrease the growth of pathogenic bacteria, viruses, and fungi. They include a large group of the following: monophenols, diphenols, 3-ethyl phenols, 3,4-dimethylphenols which are also called simple phenols. Hydroxycinnamic acids and their esterified derivatives in fruits and vegetables derive exclusively from p-coumaric acid (PCA), caffeic acid (CA), and ferulic acid (FA). They are also present in conjugated forms, usually as esters rather than glycosides. Hydroxycinnamic acid derivatives such as chlorogenic acid, coumaric acid, caffeic acid, and sinapic acid are the most essential phytochemicals in plant food powders. Subsequently, by adding these food plant powders (that are rich in bioactive phytochemicals) they have a positive impact on food reformulations helping in improving both food quality and health approval properties. By doing so will automatically improve the intake of plant-based foods as they are beneficial for human health. Flavonoids have strong antioxidant activity and are an important class of phenolic compounds. These compounds reduce the risk of serious chronic diseases and are widely used in fruits, vegetables, and other plant foods. More than 4000 different flavonoids are known yet. They also have the usual structure, usually containing an oxidized heterocycle or ring C with two aromatic rings (rings A and B) bonded by three carbon atoms. Flavonoids, flavanols (catechins), iso-flavonoids, and anthocyanins belong to different types of flavonoids [17].

2.5.2 Organosulfur Compounds

Organic sulfur compounds are organic in origin. And can be identified by its sulfur-containing functional group. Regular use of organic sulfur compounds has biological activity, which is mainly related to the health of the cardiovascular system. Wattenberg et al. have evaluated the ability of many organosulfur compounds to prevent cancer. They are stimulated by N-Nitrosodiethylamine, and the strongest organic taurine compound is diallyl-disulfide. To prevent cancer, the ability of natural products from cruciferous plants and allium members is considered significant. Furthermore, these vegetables have been extensively studied in many studies. Watercress, broccoli, and Chinese cabbage are some examples of vegetables rich in organic sulfur compounds (OSC) [18].

2.5.3 Carotenoids

Carotenoids are the most important natural pigments and are widely noted for their pro-vitamins and antioxidant properties. Over 600 carotenoids are found in nature. They can come from animals, microbes, or plants. Carotenoids have an isoprene-based skeleton containing 40 carbon atoms. Their structures have multiple degrees of hydrogenation and can be cyclized at one or both ends that maintain oxygen-containing functional groups. Usually, carotenoid compounds are found in "*trans*" form in nature. The long sequence is their most typical feature. In the center of the molecule, conjugated double bonds are observed. The shape, chemical reactivity, and light absorption properties of this compound are impressive. Carotenoids can react with free radicals and can generate further free radicals by themselves. The presence of sufficient amounts of carotenoids can inhibit lipid oxidation and related oxidative stress [19, 20].

2.5.4 Alkaloids

These are the group of ring structures composed of nitrogen-containing organic compounds with a wide range of anticancer effects. They play a role as tumor suppressors by inhibiting topoisomerase activity. This activity is involved in apoptosis, DNA mimicry, and induction of p53 gene expression. However, alkaloids existed even before the appearance of mankind. Furthermore, some of them are similar in structural composition to the neurotransmitters of the human central nervous system. Given the therapeutic value of alkaloids and explaining their role in cell replication in nature, they will be used as effective chemopreventive agents in modern drug invention [21]. Here are the main categories of Alkaloids: *Betalain alkaloids, diterpenoid alkaloids, indole alkaloids, iso-quinoline alkaloids, lycopodium alkaloids, peptide alkaloids, quinoline alkaloids, pyrrolizidine alkaloids, steroidal alkaloids, tropane alkaloids,* and *miscellaneous alkaloids* [22].

2.5.5 Flavonoids

These compounds are a group of natural substances with different phenolic structures. Mainly found in fruits, vegetables, grains, bark, roots, stems, flowers, tea, and wine. These natural products are widely known for their benefits, and efforts have been made to isolate specific components called flavonoids. It is known to be an essential ingredient in various dietary supplements, pharmaceuticals, medical purposes, and a wide range of cosmetic applications. This is because flavonoids show antioxidant, anti-inflammatory, anti-mutagenic, and anticancer properties and also have the ability to regulate the activity of major cell enzymes [23, 24].

Low mortality from cardiovascular disease and the discovery of cancer prevention drugs have fueled research on flavonoids. The information on present procedures of flavonoids is still not understood well. Though this has been broadly recognized for decades and plant-based derivatives have a wide range of biological activities. Current trends in flavonoid research and development include the isolation, detection, characterization, action of flavonoids, and ultimately, their health benefits. The knowledge of molecular docking and bioinformatics is also used to predict potential applications and is applied in various industries. Flavonoids are secondary metabolites of plants, which can cause color and fragrance of flowers and have antiviral, antibacterial, anti-inflammatory, anti-allergic, and antioxidant properties. In the process of carcinogenesis, flavonoids interfere with a variety of signal transduction pathways, leading to limited proliferation, metastasis, angiogenesis, and apoptosis promotion [25]. The different phytochemicals and natural products and their therapeutic uses in various cancers are shown in Table 1 and other plant-based derivatives against the cancerous cells are also shown in Table 2.

Table 1 The different phytochemicals and natural products and their therapeutic uses in various cancer

S. No.	Phytochemicals/natural product	Phytochemical categories	Source/plant/ Scientific name	Therapeutic uses	References
1	Vindesine	Alkaloids	*Catharanthus roseus*	Leukemias, testicular, breast, and lung cancer	[26]
2	Vincristine, Vinblastine	Alkaloids	*Catharanthus roseus*	Lymphocytic leukemia	[26]
3	5-Fluorouracil	Flavonoids	*Withania somnifera*	Human cervical cancer cell	[27]
4	Skimmianine, Colchicine	Alkaloids	*Colchicum autumnale, Aegle marmelos*	Hodgkin's lymphoma, chronic granulocytic leukemia cancers cells, and liver cancer	[28]
5	Harmine, Bullatacin	Alkaloids	*Annona squamosa, Peganum harmala*	Breast, Liver cancer	[29]
6	Larotaxel, Cabazitaxel, Paclitaxel	Alkaloids	*Taxus baccata*	Breast, bladder, Prostate cancer, and pancreatic ovarian cancer	[29, 30]
7	Solamargine	Alkaloids	*Solanum nigrum*	Breast, liver, lung, and skin cancer	[31]
8	Bryophyllin A	Alkaloids	*Bryophyllum pinnatum*	Cervical cancer	[32]
9	Artemisinin	Flavonoids	*Artemisia annua*	Liver, breast, and pancreatic cancer	[37]
10	Silymarin, Luteolin, Chrysin	Flavonoids	*Sylibum marianum, Capsicum annuum, Passiflora caerulea*	Colorectal cancer	[33, 34]
11	Psoralidin	Alkaloids	*Psoralea corylifolia*	Stomach and prostate cancer	[35]
12	Silibinin	Alkaloids	*Sylibum marianum*	Ovary, cervix, colon, liver, skin, prostate, and urinary cancer	[36]
13	Prunol, Ursolic acid	Terpenoids	*Oldenlandia diffusa*	Uterus, stomach, liver, colon, ovary, rectum, prostate esophagus, and brain cancer	[37]

(continued)

Table 1 (continued)

S. No.	Phytochemicals/natural product	Phytochemical categories	Source/plant/ Scientific name	Therapeutic uses	References
14	Cyanidin, Gallic acid	Phenolics	*Leea indica, V. vinifera*	Ehrlich ascites carcinoma cancer types,	[38]
15	Thymoquinone, Withaferin D, A	Flavonoids	*Nigella sativa, Withania somnifera*	Colon, prostate, breast, and pancreas cancer	[39]
16	Podophyllotoxin	Alkaloids	*Podophyllum peltatum*, hexandrum	Non-small-cell lung carcinoma, testis, bladder cancer	[40]
17	Betulinic acid	Terpenoids, Alkaloids	*M. oliefera*	Malignant melanoma cancer, Blood Cancer	[41]
18	Colchicine	Alkaloids	*Colchicum autumnale, Gloriosa superba*	Anticancer	[42]
19	Phenolic based	Phenols	Hydroxybenzene	Chemical carcinogens, chemical nucleophiles, promotion inhibitors	[43]
20	Vitex, Schizophyllan	Alkaloids	Vitexagnus-castu, *S. commune*	Human uterine, head, and neck cancer	[44, 45]
21	Carotenoids, nitrogen-based compounds	Terpenoids	Tetraterpenoids	Metabolic inhibitors	[46]
22	Resveratrol	Phenols	Polyphenol	Pancreatic cancer stem cell-breast-cancer	[47]
23	Vinblastine, Vincristine	Alkaloids	Periwinkle plant *Catharanthus roseus*	Anticancer	[26]
24	Alkaloids	Alkaloids	*Trychnos nux-vomica* L.	Tumor metabolism, inhibitor of cell growth	[48]
25	Podophyllotoxin	Phenols	Podophyllum species	Anticancer	[49]

3 Conclusion

In the phytochemical-based study, we conclude as potential anticancer therapeutics with the help of previous studies has demonstrated infesting way, however the devolution of the natural-based products on drug discovery, delivery, and expansion ways via regularized well documented, and modernized study according to

Table 2 The plant derivatives, extracted compounds, their target cancer cells and anti-proliferative

Plant species	Extracted compound	Target cancer cell line	References
Soap bark tree (*Quillaja saponaria*)	Saponin	Breast, colon, and skin cancer cells	[50]
Potato (*Solanum tuberosum*)	Gallic acid	Prostate cancer cells	[51]
Blue Berries (*Vaccinium corymbosum*)	Anthocyanin	Colon cancer cells	[52]
Cardus marianus (*Silybum marianum*)	Isosilybin A	Prostate cancer cells	[53]
Pea (*Pisum sativum*)	Cajanistilbene acid	Breast cancer cells	[54]
Ginger (*Zingiber officinale*)	Curcumin	Ovarian cancer cells	[55]
Grapes (*Vitis vinifera*)	Resveratrol	Breast cancer cells	[56]
Lemon (Citrus × sinensis)	Naringenin	Hepatocellular carcinoma cells	[57]
Pigeon pea (*Canjanus cajan*)	Cajanin stilbene acid	Breast cancer cells	[58]

research system requirements through literature. In this review, we will take the maximum possibilities for a researcher, biologists from the prehistory of herbal, traditional phytochemical-based medicinal work to the modern era including; purification, depth study roots, isolation of the phytochemicals, identification, production of biosynthesis compounds, via *in-silico, in-vivo, in-vitro*, drug delivery system analysis and also efficient and therapeutics agents against different types of cancer and tumor.

References

1. Tay, K.-C., et al. (2019). Formononetin: A review of its anticancer potentials and mechanisms. *Frontiers in Pharmacology, 10*.
2. Shahriyari, L., & Komarova, N. L. (2013). Symmetric vs. asymmetric stem cell divisions: an adaptation against cancer? *PloS One, 8*(10), e76195.
3. Park, C., et al. (2019). Induction of G2/M cell cycle arrest and apoptosis by genistein in human bladder cancer T24 cells through inhibition of the ROS-dependent PI3k/Akt signal transduction pathway. *Antioxidants, 8*(9), 327.
4. Rayan, A., Raiyn, J., & Falah, M. (2017). Nature is the best source of anticancer drugs: Indexing natural products for their anticancer bioactivity. *PloS One, 12*(11), e0187925.
5. Fridlender, M., Kapulnik, Y., & Koltai, H. (2015). Plant derived substances with anti-cancer activity: From folklore to practice. *Frontiers in Plant Science, 6*, 799.
6. Manara, A. (2012). Plant responses to heavy metal toxicity. *Plants and heavy metals* (pp. 27–53). Springer.
7. Gohlke, J., & Deeken, R. (2014). Plant responses to Agrobacterium tumefaciens and crown gall development. *Frontiers in Plant Science, 5*, 155.

8. Ashraf, M. A. (2020). Phytochemicals as potential anticancer drugs: time to ponder nature's bounty. *BioMed Research International, 2020*.
9. Efferth, T., et al. (2007). From traditional Chinese medicine to rational cancer therapy. *Trends in Molecular Medicine, 13*(8), 353–361.
10. Vilar, S., Cozza, G., & Moro, S. (2008). Medicinal chemistry and the molecular operating environment (MOE): Application of QSAR and molecular docking to drug discovery. *Current Topics in Medicinal Chemistry, 8*(18), 1555–1572.
11. Kelly, K. (2009). *History of medicine, facts on file* (p. 10001). New York NY.
12. Rowinsky, E. K., & Donehower, R. C. (1995). Paclitaxel (taxol). *New England Journal of Medicine, 332*(15), 1004–1014.
13. Gouyette, A. (1988). Synthesis of deuterium-labelled elliptinium and its use in metabolic studies. *Biomedical & Environmental Mass Spectrometry, 15*(5), 243–247.
14. Langer, R. (1990). New methods of drug delivery. *Science, 249*(4976), 1527–1533.
15. Liu, R. H. (2004). Potential synergy of phytochemicals in cancer prevention: Mechanism of action. *The Journal of Nutrition, 134*(12), 3479S-3485S.
16. King, A., & Young, G. (1999). Characteristics and occurrence of phenolic phytochemicals. *Journal of the American Dietetic Association, 99*(2), 213–218.
17. Decker, E. A. (1997). Phenolics: Prooxidants or antioxidants? *Nutrition Reviews, 55*(11), 396–398.
18. Reddy, B. S., et al. (1993). Chemoprevention of colon carcinogenesis by organosulfur compounds. *Cancer Research, 53*(15), 3493–3498.
19. Britton, G. (1996). Carotenoids. *Natural food colorants* (pp. 197–243). Springer.
20. Britton, G., Liaaen-Jensen, S., & Pfander, H. (2012). *Carotenoids: Handbook*. Birkhäuser.
21. Robinson, T. (1974). Metabolism and function of alkaloids in plants. *Science, 184*(4135), 430–435.
22. Herbert, R. B. (2001). The biosynthesis of plant alkaloids and nitrogenous microbial metabolites. *Natural Product Reports, 18*(1), 50–65.
23. Iwashina, T. (2000). The structure and distribution of the flavonoids in plants. *Journal of Plant Research, 113*(3), 287.
24. Samanta, A., Das, G., & Das, S. K. (2011). Roles of flavonoids in plants. *Carbon, 100*(6), 12–35.
25. Abotaleb, M., et al. (2019). Flavonoids in cancer and apoptosis. *Cancers, 11*(1), 28.
26. Cragg, G. M., & Newman, D. J. (2005). Plants as a source of anti-cancer agents. *Journal of Ethnopharmacology, 100*(1–2), 72–79.
27. Yadav, B., et al. (2010). In vitro anticancer activity of the root, stem and leaves of *Withania somnifera* against various human cancer cell lines. *Indian Journal of Pharmaceutical Sciences, 72*(5), 659.
28. Lin, X., Peng, Z., & Su, C. (2015). Potential anti-cancer activities and mechanisms of costunolide and dehydrocostuslactone. *International Journal of Molecular Sciences, 16*(5), 10888–10906.
29. Biba, V., Jeba, M., & Remani, P. (2013). Differential effects of Annona Squamosa seed extracts: Antioxidant, antibacterial, cytotoxic and apoptotic study. *International Journal of Pharma and Bio Sciences, 4*, 899–907.
30. Atkinson, J. M., et al. (2010). Development of a novel tumor-targeted vascular disrupting agent activated by membrane-type matrix metalloproteinases. *Cancer Research, 70*(17), 6902–6912.
31. Al Sinani, S. S., et al. (2016). Solamargine triggers cellular necrosis selectively in different types of human melanoma cancer cells through extrinsic lysosomal mitochondrial death pathway. *Cancer Cell International, 16*(1), 1–12.
32. Mahata, S., et al. (2012). Anticancer property of *Bryophyllum pinnata* (Lam.) Oken. leaf on human cervical cancer cells. *BMC Complementary and Alternative Medicine, 12*(1), 15.
33. Osman, N. H., et al. (2015). Luteolin supplementation adjacent to aspirin treatment reduced dimethylhydrazine-induced experimental colon carcinogenesis in rats. *Tumor Biology, 36*(2), 1179–1190.

34. León, I. E., et al. (2015). Oxidovanadium (IV) complexes with chrysin and silibinin: Anticancer activity and mechanisms of action in a human colon adenocarcinoma model. *JBIC Journal of Biological Inorganic Chemistry, 20*(7), 1175–1191.
35. Pahari, P., et al. (2016). Synthesis of psoralidin derivatives and their anticancer activity: First synthesis of Lespeflorin I1. *Tetrahedron, 72*(23), 3324–3334.
36. Rastogi, N., et al. (2015). Proteasome inhibition mediates p53 reactivation and anti-cancer activity of 6-gingerol in cervical cancer cells. *Oncotarget, 6*(41), 43310.
37. Woźniak, Ł, Skąpska, S., & Marszałek, K. (2015). Ursolic acid—A pentacyclic triterpenoid with a wide spectrum of pharmacological activities. *Molecules, 20*(11), 20614–20641.
38. Lim, D. Y., & Park, J. H. Y. (2009). Induction of p53 contributes to apoptosis of HCT-116 human colon cancer cells induced by the dietary compound fisetin. *American Journal of Physiology-Gastrointestinal and Liver Physiology, 296*(5), G1060–G1068.
39. Tu, L.-Y., et al. (2016). Synthesis, characterization and anticancer activity of kaempferol-zinc (II) complex. *Bioorganic & Medicinal Chemistry Letters, 26*(11), 2730–2734.
40. Liu, Y. Q., et al. (2015). Recent progress on C-4-modified podophyllotoxin analogs as potent antitumor agents. *Medicinal Research Reviews, 35*(1), 1–62.
41. Mishra, S., et al. (2014). Phytochemical, therapeutic, and ethnopharmacological overview for a traditionally important herb: *Boerhavia diffusa* Linn. *BioMed Research International, 2014.*
42. Bundela, S., Sharma, A., & Bisen, P. S. (2015). Potential compounds for oral cancer treatment: Resveratrol, nimbolide, lovastatin, bortezomib, vorinostat, berberine, pterostilbene, deguelin, andrographolide, and colchicine. *PloS One, 10*(11), e0141719.
43. Rice-Evans, C., Miller, N., & Paganga, G. (1997). Antioxidant properties of phenolic compounds. *Trends in Plant Science, 2*(4), 152–159.
44. Mukherjee, A. K., et al. (2001). Advances in cancer therapy with plant based natural products. *Current Medicinal Chemistry, 8*(12), 1467–1486.
45. Smith, J., Rowan, N., & Sullivan, R. (2002). *Medicinal mushrooms: Their therapeutic properties and current medical usage with special emphasis on cancer treatments.* Cancer Research UK London.
46. Gil, M. I., et al. (2002). Antioxidant capacities, phenolic compounds, carotenoids, and vitamin C contents of nectarine, peach, and plum cultivars from California. *Journal of Agricultural and Food Chemistry, 50*(17), 4976–4982.
47. Athar, M., et al. (2007). Resveratrol: A review of preclinical studies for human cancer prevention. *Toxicology and Applied Pharmacology, 224*(3), 274–283.
48. Floss, H. G. (1976). Biosynthesis of ergot alkaloids and related compounds. *Tetrahedron, 32*(8), 873–912.
49. Imbert, T. (1998). Discovery of podophyllotoxins. *Biochimie, 80*(3), 207–222.
50. Shaker, K. H., et al. (1999). Triterpenoid saponins from Fagonia indica. *Phytochemistry, 51*(8), 1049–1053.
51. Yang, S.-A., et al. (2006). α-Chaconine, a potato glycoalkaloid, induces apoptosis of HT-29 human colon cancer cells through caspase-3 activation and inhibition of ERK 1/2 phosphorylation. *Food and Chemical Toxicology, 44*(6), 839–846.
52. Waring, P. (1990). DNA fragmentation induced in macrophages by gliotoxin does not require protein synthesis and is preceded by raised inositol triphosphate levels. *Journal of Biological Chemistry, 265*(24), 14476–14480.
53. Engelman, J. A. (2009). Targeting PI3K signalling in cancer: Opportunities, challenges and limitations. *Nature Reviews Cancer, 9*(8), 550–562.
54. Musgrove, E. A., & Sutherland, R. L. (2009). Biological determinants of endocrine resistance in breast cancer. *Nature Reviews Cancer, 9*(9), 631–643.
55. Azuine, M. A., & Bhide, S. V. (1992). Protective single/combined treatment with betel leaf and turmeric against methyl (acetoxymethyl) nitrosamine-induced hamster oral carcinogenesis. *International Journal of Cancer, 51*(3), 412–415.
56. Hodnick, W. F., Ahmad, S., & Pardini, R. S. (1998). *Induction of oxidative stress by redox active flavonoids. Flavonoids in the Living System*, pp. 131–150.

57. Arul, D., & Subramanian, P. (2013). Naringenin (citrus flavonone) induces growth inhibition, cell cycle arrest and apoptosis in human hepatocellular carcinoma cells. *Pathology & Oncology Research, 19*(4), 763–770.
58. Wu, N., et al. (2009). Antioxidant activities of extracts and main components of pigeonpea [*Cajanus cajan* (L.) Millsp.] leaves. *Molecules, 14*(3), 1032–1043.

Drug Response Prediction Using Machine Learning

Sarra Akermi, Sagarika Sahoo, Rishabh Panesar, Jean Bernard, Abira Dey, Ritushree Biswas, Surabhi Johari, Subrata Sinha, Chandramohan Jana, Ria Puri, Mitali Tarika, Sunil Jayant, and Anshul Nigam

Abstract The development of anti-cancerous drugs for the treatment of cancer is always a challenging task due to long-term drug-induced toxicological responses in the patients. Due to long-term chemotherapy, to treat cancer, the patients get drug overload, and therefore, it is particularly important to understand the medication, dosage, pharmacokinetics, and pharmacodynamics in the patient's body to avoid drug-induced toxicological and adverse drug reactions. In-vitro methods can provide valuable inputs regarding the nature of cancerous cells, that is the idea about gene expression and its modulation during treatment, but long-term monitoring is expensive. Therefore, there is a need to implement a low-cost method that takes care

---

Sarra Akermi, Sagarika Sahoo, Rishabh Panesar, Jean Bernard Idoipe authors contributed equally.

S. Akermi · R. Biswas · S. Jayant
Annotation Analytics Pvt. Ltd., 36, Ward no. 14, Biswa, Amarpura, Gurgaon, Haryana 122001, India

S. Sahoo · R. Panesar · A. Nigam (✉)
Amity University Mumbai, Bhatan Post-Somathne, Panvel, Mumbai, Maharashtra 410206, India
e-mail: anigam@mum.amity.edu

J. Bernard
Insight Biosolutions, 35000 Rennes, France
e-mail: jean.idoipe@insight-biosolutions.com

A. Dey
Indian Science and Technology Foundation (ISTF), C-1/131, Yamuna Vihar, New Delhi 110053, India
e-mail: abira.dey@isto-india.org

S. Johari · R. Puri · M. Tarika
Institute of Management, Studies University Courses Campus Ghaziabad, Ghaziabad, Uttar Pradesh 201002, India

S. Sinha
Centre for Biotechnology and Bioinformatics, Dibrugarh University, Dibrugarh, Assam 786001, India

C. Jana
Department of Chemistry, Michael Madhusudan Memorial College, Durgapur, West Bengal 713216, India

K. Raza (ed.), *Computational Intelligence in Oncology*, Studies in Computational Intelligence 1016, https://doi.org/10.1007/978-981-16-9221-5_20

of treatment, side effects, and drug-drug interaction in the cancer patient. Machine learning and artificial intelligence integrate the in-vivo patient data, chemical properties of the drugs, and cell culture studies which help in decision making to narrow down prescription and research.

Keywords Anti-cancerous · Chemotherapy · Drug · Artificial intelligence (AI) · Machine learning (ML)

1 Introduction

Cancer is one of the major diseases, which is responsible for the death of millions worldwide. Pharmaceutical industry and academia have developed many drugs targeting different cancers and approved by FDA [1]. Scientists from different R&D laboratories still working to understand the function and mechanism of these drugs to reduce the severe side effects caused by them. These drugs are designed to target specific proteins that are mutated to cause cancer. The development of these drugs takes a long time, where the first step is to identify the potential target. Once we validate the target, then the next step is to identify the lead compounds against the target that is responsible to cause cancer. The lead identification process involves the usage of computational methods such as high throughput computational screening by molecular docking and selection of best lead compounds by quantitative structure–activity relationship (QSAR) (Fig. 1). These leads are converged from millions of the compounds and hot leads after finding their good affinities with the targets. Prior to the advent of computational methods, entire screening was done in real-time, which was not only cumbersome, time-consuming, and expensive.

After the selection of the hot leads, the most crucial step in the drug response prediction is at the pre-clinical and clinical stages. At the pre-clinical stage, the drug is evaluated for its metabolism and toxicity at the in vitro or in vivo. However, these in-vitro assays are not cost-effective and consume lots of money to execute. Moreover, it

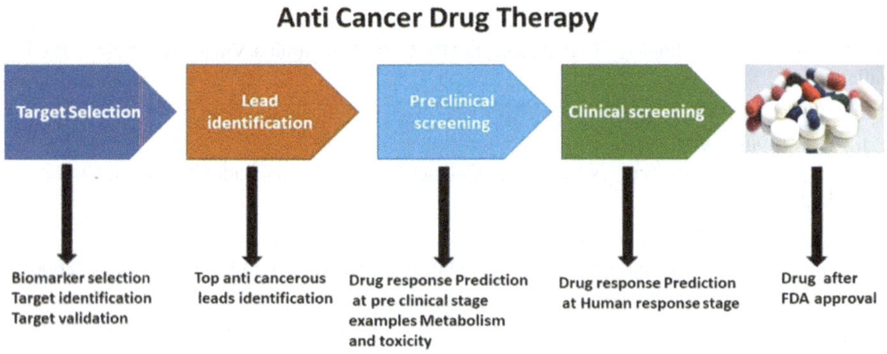

Fig. 1 Flow of anti-cancerous drug discovery

is very difficult to estimate the response of all the drug candidates. Another roadblock encountered during the treatment is due to drug-to-drug interaction which can be agonistic or antagonistic.

Therefore, there was a need to implement other alternative methods over existing computational methods. There has been an increasing trend to apply principles of ML and AI to predict the response of anti-cancerous drugs, over and above their targets while predicting side effects [2–6]. Due to the generation of a large amount of data during pre-clinical screening and at clinical trials stages, it is very difficult to draw a conclusion from it. Thanks to the application of ML and AI, the big amount of pre-clinical, clinical, and human patient data along with chemo-informatics can be integrated to develop powerful computational models that predict drug response and help in personalizing the treatment. Once the training model has been developed, then it could be validated by predicting drug response for the known anti-cancerous compounds and then extrapolated for mono or combinatory therapies for the treatment of cancer (Fig. 2).

The ML and AI are not only able to integrate a large amount of data (as mentioned above) but are also able to assemble data generated from genomic analysis, transcriptomics analysis, metabolomic analysis following the treatment with drug(s). ML and AI help in calculating drug response in terms of treatment and side effects which are crucial parameters in our fight against cancer (Fig. 3) [8].

There are several algorithms that have been developed for the implementation of ML and AI methods to predict drug response. These algorithms are an integral part of various software. In Table 1, the mathematical basis of a few algorithms that are used for analyzing drug response is mentioned.

These different methods are implemented in different software. Few important software's are based on machine learning algorithms (Table 2).

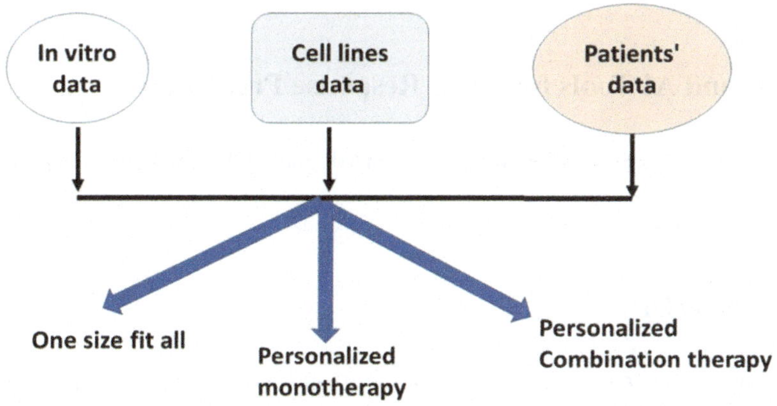

Fig. 2 Integration of the cell lines data for metabolisms and toxicity, and patient data for drug response in order to derive prediction models for designing monotherapies or a combination of the therapies [7]

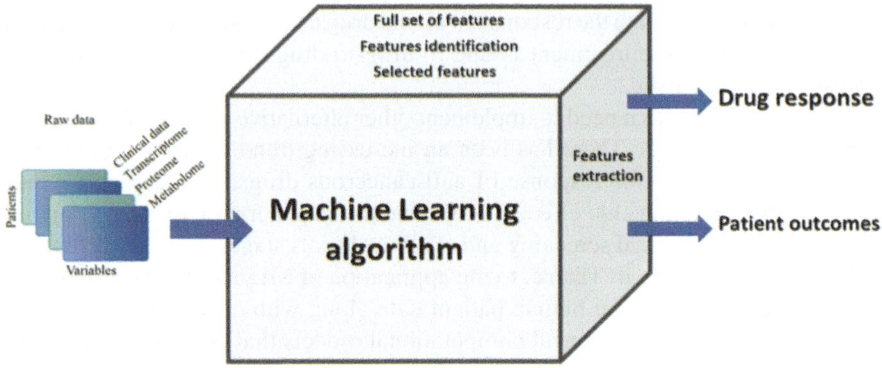

Fig. 3 Flow of data from the in-vitro end-points and patients' data to drug response prediction by integration using machine learning algorithms

Table 1 Machine learning methods for prediction of drug response

Methods	Advantage	Algorithms used	References
Linear regression model	Simple and significant precision and easy interpretation	Linear and logistic regression	[9]
Decision trees model (nonlinear)	Able to determine variability in the data interactions	CART and classification trees	[10]
Ensemble models (nonlinear)	Able to determine more complex interactions	Random forest	[11]
Neural network model (nonlinear)	Can capture non-associated complex interactions	Recurrent neural networks	[12]

2 ML and AI Tools for Drug Response Prediction

We are discussing a few online tools based on ML and AI that are helpful in predicting drug response.

2.1 *CancerDP*

CancerDP (*CancerDP: Prioritization of anti-cancer drugs (osdd.net)*) is a support vector machine (SVM)-based model which uses input data from genomic features (a) mutation, (b) variation, (c) expression, and [4] copy number variation. After giving these data as input, machine learning algorithms integrate the data and provide drug responses of 24 anti-cancer drugs. The platform is divided into three features: drug

Table 2 Table showing the important machine learning software

Software	Open source or commercial	Algorithms	Website
TensorFlow	Free, open source	Deep neural networks	https://www.tensorflow.org/
Shogun	Open source	Support vector machines and hidden Markov models	https://getshogun.com/
Apache Mahout	Open source	Linear algebra	https://mahout.apache.org/
Apache Spark MLlib	Open source	Classification, Naive Bayes, logistic regression Regression—linear, survival analysis Gradient boosting, LDA, topic modeling Decision trees, random forests, etc.	https://spark.apache.org/mllib/
PyTorch	Open source	Deep neural networks and tensors	https://pytorch.org/
Weka	Open source	Classification, clustering, regression, visualization as well as data preparation	https://www.weka.fr/
KNIME	Open source	Modular data pipelining concept	https://www.knime.com/

prioritization, drug calculator, and signatures [13]. The platform for CancerDP is shown in Fig. 4.

2.2 *Cancer Drug Response Profile Scan (CDRscan)*

CDRscan is a drug response model for the prediction of the response of anti-cancer based on the principle of deep learning. CDRscan is made from a combination of five convolutional neural networks (CNN) and develops the model after integration of all data, and it predicts the half-maximal inhibitory concentration (IC_{50}) values and correlated with the genomic data to predict the fate of the drug response as oncology or non-oncology drugs [14]. It contains data from a large number of drug screening assays which includes genomic profiling from 787 human cancer cell lines along with the data from 244 drugs which contain structural and physio-chemical data. It integrates the genomic and molecular modeling feature by in silico modeling of drug treatment.

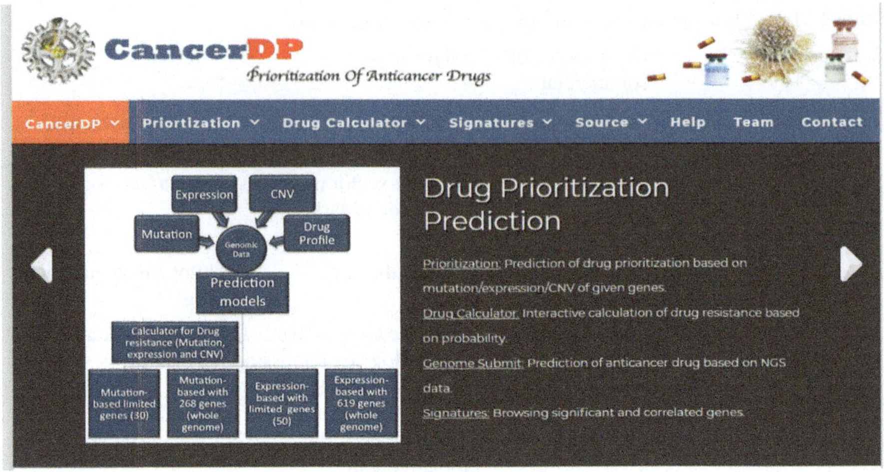

Fig. 4 Graphics of CanderDP platform [13]

2.3 DIGREM

Drug-induced genomic response models for identification of effective multi-drug combinations (DIGREM) is a Web-based platform that can enumerate drug synergies. This helps in narrowing down the most promising combinations. DIGREM assembles data coming from different models such as DIGRE, IUPUI-CCBB, gene set-based, and correlation-based models. These models are based on the principle that the drug synergy should disrupt functionally comparable genes, biological pathways, or cellular processes. DIGRE measures the relationship between drug X and drug Y. To exemplify when cell cultures are perturbed with the two drugs X and Y, how the changes in the transcriptome signatures caused by the first drug X will modify the effect of the second drug Y. The synergistic effects of two drugs can be used to simulate the effect of a medication combination. DIGREM is the first publicly available free software that uses transcriptome and dose–response data to evaluate synergistic drug pairings [15]. It will make it easier to find out the best possible medication from massive combinations available, as well as it will improve our knowledge of drug interactions (Fig. 5).

2.4 SynergyFinder

SynergyFinder is an interactive tool for assessing dosage response data for drug combinations. SynergyFinder 2.0, released in 2021, is better than its previous version as it allows for the study of both pairwise as well as multiple medications [16, 17].

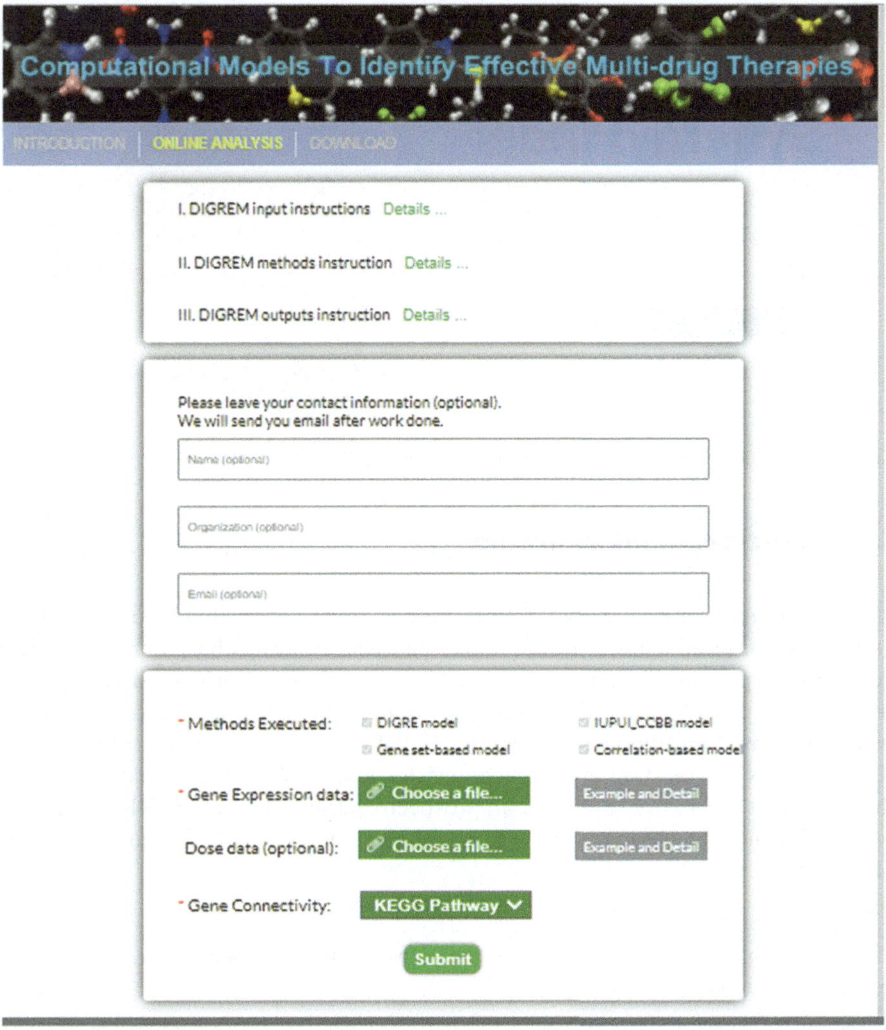

Fig. 5 DIGREM platform (https://lce.biohpc.swmed.edu/drugcombination/onlineAnalysis.php)

It includes novel and enhances multi-drug combination data analysis and visualization capabilities in response to the user demands. It calculates synergy ratings for higher-order combination data using reference synergy models HSA, Bliss, Loewe, and ZIP. These models measure synergistic and antagonistic (Loewe/ZIP) drug responses along with the independent response (HSA/Bliss). SynergyFinder has gained popularity as a tool for generating novel medications at the pre-clinical stage (Fig. 6).

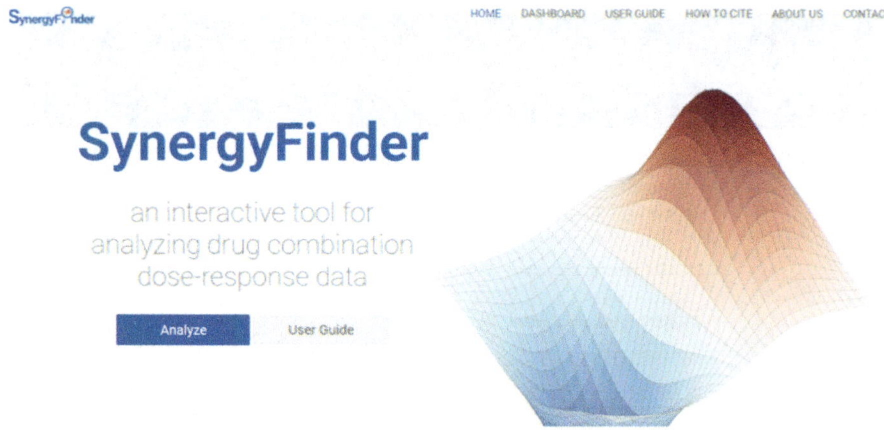

Fig. 6 SynergyFinder platform (https://synergyfinder.org/)

2.5 Kernelized Rank Learning

Kernelized rank learning (KRL) is a machine learning approach where data is integrated from several sources, differentiate, and classify drugs based on their effect per cell line (patient). It outperforms various state-of-the-art drug recommendation predictors, especially when the training dataset is sparse, and generalizes to patient data. The primary difference between KRL and other regression algorithms is that KRL predicts the top-ranking medications for a specific cell line (patient) rather than the exact sensitivity values for all prospective drugs [18]. When KRL is trained on cell line models, it can provide reasonable recommendations for cancer patients (Table 3).

Table 3 Biological-based drug response prediction models using machine learning

Models	Output	References
CancerDP	Provides drug response of 24 anti-cancer using data from different genomic features such as mutation, variation, expression, and copy number variation	[13]
CDRscan	Predicts IC_{50} values and correlated with the genomic data	[14]
DIGREM	Predicts drug synergies	[15]
SynergyFinder	Predicts enhanced multi-drug combination data analysis and visualization capabilities	[16, 17]
KRL	Predicts the top-ranking medications for a specific cell line (patient)	[18]

3 Case Study: Development of Genotoxicity Drug Response Prediction Using Machine Learning

Here, in this chapter, we are reporting a case study of a machine learning algorithm trained to predict the genotoxicity of anti-cancerous drugs.

3.1 Introduction

Genotoxins are chemicals that can cause damage to genetic materials within the cell. The genotoxins create several alterations on genetic materials, such as the mutation, chromosomal aberrations, mistimed event activation, etc. Permanent, genetic changes can influence either the organism's somatic cells or the transfer of germ cells to future generations, whereas this damage is mitigated by the cells either by repairing genetic material or by apoptosis mechanism (programmed cell death). But the damage contributed by genotoxins cannot always be prevented or fixed [19]. Damages caused by genotoxins can lead to carcinogenesis. Therefore, early detection of these genetic damages and knowledge about genotoxic chemicals is very important for taking necessary measures to counter them. Computational methods for envisaging genotoxicity on basis of chemical structures and properties are accepted as a low-cost alternative compared to expensive and rigorous laboratory tests. Therefore, we have explored machine learning algorithms to predict the genotoxicity of drugs anti-cancerous drugs.

ML and AI have the power to transform oncology by predicting the response of drugs even before they are used in real-life scenarios. The physio-chemical properties of drugs can be used to develop models which are able to find a pattern between the properties and the drug's response. Besides, ML also finds the relationship between the targets and the inputs, which will enable the researchers to understand how and what aspects of drugs needed to be altered to develop personalized drugs for best results in each case. Below we are discussing a case study of the application of ML by predicting the genotoxicity of anti-cancer drugs. ML models were prepared to classify drugs as genotoxic and non-genotoxic. In our case study work, the physio-chemical data of 442 drugs were collected from various open and reliable data sources.

3.2 Motivation

The main motivation behind this analysis is to develop a mechanism to help in predicting the potential genotoxic compounds based on their properties themselves. Several visualizations were created from the dataset, which showed that the genotoxic and non-genotoxic compounds exist in distinct clusters. Finally, a receiver operator characteristic curve was prepared to compare each model's performance.

Table 4 Features of the compounds from PubChem database

S. no.	Features	Descriptions
1	Compound name	Name of the compound, chemical formula, or SMILES
2	Molecular weight	Molecular weight of the molecules
3	XLOP3-AA	Log P-value
4	Hydrogen bond donor count	For the tendency to make Hydrogen bond formation
5	Hydrogen bond acceptor count	For the tendency to make Hydrogen bond formation
6	Rotatable bond count	For flexibility of the compound
7	Genotoxicity values (1 = Genotoxic, 0 = non-Genotoxic)	Assignment of genotoxicity classification
8	Topological polar surface area	Area of affinities

3.3 Methodology

First, we have selected a total of 442 compounds from the literature [20]. We obtained the physio-chemical properties of each compound from the PubChem database (https://pubchem.ncbi.nlm.nih.gov/).

The dataset had the following main features (Table 4):

From the above features, the genotoxicity value must be predicted or classified by the trained models. Since the target feature has two types of data, specifically 0 or 1, it is called categorical data (Figs. 7 and 8).

Data visualization: Scatter plots are plotted to compare each of the features of the dataset based on their genotoxicity value. The seaborn library of Python is used to create comprehensive visualization. After analysis of the above plot, it can be deduced that the genotoxic compounds (orange dots) and non-genotoxic compounds (blue dots) lie in distinct clusters (Fig. 9). Therefore, there is scope of classification between the two types. It is important to note that, majority of the genotoxic compounds are lighter in weight as compared to non-genotoxic compounds, genotoxic compounds have a smaller number of rotatable bond count as compared to non-genotoxic compounds and most of the non-genotoxic compounds have a high number of hydrogen bond donor and acceptor counts.

3.4 Model Selection, Training, Testing, and Prediction

Since the target feature is categorical data, the machine learning models need to perform the task of classification. There are multiple classification tasks that machine learning models can do. There are multiple classification tasks that machine learning models can do, to exemplify, classification predictive modeling, binary classification,

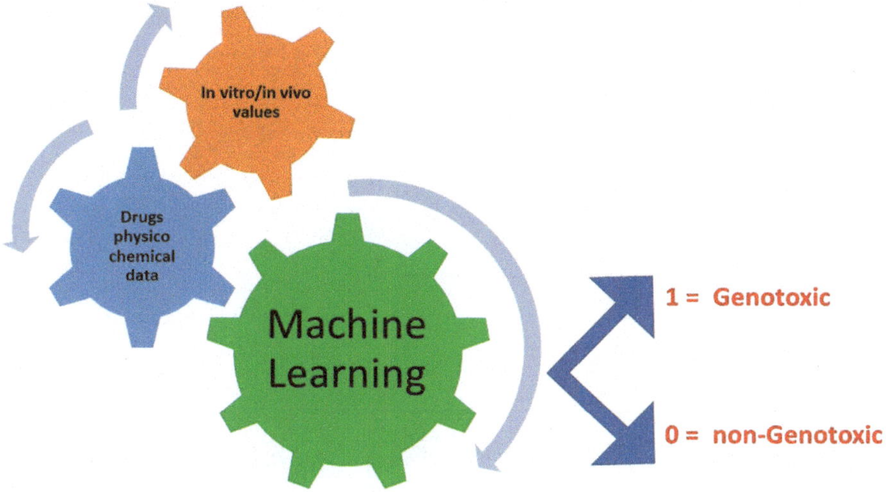

Fig. 7 Integration of in-vitro/in-vivo cell lines data, drugs physicochemical data using machine learning method to predict genotoxicity drug response prediction model

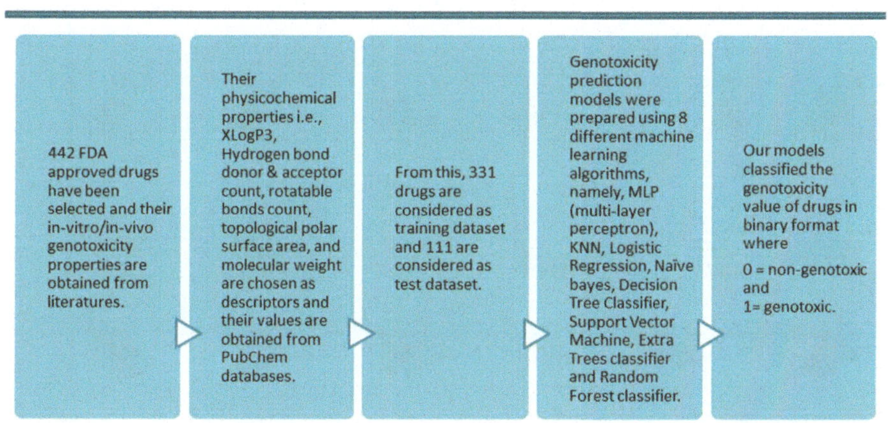

Fig. 8 Flow of methodology for developing the genotoxicity drug response prediction model

etc. Since in target features there are only two classes (0 & 1 or non-genotoxic and genotoxic) of compounds, a binary classification approach is suitable in this case. Various algorithms have been used to classify the compounds, and these are:

i. Logistic regression
ii. Multi-layer perceptron (neural network)
iii. K-nearest neighbor
iv. Naive Bayes
v. Decision tree classifier

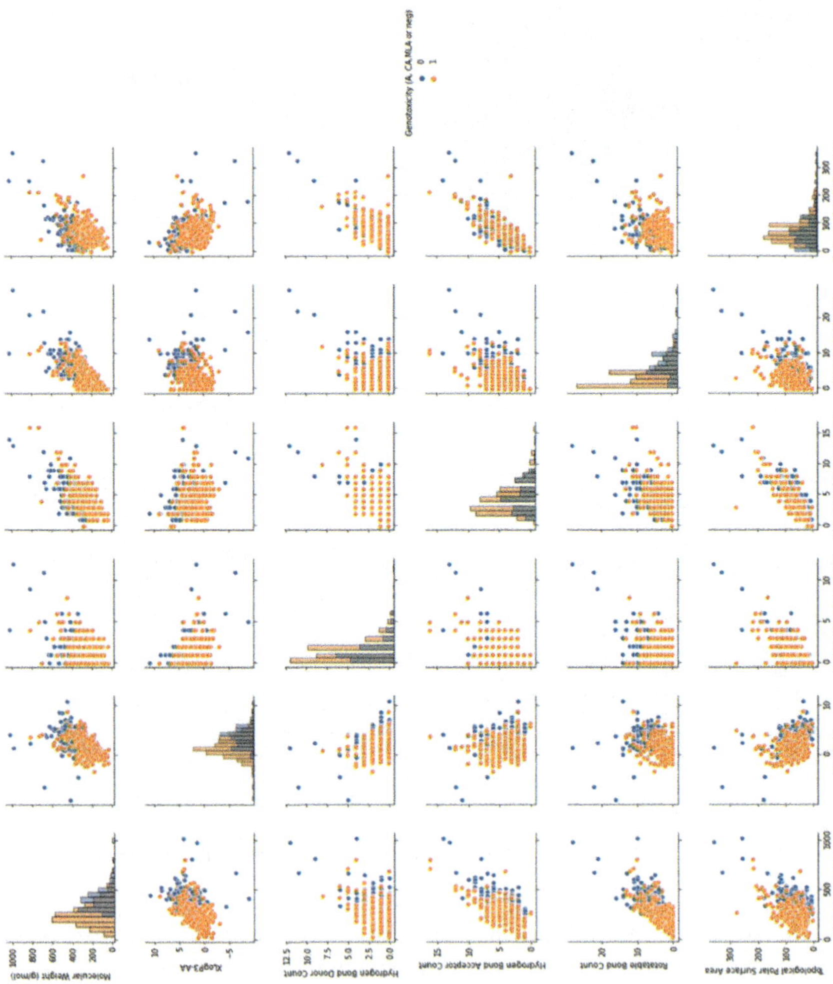

Fig. 9 Scatter plots are plotted to compare each of the features of the dataset based on their genotoxicity value

vi. Support vector machines
vii. Extra trees classifier
viii. Random forest classifier.

3.4.1 Logistic Regression Model

The logistic regression model is a popular algorithm that is taken directly from the field of statistics. This algorithm gets its name from the core function used in this model, the logistic function [22]. The logistic function is also known as the sigmoid function [21] and takes any real-valued number and maps it within the range of 0 to 1 (but never exactly equal to any of those limits) (Fig. 10).

$$\text{Logistic Function} = \frac{1}{(1 + e^{-x})}$$

Representation of logistic regression equation:

$$y = \frac{e^{(b_0 + b_1 x)}}{\left(1 + e^{(b_0 + b_1 x)}\right)}$$

where y is the prediction, b_0 is the intercept 1, and b_1 is the coefficient for the input value x.

The logistic regression model performed very well in classifying the compounds as genotoxic or non-genotoxic. The model scored an accuracy of 81.08%, specificity of 0.747, and sensitivity of 0.833. The data of sensitivity and specificity will be used further for evaluating the performance of all the models.

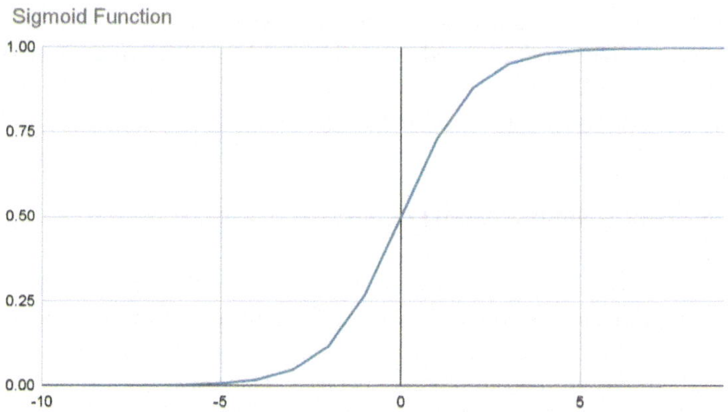

Fig. 10 Plot showing sigmoid function distribution

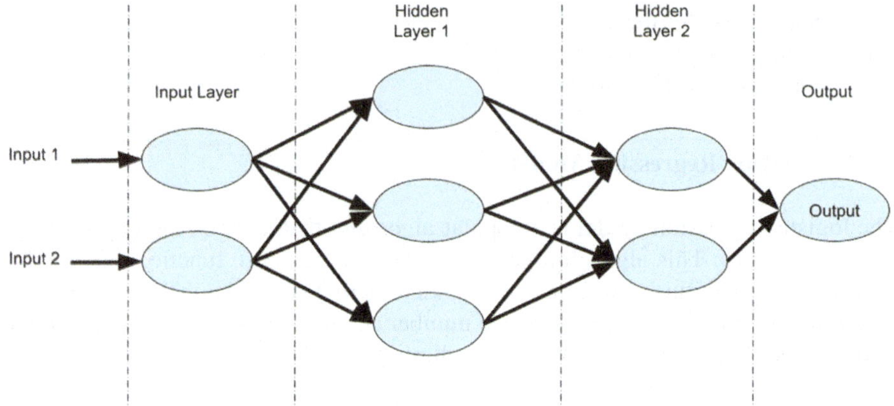

Fig. 11 Working of a multi-layer perceptron model

3.4.2 Multi-Layer Perceptron Model

This is a type of feedforward artificial neural network (ANN) model that learns from the errors made in each layer of the model and tries to correct them in the next layer. The predictions of this model depend on the learning rate, weights, and activation function (Fig. 11) [22].

The multi-layer perceptron compares the predicted value in each hidden layer with the actual value and uses the difference in predicted and actual value to correct itself and correctly predict the instances in the next layer, until it reaches the output layer where the algorithm makes the final prediction. Each layer is hidden from the other one in this algorithm, i.e., the inputs in one layer are not disclosed to the other layers.

The MLP model performed very well in classifying the compounds as genotoxic or non-genotoxic. The model scored an accuracy of 81.98%, specificity of 0.8148, and sensitivity of 0.8214. The data of sensitivity and specificity will be used further for evaluating the performance of all the models.

3.4.3 K-Nearest Neighbor Model (KNN)

KNN is ML algorithms used to classify data based on their properties. The KNN model classifies the data based on its distance from the centroid of clusters and maps it to the nearest cluster to the data point. Its advantage is that it is robust to noisy data and works effectively if the training data is large. The drawback of this algorithm is the amount of computation power that it requires because it relies on calculating the Euclidean distance between the data point and the clusters. Moreover, the number of clusters needs to be decided in advance, before starting with the clustering process.

The KNN model performed well in classifying the compounds as genotoxic or non-genotoxic. The model scored an accuracy of 79.28%, specificity of 0.8148, and sensitivity of 0.7857. The data of sensitivity and specificity will be used further for evaluating the performance of all the models.

3.4.4 Naive Bayes Algorithm

The Naive Bayes algorithm considers that each of the features is independent of each other, and there is no relation between them. It also considers that all the features have equal weights and importance in performing the classification tasks. It works by finding the probability of occurrence of an event given the probability of another event that has already occurred.

The Naive Bayes model had a fair performance in classifying the compounds as genotoxic or non-genotoxic. The model scored an accuracy of 77.48%, specificity of 0.6667, and sensitivity of 0.8095. The data of sensitivity and specificity will be used further for evaluating the performance of all the models.

3.4.5 Decision Trees Classifier

Decision tree classifier is a robust machine learning algorithm that explores both types of problems (classification and regression). This algorithm works on the principle of trees, nodes, and branches. Each tree has a root node that represents the main feature of the dataset, and each node has branches based on the decision rule for each feature. At the end of each final branch, there is a leaf node, which represents the outcome of each decision.

The decision tree classifier uses the CART algorithm, which is short for the classification and regression tree algorithm (Fig. 12).

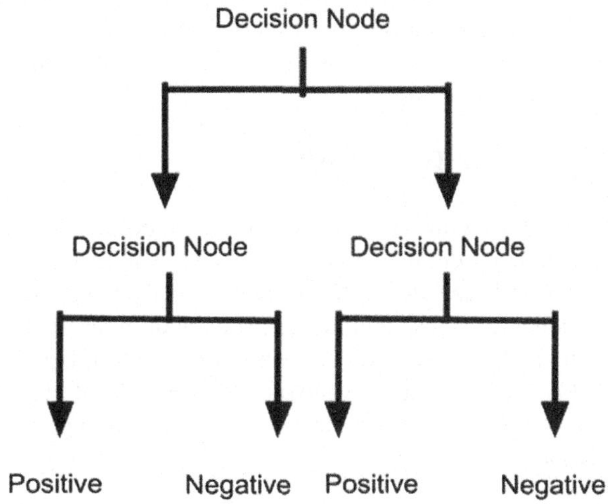

Fig. 12 Process of generating decision in decision tree classifier

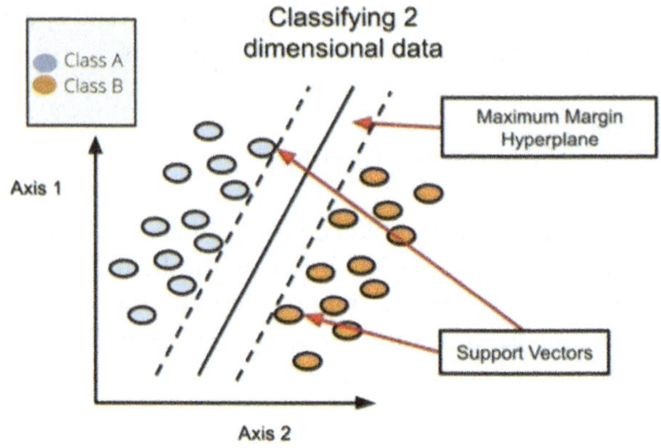

Fig. 13 Support vector machine model representation for classifying 2D data [22]

The decision tree classifier model had a fair performance in classifying the compounds as genotoxic or non-genotoxic. The model scored an accuracy of 68.47%, specificity of 0.7407, and sensitivity of 0.6667. The data of sensitivity and specificity will be used further for evaluating the performance of all the models.

3.4.6 Support Vector Machines

Support vector machine is a commonly used ML algorithm that is used for solving classification and regression problems. Its decision-making and classification process relies on the hyperplane; it generates which separates the data points belonging to different classes. Its goal is to create a maximum margin hyperplane that helps in segregating and classifying n-dimensional data (Fig. 13) [22].

The support vector classifier model performed well in classifying the compounds as genotoxic or non-genotoxic. The model scored an accuracy of 80.18%, specificity of 0.7778, and sensitivity of 0.8095. The data of sensitivity and specificity will be used further for evaluating the performance of all the models.

3.4.7 Extra Trees Classifier

Extra trees classifier or extremely randomized trees classifier algorithm is an ensemble model which aggregates the result produced by several uncorrelated decision tree classifiers in a "pool" or a "forest" to generate its output [23]. The extra trees classifier has many similarities to the random forest classifier, except in the extra trees fit several randomized decision trees on multiple sub-samples of the given dataset and apply to average to enhance its accuracy of classification and prediction while controlling over-fitting. It is also used for finding the importance of each feature in the dataset.

Table 5 Accuracy specificity and sensitivity values obtained by each model

	MLP	Logistic regression	KNN	Naive Bayes	Decision trees (criterion = gini)	SVC RS = None	Extra trees	Random forest classifier
Accuracy (%)	81.98	81.08	79.27	77.47	72.07	80.18	74.77	73.87
Specificity	0.8148	0.7407	0.8148	0.6666	0.5925	0.7777	0.7407	0.7407
Sensitivity	0.8214	0.83	0.7857	0.8095	0.7619	0.8095	0.75	0.738

In the study, extra trees were trained and used to classify the unseen compounds. The extra trees classifier produced results with an accuracy of 74.77%, specificity of 0.7407, and sensitivity of 0.75.

3.4.8 Random Forest Classifier

Random forest is a ML algorithm, and it is used for both classification and prediction tasks. A random forest algorithm is a classifier that contains several decision trees, all together called a forest. The forest is trained using a bagging or bootstrap aggregation method. It focuses on improving the accuracy of the algorithm. The building blocks of the decision trees are entropy and information gain. A high value of information gain implies that a higher degree of uncertainty has been removed, and higher are the chances of getting accurate predictions. In the case of the random forest classifier, the output chosen by many of the decision trees will be the final decision of the ensemble model. In the study, a random forest classifier model was trained and used to classify the unseen compounds. The model produced results with an accuracy of 73.87%, specificity of 0.7407, and sensitivity of 0.7381 (Table 5).

4 Receiver Operator Characteristic Curve for Model Evaluation

Accuracy and reliability of binary classification and a receiver operator characteristic curve are prepared based on the true positive rate and false = −positive rates of each model (Fig. 14).

Receiver operating characteristic (ROC) is a popular method that determines the performance of binary classification models. ROC plots the model's sensitivity or true positive rate and specificity or false positive rate and separates the "signal" from the "noise." Here, the signal is the genotoxicity value, which the models are trying to detect. Area under the curve (AUC) is the metric that summarizes a ROC plot, and it provides an aggregate measure to assess the performance of various models across

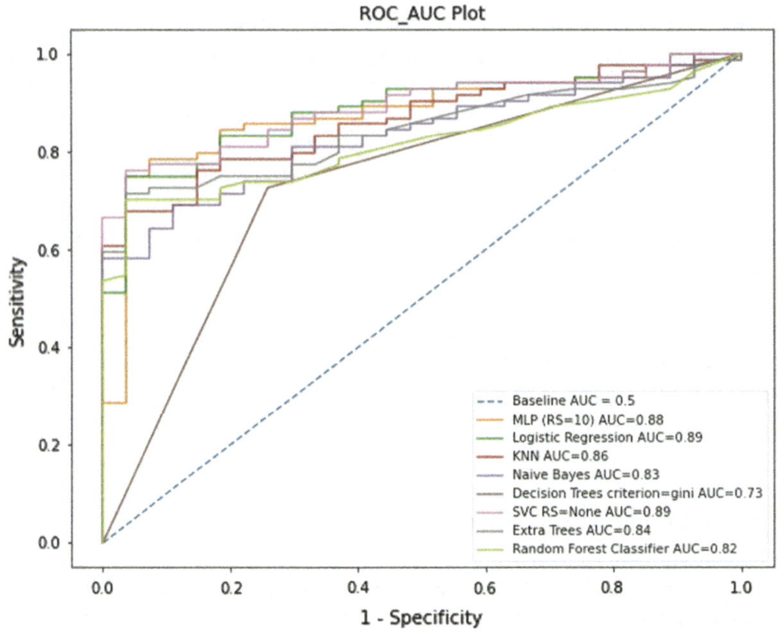

Fig. 14 ROC_AUC plot

all possible classification thresholds. AUC values are acceptable in the range of 0.5 to 1 as it indicates their ability to distinguish between positive and negative classes.

5 Conclusion

The trained models were able to distinguish and classify between the genotoxic and non-genotoxic compounds. There is a scope for increasing the classification accuracy by including more specific data which will help machine learning models and neural networks to distinguish with a higher true positive rate. This chapter gives an overview of different methods used for drug response prediction with a focus on anti-cancer drugs. Regulatory agencies such as FDA and EMA are always concerned about the side effect of anti-cancerous drugs on patients as these drugs are lifesaving drugs and always need to the consumer at regular intervals during treatment. Hence, it is always necessary to predict drug response at pre-clinical and clinical stages. Several in-vitro screening assays approved by regulatory authorities are available to predict drug cytotoxicity, genotoxicity, carcinogenicity, and mutagenicity. Although, there has been consistent progress in methods to evaluate drug response at the clinical stage. However, all these methods are very time-consuming and expensive. Therefore, there is a strong need to find alternative solutions to predict the response of anti-cancerous drugs, so that the severe side effect of the drugs can be predicted before application.

Computational tools such as molecular modeling and machine learning algorithms could be useful to provide accurate and faster drug response prediction for the anti-cancerous compounds by integration of data from a variety of sources like in-vitro assays, in vivo, and treatment, so that the developed predicted models may provide very precise and accurate results. We have discussed a few Web-based tools that can perform the above task. These machine learning models may improve the evaluation of potential drug molecules in terms of efficacy and side effects.

We have reported the case study of the application of ML to predict the genotoxicity of anti-cancerous drugs. We have chosen several anti-cancer drugs for developing training models to evaluate genotoxicity response. ML algorithm classified these drugs into genotoxic and non-genotoxic. Moreover, the highest accuracy 81.98% was obtained by MLP model, and its specificity was 81% and sensitivity was 82%. The other models also classified with accuracy >72%, sensitivity >73%, and specificity >59%. Our machine learning approach paves a path to find genotoxicity of any unknown compound from its physio-chemical properties, which is way cheaper than any in-vitro method. Thus, we conclude that ML models can support pharma companies by predicting the safety of novel anti-cancerous compounds while reducing the time and expenditure on the effective treatment of cancer. We are still improving the accuracy of our method by adding a greater number of compounds in the training and test dataset.

References

1. FalzoneL, S. S., & Libra, M. (2018). Evolution of cancer pharmacological treatments at the turn of the third millennium. *Frontiers in Pharmacology, 9*, 1300.
2. Gupta, A. (2020). *ML|extra tree classifier for feature selection*. https://www.geeksforgeeks.org/ml-extra-tree-classifier-for-feature-selection/
3. Hassanzadeh, P., Atyabi, F., & Dinarvand, R. (2019). The significance of artificial intelligence in drug delivery system design. *Advanced Drug Delivery Reviews, 151–152*, 169–190. https://www.sciencedirect.com/science/journal/0169409X/151/supp/C
4. Lipinski, C. F., Maltarollo, V. G., Oliveira, P. R., Silva, A. B. F., & Honorio, K. M. (2019). Advances and perspectives in applying deep learning for drug design and discovery. *Frontiers Robotics AI*. https://doi.org/10.3389/frobt.2019.00108
5. Iqbal, M. J., Javed, Z., Sadia, H., Qureshi, I. A., Irshad, A., Ahmed, R., Malik, K., Raza, S., Abbas, A., Pezzani, R., & Sharifi-Rad, J. (2021). Clinical applications of artificial intelligence and machine learning in cancer diagnosis looking into the future. *Cancer Cell International, 21*, 270.
6. Rafique, R., Islam, R. S. M., & Kazi, U. (2021). Machine learning in the prediction of cancer therapy. *Computational and Structural Biotechnology., 19*, 4003–4017.
7. Adam, G., Rampášek, L., Safikhani, Z., Smirnov, P., Haibe-Kains, B., & Goldenberg, A. (2020). Machine learning approaches to drug response prediction: challenges and recent progress. *NPJ Precision Oncology, 4*, 19.
8. Toh, T. S., & DondelingerF, W. D. (2019). Looking beyond the hype: Applied AI and machine learning in translational medicine. *The Lancet, 47*, 607–615.
9. Schneider, A., Hommel, G., & Blettner, M. (2010). Linear Regression Analysis. *DtschArztebl International, 107*(44), 776–782.

10. Dumitrescua, E., Hué, S., Hurlin, C., & Tokpavi, S. (2021). Machine learning for credit scoring: Improving logistic regression with non-linear decision-tree effects. *European Journal of Operational Research*, https://doi.org/10.1016/j.ejor.2021.06.053
11. Guha, R., & Jurs, P. C. (2004). Development of linear, ensemble, and nonlinear models for the prediction and interpretation of the biological activity of a set of PDGFR inhibitors. *Journal of Chemical Information and Computer Sciences, 44*(6), 2179–2189.
12. Härter, F. P., & Velho, H. F. C. (2008). New approach to applying neural network in nonlinear dynamic model. *Applied Mathematical Modelling, 32*(12), 2621–2633.
13. Gupta, S., Chaudhary, K., Kumar, R., Gautam, A., Nanda, J. S., Dhanda, S. K., Brahmachari, S. K., & Raghava, G. P. S. (2016). Prioritization of anticancer drugs against a cancer using genomic features of cancer cells: A step towards personalized medicine. *Science Report, 31*(6), 23857.
14. Chang, Y., Park, H., Yang, H. J., Lee, S., Lee, K. Y., Kim, T. S., Jung, J., & Jae-Min, S. J. M. (2018). Cancer drug response profile scan (CDRscan): A deep learning model that predicts drug effectiveness from cancer genomic signature. *Science Report 11, 8*(1):8857.
15. Zhang, M., Lee, S., Yao, B., Xiao, G., Xu, L., & Xie, Y. (2019). DIGREM: An integrated web-based platform for detecting effective multi-drug combinations. *Bioinformatics 15, 35*(10), 1792–1794.
16. Ianevski, A., Giri, A. K., & Aittokallio, T. (2020). Synergy finder 2.0: Visual analytics of multi-drug combination synergies. *Nucleic Acids Research, 48*(W1), W488–W493.
17. Ianevski, A., He, L., Aittokallio, T., & Tang, J. (2017). Synergy finder: A web application for analyzing drug combination dose-response matrix data. *Bioinformatics. 1, 33*(15), 2413–2415.
18. He, X., Folkman, L., & Borgwardt, K. (2018). Kernelized rank learning for personalized drug recommendation. *Bioinformatics. 15, 34*(16), 2808–2816.
19. Jackson, S. P., & Bartek, J. (2009). The DNA-damage response in human biology and disease. *Nature. 22, 461*(7267), 1071–1078.
20. Snyder, R. D., Holt, P. A., Maguire, J. M., & Trent, J. O. (2013). Prediction of noncovalent drug/DNA interaction using, computational docking models: Studies with over 1350 launched drugs. *Environmental and Molecular Mutagenesis, 54*(8), 668–681.
21. Swaminathan, S. (2018). Logistic regression—Detailed overview. https://towardsdatascience.com/logistic-regression-detailed-overview-46c4da4303bc
22. Brownlee, J. (2016). Deep learning with Python: Develop deep learning models on theano and tensorflow using keras. *Machine Learning Mastery.*
23. Gupta, R., Srivastava, D., Sahu, M., Tiwari, S., Ambasta, R. K., & Kumar, P. (2021). Artificial intelligence to deep learning: machine intelligence approach for drug discovery. *Molecular Diversity, 25*, 1315–1360.

The Incipient Role of Computational Intelligence in Oncology: Drug Designing, Discovery, and Development

Ritu Karwasra, Kushagra Khanna, Surender Singh, Shaban Ahmad, and Saurabh Verma

Abstract Computational intelligence (CI) approaches are multi-layered neural networks having robust reasoning, logical, and self-regulating capability to learn that highly simulate the human cognitive process. CI technologies such as machine learning (ML), deep learning (DL), and artificial intelligence (AI) algorithms appeared to be the promising solution that overcome the obstacle and problems in designing and discovering drugs. Drug designing, discovery, and development are associated with certain hurdles and challenges such as off-target delivery, inappropriate dosage, less efficacy, production costs, and time consumption. Additionally, the complex and enormous data from proteomics, microarray, genomics data, and clinical trials impact the drug discovery pipeline. In oncology, the drug discovery process is more crucial as there are approximately three hundred variant forms of cancers that affect people of all age groups. Even though understanding disease pathogenesis and progress is in developing innovative small molecule drugs, successful discovery and development require 13–14 years and expensive investment. Therefore, the CI can envisage oncology drug discovery and development and further aid in addressing resistance in oncology drugs by learning and analyzing data. Oncology remains at the forefront to reap the profits of CI for the overall management of cancer, including identifying the target, hit identification, optimization of the lead compound, preclinical or clinical trials, and then regulatory approvals. This study described the current advancement of CI in the arena of oncology, with the simultaneous prospect of anticancer drug development and therapeutic approaches. CI tools and techniques such as machine and deep learning can profoundly augment the prevailing method of oncology drug research.

R. Karwasra · S. Verma (✉)
ICMR-National Institute of Pathology, Safdarjung Hospital Campus, New Delhi 110029, India

K. Khanna
Department of Pharmacy, Lloyd Institute of Management and Technology (Pharm), Greater Noida 201306, India

S. Singh
Department of Pharmacology, All India Institute of Medical Sciences, New Delhi 110029, India

S. Ahmad
Department of Computer Science, Jamia Millia Islamia, New Delhi 110025, India

K. Raza (ed.), *Computational Intelligence in Oncology*, Studies in Computational Intelligence 1016, https://doi.org/10.1007/978-981-16-9221-5_21

Keywords Anticancer · Computational intelligence · Drug discovery · Drug development · Deep learning

1 Introduction

Computational intelligence paradigms (CI) in this pandemic era present tremendous benefits in vast areas, including engineering, healthcare, science, and management [35]. A significant advancement in high computing technologies plays an imperative role in drug discovery [7]. In addition, the progress of superior algorithms, high-performance computing, computer-assisted drug design technology, and accumulation of enormous chemical and biological data with benefits of fast speed, high efficiency, and low cost paved a way to develop oncology cargos [20]. CI has transformed the oncology drug discovery process, as oncology therapeutics cost approximately 2.6 billion USD and took almost a decade to develop [42]. But with the help of CI, we may be able to reduce the cost and time involved in discovering, designing, and developing effective oncology therapeutic drugs (cargos) [2]. Recent advancement in CI technologies enables the possibility of eliminating the soaring costs invested in 92% of candidate molecules that eventually fail at later phases of the drug development process before drug regulatory approval [1]. CI framework involves artificial intelligence (AI), in which machines perform the tasks associated with the human thinking process and machine learning (ML) is a subdivision of AI. Machines interpret the data for the investigation of intricate, distinct datasets. CI in the oncology drug development process will revolutionize and change how cargos are discovered. Thus, it helps in CI-aided organic synthesis, discovery of compounds, tumor classification, assays development, and target and biomarkers discoveries (Fig. 1) [22].

CI, thus, in particular, intended to optimize and automate the drug discovery processes and, in turn, speed up the research and development of drug designing, identification, and development methodologies [40]. Beginning with the introduction of the AI platform, Pfizer in 2016 united with IBM Watson Health to improve their quest for immune-oncology treatments [8]. In 2021, a German biotechnologist firm Evotech started their clinical trial (Phase I) of a new anticancer candidate molecule. They discovered it in partnership with Exscientia, Oxford, UK, which applied CI techniques in the drug discovery of small molecules. Several other pharmaceutical firms collaborated with AI platforms to discover the drugs of different indications. Numerous tech companies also investigating in drug discovery process with the aid of CI platform. AlphaFold, an Alphabet's subsidiary DeepMind, developed CI Platform, and it predicts the 3D protein structure depending upon the genomic data [26]. Lantern Pharma (LTRN) is a clinical division of oncology-focused biopharmaceutical corporation which uses RADR® AI platform and ML to discover the oncology drug candidates. Currently, Lantern is in process of developing four new drug candidates and also explored seven disclosed tumor targets. RADR® AI platform surpasses 4.6 billion data points and aid in advancing the company strategy in developing AI

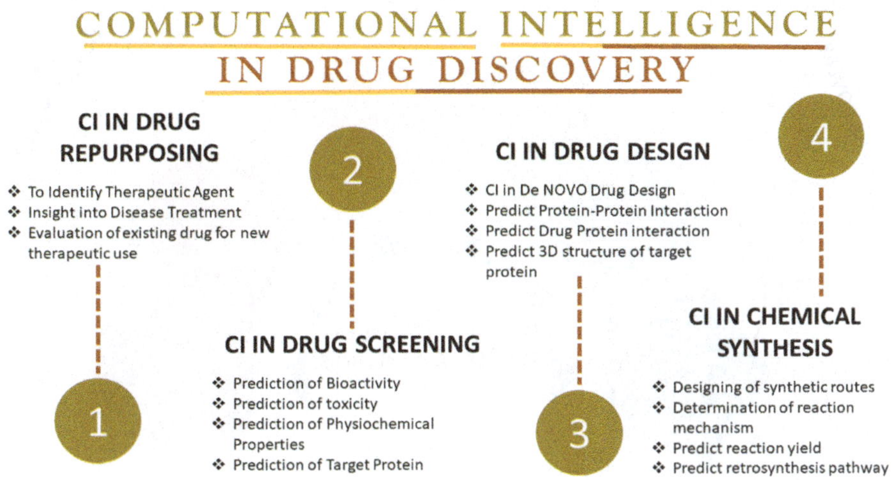

Fig. 1 Computational intelligence framework in drug screening, drug design, and synthesis

platform for oncology-focused drug development. Keeping this overview in mind, we initiate with introduction of some vital components of traditional oncology drug discovery and its accompanying pitfalls. Afterward, a brief introduction of some of the fundamental CI concepts is addressed along with the historical and modern advancements. Petite overview of applications of CI in target discovery, biomarker discovery, and patient stratification is given. In the last, forthcoming potential and challenges of CI in oncology are also addressed.

2 Conventional Oncology Drug Design, Discovery and Development

Conventional drug discovery program is long and arduous; it begins with the designing of the drug, its discovery phase, and development phases (Fig. 2). The pipeline has key components, including target identification, drug design, lead molecule discovery, preclinical and clinical development processes, and regulatory approval (IND submission) [26]. The first step is biological target identification, accompanied by numerous entities (small molecule or large biologics) that elicit a response [14]. Methods such as proteomics, gene expression, phenotype screening, and genomics analysis exist to identify the biological targets. While identifying the target, either of these methods is employed, but it, later on, be validated, and this step requires several processes [15]. A multi-validation approach augments the identification of biological targets and simultaneously aid in drug candidate success.

The study has numerous target validation parameters like protein expression, functional analysis, in vitro/in vivo genetic manipulation, animal disease models,

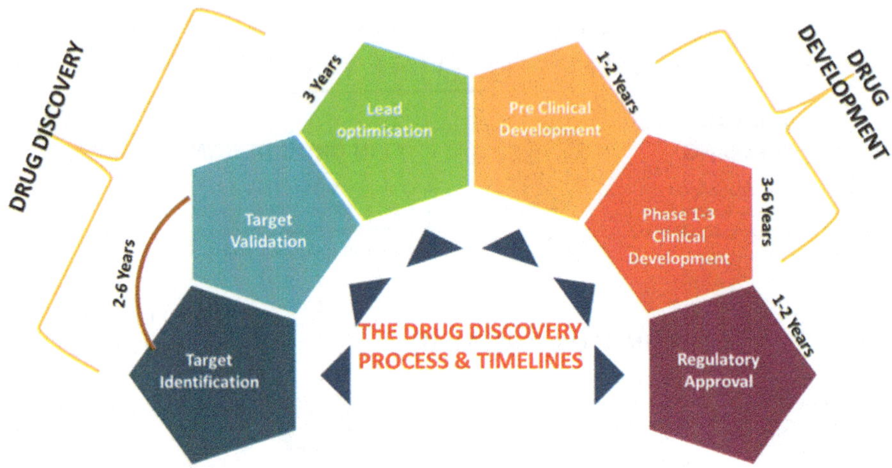

Fig. 2 Conventional oncology drug discovery and development process

biomarkers, etc., though these steps require target expression in disease-oriented tissues and cells.

Classical validation protocol requires measurement of mRNA or protein expression in patients. In drug development, in vivo studies play a pivotal role, and, therefore, transgenic animal models are often employed to study phenotypic observations [12]. Several knock-out, knock-in, or genetic models are there to investigate the efficacy and therapeutic side effects. Recently, an emerging technique that augments target validation is organ-on-chips (3D-microfluidic cell culture chip). These chips mimic our body's physiology and organ functionality and are used to assess efficacy and response to therapeutic drugs [21].

To sum up, several measures validate targets, which ultimately evaluate target cellular functionality and thus aid in screening drug candidates. After the identification of the biological target, its validation and then comes the lead identification phase. This segment is composed of identification of hit compound, hit-to-lead stage, and lead optimization. In the first phase of hit identification, the drug compound screening assays such as high throughput screening, fragment screening, and focused screening are developed. High-throughput screening employs a compound library and evaluates the activity of each substance on a biological target. Focus-based screening opts compounds from the library and literature, and patents and publications derive the desired target activity. So, it is also termed as a knowledge-based screening assay. Fragment screening employs the libraries (small molecular weight) and evaluates them at high concentrations. The following fundamental step in the conventional drug discovery process is the hit-to-lead and lead optimization phase [44]. This process aims to obtain the compounds with optimum metabolic, structural, and pharmacokinetic properties [45]. The drug discovery and development pipeline include preclinical and clinical investigations of the lead compound. Preclinical experimentation is conducted with the aid of laboratory animal models [37]. These preclinical studies determine a safe dose, pharmacodynamics, pharmacokinetics, mechanism of action, and potential drug–drug interactions. From these experiments, we investigate the safe amount to be used for human studies [36]. In this notion, approximately, 1 in 5000 preclinical drug candidates passed the preclinical stage and got regulatory approval. Phase I clinical studies were conducted on a few healthy volunteers to determine the safety profile and dose–response relationship. Phase II and III are exploratory trials and involve investigation on a large number of diseased individuals. These phases determine the effectiveness, side effects, and associated risk factors. After drug approval, phase IV (post-marketing surveillance) studies warrant a more significant population-scale safety profile of drugs.

3 Challenges in the Drug Development Pipeline

Cargos (therapeutic drugs) failed because of three main reasons, and out of which, the foremost one is they are ineffective, or they are not safe, and secondly, they are unsafe on clinical administration. The last one is due to poor clinical trial structure. In the conventional drug development pipeline, the cost soars largely, and 92% fail during the process or before the approval. As we discussed, the prime source of trial failure is the ineffectiveness of the lead compound. A phase III study conducted by [16] investigated 640 trials, and from which, 54% failed due to ineffectiveness [16]. This includes poor study design, having fewer samples in a problem, which affects statistical power and not being able to reject the null hypothesis, and, most importantly, the propagation of error due to flaws in the validation of the target. One such example is the Drug Olaparib, a PARP inhibitor (poly ADP ribose polymerase) designed for ovarian cancer, which failed in its Phase I trial due to improper clinical trial structure. In the same problem at the initial stage, it is seen that Olaparib in platinum-sensitive and BRCA mutation recurrent ovarian tumor delayed the recurrence time from 11.2 months to 4.3 months. Though, the median death time in the control group was 31.9 months and 34.9 months in the test group. Later, in 2014, Kaufman and colleagues presented a response rate of greater than 30% with Olaparibmono therapy in patients with three or more chemotherapy cycles [19]. FDA approved Olaparib in 2014 for women with recurrent ovarian tumors with BRCA mutation [19]. Safety is another challenge for conventional drug development programs. In the same study, Hwang et al. tested 640 compounds, 17% failed due to safety [16].

Though safety is a pressing concern in every stage of a clinical trial, major problem lies with a large population. Patients will report the adverse event that concerns them, and safety may not align with the administering physician [5]. The cost of determining safety concerns also soars the expense of the drug development process. An example of this is sulfanilamide, marketed in bolus and elixir formulations. In 1930, this drug was sold in both formulations, and safety was not established in elixir formulations; and due to this, approximately 100 people died. This was due to the poisoning of diethylene glycol in elixir formulations, which led to the emergence of the two most influential acts, i.e., Drug and cosmetics act and the Food, Drug, and Cosmetic Act [4].

4 Historical Progression of CI

The historical progression of CI is noteworthy in the drug discovery process in the notion that it was inbred in 1950 and employed in effect after the QSAR presentation in 1960 [30]. In 1950, a test was known as the Turing test proposed by Alan Turing, and that verified machine ability to exhibit intelligence behaviors (equivalent to human brains). Later, in the year 1955, there was the creation of the first artificial intelligence program, i.e., Logic Theorist, and this program proved 38 out of 52 mathematics theorems. The golden years begin in the era 1956–1974 [32]. Joseph Weizenbaum created the first chatbot algorithm that solved mathematical problems in the year 1966, named ELIZA. The first intelligent humanoid robot was constructed in the year 1972 and named WABOT-1. In 1980, CI was programmed to simulate the decision-making ability of human experts. Earlier, the linear regression models (limited to chemical structural descriptors) were employed for drug discovery studies in 1990. In 2011, IBM Watson proved the intelligence of CI networking in solving tricky questions in a quiz and established that it has intelligence like the human thinking process [3]. In 2018, the project debate launched by the IBM group gained widespread attention based on intelligence like human beings. In recent years, CI has developed remarkably, and several companies (tech, pharmaceutical, Google, Amazon, and IBM) have started investing in CI platforms. In the long term, CI may surpass human cognitive abilities and permeate deeper into many other companies for the foreseeable future (Table 1).

5 Applications of CI in Pharmaceutical Drug Discovery and Development Process

Search for a new drug for any ailment is daunting and primarily the most challenging part of drug development. There are vast sizes of chemical space involving 10^{60} molecules. CI technologies became versatile tools and ubiquitously engaged in each stage of the drug development process, such as designing of new drug candidates, aiding in refining the decision-making process for recruitment of patients in clinical trials, drug target identification and validation, aggregation, and analysis of biomedical information, repurposing of drugs, and improvement in R&D efficiency [31]. These latent benefits of CI provide the opportunity to combat the inefficiency and uncertainty associated with conventional drug development programs while curtailing human intervention and bias minimization. Other application in drug discovery methods includes the association of drug targets, pharmacological activities, prediction of feasible synthetic routes for drug candidates, repurposing of drugs, characteristics of proteins, mRNA, a combination of drugs, efficacy measurement, discovering relation between diseases and drugs, precision medicine based on omics biomarkers, and lastly, also aid in the identification of novel signaling pathways or targets using omics analysis [24]. DL circumvent various problems in conventional

Table 1 Historical progression of CI technologies

S. No.	Year	Events for advancement in CI
1	1642	Blaise Pascal developed the first mechanical calculating machine
2	1837	Charles Babbage, along with Ada Lovelace, designed programmable machine
3	1943	Warren McCulloch and Walter Pitts founded a neural network
4	1950	Alan turning established a machine intelligence test known as turning test
5	1955	Artificial intelligence term was coined
6	1965	A natural language program was developed, which was named ELIZA
7	1980	Edward Feigenbaum designed a system that imitates the decision of human experts
8	1997	World chess champion Garry Kasparov lost a game against computer-based learning software
9	2009	A self-driven car was developed by google
10	2011	Watson, an IBM AI software, wins the US game show
11	2011–2014	Personal assistance like Google now, Siri, etc., were developed to recognize the voice and answer the question
12	2014	Ian good fellow developed a generative adversarial network
13	2018	A considerable number of universities globally started a course on AI
14	2020	Using CI the vaccine research and development was initiated just after the first case of COVID-19 was reported and by March 2020, vaccine to fight was undergoing human trials
15	2020	Automated driving robotaxis and quantum computing
16	2021	University of Liverpool designed a CI tool that can predict unknown acquaintances between mammals and viruses
17	2021	CI can predict healthy stem cells and can also speed up the process for evaluating stem cell quality
18	2021	A new advancement in CI can predict the stress and strain on material just by analyzing its photo
19	2021	Prediction of bacterial infection outcomes for new treatment processes and its optimization

drug development method, and it demonstrated outstanding success in proposing suitable drug candidates while predicting their effectiveness and associated possible toxicity risks. Analysis of large datasets, laborious screening of lead compound, and minimization of the standard error are encountered in the conventional drug development process. Still, with the emergence of DL, the cost and time are reduced. With the advent of CI technologies, one may design new studies in which assistance is provided in novel drug targets, rational drug designing, and repurposing of drugs. CI transformed the methods or the pathway of identifying targets by incorporating either genomic, biochemical information, or traceability of targets. A study conducted by Ferroro et al. in 2017 predicts the therapeutic targets with the aid of CI, known as open targets, a platform for gene–disease association data with more than 71% prediction power [11]. For drug discovery, an AI platform named IBM Watson has identified five novel RNA-binding proteins and assessed the linkage in amyotrophic lateral sclerosis. Incorporation of in silico prediction enables profile selection and reduces attrition and R&D costs. The virtual ligand or structure-based designs approaches are primarily used in in silico predictions on small molecule modulator probes. Currently, numerous computer-aided organic compound synthesis (CAOCS) systems are available to select synthesis routes [28].

6 Incipient Role of CI in Oncology Drug Discovery

CI is used to predict oncology drug activity including Genomics of Drug Sensitivity dataset in cancer and assist in the oncology drug discovery and development process through various domains of machine learning, deep learning, and artificial neural network. There are variant forms of tumors, i.e., benign (non-cancerous), premalignant, the cells are not yet cancerous, but they have the potential to become malignant, and lastly, the malignant tumor (cancerous cells); for this, different drugs like 5-fluorouracil, gemcitabine, methotrexate, and 6-mercaptopurine, etc., are used with varying mechanisms of action. Generally, the high-throughput screening reveals the relationship of drug activity with the genomic variability of tumor cells. A study conducted by Wang et al. developed a machine learning model known as the drug sensitivity prediction model (based on elastic net regression). It predicts the sensitivity of drugs in patients with endometrial tumors, ovarian, and gastric tumors. This model predicted the drug resistance in which tamoxifen was given to ovarian tumor patients, 5-fluorouracil was given to gastric tumor patients, and paclitaxel was administered to endometrial tumor patients showed poor prognosis. The study depicts that CI has the potential in addressing drug resistance in tumors. The machine learning tools quickly predict the mechanism of how tumor cells became resistant to oncology drugs. CI analyzes and learns the data on tumor-resistant cells and further help in improving drug development method (Fig. 3).

Lind et al., in 2019, developed a random forest model with the aid of integrating machine learning and screening data. This model predicts oncology drugs' efficacy following the tumor cell genome [25]. ML algorithms in high-throughput screening are trained to predict the drug response on in vitro (tumor cell lines) and in vivo (patients) in oncology drug research. It also aids in investigating or speeding up the drug repurposing, newer drugs, or a combination of medications for anticancer activity. Researchers augment the drug discovery process with the assistance of ML by generating or creating reverse synthesis pathways for molecules. The creation of a new drug produces a lot of data, so this ML offers a prospect to processing the chemical synthesis data congregated in years and even in decades in a short period. The creation of results by ML helps accelerate the drug development process, and additionally, it will help us make more informed decisions rather than be made through experimentation. In the same context, DL is also a machine algorithm responsible for

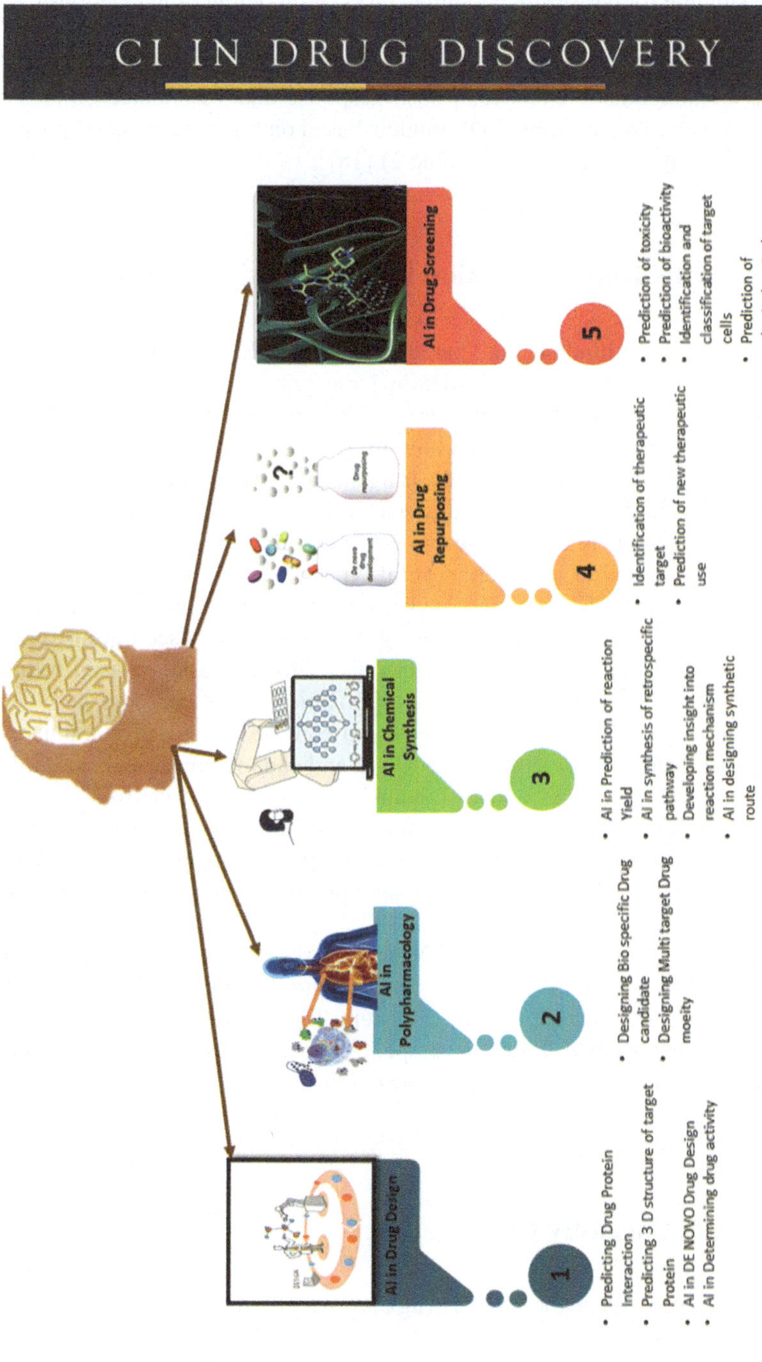

Fig. 3 Role of CI in oncology drug discovery

the drug discovery process. These models are used to predict drug response prediction and are suitable for performing complex tasks of modeling drug reactions based on biological and chemical data. Currently, DL makes unprecedented advancement in extracting information from computers. Reference [18] developed the DL method by applying an antagonistic encoder in dose–response data (calculated on NCI-60 cell line). This type of generation of DL models based on big-scale datasets presents avenues in new drug reuse prospects (Table 2) [18].

7 CI Platforms Implementation in Drug Designing Pipeline

CI involves numerous fundamental paradigms (AI, ML, and DL) and domain methods (reasoning, solution search, and knowledge representation). ML algorithms recognize patterns within the dataset that are further classified. DL engages ANN and comprises interconnected sophisticated computing elements (perceptions) analogous to human biological neurons and mimic the transmission of electronic impulses to the human brain. ANN includes a set of nodes; each one receives a separate input and is converted into the output either in single or multilinked algorithms to resolve a particular problem. In this notion, there are several types of ANN, including multilayer perceptron networks (MLP), convolutional neural networks (CNN), and recurrent neural network (RNN), that utilize either unsupervised or supervised training procedures [26]. Network deploying MLP are usually trained in a supervised training program that operates unidirectional and has applications such as optimization aids, pattern recognition, identification of process, and controls. It is used as a universal pattern classifier. RNN networks are closed-loop and can memorize and store information like Hopfield networks and Boltzmann constants. CNN networks involve a series of dynamic systems with local connections. They will be characterized on basis of topology, pattern recognition, image or video processing, processing complex brain functions, biological system modeling, and processing of sophisticated signals (Table 3).

RBF networks, Kohonen networks, LVQ networks, ADALINE networks, and counter-propagation networks. There are numerous tools based on this networking that forms the core architecture of the CI system. International Business Machine Watson supercomputer (IBM, USA) developed AI-based tools, and it was designed to assist in analyzing patient medical information and its correlation with a vast database.

8 Challenges Faced by CI

CI plays an imperative role in the current drug discovery process as it manifests recognition in the extraction of traits from big, complex, and heterogeneous noisy data. Though, it faces many challenges that are not yet resolved [9]. First and foremost,

Table 2 Current companies involved in AI-based drug development programs

CI technologies	Companies	Integration of AI platforms with drug development companies
Numedii	Astellas	The AI-based patient monitoring platform
BioVista	Astellas	Drug repurposing
Xbird	Bayer	Tracking of real-time data
Turbine	Bayer	Prediction of treatment response on cancer cells
Bina	RocheT Berg Biogen	Genomics
Exscientia	GSK	Discovering small molecules
Benevolent AI	Janssen	Develop, manufacture, and commercialize drug molecules functional at clinical stages
Exscientia	Evotec	Bio-specific drug molecule for therapies related to immune-oncology
Insilico medicine	GSK	New pathway and biological targets
GNS healthcare	Genentech	Discover novel targets for cancer drugs
Cancer outcomes tracking and analysis	Novartis	New therapies for clinical development in breast cancer
IBM Watson health	Novartis	Better outcomes for breast cancer
IBM Watson health	TEVA	Develop novel treatment options and improve the management of chronic disease
IBM Watson health	Johnson & Johnson	Augment drug discovery of immuno oncology
IBM Watson health	Pfizer	Predict new combination therapies, patient selection, and novel drug targets in immuno oncology
TBerg	AstraZeneca	Identification of new targets for neurodegenerative disease
TBerg	Sanofi	Biomarkers for flu vaccine

(continued)

Table 2 (continued)

CI technologies	Companies	Integration of AI platforms with drug development companies
Numerate	Merck	New drug candidate development from unnamed cardio targets
AiCure	Abbvie	AI-centered monitoring of patients
Hitachi	Mitsubishi Tanabe Pharma	Planning of clinical trial using AI
Numerate	Takeda	To discover drug moieties for oncology, CNS disease, and gastroenterology
twoXAR	Santen	Newer drug for glaucoma
Numerate	Servier	Modulators of ryanodine receptor 2
Exscientia	Sumitomo Dainippon Pharma	A newer treatment for psychiatric disorders

Table 3 CI tools used in the drug discovery process

S. No.	Tools	Details	References
1	AlphaFold	Predict 3D protein structure	https://alphafold.ebi.ac.uk/
2	Chemputer	Report chemical synthesis procedure in a standardized format	[13]
3	DeepChem	Python-based CI system to discover lead compound	[34, 43]
4	DeepNeural net QSAR	Python-based CI tools that detect molecular activity	[27]
5	DeepTox	Predict toxicity of 12,000 drugs	[23, 29]
6	DeltaVina	Rescoring drug–ligand binding affinity	[41]
7	Hit dexter	Predict molecules based on biochemical assays	[38]
8	PotentialNet	Use of ANN to predict ligand-binding affinity	[10]
9	Neural graph fingerprint	Predict novel molecule properties	[17]

one is difficult and ambiguous in the CI model mechanism. Secondly, the availability of essential data from database providers and access to this require extra cost to the company. Another challenge encountered during the deployment of CI is the lack of skilled personnel to operate CI platforms. The lack of data is the major problem experienced by every industry that invests in AI platforms. The machine learning algorithms need to be trained on hundreds or thousands of sample data points to perform well. Instead, the minimum number of samples in conventional biologic studies should be six to be valid [39].

Furthermore, obtaining labeled data is also a challenge as it requires manual input. In oncology research, large databases such as The Cancer Genome Atlas Program (TCGA) are open and aggregating sources and provide ample amounts of data from numerous research institutions [33]. Though often, the data or the extensive database may not exist. To combat this situation, there is a process of creating artificial data from accurate data, known as data augmentation. Varied data augmentation approaches increase the data for training models without the need for new dataset collection. Lack of interpretability is another set of challenges faced by CI algorithms. The black box model is often employed to describe the complex behavior of machine learning. Though, a number of tools are being developed such as Local Interpretable Model-Agnostic explanations (LIME) and Shapley Additive Explanations (SHAP) in order to elucidate explainability. LIME, SHAP, and other strategies are projected as common practice in CI learning [6]. LIME displays a local linear approximation of model behavior, and SHAP employs theory-based output to explain model output. A major recurring challenge with CI in medical data is that multi-dimensionality and sparse data. Particularly, in omics study, the datasets used are small with countless features (typically, in less than 100 samples, containing thousands of features) and, therefore, complicating the data. This can be addressed with an array of dimensionality reduction techniques. On the whole, there are series of challenges that meant to be discussed for CI. In this context, we have described few of the obstacles. Still, they can be addressed with advancements in machine learning tools and techniques such as feature reduction techniques, repositories, and augment explainability [26].

9 Concluding Remarks

In the oncology drug development and discovery process, taking a drug from concept to the clinic stage is a long, varied process that involves a considerable cost (over 2.6 billion dollars) and approximately 13–14 years. In the whole process, numerous drugs fail at the last stage of drug development, before the regulatory approval or before IND submission. This, in turn, creates a loss of time and money, and, in addition, the conventional methods are also less suitable to handle heterogeneous and complex data of this era. Therefore, the introduction of CI platforms emerged drug designing with the desired properties and upgraded the approval success rate of new chemical entities. These CI-based technologies have strong data mining capability that enables computer-assisted drug designing of current era data. CI made a significant contribution in oncology drug development and treatment as their level of knowledge limits the humans. CI provides the imperative insights and information that is difficult for humans to identify and provide personalized treatment to each tumor patient. In this domain, CI improved the discovery of new compounds and diagnostics to accelerate the discovery process. Consequently, it is believed that CI, in the future, will be a powerful, driven force for oncology research and will bring insightful variation in medical knowledge in upcoming years.

References

1. Ali, D., & Frimpong, S. (2020). Artificial intelligence, machine learning and process automation: Existing knowledge frontier and way forward for mining sector. *Artificial Intelligence Review, 53*, 6025–6042. https://doi.org/10.1007/s10462-020-09841-6
2. Avorn, J. (2015). The $2.6 billion pill—Methodologic and policy considerations. *New England Journal of Medicine, 372*, 1877–1879. https://doi.org/10.1056/nejmp1500848
3. Bakkar, N., Kovalik, T., Lorenzini, I., et al. (2018). Artificial intelligence in neurodegenerative disease research: Use of IBM watson to identify additional RNA-binding proteins altered in amyotrophic lateral sclerosis. *Acta Neuropathologica, 135*, 227–247. https://doi.org/10.1007/s00401-017-1785-8
4. Chen, C., & Wong, R. (2018). *Black patients miss out on promising cancer drugs.* ProPublica
5. Crowther, M. (2013). Phase 4 research: What happens when the rubber meets the road? *Hematology. American Society of Hematology. Education Program, 2013*, 15–18. https://doi.org/10.1182/asheducation-2013.1.15
6. de Sousa, I. P., Vellasco, M. M. B. R., & da Silva, E. C. (2019). Local interpretable model-agnostic explanations for classification of lymph node metastases. *Sensors (Switzerland), 19.* https://doi.org/10.3390/s19132969
7. Deloitte (2018) *Artificial intelligence innovation report.*
8. Dlamini, Z., Francies, F. Z., Hull, R., & Marima, R. (2020). Artificial intelligence (AI) and big data in cancer and precision oncology. *Computational and Structural Biotechnology Journal, 18*, 2300–2311.
9. Fahimirad, M. (2018). A review on application of artificial intelligence in teaching and learning in educational contexts. *International Journal of Learning and Development, 8*, 106. https://doi.org/10.5296/ijld.v8i4.14057
10. Feinberg, E. N., Sur, D., Wu, Z., et al. (2018). PotentialNet for molecular property prediction. *ACS Central Science, 4*, 1520–1530. https://doi.org/10.1021/acscentsci.8b00507
11. Ferrero, E., Dunham, I., & Sanseau, P. (2017). In silico prediction of novel therapeutic targets using gene-disease association data. *Journal of Translational Medicine, 15.* https://doi.org/10.1186/s12967-017-1285-6
12. Golka, K., Prior, V., Blaszkewicz, M., & Bolt, H. M. (2002). The enhanced bladder cancer susceptibility of NAT2 slow acetylators towards aromatic amines: A review considering ethnic differences. *Toxicology Letters, 128*, 229–241.
13. Gromski, P. S., Granda, J. M., & Cronin, L. (2020). Universal chemical synthesis and discovery with "The Chemputer." *Trends Chemistry, 2*, 4–12.
14. Guedes, R. C., & Rodrigues, T. (2019). Drug target prediction using chem- and bioinformatics. *Physics Science Review, 3.*
15. Hein, D. W. (2002). Molecular genetics and function of NAT1 and NAT2: Role in aromatic amine metabolism and carcinogenesis. *Mutation Research—Fundamental Molecular Mechanisms Mutagenesis, 506–507*, 65–77. https://doi.org/10.1016/S0027-5107(02)00153-7

16. Hwang, T. J., Carpenter, D., Lauffenburger, J. C., et al. (2016). Failure of investigational drugs in late-stage clinical development and publication of trial results. *JAMA Internal Medicine, 176*, 1826–1833. https://doi.org/10.1001/jamainternmed.2016.6008
17. Ishida, S., Miyazaki, T., Sugaya, Y., & Omachi, S. (2021). Graph neural networks with multiple feature extraction paths for chemical property estimation. *Molecules, 26*. https://doi.org/10.3390/molecules26113125
18. Kadurin, A., Nikolenko, S., Khrabrov, K., et al. (2017). DruGAN: An advanced generative adversarial autoencoder model for de novo generation of new molecules with desired molecular properties in silico. *Molecular Pharmaceutics, 14*, 3098–3104. https://doi.org/10.1021/acs.molpharmaceut.7b00346
19. Kaufman, B., Shapira-Frommer, R., Schmutzler, R. K., et al. (2015). Olaparib monotherapy in patients with advanced cancer and a germline BRCA1/2 mutation. *Journal of Clinical Oncology, 33*, 244–250. https://doi.org/10.1200/JCO.2014.56.2728
20. Kaur, P., & Khatik, G. (2020). An overview of computer-aided drug design tools and recent applications in designing of anti-diabetic agents. *Current Drug Targets, 22*, 1158–1182. https://doi.org/10.2174/1389450121666201119141525
21. Kefallinou, D., Grigoriou, M., Boumpas, D. T., Gogolides, E., Tserepi, A. (2020). Fabrication of a 3D microfluidic cell culture device for bone marrow-on-a-chip. *Micro Nano Engineering, 9*. https://doi.org/10.1016/j.mne.2020.100075
22. Khong, J., Wang, P., & Gan, T. R. X., et al. (2019). The role of artificial intelligence in scaling nanomedicine toward broad clinical impact. In *Nanoparticles for biomedical applications: Fundamental concepts, biological interactions and clinical applications*, (pp. 385–407).
23. Klambauer, G., Unterthiner, T., Mayr, A., & Hochreiter, S. (2017). DeepTox: Toxicity prediction using deep learning. *Toxicology Letters, 280*, S69. https://doi.org/10.1016/j.toxlet.2017.07.175
24. Koromina, M., Pandi, M. T., & Patrinos, G. P. (2019). Rethinking drug repositioning and development with artificial intelligence, machine learning, and omics. *Omi A Journal Integrative Biology, 23*, 539–548. https://doi.org/10.1089/omi.2019.0151
25. Liang, G., Fan, W., Luo, H., & Zhu, X. (2020). The emerging roles of artificial intelligence in cancer drug development and precision therapy. *Biomedicine Pharmacother, 128*.
26. Linton-Reid, K. (2020). Introduction: An overview of AI in oncology drug discovery and development. In *Artificial Intelligence in Oncology Drug Discovery and Development*.
27. Ma, J., Sheridan, R. P., Liaw, A., et al. (2015). Deep neural nets as a method for quantitative structure-activity relationships. *Journal of Chemical Information and Modeling, 55*, 263–274. https://doi.org/10.1021/ci500747n
28. Mak, K. K., & Pichika, M. R. (2019). Artificial intelligence in drug development: Present status and future prospects. *Drug Discovery Today, 24*, 773–780.
29. Mayr, A., Klambauer, G., Unterthiner, T., Hochreiter, S. (2016) DeepTox: Toxicity prediction using deep learning. *Front Environmental Science, 3*. https://doi.org/10.3389/fenvs.2015.00080
30. Muthukrishnan, N., Maleki, F., Ovens, K., et al. (2020). Brief history of artificial intelligence. *Neuroimaging Clinics of North America, 30*, 393–399.
31. Nagarajan, N., Yapp, E. K. Y., & Le, N. Q. K., et al. (2019). Application of computational biology and artificial intelligence technologies in cancer precision drug discovery. *Biomedicine Research International, 2019*.
32. Nakahara, R. (2020). The history of artificial intelligence. *Okayama Igakkai Zasshi (Journal of Okayama Medical Association), 132*, 144–147. https://doi.org/10.4044/joma.132.144
33. National Cancer Institute. (2020). The cancer genome atlas program. In *Bethesda*.
34. Ramsundar, B., Liu, B., Wu, Z., et al. (2017). Is multitask deep learning practical for pharma? *Journal of Chemical Information and Modeling, 57*, 2068–2076. https://doi.org/10.1021/acs.jcim.7b00146
35. Raza, K., & Qazi, S. (2021). An introduction to computational intelligence in COVID-19: Surveillance, prevention, prediction, and diagnosis. In *Studies in computational intelligence, 923*, 3–18. https://doi.org/10.1007/978-981-15-8534-0_1
36. Reddy, A. S., & Zhang, S. (2013). Polypharmacology: Drug discovery for the future. *Expert Review of Clinical Pharmacology, 6*, 41–47.

37. Scannell, J. W., Blanckley, A., Boldon, H., & Warrington, B. (2012). Diagnosing the decline in pharmaceutical R&D efficiency. *Nature Reviews. Drug Discovery, 11*, 191–200.
38. Stork, C., Chen, Y., Šícho, M., & Kirchmair, J. (2019). Hit dexter 2.0: Machine-learning models for the prediction of frequent hitters. *Journal of Chemical Information and Modeling, 59*, 1030–1043. https://doi.org/10.1021/acs.jcim.8b00677
39. Sunarti, S., Fadzlul Rahman, F., Naufal, M., et al. (2021). Artificial intelligence in healthcare: Opportunities and risk for future. *Gaceta Sanitaria, 35*, S67–S70. https://doi.org/10.1016/j.gaceta.2020.12.019
40. Vyas, M., Thakur, S., Riyaz, B., et al. (2018). Artificial intelligence: The beginning of a new era in pharmacy profession. *Asian Journal Pharmaceutica, 12*, 72–76.
41. Wang, C., & Zhang, Y. (2017). Improving scoring-docking-screening powers of protein–ligand scoring functions using random forest. *Journal of Computational Chemistry, 38*, 169–177. https://doi.org/10.1002/jcc.24667
42. Wang, Y., Wang, Z., & Xu, J., et al. (2018). Systematic identification of non-coding pharmacogenomic landscape in cancer. *Nature Communications, 9*. https://doi.org/10.1038/s41467-018-05495-9
43. Wu, Z., Ramsundar, B., Feinberg, E. N., et al. (2018). MoleculeNet: A benchmark for molecular machine learning. *Chemical Science, 9*, 513–530. https://doi.org/10.1039/c7sc02664a
44. Yuan, Y., Pei, J., & Lai, L. (2011). LigBuilder 2: A practical de novo drug design approach. *Journal of Chemical Information and Modeling, 51*, 1083–1091. https://doi.org/10.1021/ci100350u
45. Zhu, T., Cao, S., Su, P. C., et al. (2013). Hit identification and optimization in virtual screening: Practical recommendations based on a critical literature analysis. *Journal of Medicinal Chemistry, 56*, 6560–6572.

Gene Expression, Multi-omics Analysis, and Blockchain

Computational Intelligence-Based Gene Expression Analysis in Colorectal Cancer: A Review

Ankit Srivastava, Sandhya Rai, Manish Pratap Singh, and Sameer Srivastava

Abstract Key challenges in cancer gene expression analysis are to collectively identify the gene (tumor suppressor, proto-oncogenes, and mismatch repair) or sets of genes that are differentially expressed significantly in cancer and normal samples. High throughput expression techniques provide quantitative data about the expression of thousands of genes per biological sample. However, such technologies have some common problems including but not limited to dataset complexity, data integration, and noise. Data generated from the latest technologies are growing at an explosive rate; therefore, it becomes essential to dig out useful information from this data and create biological knowledge. Moreover, traditional data analysis is sometimes not effective to extract valuable information from biological datasets. More recently, to overcome these issues, computational intelligence methods such as artificial intelligence (AI) and machine learning (ML) have been widely applied to study gene co-expression networks, differential gene expression analysis, pathway analysis, and predicting biomarkers and therapeutic targets in cancer. In this chapter, we attempt to describe how computational intelligence-based algorithms can contribute to this field to generate quality knowledge needed in cancer biology. Special emphasis is given on colorectal cancer (CRC) studies, wherein apart from expression biomarkers, diagnostic potential of AI-based analysis has also been investigated. We have highlighted algorithms widely used in identifying unique gene expression signatures in CRCs. AI and ML-based methodologies could help us identify high-risk genes or gene sets and their aberrant expression associated with them. In the future, this would help us improve diagnosis and prognosis for better monitoring and management of CRC.

Keywords Colorectal cancer · Artificial intelligence · Gene expression · High-throughput technologies · Machine learning

A. Srivastava · S. Rai · M. P. Singh · S. Srivastava (✉)
Department of Biotechnology, Motilal Nehru National Institute of Technology, Allahabad 211004, India
e-mail: sameers@mnnit.ac.in

M. P. Singh
e-mail: manish.biophd@mnnit.ac.in

K. Raza (ed.), *Computational Intelligence in Oncology*, Studies in Computational Intelligence 1016, https://doi.org/10.1007/978-981-16-9221-5_22

Abbreviations

AB	Ada boost
AI	Artificial intelligence
ANN	Artificial neural network
BRAF	v-Raf murine sarcoma viral oncogene homolog B1
CRC	Colorectal cancer
DT	Decision tree
DL	Deep learning
FNN	Fuzzy neural network
LR	Logistic regression
LDA	Linear discriminant analysis
ML	Machine learning
NB	Naive Bayes
SOM	Self-organizing map
SVM	Support vector machine

1 Introduction

Cancer is the second deadliest disease and cause of death globally. There are several types of cancers, but among all, lungs, breasts, prostate, ovarian, and colorectal cancer (CRC) are highly acknowledged due to their notorious nature. CRC is a heterogeneous disease and one of the most common malignancies ranked third in incidence and second in mortality worldwide [1]. Despite a lot of advancement in detection methods, screening programs and healthcare equipment, increasing global burden, and early diagnosis are still a matter of concern throughout the world. Currently, diagnosis at an early stage of CRC is usually not possible in all cases of incidence and is often handled with conventional treatment such as surgical resection, chemotherapy, and radiotherapy. However, this treatment regimen is sometimes not suitable for all patients and is often also associated with poor median overall survival (OS) and progression-free survival (PFS) [2]. Early detection of CRC is limited by many factors; however, accurate treatment is something that can be offered to CRC patients who have been diagnosed late. Considering the heterogeneous nature of CRC, which is attributed to a myriad of genes and pathways being altered in each molecular type, for accurate treatment, it is more important to identify the candidate genes/pathways responsible for it to suitably stratify the patient and decide the treatment regimen. In recent years, the popularity of translational research in the field of molecular oncology has grown immensely, and it offers accurate diagnosis/prognosis and selective treatment by modulating specific gene/protein functions. These specific genes/proteins could function as novel therapeutic targets or diagnostic/prognostic biomarkers which are an invaluable tool for CRC disease management. Extensive research on CRC has identified a large number of genes (tumor suppressor, proto-oncogenes, and mismatch repair or set of other genes) that are differentially regulated or show impaired expression during progression. Previous studies have reported the occurrence of genes such as KRAS, BRAF, APC, TP53, PIK3CA, and TGF-β, MAPK, and certain Wnt pathway genes that acquire early alterations (mutation or aberrant expression) are possibly the driving factor for CRC progression [3]. Likewise, many other genes have already been discovered, and some are still under investigation for the CRC onset. But, the major challenges faced in today's scenario are to collect and precisely identify the candidate driver genes which are differentially expressed in CRC and its normal sample.

In present times, health informatics has become a modern healthcare tool that is clinically important to manage any disease including cancer progression [4]. Modern High-throughput gene expression analysis techniques help to identify cancer-related genes and elucidate the relationship between genes and disease with all the clinical information [5–7]. Several studies have shown the effectiveness of high-throughput technologies such as microarray gene expression and next-generation sequencing analysis, in stratifying the CRC patients harboring unique molecular gene signatures as low-risk and high-risk groups as well as discriminating them from the control group have different survival outcomes [8–10]. In this context, our lab has recently reported that CXCL3, IL1B, MET, and TNS1 genes ($p = 0.015$, 0.038, 0.049, and 0.011 respectively) were found to be differentially expressed in early age onset colorectal cancer (EOCRC) tumors and were associated with overall survival and may function as biomarkers in EOCRCs. Moreover, this study also reported the deregulated genes and pathways implicated in EOCRC by following the high-throughput transcriptome analysis [11]. Similarly, DNA microarray analyses allow examining the hidden pattern of the expression level of thousands of genes simultaneously in a single experiment. However, the data analysis of biological datasets generated using traditional and new-generation technologies such as microarray, next-generation sequencing is not robust and accurate and therefore are believed to be unsuitable in some cases. Some general issues, identified in data analysis but not limited to the following list, are listed below:

(a) A small sample size produces poor results.
(b) Sometimes, sets of data generated are complex and noisy.
(c) Data integration due to protocol complexity.
(d) Various preprocessing steps lead to dissimilar results.
(e) High-dimensionality comes with poor diagnostic results.
(f) Tumor of different origin.
(g) A large number of genes limit the accuracy and speed of classification.
(h) Lack of standard methodology for the processing and analysis of data.
(i) The difference in the platform used to generate data from tumor samples and their comparison is always not possible.

Consequently, there is a need for more effective and dedicated techniques for data analysis to overcome the above complications in gene expression classification in cancer datasets. In recent years, computational intelligence methods such as artificial intelligence (AI) have been immensely used in high-throughput data analysis for various cancers including CRC with high accuracy. Particularly, machine learning (ML) and deep learning (DL) technologies include a wide range of algorithms to detect the most significant gene or gene sets from the dataset which might be important for cancer progression or may serve as potential diagnostic and prognostic markers in the future. In spite of that some ML-based algorithms classify the expressed gene with low accuracies such as fuzzy neural network (FNN) [12], hierarchical clustering [13], K-means clustering [14], self-organizing map (SOM) [15], and decision tree (DT) method [16], while support vector machine (SVM) [17], artificial neural network (ANN) [18] and genetic algorithm [19] are noted to have higher accuracy. Here, we have described the computational intelligence-based applications used to identify and classify the genes which are significantly differentially expressed between control and CRC. A proposed design of such a study has been demonstrated with the help of a flow diagram in (Fig. 1).

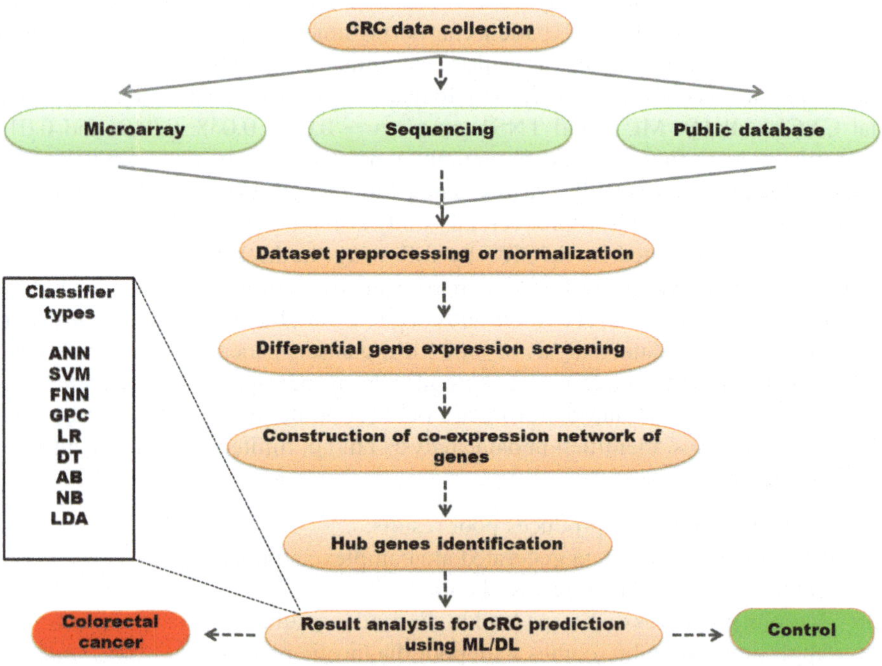

Fig. 1 Flow diagram for analysis: customizes the gene expression data classification using computational intelligence-based classifier

2 Computational Intelligence-Based Models: Application in CRC

Computational intelligence incorporates artificial intelligence, machine learning, neural network, and deep learning approaches for the identification of gene targets in cancer [20]. This is schematically shown in Figure 2. AI is a computing program, which requires specific software and/or hardware to emulate human intelligence. AI is a rapidly growing technology, which covers almost every area from health care, environment, and agriculture to gaming, education, robotics, travel, entertainment, and many more. Primarily, it covers a wide range of applications from imaging of medical specimens, clinical diagnosis and treatment, drug development, to the area of surgical and nursing robots [21].

2.1 *Artificial Intelligence*

Artificial intelligence (AI) mimics human intelligence and focuses on creating intelligent computers [22, 23]. AI provides better opportunities in the diagnosis, prognosis, and clinical response against the treatment of diseases that help the doctors to accurately analyze the patients. AI system-specific natural language processing (NLP) was utilized by Imler et al. [24] to monitor the results of colonoscopy. This diagnostic method has the potential to serve as the gold standard for CRC screening and monitoring. ColorApp is another application that was developed by Marzuki et al. [25]. It is an AI-based application that is integrated with a mobile device. It shares information about educating the public on CRC and is able to get the current information for CRC prevention. Several other AI-based applications are all around us, and they find their application in a wide range of areas. In general, there are two types of AI applications in the medical field: virtual and physical. The virtual component of AI is made up of machine learning (ML) and deep learning (DL, a subset of ML). There are three types of machine learning algorithms: supervised, unsupervised, and reinforcement learning. These are classified based on predictive modeling, in which a class label is defined depending on the input data. In general, there is no proper definition of ML algorithms; however, the broader and comprehensive description of supervised learning refers to an algorithm that is trained using input/labeled data, and the best model is built independently, while an unsupervised algorithm is used to train with an unlabeled input dataset for preparing the best model The concept of AI technology, especially deep learning (DL), helps us to understand the CRC at the molecular level through image analysis of tumor samples and has resulted in further improvements in the surveillance, diagnosis, prognosis, staging, and treatment of CRC. In addition, AI-based analysis could be also useful in terms of providing insights for drug design through screening at the clinical level and offers great opportunity in the development of personalized drugs to treat patients [26]. One of the important features of AI is its

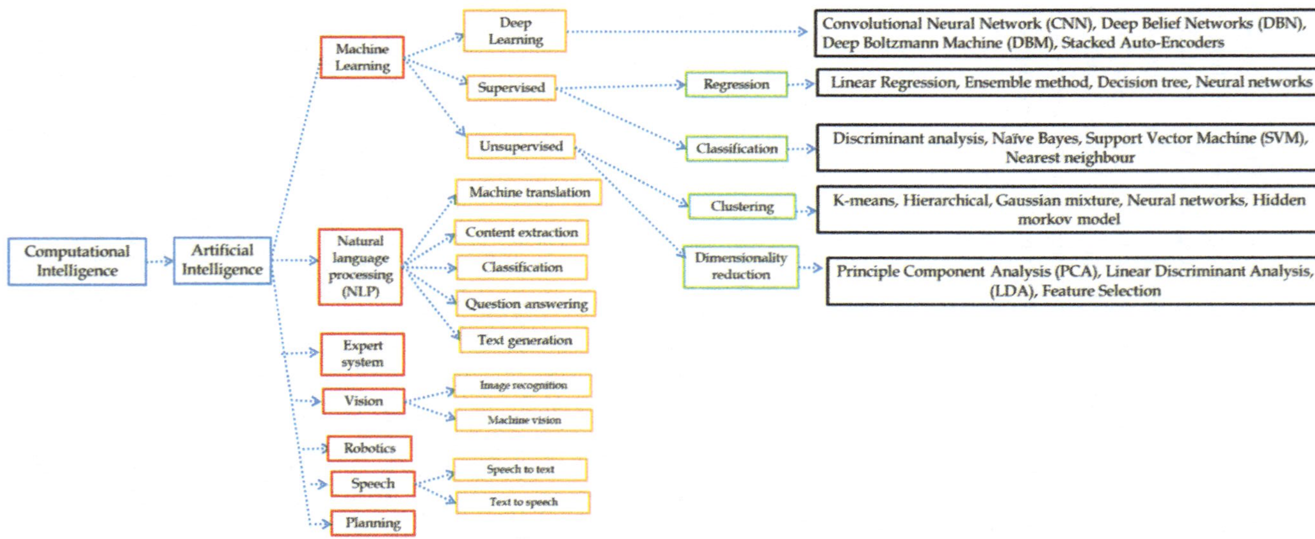

Fig. 2 This provides an overview of the model involved in computational intelligence

ability to serve as the optimal solution for drug target validation and drug design optimization for successful treatment to selectively fight diseases like cancer, along with its high-rated features such as predicting drug-protein interaction, the 3D structure of target protein and determination of drug activity. These properties can aid in making the AI more efficient for cancer therapeutics, including CRC. Recent advancements of AI in drug formulation and designing have led to the development of software and Web-based tools such as Targethunter (https://www.cbligand.org/TargetHunter3D/), PharmMapper (http://lilab-ecust.cn/pharmmapper/), TarPred (http://www.dddc.ac.cn/tarpred/), Swiss Target Prediction (http://www.swisstargetprediction.ch/), and ChemMapper (http://lilab.ecust.edu.cn/chemmapper/). Among the aforementioned Web-based tools, PharmMapper is widely used to prioritize potential therapeutic drug targets for colorectal cancer research with optimal accuracy.

2.2 *Machine Learning*

Machine learning (ML) is an interdisciplinary field of AI that contains various statistical, mathematical, and optimization tools. It could help in the prediction/identification of novel targets by using genomics, proteomics, and transcriptomics data of different patients [27]. ML has several applications in CRC such as establishing a good or bad prognosis, early diagnosis, and personalized therapy. It helps in the discovery of biomarkers by detecting the target biomarker genes in the patients; however, choosing the most appropriate biomarker is generally based on its stability and prediction accuracy [28]. ML-based strategies like unsupervised clustering methods were applied to monitor the clinical outcome of the panitumumab-based therapy in metastatic CRC. Clustering generated seven distinct subtypes of the patients that had different survival outcomes and shared genetic characters. Clustering of cancer patients based on their shared genetic characteristics is an essential need to predict the anticancer drug response for a better understanding of the therapeutic outcome. However, AI-based prediction of the drug response could be ambiguous that led to identifying the robust translational biomarkers from preclinical models and merging them with the pharmacogenomics data of the 3D organoid models. The screened biomarkers were able to accurately predict the drug response of about 114 CRC patients receiving 5-FU, and this model was also able to distinguish between drug-resistant and drug-sensitive isogenic cancer cell lines. In CRC, colonoscopy is the best diagnostic method to detect the polyps; however, sometimes, small polyps are hard to detect, nevertheless, and training machine learning algorithms on imaging data can be used to increase the polyp detection rate and eventually leading to early detection and treatment [29]. Researchers recently developed AI models to improve CRC screening outcomes and lower the percentage of missed adenomas and the risk of getting cancer [24–26]. Computer-assisted detection and characterization systems are generating a lot of buzz these days. Endoscopists may be able to make more accurate and fast diagnoses using AI aid for colorectal polyp identification and visual diagnosis during colonoscopy [30–32]. It was also shown that the accuracy of the machine learning approach is high, which suggests that ML has the potential and can improve the adenomas detection rate, ultimately reducing the rate of mortality due to CRC [33]. Furthermore, robotic surgery and innovative computer-assisted medication administration techniques usher in a new era in CRC therapy. Health care, on the other hand, is quickly heading toward precision or customized treatment.

2.3 *Artificial Neural Networks*

Artificial neural networks (ANNs) are recognized as very useful in big data analysis. Other networks like convolutional neural networks (CNNs) are used in image analysis [34]. AI-based techniques are very advanced, and the ultimate goal of these techniques is to increase early detection in CRC, fast and accurate diagnosis. As per the earlier work of Burke et al., 1997, ANN and multiLayer perceptrons (MLPs) are considered to be best suited for the prognostic system and survival prediction for patients with CRC over other methods [18]. Further, studies consistently report a close and strong association between neural network and survival prediction in patients with CRC [35, 36].

Apart from the above-discussed applications of AI, a subclass of AI such as ML, DL, and ANN can also be used on gene expression data to analyze and precisely identify unique molecular signatures for cancer subtyping, identifying molecular features responsible for clinical response against therapy and associating gene or set of genes having significant prognostic and diagnostic biomarker potential. Nasarian et al., 2020, reported that expression-based studies on colon cancer using statistical as well as AI-based (ANN) methods precisely cluster the CRC patients into two major clusters displaying 20 signature genes; some of these genes are novel and are supposed to be involved in the early age onset of CRC [37]. Similarly, soft tissue sarcomas having divergent clinical features are considered to be hard to treat, so David et al. explored the problem using gene expression data available on the TCGA database using a machine learning approach. They have identified three clusters overlapping the clinical as well as molecular features. Therapeutic response analysis based on these clusters was analyzed for the HDAC inhibitor and shows that leiomyosarcoma and synovial sarcoma are significantly responded with HDAC inhibitor [38]. These techniques are elaborated in the following sections.

3 Significance of Gene Expression Profiling in Cancer Research

"Expression of gene" or "Gene Expression" generally refers to transcription of mRNA from the DNA (encoding a gene) which ultimately is translated to the product of the gene that is protein. Gene expression is a tightly regulated process that governs the cell behavior against its changing environment. Change in regulatory mechanisms that control gene expression also results in a change in gene expression. Any alteration in the gene expression pattern of a cell could lead to a different phenotype of the cell. Gene expression is dynamic in nature, and measuring aberrant expression is vital for understanding the various underlying informations which differentiates the cancer cell from normal cells. Changes in the expression level of genes can usually be measured at two stages: transcript and protein level. Numerous tools such as Alexa-Seq, Bit-Seq, ExAtlas, ExpressionSuite, DEGSeq, NetworkAnalyst, GeneCluster, and bioconductor are available that are specifically designed to analyze the variability of gene expression either at the transcript or protein level. However, measuring the expression level of proteins is sometimes not appropriate due to modification, varying location, and incompleteness of the proteome. Moreover, measuring the whole proteome is more complex and cumbersome than measuring the transcriptome. For instance, it is easier to measure the expression of genes products at transcript level using methods such as northern blotting, serial analysis of gene expression, RNA-Seq., microarray, and quantitative polymerase chain reaction, often with the better approximation but with less biological relevance (Fig. 3).

Gene expression provides an insight into the cellular responses at different cellular states and conditions. It has been found that several common sources can influence gene expressions such as gender, age, tissue specificity, environment, and heritable changes that may be associated with the adverse consequences of tumorigenesis and its progression. The occurrence of cancer is usually due to aberrant expression of multiple gene signatures of its own or sometimes driven by sources such as the presence or absence of certain signaling molecules in the external environment of cell or tissue, UV irradiation, toxins, and carcinogens that are pathogenic [39].

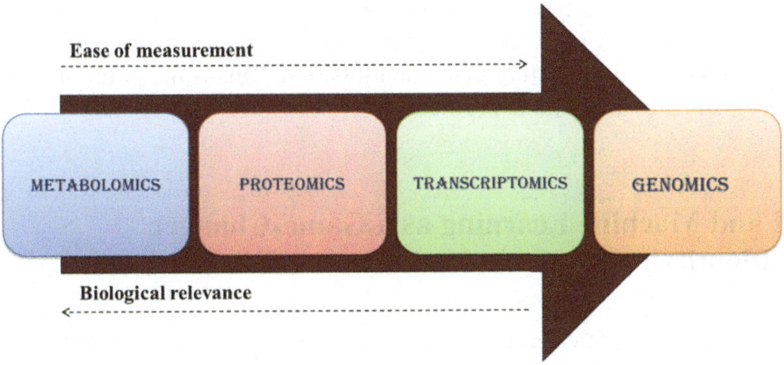

Fig. 3 High-throughput analysis: ease of measurement and its biological relevance

4 Gene Expression Classification: A Framework

Alteration in gene expression is due to changes in regulatory mechanisms. Our increased knowledge of the regulatory processes of gene expression has strengthened our understanding of cancer progression including CRC [40]. Measuring the gene expression and associating the aberrant expression to the cancer susceptibility is a nontrivial task. Although to characterize significantly differentially expressed genes, it is critical to perform variable screening-based analysis, by employing the high-throughput gene expression analysis tools. These tools vary with the type of platform used to generate the transcriptomics data. In the case of NGS platforms generating short reads, tools such as DESeq2 [41], EdgeR [42], and limma [43] are of choice. Similarly, affy [44], bead array [45], illuminaio [46], and Biobase [47] are other tools that deal with data from various other new-generation platforms using the expression data. Once the relevant network of expressed genes associated with cancer is identified, the next step is to understand the biological correlations and co-expression among identified genes (Fig. 1). The construction of a co-expression network could be best explained by using the algorithms such as "Weighted gene co-expression network analysis (WGCNA), hierarchical clustering tree, and dynamic tree cut method" that could more accurately identify biologically relevant co-expressed gene sets [48, 49]. Finally, screening of the top hub genes (having high gene significance) has received great consideration in reducing the curse of high dimension that often interferes with the analysis. It is worth noting that various authors in the past have used other methodologies such as ranksum [13], chi-square [14], principle component analysis (PCA) [10], and kruskal Wallis (KW) [13] test and identified the most significant set of genes in cancer. Nonetheless, these entire gene expression data analysis modules provide a flexible option for gene expression analysis. The typical structure of such a model is shown graphically in (Fig. 4). On a different note, this alternative method results in a simpler approach but is less sensitive in predicting gene identification. This is the point of view from where we will be looking at the problem.

5 AI and Machine Learning as a Game-Changer in Identifying the Gene Signatures in CRC

Cancer subtyping is critical for identifying patients who would benefit most from specific treatments and for developing new targeted medicines. Cancer subtyping has traditionally been based mostly on histological and clinical features, which makes it difficult to adopt universally because pathologist expertise is often a key aspect in subtyping. Although these categories have undeniable prognostic value, their ability to predict medication effectiveness is limited due to a lack of a clear molecular foundation. In CRC, KRAS mutation and microsatellite instability (MSI) have been

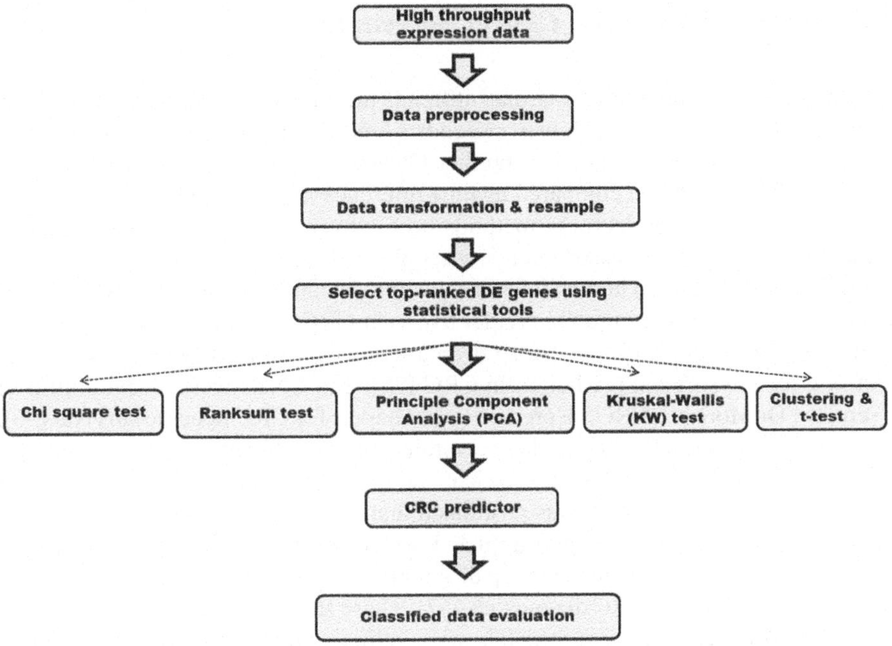

Fig. 4 This illustrates the basic model of the differentially expressed cancer gene classification system

shown to predict the therapeutic efficacy of anti-EGFR and 5-FU [50]. However, classifications based on such molecular features fail to account for a significant amount of cancer heterogeneity that exists above KRAS and MSI alterations. In recent years, cancer subtyping based on transcriptome analysis has been demonstrated to be an effective method for establishing cancer heterogeneity. DL for cancer classification has shown a lot of promise in recent developments in the machine learning field [51]. Deep convolutional neural networks have been shown to increase tumor classification accuracy and repeatability using histological or radiographic data. D-GEX, DeepChrome, and DeepSEA are examples of deep learning-based platforms for determining gene expression or noncoding variation effects related to higher genomic or epigenomic profiles [52, 53]. Furthermore, numerous algorithms based on supervised and unsupervised deep learning classification for cancer screening and prevention have been suggested, and their performance has been proven to be superior to traditional approaches like support vector machines (SVM) and random forests (RF) [22].

5.1 Applications of AI: Cancer Screening

Recent cancer research suggests that utilizing the image of histopathology slides as input DL may predict diagnosis, prognosis, and therapy response. For example, a DL system had been created to predict Gleason score in prostate cancer based on histology [54]. When compared against reference ratings supplied by genitourinary pathologists, deep learning methods beat conventional pathologists, although accuracy in assigning Gleason scores was only 0.70. From spot pictures of hematoxylin and eosin (H&E) tumor slides, a convoluted neural network-based (CNN) DL method was shown to accurately predict five-year CRC-specific survival, regardless of tumor stage or grade [55]. A "deep stroma score" was created using CNN transfer learning for the survival prediction in CRC [55]. Ten CNNs were recently utilized to create "DoMore-v1-CRC," a predictive biomarker for CRC-specific survival [56]. To improve accuracy, this biomarker was trained using different resolutions of H&E images and was linked with many clinical and molecular characteristics. In a recent report by Zhang et al. [57], it was postulated that key genes are significantly associated with CRC in 378 histology samples. Further, integrated analysis of oncogenic networks was applied to screen the top differently expressed genes and hub genes for the biomarker study on CRC diagnostics [57]. These studies justify the application of AI and ML in CRC screening, which is more in line with the approach used in Table 1. Deep learning is now being used to anticipate cancer molecular characteristics like genomes, transcriptomics, and proteomics. Recently, researchers classified non-small cell lung cancer into various histological categories and identified the mutation status of numerous genes using a CNN algorithm [58].

5.2 Applications of Artificial Intelligence: Biomarker Discovery

The discovery of biomarkers is a prevalent area of concern and research interest in the early diagnosis of patients with CRC. Over the past year, AI and ML have introduced an impressive new technology for identifying the biomarkers using the microarray data, sequencing data, and the public database, and have made significant advances in research into the underlying molecular mechanism. Some experts have started applying these techniques to the real world, in the case of early CRC diagnosis and treatment. The S-Kohonen, back propagation (BP), and SVM neural networks were tested for classification accuracy. Hu et al. [71] claimed that the S-Kohonen neural network (91%) was more successful in classifying colon cancer than BP (66%) and SVM (70%) [71]. Xu et al. [72] used SVM analysis to discover differentially expressed genes (DEGs) that may be used to differentiate individuals with a high risk of colon cancer recurrence. They discovered a 15-gene signature that may be used to predict the likelihood of recurrence and prognosis in colon cancer patients [72]. Zhang et al. [57] presented a sensitive and low-cost approach

Table 1 Summarized studies for the gene expression classification by employing the ML and DL classifier in colorectal cancer

S. No.	Sample size	Array type	Classifier method	Statistical method	Number of genes or events	References
1	434	Data extracted from two public database	Artificial neural network (ANN)	Odds likelihood ratio test and McNemar test, (non-parametric test)	Death prediction	[59]
2	62	Affymetrix Hum6000 array	Two-way clustering algorithm	Distribution correlation coefficients	~6500	[60]
3	Random selection from database	Data extracted from National Cancer Database (NCDB)	Regression analysis, artificial neural network, and fuzzy logic system,	Kaplan–Meier and cox model	5-year survival prediction	[61]
4	25	Pyrosequencing (454 GS20 genome sequencer) and serial analysis of gene expression (SAGE)	Logistic regression	Bonferroni correction and pairwise comparison	31	[62]
5	66	Affymetrix HG U133 Plus 2.0 GeneChips (Affymetrix, Santa Clara, CA) and Immunohistochemical analysis (IHC)	Hierarchical clustering	Chi-square test	1377	[63]
6	–	Microarray	Boolean logic and guilt-by-association algorithm (GBA)	Parsimonious mixed-effect ANOVA	749	[64]

(continued)

Table 1 (continued)

S. No.	Sample size	Array type	Classifier method	Statistical method	Number of genes or events	References
7	26	Illumina Ref-8 whole genome expression BeadChip	STRING (Search tool for the retrieval of interacting genes), mRMR (Maximum relevance minimum redundancy), nearest neighbor algorithm (NNA) and Dijkstra's algorithm	Independent dataset test, subsampling test, and jackknife test	41	[65]
8	11,541	Data extracted from national cancer institute's surveillance, epidemiology, and end results (SEER) and hospital of China medical university	Back propagation network (BP), Radial basis function (RBF), Artificial neural network (ANN), General regression neural network (GRNN), Adaptive-network-based fuzzy inference system (ANFIS), Support vector machines (SVMs), Naive Bayes (NB), Bayesian networks (BNs), Classification and regression tree (CART), and Logistic regression (LR)	Random sampling and K-fold cross-validation model	TNM staging for CRC	[66]

(continued)

Table 1 (continued)

S. No.	Sample size	Array type	Classifier method	Statistical method	Number of genes or events	References
9	62	Microarray	Linear discriminant analysis (LDA), Quadratic discriminant analysis (QDA), Naïve Bayes (NB), Gaussian process classification (GPC), Logistic regression (LR), SVM, ANN, Adaboost (AB), Decision tree (DT), and Random forest (RF)	Kruskal Wallis (KW), and F-test, *t* test Wilcoxon sign rank sum (WCSRS)	2000	[67]
10	181	Illumina Hiseq 2000/2500 (Illumina San Diego, USA)	Logistic regression (LR) and SVM	Matthews correlation coefficients	–	[68]
11	378	Microarray data GSE68468	Weighted correlation network analysis (WGCNA)	Pearson correlation coefficients and Kaplan–Meier plot	400	[57]
12	238	Affymetrix Human Genome U133 Plus 2.0 Array	Variational autoencoder (VAE) support vector machines (SVM)	Pearson correlation coefficient (PCC)	13,487	[69]
13	–	Immunohistochemical analysis and PCR-based assay	Deep learning (convolutional neural network) CNN	–	Mismatch repair genes (MMR)	[70]

for identifying BRAF-V600E gene mutation. The present model exhibited 100% diagnostic sensitivity, 87.5% diagnostic specificity, and 93.8% diagnostic accuracy when employed to screen for the v-Raf murine sarcoma viral oncogene homolog B1 (BRAF) V600E mutation in colorectal carcinomas [73]. Coppedè et al. [54] used artificial neural networks 2015 to look at the relationship between hereditary and environmental variables and DNA methylation in CRC [74]. Wang et al. [75] used The Cancer Genome Atlas (TCGA) gene expression data and AI algorithms to enhance CRC detection a few years later [75]. Furthermore, utilizing tumor-derived cell-free DNA, Wan et al. [75] presented a machine learning technique with excellent sensitivity and specificity for early diagnosis [76]. Their method might be a potential new path for early-stage CRC detection studies in the future. In a recent study, Ai et al. [69] identified the most suitable biomarkers from the hub genes by extracting the information from microarray data for 238 CRC and normal samples. They consider the variational autoencoder (VAE) and SVM for the CRC classifier followed by a screening of the hub genes by considering the module membership, gene significance, and intramodular connectivity [69]. Similar microarray data analysis had been performed using ML/DL-based algorithms such as Naïve Bayes (NB), linear discriminant analysis (LDA), Gaussian process classification (GPC), quadratic discriminant analysis (QDA), SVM, ANN, logistic regression (LR), AdaBoost (AB), decision tree (DT), and random forest (RF) [57, 60, 63, 64, 67]. In addition, Table 1 discusses best practices and emerging novel techniques of AI and ML-based models in the detection of biomarkers for the early CRC diagnosis for data generated using next-generation sequencing methods as well [62, 65, 68].

Identifying particular noncoding RNA (ncRNA), expression changes in colon tissue and plasma/serum samples may prove useful in early CRC diagnosis, prognosis prediction, and targeted therapy, since recent research sheds light on ncRNAs' function in cancer diagnosis and treatment [77]. Chang et al. [78] identified differentially expressed micro-RNAs (miRNAs) by comparing the expression patterns of 380 miRNAs in stage II colorectal tumors and normal tissues using artificial neural network analysis. They discovered three miRNA signatures (miR-139-5p, miR-3, and miR-17-92) that may be used to predict the tumor status in stage II CRC patients [78]. A team of researchers developed a unique computational approach for miRNA-target prediction in CRC employing a Naive Bayes classifier with the goal of refining this method and increasing prediction accuracy. CRC miRTar, the current model, was also able to decipher the CRC-specific interactions between miRNAs and target messenger RNAs (mRNAs) [79].

Currently, AI technologies also allow physicians to estimate the prognosis of CRC patients. In a study, the researchers discovered 40 SVM-classified signature genes in metastatic colorectal neoplasms with AMPK signaling and ubiquitin-mediated proteolysis pathways significantly enriched in metastatic colorectal neoplasms [80]. To detect aberrant tissue that might be suggestive of a premalignant precursor lesion or an early-stage tumor, effective screening techniques have been developed. Machine learning algorithms might be used to test for CRC risk in large populations in a non-invasive and cost-effective manner [81].

6 Case Studies

Case study #1: Machine learning improves the accuracy of stage II CRC prognosis [82].

Machine learning is widely investigated as a promising AI tool for CRC. It is believed that an accurate prognosis is key to successful therapy for CRC patients. However, several problems are associated with classifying the CRC patients primarily on the basis of stages that have higher variability in survival. In a recent study, researchers explored various ML approaches to extract the histopathological data that were useful in predicting survival for 2nd stage CRC patients. A setup has been developed to support the development and testing of this approach. 180 2nd stage patients diagnosed with CRC were recruited to undergo surgical resection, and their tissue samples were used to obtain the clinical data. The tumor samples were subjected to immunofluorescence with D2-40 antibodies, followed by staining with a DAPI reagent. The whole slide image was captured at 40X magnification to properly visualize the lymphatic vessels, cell nuclei, and epithelial cells, resulting in collecting the histopathological features (not mentioned here) associated with each patient. The baseline classifiers such as support vector machine, k-nearest neighboring, and Naïve Bayes were used both for the classification task and for the survival analysis. All of the classifiers used in this study maximized the average curve, yielding a value of 0.89 for both the 5-year and 10-year prognosis, which was approximately higher than when using the simple statistical approach of both for the 5 and 10-year prognosis observed was 0.82. Moreover, employing ML improved the prediction of the mortality rate in stage II CRC patients (AUROC = 0.94). Therefore, the introduction of the ML approach has the potential to provide convenient and multidimensional data, assist in fast and accurate medical image processing, and to improve the better prognosis of stage II CRC patients [82].

Case Study #2: Classification of colon microarray gene expression data using multiple machine learning paradigm [83].

In this study, the aim of the researcher was to identify the candidate genes responsible for cancer progression. ML approach was used to classify the high-risk genes. 2000 gene sets were extracted from 62 samples (including 40 cancer and 22 control samples) and were classified using different classifiers namely NB, SVM, LR, and AB. The novelty of this study was assessed with standardized accuracy and area under the curve, which showed an accuracy of 90.50%. However, a significant outcome was observed with RF and WCSRS classifiers showing an improved accuracy of 99.81%. With these results, the authors concluded that among all the classifiers discussed, RF-based models fulfill two functions that can accurately detect the high-risk gene associated with colon cancer [83].

Here, we have discussed the two recent computational intelligence-based studies that identified accurately the prognosis/diagnosis of CRC. Although, a large number of experimental studies have been carried out; however, careful consideration is required in order to accommodate this knowledge to be translated into important clinical insights.

Study limitation and challenges of Computational Intelligence

In recent years, the idea of computational intelligence learning has found its utility in various research fields including mathematics, physics, computer science, and life science. Despite the reported successes of computational intelligence (AI/ML/DL) in the field of life science particularly in cancer research, it suffers from a series of limitations/challenges which are discussed in the following section.

(a) Several studies demonstrated that artificial intelligence algorithms such as artificial neural networks, support vector machines, Bayesian networks, clustering, and many others to aid in gene expression analysis, however, sometimes due to heterogeneous data and varying data form across various databases cancer-associated gene classification are always not possible.
(b) Overfitting is always posing a problem resulting in limitations with data access and quality with degraded performance. Thus, computational intelligence (ML/AI) often involves a trade-off between accuracy and intelligibility.
(c) The use of mathematical and statistical algorithms may not discover interesting facts from the generated datasets.
(d) Currently, most clinicians, data scientists, and bioinformaticians have lacked proper training and experience with cancer research and its data management, limiting the ability to better elucidate and identify the potential drug development and biomarkers discovery.

Recognizing and overcoming the limits of computational intelligence are a great challenge. However, there is a number of innovative approaches that optimize processes and enable accelerated data management. The following assumption can aid to overcome the constraints:

(a) Data biases: The AI recruiting system should be trained with unbiased data
(b) AI human interface—more trained professionals will replace the manpower shortage to get maximum output from the technology.
(c) Data security—a huge volume of data generated using the traditional approach is often sensitive and can be lost. Therefore, computational intelligence-based algorithms are available that minimize data loss with enhanced security.
(d) Short of complexity—the datasets generated with AI and ML algorithms are more interesting and inventive that aid to solve complex problems.
(e) Zero fault diagnosis—with the implementation of new technology such as the Internet of Things (IoT), big data, and intelligent manufacturing, it is easy to develop robust methods for condition and real-time monitoring and zero fault diagnosis system.

7 Important Advantages of Computational Intelligence

(a) It provides a better interface for human interaction with improved programming and software.

(b) Rapid development in the application of computational intelligence leads to the collection and aggregation of a large volume of data information and convert it into meaningful knowledge.
(c) Through AI, significant progress has been made in terms of operational reliability and management, production efficiency, and cost-effective maintenance of the system.
(d) Computational intelligence approaches would be an ideal method of choice to address complex problems. This approach has the lowest error out of all the methods employed to handle large-scale and complex problems.
(e) Computational intelligence technique has an option of "fusion" demonstrating its critical advantage in decision-making and problem-solving. However, the fusion of networks (neural network, fuzzy system, genetic algorithm, approximate reasoning, etc.) comprehensively demonstrates its role in the handling of complexity and managing uncertainty and imprecision.

8 Conclusion and Future Scope

Analyzing gene expression in CRC is a complex and multifaceted process. Understanding the aberrant expression of candidate genes in CRC helps in diagnosis, prognosis, and even underlying mechanisms and identifies patients at higher risk for adverse events from specific treatments. For this reason, multiple AI/ML-based algorithms are available that can be used for several purposes such as to identify the expressed genes, classify gene expression data according to associated risk factors and identify potential biomarkers. Since ML and AI applications continue to assist in oncologic research, more labor requires attention to translate this work into meaningful clinical application. More advancement and development in the ML and AI applications requires a multidisciplinary and collaborative approach in cancer research. Therefore, to maximize the impact of ML and AI technology in oncology, some knowledge gaps need to be addressed, such as: providing periodic training to the clinicians, physicians, scientists, researchers to adopt these algorithms and conduct research, collaborate with an oncologist, data scientist, and bioinformatician and promote the dissemination of these AI-based methods in cancer research.

References

1. Bray, F., Ferlay, J., Soerjomataram, I., Siegel, R. L., Torre, L. A., & Jemal, A. (2018). Global cancer statistics 2018: GLOBOCAN estimates of incidence and mortality worldwide for 36 cancers in 185 countries. *CA: A Cancer Journal for Clinicians, 68*(6), 394–424.
2. Colorectal Cancer Survival Rates, Colorectal Cancer Prognosis. Retrieved 20 August 2021, from https://www.cancer.org/cancer/colon-rectal-cancer/detection-diagnosis-staging/survival-rates.html

3. Singh, M. P., Rai, S., Suyal, S., Singh, S. K., Singh, N. K., Agarwal, A., & Srivastava, S. (2017). Genetic and epigenetic markers in colorectal cancer screening: Recent advances. *In Expert Review of Molecular Diagnostics, 17*(7), 665–685.
4. Ng, R. T., & Pei, J. (2007). Introduction to the special issue on data mining for health informatics. *ACM SIGKDD Explorations Newsletter, 9*(1), 1–2.
5. Chen, H. Y., Yu, S. L., Chen, C. H., Chang, G. C., Chen, C. Y., Yuan, A., Cheng, C. L., Wang, C. H., Terng, H. J., Kao, S. F., Chan, W. K., Li, H. N., Liu, C. C., Singh, S., Chen, W. J., Chen, J. J. W., & Yang, P. C. (2007). A five-gene signature and clinical outcome in non-small-cell lung cancer. *New England Journal of Medicine, 356*(1), 11–20.
6. Rosenwald, A., Wright, G., Wiestner, A., Chan, W. C., Connors, J. M., Campo, E., Gascoyne, R. D., Grogan, T. M., Muller-Hermelink, H. K., Smeland, E. B., Chiorazzi, M., Giltnane, J. M., Hurt, E. M., Zhao, H., Averett, L., Henrickson, S., Yang, L., Powell, J., Wilson, W. H., & Staudt, L. M. (2003). The proliferation gene expression signature is a quantitative integrator of oncogenic events that predicts survival in mantle cell lymphoma. *Cancer Cell, 3*(2), 185–197.
7. Dressman, H. K., Berchuck, A., Chan, G., Zhai, J., Bild, A., Sayer, R., Cragun, J., Clarke, J., Whitaker, R. S., Li, L., & Gray, J. (2007). An integrated genomic-based approach to individualized treatment of patients with advanced-stage ovarian cancer. *Journal of Clinical Oncology, 25*(5), 517–525.
8. Sabates-Bellver, J., Van der Flier, L. G., de Palo, M., Cattaneo, E., Maake, C., Rehrauer, H., Laczko, E., Kurowski, M. A., Bujnicki, J. M., Menigatti, M., & Luz, J. (2007). Transcriptome profile of human colorectal adenomas. *Molecular cancer research, 5*(12), 1263–1275.
9. Qin, L., Zeng, J., Shi, N., Chen, L., & Wang, L. (2020). Application of weighted gene co-expression network analysis to explore the potential diagnostic biomarkers for colorectal cancer. *Molecular Medicine Reports, 21*(6), 2533–2543.
10. Lenz, M., Müller, F. J., Zenke, M., & Schuppert, A. (2016). Principal components analysis and the reported low intrinsic dimensionality of gene expression microarray data. *Scientific Reports, 6*(1), 1–11.
11. Singh, M. P., Rai, S., Singh, N. K., & Srivastava, S. (2021). Transcriptomic landscape of early age onset of colorectal cancer identifies novel genes and pathways in Indian CRC patients. *Scientific Reports, 11*(1), 1–11.
12. Cortes, C., & Vapnik, V. (1995). Support-vector networks. *Springer, 20*, 273–297.
13. Chen, D., Liu, Z., Ma, X., & Hua, D. (2005). Selecting genes by test statistics. *Journal of Biomedicine and Biotechnology, 2005*(2), 132.
14. Dahiru, T. (2008). P-value, a true test of statistical significance? A cautionary note. *Annals of Ibadan Postgraduate Medicine, 6*(1), 21–26.
15. Sun, G., Dong, X., & Xu, G. (2006). Tumor tissue identification based on gene expression data using DWT feature extraction and PNN classifier. *Neurocomputing, 69*(4–6), 387–402.
16. Hsu, Y. C., Yuan, S., Chen, H. Y., Yu, S. L., Liu, C. H., Hsu, P. Y., Wu, G., Lin, C. H., Chang, G. C., Li, K. C., & Yang, P. C. (2009). A four-gene signature from NCI-60 cell line for survival prediction in non-small cell lung cancer. *Clinical Cancer Research, 15*(23), 7309–7315.
17. Ramaswamy, S., Tamayo, P., Rifkin, R., Mukherjee, S., Yeang, C. H., Angelo, M., Ladd, C., Reich, M., Latulippe, E., Mesirov, J. P., & Poggio, T. (2001). Multiclass cancer diagnosis using tumor gene expression signatures. *Proceedings of the National Academy of Sciences, 98*(26), 15149–15154.
18. Burke, H. B., Goodman, P. H., Rosen, D. B., Henson, D. E., Weinstein, J. N., Harrell, F. E., Jr., Marks, J. R., Winchester, D. P., & Bostwick, D. G. (1997). Artificial neural networks improve the accuracy of cancer survival prediction. *Cancer, 79*(4), 857–862.
19. Rothberg, B. E. G., Berger, A. J., Molinaro, A. M., Subtil, A., Krauthammer, M. O., Camp, R. L., Bradley, W. R., Ariyan, S., Kluger, H. M., & Rimm, D. L. (2009). Melanoma prognostic model using tissue microarrays and genetic algorithms. *Journal of Clinical Oncology, 27*(34), 5772.
20. Dimitrakopoulos, C. M., & Beerenwinkel, N. (2017). Computational approaches for the identification of cancer genes and pathways. *Wiley Interdisciplinary Reviews: Systems Biology and Medicine, 9*(1), e1364.

21. Wang, K. W., & Dong, M. (2020). Potential applications of artificial intelligence in colorectal polyps and cancer: Recent advances and prospects. *World Journal of Gastroenterology, 26*(34), 5090.
22. Mitsala, A., Tsalikidis, C., Pitiakoudis, M., Simopoulos, C., & Tsaroucha, A. K. (2021). Artificial intelligence in colorectal cancer screening, diagnosis and treatment. A New Era. *Current Oncology, 28*(3), 1581–1607.
23. Shalev-Shwartz, S., & Ben-David, S. (2014). *Understanding machine learning: From theory to algorithms*. Cambridge University Press.
24. Imler, T. D., Morea, J., Kahi, C., Cardwell, J., Johnson, C. S., Xu, H., & Imperiale, T. F. (2015). Multi-center colonoscopy quality measurement utilizing natural language processing. *Official Journal of the American College of Gastroenterology, ACG, 110*(4), 543–552.
25. Marzuki, M. F. M., Yaacob, N. A., bin Yaacob, N. M., Hassan, M. R. A., & Ahmad, S. B. (2019). Usable mobile app for community education on colorectal cancer development process and usability study. *JMIR Human Factors, 6*(2), e12103.
26. Wang, Y., He, X., Nie, H., Zhou, J., Cao, P., & Ou, C. (2020). Application of artificial intelligence to the diagnosis and therapy of colorectal cancer. *American Journal of Cancer Research, 10*(11), 3575.
27. Cruz, J. A., & Wishart, D. S. (2006). Applications of machine learning in cancer prediction and prognosis. *Cancer Informatics, 2*, 117693510600200030.
28. Kourou, K., Exarchos, T. P., Exarchos, K. P., Karamouzis, M. V., & Fotiadis, D. I. (2015). Machine learning applications in cancer prognosis and prediction. *Computational and Structural Biotechnology Journal, 13*, 8–17.
29. Mori, Y., Kudo, S. E., Misawa, M., & Mori, K. (2019). Simultaneous detection and characterization of diminutive polyps with the use of artificial intelligence during colonoscopy. *VideoGIE, 4*(1), 7.
30. Ruffle, J. K., Farmer, A. D., & Aziz, Q. (2019). Artificial intelligence-assisted gastroenterology—Promises and pitfalls. *Official Journal of the American College of Gastroenterology, ACG, 114*(3), 422–428.
31. Kudo, S. E., Mori, Y., Misawa, M., Takeda, K., Kudo, T., Itoh, H., & Mori, K. (2019). Artificial intelligence and colonoscopy: Current status and future perspectives. *Digestive Endoscopy, 31*(4), 363–371.
32. Mori, Y., Kudo, S. E., Berzin, T. M., Misawa, M., & Takeda, K. (2017). Computer-aided diagnosis for colonoscopy. *Endoscopy, 49*(08), 813–819.
33. Nazarian, S., Glover, B., Ashrafian, H., Darzi, A., & Teare, J. (2021). Diagnostic accuracy of artificial intelligence and computer-aided diagnosis for the detection and characterization of colorectal polyps systematic review and meta-analysis. *Journal of Medical Internet Research, 23*(7), e27370.
34. Dash, S., Shakyawar, S.K., Sharma, M., & Kaushik, S. (2019). Big data in healthcare: Management, analysis and future prospects. *Journal of Big Data, 6*(1).
35. Bottaci, L., Drew, P. J., Hartley, J. E., Hadfield, M. B., Farouk, R., et al. (1997). Artificial neural networks applied to outcome prediction for colorectal cancer patients in separate institutions. *Lancet, 350*, 469–472.
36. Grumett, S., Snow, P., & Kerr, D. (2003). Neural networks in the prediction of survival in patients with colorectal cancer. *Clinical Colorectal Cancer, 2*, 239–244.
37. Nasarian, E., Abdar, M., Fahami, M. A., Alizadehsani, R., Hussain, S., Basiri, M. E., Zomorodi-Moghadam, M., Zhou, X., Pławiak, P., Acharya, U. R., & Tan, R. S. (2020). Association between work-related features and coronary artery disease: A heterogeneous hybrid feature selection integrated with balancing approach. *Pattern Recognition Letters, 133*, 33–40.
38. van IJzendoorn, D. G., Szuhai, K., Briaire-de Bruijn, I. H., Kostine, M., Kuijjer, M. L., & Bovée, J. V. (2019). Machine learning analysis of gene expression data reveals novel diagnostic and prognostic biomarkers and identifies therapeutic targets for soft tissue sarcomas. *PLoS Computational Biology, 15*(2), e1006826.
39. Bärlund, M., Monni, O., Kononen, J., Cornelison, R., Torhorst, J., Sauter, G., Kallioniemi, O. P., & Kallioniemi, A. (2000). Multiple genes at 17q23 undergo amplification and overexpression in breast cancer. *Cancer Research, 60*(19), 5340–5344.

40. Koleck, T. A., & Conley, Y. P. (2016). Identification and prioritization of candidate genes for symptom variability in breast cancer survivors based on disease characteristics at the cellular level. *Breast Cancer: Targets and Therapy, 8*, 29.
41. Love, M. I., Huber, W., & Anders, S. (2014). Moderated estimation of fold change and dispersion for RNA-seq data with DESeq2. *Genome Biology, 15*(12).
42. Robinson, M. D., McCarthy, D. J., & Smyth, G. K. (2010). edgeR: A bioconductor package for differential expression analysis of digital gene expression data. *Bioinformatics, 26*(1), 139–140.
43. Ritchie, M. E., Phipson, B., Wu, D. I., Hu, Y., Law, C. W., Shi, W., & Smyth, G. K. (2015). limma powers differential expression analyses for RNA-sequencing and microarray studies. *Nucleic Acids Research, 43*(7), 47–47.
44. Gautier, L., Cope, L., Bolstad, B. M., & Irizarry, R. A. (2004). Affy—Analysis of affymetrix genechip data at the probe level. *Bioinformatics, 20*(3), 307–315.
45. Dunning, M. J., Smith, M. L., Ritchie, M. E., & Tavaré, S. (2007). Beadarray: R classes and methods for Illumina bead-based data. *Bioinformatics, 23*(16), 2183–2184.
46. Smith, M. L., Baggerly, K. A., Bengtsson, H., Ritchie, M. E., & Hansen, K. D. (2013). Illuminaio: An open source IDAT parsing tool for illumina microarrays. *F1000Research, 2*.
47. Huber, W., Carey, V. J., Gentleman, R., Anders, S., Carlson, M., Carvalho, B. S., Bravo, H. C., Davis, S., Gatto, L., Girke, T., Gottardo, R., & Morgan, M. (2015). Orchestrating high-throughput genomic analysis with bioconductor. *Nature Methods, 12*(2), 115–121.
48. Langfelder, P., Zhang, B., & Horvath, S. (2008). Defining clusters from a hierarchical cluster tree: The dynamic tree cut package for R. *Bioinformatics, 24*(5), 719–720.
49. Wani, N., Barh, D., & Raza, K. (2021). Modular network inference between miRNA-mRNA expression profiles using weighted co-expression network analysis. *Journal of Integrative Bioinformatics, 18*(4), 20210029. https://doi.org/10.1515/jib-2021-0029
50. Battaglin, F., Puccini, A., Naseem, M., Schirripa, M., Berger, M. D., Tokunaga, R., & Lenz, H. J. (2018). Pharmacogenomics in colorectal cancer: Current role in clinical practice and future perspectives. *Journal of Cancer Metastasis and Treatment, 4*.
51. Gao, F., Wang, W., Tan, M., Zhu, L., Zhang, Y., Fessler, E., & Wang, X. (2019). DeepCC: A novel deep learning-based framework for cancer molecular subtype classification. *Oncogenesis, 8*(9), 1–12.
52. Chen, Y., Li, Y., Narayan, R., Subramanian, A., & Xie, X. (2016). Gene expression inference with deep learning. *Bioinformatics, 32*(12), 1832–1839.
53. Singh, R., Lanchantin, J., Robins, G., & Qi, Y. (2016). DeepChrome: Deep-learning for predicting gene expression from histone modifications. *Bioinformatics, 32*(17), 639–648.
54. Nagpal, K., Foote, D., Liu, Y., Chen, P. H. C., Wulczyn, E., Tan, F., & Stumpe, M. C. (2019). Development and validation of a deep learning algorithm for improving gleason scoring of prostate cancer. *NPJ Digital Medicine, 2*(1), 1–10.
55. Kather, J. N., Krisam, J., Charoentong, P., Luedde, T., Herpel, E., Weis, C. A., & Halama, N. (2019). Predicting survival from colorectal cancer histology slides using deep learning: A retrospective multicenter study. *PLoS Medicine, 16*(1), e1002730.
56. Skrede, O. J., De Raedt, S., Kleppe, A., Hveem, T. S., Liestøl, K., Maddison, J., & Danielsen, H. E. (2020). Deep learning for prediction of colorectal cancer outcome: A discovery and validation study. *The Lancet, 395*(10221), 350–360.
57. Zhang, H., Du, Y., Wang, Z., Lou, R., Wu, J., & Feng, J. (2019). Integrated analysis of oncogenic networks in colorectal Cancer identifies GUCA2A as a molecular marker. *Biochemistry Research International*, 2019.
58. Coudray, N., Ocampo, P. S., Sakellaropoulos, T., Narula, N., Snuderl, M., Fenyö, D., & Tsirigos, A. (2018). Classification and mutation prediction from non-small cell lung cancer histopathology images using deep learning. *Nature Medicine, 24*(10), 1559–1567.
59. Bottaci, L., Drew, P. J., Hartley, J. E., Hadfield, M. B., Farouk, R., Lee, P. W., & Monson, J. R. (1997). Artificial neural networks applied to outcome prediction for colorectal cancer patients in separate institutions. *The Lancet, 350*(9076), 469–472.
60. Alon, U., Barkai, N., Notterman, D. A., Gish, K., Ybarra, S., Mack, D., & Levine, A. J. (1999). Broad patterns of gene expression revealed by clustering analysis of tumor and normal colon

tissues probed by oligonucleotide arrays. *Proceedings of the National Academy of Sciences, 96*(12), 6745–6750.
61. Snow, P. B., Kerr, D. J., Brandt, J. M., & Rodvold, D. M. (2001). Neural network and regression predictions of 5-year survival after colon carcinoma treatment. *Cancer: Interdisciplinary International Journal of the American Cancer Society, 91*(S8), 1673–1678.
62. Meeh, P. F., Farrell, C. L., Croshaw, R., Crimm, H., Miller, S. K., Oroian, D., & Buckhaults, P. J. (2009). A gene expression classifier of node-positive colorectal cancer. *Neoplasia, 11*(10), 1074-IN12.
63. Uddin, S., Ahmed, M., Hussain, A., Abubaker, J., Al-Sanea, N., AbdulJabbar, A., & Al-Kuraya, K. S. (2011). Genome-wide expression analysis of middle eastern colorectal cancer reveals FOXM1 as a novel target for cancer therapy. *The American Journal of Pathology, 178*(2), 537–547.
64. Nagaraj, S. H., & Reverter, A. (2011). A Boolean-based systems biology approach to predict novel genes associated with cancer: Application to colorectal cancer. *BMC Systems Biology, 5*(1), 1–15.
65. Li, B. Q., Huang, T., Liu, L., Cai, Y. D., & Chou, K. C. (2012). Identification of colorectal cancer related genes with mrmr and shortest path in protein-protein interaction network. *PLoS ONE, 7*(4), e33393.
66. Gao, P., Zhou, X., Wang, Z. N., Song, Y. X., Tong, L. L., Xu, Y. Y., Yue, Z. Y., & Xu, H. M. (2012). Which is a more accurate predictor in colorectal survival analysis? Nine data mining algorithms versus the TNM staging system. *PLoS ONE, 7*(7), e42015.
67. Maniruzzaman, M., Rahman, M. J., Ahammed, B., Abedin, M. M., Suri, H. S., Biswas, M., & Suri, J. S. (2019). Statistical characterization and classification of colon microarray gene expression data using multiple machine learning paradigms. *Computer Methods and Programs in Biomedicine, 176*, 173–193.
68. Zhao, D., Liu, H., Zheng, Y., He, Y., Lu, D., & Lyu, C. (2019). A reliable method for colorectal cancer prediction based on feature selection and support vector machine. *Medical and Biological Engineering and Computing, 57*(4), 901–912.
69. Ai, D., Wang, Y., Li, X., & Pan, H. (2020). Colorectal cancer prediction based on weighted gene co-expression network analysis and variational auto-encoder. *Biomolecules, 10*(9), 1207.
70. Hildebrand, L. A., Pierce, C. J., Dennis, M., Paracha, M., & Maoz, A. (2021). Artificial intelligence for histology-based detection of microsatellite instability and prediction of response to immunotherapy in colorectal cancer. *Cancers, 13*(3), 391.
71. Hu, H. P., Niu, Z. J., Bai, Y. P., & Tan, X. H. (2015). Cancer classification based on gene expression using neural networks. *Genetics and Molecular Research, 14*(4), 17605–17611.
72. Xu, G., Zhang, M., Zhu, H., & Xu, J. (2017). A 15-gene signature for prediction of colon cancer recurrence and prognosis based on SVM. *Gene, 604*, 33–40.
73. Zhang, X., Yang, Y., Wang, Y., & Fan, Q. (2019). Detection of the BRAF V600E mutation in colorectal cancer by NIR spectroscopy in conjunction with counter propagation artificial neural network. *Molecules, 24*(12), 2238.
74. Coppedè, F., Grossi, E., Lopomo, A., Spisni, R., Buscema, M., & Migliore, L. (2015). Application of artificial neural networks to link genetic and environmental factors to DNA methylation in colorectal cancer. *Epigenomics, 7*(2), 175–186.
75. Wang, Q., Wei, J., Chen, Z., Zhang, T., Zhong, J., Zhong, B., & Cao, J. (2019). Establishment of multiple diagnosis models for colorectal cancer with artificial neural networks. *Oncology Letters, 17*(3), 3314–3322.
76. Wan, N., Weinberg, D., Liu, T. Y., Niehaus, K., Ariazi, E. A., Delubac, D., Kannan, A., White, B., Bailey, M., Bertin, M., Boley, N., & Haque, I. S. (2019). Machine learning enables detection of early-stage colorectal cancer by whole-genome sequencing of plasma cell-free DNA. *BMC Cancer, 19*(1), 1–10.
77. Galamb, O., Barták, B. K., Kalmár, A., Nagy, Z. B., Szigeti, K. A., Tulassay, Z., & Molnár, B. (2019). Diagnostic and prognostic potential of tissue and circulating long non-coding RNAs in colorectal tumors. *World Journal of Gastroenterology, 25*(34), 5026.

78. Chang, K. H., Miller, N., Kheirelseid, E. A., Lemetre, C., Ball, G. R., Smith, M. J., & Kerin, M. J. (2011). MicroRNA signature analysis in colorectal cancer: Identification of expression profiles in stage II tumors associated with aggressive disease. *International Journal of Colorectal Disease, 26*(11), 1415–1422.
79. Amirkhah, R., Farazmand, A., Gupta, S. K., Ahmadi, H., Wolkenhauer, O., & Schmitz, U. (2015). Naive Bayes classifier predicts functional microRNA target interactions in colorectal cancer. *Molecular Biosystems, 11*(8), 2126–2134.
80. Zhi, J., Sun, J., Wang, Z., & Ding, W. (2018). Support vector machine classifier for prediction of the metastasis of colorectal cancer. *International Journal of Molecular Medicine, 41*(3), 1419–1426.
81. Nartowt, B. J., Hart, G. R., Muhammad, W., Liang, Y., Stark, G. F., & Deng, J. (2020). Robust machine learning for colorectal cancer risk prediction and stratification. *Frontiers in Big Data, 3*, 6.
82. Dimitriou, N., Arandjelović, O., Harrison, D. J., & Caie, P. D. (2018). A principled machine learning framework improves accuracy of stage II colorectal cancer prognosis. *NPJ Digital Medicine, 1*(1), 1–9.
83. Maniruzzaman, M., Rahman, M. J., Ahammed, B., Abedin, M. M., Suri, H. S., Biswas, M., El-Baz, A., Bangeas, P., Tsoulfas, G., & Suri, J. S. (2019). Statistical characterization and classification of colon microarray gene expression data using multiple machine learning paradigms. *Computer Methods and Programs in Biomedicine, 176*, 173–193.

Multi-omic Approaches to Improve Cancer Diagnosis, Prognosis, and Therapeutics

Diksha Singla and Manjeet Kaur Sangha

Abstract Cancer can arise as a consequence of a wide range of genomic aberrations including mutations, copy number alterations, expression changes, and epigenetic modifications encompassing multiple omic layers. While cost-efficient high-throughput technology provides a rising amount of data, single-layer data analysis rarely provides a causal relationship. Multi-omic data integration techniques at all levels of cellular function include genome, epigenome, transcriptome, proteome, metabolome, and microbiome which present unequaled opportunities to know the development and progression of cancer. This chapter aims to discuss a number of the most widely used data integration strategies and describe areas of research where multiple omics approaches greatly benefit the understanding of procedures and result of the malignant transformations. It also includes "algorithmic frameworks" designed to identify subtypes of cancer and methods to identify driver genomic changes and to consider the importance of integrated multiple omic approaches in improving cancer diagnosis, prognosis, and therapeutics. This chapter mainly focuses on providing a comprehensive outline of the progress of each omics strategy within the medical framework and discusses the major challenges facing their medical implementation. In addition to its incomparable benefits, multi-omics data integration delays access to daily clinics. One main problem is the unequal maturity of each omic technique and the increasing gap among the productions of large amounts of data as compared to its processing ability. Hence, analysis of integrative multi-omics will soon be the benchmark for studying complex systems. Thus; this chapter will help advance new computational advancements to deal with data heterogeneity, computational efficiency, and result analysis which can eventually push forward the oncology sector.

Keywords Cancer · Genome · Transcriptome · Multi-omics · Data integration

D. Singla (✉) · M. K. Sangha
Department of Biochemistry, Punjab Agricultural University, Ludhiana 141004, India

M. K. Sangha
e-mail: manjeet_kaursangha@pau.edu

K. Raza (ed.), *Computational Intelligence in Oncology*, Studies in Computational Intelligence 1016, https://doi.org/10.1007/978-981-16-9221-5_23

1 Introduction

Despite current advances in cancer treatment, it continues to dominate as one of the world's leading causes of death. In 2019, more than 17 lacs cases and more than 60,000 deaths were there in the US alone [1]. Cancer can be considered an extremely assorted set of diseases, whereas some tumors might have a good prediction and are curable, others are somewhat aggressive, lethal, or lack normal care [2]. The growth of malignant mutations needs cellular alterations at several levels. Changes in DNA, RNA, protein, metabolite, and medical imaging levels create a host of malignant molecular networks that make cancer a complex biological system. Any individual-level study is not sufficient to determine the complex pathogenesis of cancer. Single-level omic techniques test the whole pool of genome, epigenome, transcriptome, proteome, microbiome, and metabolome with affordable technology to unravel the mechanisms of cancer progression [3]. The continuous reduction in the processing time and expenditure of omics has led to the explosion of large data in every sector and has converted the "hypothesis-driven" targeted research toward addressing unintended data analysis. However, single-level omic technologies do not have the potential to resolve the causal relationship between phenotypic expressions and molecular modifications. In comparison, "systems biology" encompasses a wide range of data and offers a good promise to know the biological interactions completely and systematically [4]. The data integration of multiple omics plays a crucial function in determining the molecular means of tumorigenesis and the finding of novel biomarkers as well as drug targets [5]. The measurement of biological trial samples on different levels of omics provides an improved understanding of the genetic diversity; the nature as well as the interaction of two complex systems of biology. The data analysis of multi-omics makes sample clustering better in genetic groups, thereby providing a better understanding of predictive and prognostic phenotypes, disseminating molecular responses to treatment, and facilitating translational research through integrated methods [6].

The "class imbalance" distribution is also a common problem in the analysis of cancer data. Of particular concern is the use of data analysis for diagnosis, and treatment is the unequal quality of many and small classes. Analyzing data sets on the unequal distribution of classes is a fundamental challenge of learning dividers [7]. In unequal data sets, representative samples are distributed evenly over the comparison categories. The minority class is often regarded as the best class, while the majority class is considered the worst. Data retrieval is a common way to solve classroom inequality. To achieve the optimal balance (50:50, e.g.), the actual data structure is changed [8]. Incorporating a standard flexible learning algorithm into a training data set is an advantage over-refinement. The independence of these methods from learning the algorithm makes them very useful.

In recent times, a few studies have shown that combining sets of omics data sets a better understanding and a clearer picture of the system under investigation. For example, a combined analysis of ChIP-Seq and RNA-Seq data for lines of the head and neck squamous cell carcinoma (HNSCC) revealed that specific cancer markers, H3K4me3 and H3K27ac, which were associated with genetic mutations in the HNSCC gene, growth epidermal factor receptor (EGFR), FGFR1, and FOXA1 [6]. Zhang et al. [9] demonstrated the importance of combining proteomics data with genomic and transcriptomic data to prioritize cancer genes in the colon and rectal colonies. Their results showed that the 20q amplicon chromosome was associated with the world's largest mutations in both messenger RNA (mRNA) and protein levels. The compilation of proteomics data has helped identify 20q people, including hepatocyte nuclear factor 4 alpha (HNF4A), translocase of outer mitochondrial membrane 34 (TOMM34), and SRC proto-oncogene, non-receptor tyrosine kinase 0.5. In another study, a combination of metabolomics and transcriptomics revealed cellular cancer-causing cells. The metabolite sphingosine has shown high specificity and sensitivity to differentiate prostate cancer from benign prostatic hyperplasia, as reported in this study. Downstream of the sphingosine stream, the non-invasive sign of sphingosine-1-phosphate receptor 2 represents a genetic loss of tumor suppression and a potential oncogenic pathway to medical guidance [10].

These studies have further demonstrated the importance of combining multiple omics data into a single analysis. Multi-purpose hiring has led to the creation of various tools, methods, and platforms to provide omics data analysis, visualization, and translation. Yan et al. [4] summarize the network-based methods used for data analysis of multiple omics, and Tini et al. [11] provide a measurement of non-targeted collection methods in data collection. Therefore, a drastic shift in the treatment of cancer is taking place in the terms of "predictive," "preventive," and "personalized" medicine [12]. This chapter highlights a number of the most widely used methods of data integration in the field of tumors and examines the power of multiple approaches of omics in the effective detection of driver genomic mutations, tumor classification, prognosis, and diagnosis.

2 Multi-omics Paradigm

'Multi-omics' is the term given to the novelization approach in biological hats which utilizes more than one omic technique to visualize biological systems at the natural level [13]. The chief purpose of this multidisciplinary approach is to identify multi-omic signatures that can be "diagnostic" (healthy versus diseased), "prognostic" (good versus poor patient result), or "predictive" (positive versus negative response to healing interventions). The choice of the optimum signature size, which is the number of molecular characters required to differentiate patients, is not small. Generally, the smaller the size of the signature, the easier is its clinical applicability, but the lesser its accuracy, due to heterogeneous patients. The systematic cancer research provided by different omics is based on the acceptance of involvement of a wide range of aspects in the growth and preservation of the malignancies, together with genetic disorders, epigenetic mutations, changes in cell signaling, changes in metabolism, and ahead of [14].

In fact, the basic premise of "systems biology" is that it views organisms as systems, that is, structures that are made up of a huge number of multifaceted molecular as well as natural components that interact at many levels to form the efficient elements of the stated system. For example, the behavior of the tumor is decided by the combination of alterations in the genomic data that can or cannot be related with abnormal profiles of gene expression; affects protein abundance, however, also changes the structure of proteins, along with modifications in protein folding and supramolecular assembly. Modifications in control patterns can also influence cellular signaling processes and its reactions. Complex interactions of nucleic acids (DNA and RNA), as well as proteins in the process of duplication, transcription, metabolism, and cell signaling networks, are thus considered to be the crucial reasons for the functioning of the tumor cell [15]. These are inter-dependent conditions that cannot be treated individually; thus, there is a need for data integration methods. So the other important challenge in modern studies is data integration. Integrated data permits for the understanding of the largest database created by experimental multiple omic technologies. Truly, this is not a small task, because the mere handling of such huge information represents a challenge that is known as the "big data paradigm."

3 Methods for Data Integration to Improve Cancer Diagnosis, Prognosis, and Therapeutics

3.1 Multivariate Methods

One of the latest and main efforts in this area has led to an "R package" called "mixOmics" [16]. This method permits multivariate analysis of the omics data comprising exploration of data, reduction in dimension, and visualization. It can be used in many studies for a variety of purposes, e.g., integration and identification of biomarkers from multiple omics approaches. The R package involves two different kinds of multi-omics combinations. One aims to integrate different omic data for the identical biological samples, whereas the second one focuses on compiling autonomous data which is calculated on similar forecasters to enhance the size of the sample as well as statistical power. Both of these frameworks target extracting appropriate biological factors (e.g., molecular marks, using FT techniques). Rohart et al. [16] reported the results in 150 mRNA samples, micro-RNA, and breast cancer information and demonstrated its capability to effectively differentiate between three kinds of breast cancer.

"MiBi-Omics" is a Web-based (and independent) collaborative application to easily and efficiently scrutinize organizations on omics databases. By using a network-based integration strategy, it can help biologists identify potential ways of communicating and generate new novel ideas. The essence of the application lies in the reduction of the size of the omics databases to properly link them to the cellular level, and to identify biomarkers associated with a specific practice or phenotype [17]. The MiBi-omics pipeline facilitates the analysis, integration, and analysis of a wide range of omics data for a wide audience by providing scientists with a powerful way to predict and test molecular mechanisms that subordinate complex phenotypes to a wide range of scales and biological systems.

"MoCluster" can find combined patterns across multi-omics data by means of "multi-block multivariate analysis," followed by integration. By combining the data of messenger RNA, protein, and DNA methylation, this method distinguished microsatellite high-grade unstable tumors together with three new subtypes in colorectal carcinoma [18]. In conclusion, the common feature of the above-mentioned methods is that they all put the data set of multiple omic techniques into a stacked matrix which ultimately contributes to the consequent cluster analysis.

3.2 Statistically-Based Methods

General uses of statistical methods in the milieu of clinics are the prediction of vulnerability, reappearance, as well as survival [19]. In addition, models of classification and relationships are often used in the interpretation of molecular cancer studies. For example, the discovery of a biomarker [20] is a commonly sought aim for modeling based on the analysis of biochemical as well as multiple omics techniques. This is an essential field to study, because biomarkers are not very common, because biomarkers are molecular measures of cell activity in the form of living systems. These biomolecules are in the tightly linked pathways of biology that provide information flow and thus can produce basic biology. The comprehensive analysis provides an important opportunity to identify reliable biomarkers based on data from multiple cellular events [19]. Since the validation of biomarkers is time-consuming, the promotion of information based on the in-silico process of the biomolecule may work.

Identifying biomarker-related clinical outcomes, the integrative "Bayesian analysis of genomics" (iBAG) data, a multidisciplinary monitoring process, looking at the biological correlations across the data from various omic platforms, and applying a sequential model. The very first step is the "regression model" which partitions the data into its main components. The medical, as well as survival information, is involved in the mutual regression, comprising the features from the first step. Integrating the data of gene expression plus DNA methylation with the iBAG in the samples of glioblastoma facilitated the description of new methylation-controlled genes related to the survival of patients [21].

Among the widely distributed biomarkers of immunotherapy are death-ligand 1 (PD-L1), microsatellite instability/misalignment correction (MSI/dMMR), and tumor modification load (TMB). MSI/dMMR is approved for clinical use regardless of the type of tumor, and PD-L1 is only approved for use in certain types of cancer (e.g., predicting response to first-line pembrolizumab monotherapy for non-small cell lung cancer). PD-L1 (CD274, B7-H1) was the first and remains the most predictable biomarker for immune response point inhibitor (ICI). PD-L1 is present in a variety of cell types, including cancer cells, dendritic cells, activated T lymphocytes, and macrophages. PD-L1 often plays a role in protecting tissues from overexertion and autoimmune reactions. As a predictive biomarker of the PD-L/PD-L1 antibody, PD-L1 is probably best confirmed in patients with NSCLC (adenocarcinoma and squamous cell carcinoma). Therefore, in a first-phase trial, Reck et al. [22] reported that patients with high NSCLC who showed a high concentration of PD-L1 (50% skin cell tumor) received an overall response rate of 45.2% [22].

3.3 Network-Based Methods

A network viewpoint can improve all aspects of multiple omics studies. For example, mapping omic details to route the networks may give a chance to biologically set up the information. An old tool for this is the "*path view*" [23] package. The "*Graphite*" package [24] is a flexible approach, as it permits for the detection of paths from a variety of data resources and thereby offers appropriate graph elements that may be used by utilizing network detection tools. GRAPH interaction from the topological environment (Graphite) is a bioconductor package that provides networks from four data pathways (Biocarta; KEGG, KEGG, NCI/Nature Pathway Interaction Database, and Reactome). It discriminates between different types of genetic groups; spreads genetic communication through chemical compounds; allows the selection of edges by contact type; similarly converts heterogeneous node IDs into EntrezGene IDs and HUGO symbols; and ultimately allows the user to directly use SPIA, DEGraph, and topologyGSA which analyzes over the provided networks [24]. Currently, the "*metaGraphite*" package gave a main update to the first tool, successfully integrating the different omics by adding a layer of metabolomics [19].

"iOmicsPASS" uses a network-based approach to integrate multiple omics profiles above genome-level biological systems [25]. This tool offers analytical components to convert qualitative data of multi-omics into the scores for biological interactions and subsequently utilizes the resultant scores as an effort to choose predictive networks; lastly, it opts for the predictive edges of the phenotypic groups by means of a "modified shrunken centroid algorithm." Koh and coworkers [25] validated "iOmicsPASS" on "Breast Invasive Ductal Carcinoma" data, combining the messenger RNA expression as well as protein abundance, with or without the data normalization of messenger RNA by DNA "copy number variation." When compared to the actual closest shrunken centroid system algorithm, this method surpasses the basic system, which demonstrates the significance of choosing speculative signature types that are closely linked to smaller networks, thereby reducing the research space for prognostic features in well-known interactions.

3.4 Fusion-Based Methods

"Pattern Fusion Analysis" knows how to recognize important sample patterns from various omic profiles with automatic information arrangement as well as bias correction. This method incorporates local sample patterns from every data type to a worldwide pattern related to phenotypes. It measures the contributions of each type of data and reveals the key sample prototypes from various omic profiles to reflect joint sample patterns. This fusion method has been able to detect different clinical subtypes in lung squamous carcinoma, clear cell carcinoma along with the samples of samples from TCGA with identical combinations of similarity network fusion and iCluster, but with greater predictive efficacy [26]. Conversely, identifying a new biomarker is not possible with this fusion method and could not describe insight into the underlying tumorigenesis mechanisms.

3.5 Similarity-Based Methods

Such methods are based on inter-patient similarity. "Similarity network fusion" (SNF) creates single networks for each omic and renews them with the aim of increasing their resemblance until they become a single network [27]. The study of methylation, gene expression patterns of messenger RNA, and micro RNA with SNF in all 215 glioblastoma samples completed one type of data analysis and discovered three different groups, with one in younger patients with IDH subtype and positive prediction and one more subtype with the positive reaction to temozolomide. This method aids to detect subtypes of cancer but cannot be used to identify biomarkers.

"Neighborhood-based multi-omics clustering" (NEMO) is a tool that figures out "inter-patient similarity matrices" for each omic via "radial basis function kernel" (RBF) [28]. RBF kernel is a kernel function that is used in machine learning to find a nonlinear classifier or regression line. This method addresses the difficulty of partial information stocks, in which all the omic techniques can be computed for all the patients and the final mean number is calculated on the observed omic values, without making imputations. This clustering represents greater performance as compared to the similar method with the data set, whereas in TCGA cancer databases, it finds considerable differences in the survival of 6 out of 10 types of cancer.

3.6 Correlation-Based Methods

The development of breast cancer treatments and the development of cancer research centers have required the collection of many variations in patients with breast cancer. Finding important variables such as prediction and results between them, without using the correct mathematical method is a very difficult task. Due to the frequent recurrence of breast cancer that occurs at different times, there is often more than one variation in the set of outcomes. With the prevention of this multicollinearity problem, a mathematical method called canonical correlation analysis (CCA) is a good solution.

Canonical correlation analysis (CCA), developed by Hotelling (1936), is a method for applying structure coefficients as indices for choosing essential predictors. It is characteristically utilized to evaluate the relationship across copy number variation, DNA methylation, as well as gene expression data and may possibly offer a vision into the processes of carcinogenesis. It makes a selection for each factor while incorporating group effects of factors in the analysis [29, 30]. This method selected inequitable characters from multiple omics data resources to foresee the survival of renal kidney cell carcinoma [31] but has lower effectiveness in molecular subtype testing and choice of the biomarker.

In a study, Sadoughi et al. [32] used the CCA to identify key risk factors leading to the recurrence of breast cancer in Iranian women. The analysis showed seven important predictions that led to the recurrence of breast cancer at different times. Family history and loco-regional recurrence over 5 years after diagnosis were the most important variables between prediction and set results, respectively. Therefore, their research concluded that the CCA could be used as a useful tool for managing and modifying medical data for access to confidential information.

3.7 Machine Learning Model

Machine learning (ML) has the power to transform oncology and, in general, medicine 1. The introduction of ML to health care is enhanced by the digital integration of patient data, including the receipt of electronic medical records (EMRs). This change provides an unprecedented opportunity to obtain clinical data from a comprehensive analysis of patient data. Machine learning has the ability to detect image features without previous training using neural networks that can integrate different sets of clinical data. The resulting algorithms can then be used in the same, new clinical information to predict individual patient responses according to large groups of previous patients. Alternatively, the same techniques can be used in photographs to identify less-than-difficult people. In addition, machine learning can play a role in producing a hypothesis by identifying unknown, distinct features of images, or a combination of factors related to disease progression or outcome. For example, a subset of patients with memory loss who may be prone to dementia may have features found prior to symptom development [33]. This approach allows for a larger population study by subsequent clinical follow-up and identification of clinically relevant fingerprints, rather than data analysis of low volume recovery in patients who have already developed cerebral palsy. In-depth learning is part of a wider family of machine learning methods based on artificial neural networks with representative learning. In-depth learning is a modern variation related to the unlimited number of layers of bonded size, which allows for efficient use and implementation while being kept everywhere under minimal conditions. In deep learning, the layers are also allowed to separate and deviate significantly from knowledgeable connecting models, in order to be efficient, trained, and understandable, where the "structured" part emerges.

Deep learning methods have greatly improved our ability to detect control factors [34, 35] and to predict the effect of genetic variation on those objects. DeepSEA, a multidisciplinary CNN trained in large-scale genomics operations [36], was able to study the sequence dependence on multiple scales and simultaneously produced DNase hypersensitive sites, factor-binding sites, histone markers, and the effect of genetic variation on those control items, with a higher accuracy level than other tools for prioritizing differential performance without coding [37].

4 Methods for the Detection of Driver Genomic Mutations and Cancer Biomarkers

In a combination of multiple omics, the flexible choice to decrease the size of the omics database plays a major role. Elimination of repetitive traits was exploited to choose the subsets of expressed genes as well as the data of methylation to categorize the subtypes of breast cancer by "Random Forest" [38]. Gene priorities allowed for the prediction of cancer in a variety of cancers from genomics, epigenomics and transcriptomics data [39], and the discovery of biomarkers in prostate cancer [40].

"netDx" enables the choice of features on "Patient Similarity Networks" that categorize patients into several predictive groups [41]. It is designed for each omic approach that the "nodes" signify the patients and the "edges" represent the resemblance of the two notes in the given sight. It subsequently detects which omic approach strongly links low-risk and high-risk patients with the "GeneMANIA" algorithm [42], which solves the problem of relapse to amplify the links that connect uncertain patients. As a final point, each of the networks is rated according to its capability to define patients of a similar group, and networks that have a number that exceeds the specified threshold are [41] preferred and integrated into a single network by measuring their similarity scores. Pai and coworkers have benchmarked the netDx method against numerous machine learning procedures to foresee the survival results in "PanCancer" TCGA multi-omics data sets, showing similar outcomes. In the breast cancer database, the selected characters of netDx are in line with the known uncontrollable mechanisms for this type of cancer.

"DrugComboExplorer" [43] identifies a combination of drugs designed to target the networks of cancer driver genome signaling by analyzing DNA sequences, methylation, RNA-seq, and copy number variation data from each cancer patient with pipeline combined algorithms. This algorithm is based on two components—the first component isolates the dysregulated arrangements from transcriptome along with methylation profiles of particular patients via "bootstrapping-based simulated annealing" and "weighted co-expression network analyses." The second part produces driver network marks for every drug, examines the effect of drug combinations, and introduces drug combinations based on interaction results. Huang et al. [43] used this method in the spread of major prostate cancer and B-cell-lymphoma demonstrating the tool's capability to detect synergistic combinations of drugs and its high predictive precision against existing computational methods.

5 Clinical Translation of "Single Omics" Techniques in Cancer

5.1 *Genomics*

Genomics has contributed to the detection of major subtypes of disease through consequent genetic mutations and supports the discovery of effective therapeutic objectives predicting the effectiveness of targeted interventions and daily treatment modalities [44]. In addition to the individualized mutations, genomics can test mutation signatures as well as mutation load to predict the "immune-checkpoint inhibitors" (ICI) efficiency [45]. The various ICIs are as ipilimumab, tremelimumab, pembrolizumab, avelumab, etc. The use of genomic methods is increasing in clinical areas like monitoring the response to treatment and depiction of resistance methods. However, genetic details focus mostly on exome information, single nucleotide polymorphism (SNPs), and the pharmaco-genomic risk variants which make up only around 3% of the genome [46]. In multifaceted diseases, it is hard to create a clear relation with certain genetic variants; therefore, genomics is just the beginning of tackling the cancer challenge.

5.2 *Transcriptomics*

The transcriptomic analysis is used to evaluate the presence and quantity of RNA in a given physical environment [47]. Possibly, the most frequent use of transcriptomics is to determine gene expression. The gene expression report of the phenotype can thus be able to be utilized as a barcode for its natural state. These barcodes can then be compared via differential gene expression analysis, to identify the molecular changes in cancer. The gene expression profile is the result of the gene control system embedded in the epigenome and genome. By assessing gene expression, one can indirectly record the regulatory alterations that are at the center of the disease.

5.3 *Proteomics*

Proteomic analysis is used to discover and measure a set of proteins there within the genetic system [48]. Research on cancer proteomics is capable as a means of discovering biomarkers and curative targets [49]. This is not shocking as proteins are the cellular units from which the cell's structure and function arise. During the acquisition of data, the observed cell fragments must be detected. This is usually done by comparing the fragments with the database in actual time. Later, the protein aggregation from discovered peptide fragments needs one more set of calculation methods [50]. The advancement of these methods remains a dynamic research area [51]. "*Bioconductor*" provides systematic data management tools for proteomics, from data processing to functional analysis [52]. Another way to measure protein is "*maxquant*" toolset [53].

5.4 *Metabolomics*

Metabolic mutations are an important factor in the development of cancer. "Cancer metabolomics" has become an essential topic of research in the field of oncology [54], with the assurance of providing new information on cancer progression and possible treatment options. "Lipidomics" is essentially a subset of metabolomics. Cancer lipidomics research can lead to the discovery of important biomedical findings, like novel biomarkers [55].

5.5 *Microbiomics*

Microbiomics is a promising area that focuses on microbial populations colonizing our bodies [56]. The gut microbiome is quickly transformed through drugs, diet, or other ecological signals which alters metabolism and represents direct contact with nature. The whole microbial structure of a given body site can be studied with "16S amplicon" and "shotgun metagenomic sequencing." In the framework of accurate medicine, different researches have proved that inhabitant gut bacteria can influence cancer immunotherapy reactions. Routy and coworkers [57] reported the use of antibiotics altered the response to PD-1 inhibition in patients with kidney and lung cancer [57], and a decrease in PD-1 inhibition in melanoma was associated with unbalanced intestinal flora [58, 59]. The results suggested that preservation of the healthy commensal microbiome contributes to the anti-tumor immunity, though the microbial taxa-related with reaction to immune checkpoint inhibition differ between studies.

5.6 Multi-omics Data Integration in Cancer Research

Cancer is a multifaceted disease and entails a down-regulation in several levels of nucleic acids (DNA and RNA), proteins, and metabolites; and those different levels of molecules are equally related [60–62]. Any individual study at a different level is not enough to determine the complex pathogenesis of cancer. The multi-omics data integration is important in cancer study and is consistent with the actuality of cancer [60] which will give a complete overview of what actually happens during harmful cell mutations and tumor progression, and can be effective in improving targeted therapeutic and functional therapies, in the elucidation of cancer therapeutic resistance, and also in the discovery of new biomarkers and targeted drugs (Fig. 1).

5.6.1 Importance and Scientific Merit of Integrating Multi-omics Data Analysis in Cancer Studies

The integrated multi-omics have been extensively used in cancer studies. Compared to post-analysis integration, the integrated data analysis strategy takes advantage of specialized algorithms and tools for integrating pre-analyzed data sets on different

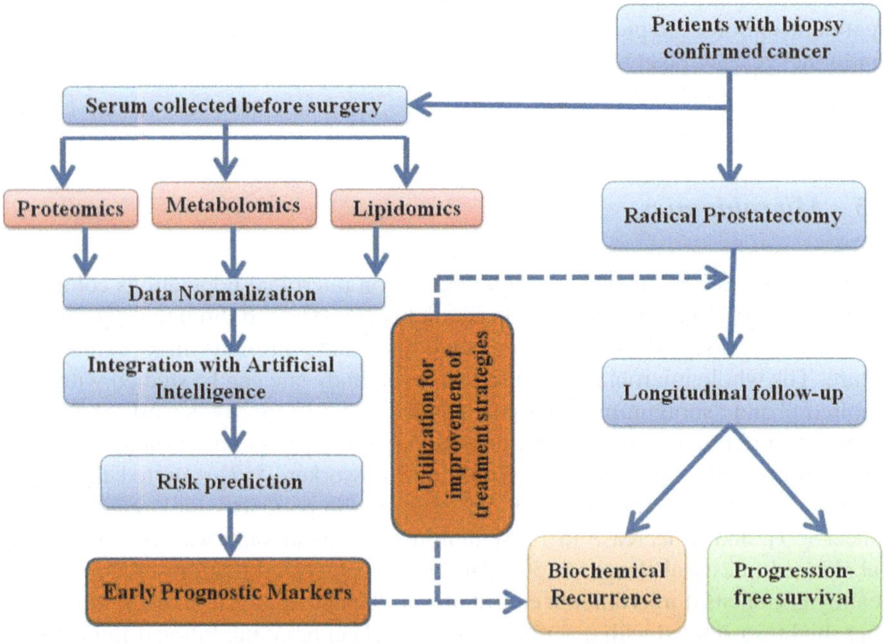

Fig. 1 Conceptual schematic describes approaches for integrating multi-omics and artificial intelligence for biomarker discovery from presurgical serum for prognosis of cancer progression

omics platforms before committing to data analysis. For example, a combined analysis of transcriptomic and proteomic data representing 65 breast cancer and 53 nearby non-cancerous tissues revealed concordance of a high RNA-to-protein messenger in the gut where increased concordance between mRNA and protein levels was linked to severe breast cancer, including basal-like/triple-negative breast cancer, and reduced survival [63]. In addition to the strengths and weaknesses associated with background analysis and integrated approaches, these techniques are currently being used as experimental tools to create a new hypothesis or to provide some definition of cancer-specific phenotypes.

Curtis and coworkers [64] reported a combined analysis of genome as well as transcriptome data and long-lasting clinical results analyzing the alterations in gene expression based on the "somatic gene copy number aberrations" discovered some possibly significant targeted curative reaction-associated events and suggested a novel molecular categorization of breast cancer patients [64]. Stemke et al. [65] studied another integrated analysis of genomics and proteomics data which showed that PI3K route disruption is more frequent in hormone receptor-positive breast cancer, which may be significant in the clinical choice of targeted therapies [65]. Another study by Nam and co-workers for integrative analysis of "tissue transcriptomic"' and "urine metabolomics" identified four highly reliable urinary biomarkers compared to biomarkers found in a single approach of omics [66]. Analysis of the combination of proteomics, transcriptomics, and clinical effect on HER2-positive breast cancer-resistant lapatinib discovered that EGFR/HER2 signaling was still obstructed, and inhibition was reduced due to reduced glucose metabolism and endoplasmic reticulum pathways [67]. The integrative analysis of proteomic and transcriptomic data in glioblastomas exposed a significant increase in the expression of gonadotropin-releasing hormone (GnRH) that was not deciphered in single omic data sets, showing promise for the research on multi-omics and its analysis to better understand the complexity of cancer [68].

"Multimodal omics" can be integrated *in silico* to answer the difficult biological queries that need a "systems biology approach." One such example is the prediction of "tumor neoantigens," i.e., mutated peptides that are bound to MHC molecules of cancerous cells and may trigger immune anticancer reactions. Schrors and coworkers [69] derived a combined map of the genome, transcriptome plus neoantigen landscape of the most extensively utilized models of breast cancer—"4T1 murine mammary cancer cell line." They observed that the 4T1 cells shared molecular characters with triple breast cancer and, therefore, represented a potential model for prenatal studies. Additionally, they confirmed the antigenic activity of 23 mutated peptides that were chosen from a neoantigens pool observed in silico using "IFNγ-ELISpot assays" [69].

6 Clinical Applications of Multi-omics

6.1 *Multi-omics Can Diagnose the Earlier Undiagnosed Patients with Unusual Phenotypes*

Escape from the diagnostic excursion is the main obstacle for lots of patients with unusual diseases. With the integration of complete "WES," "chromosome microarray," "linkage analysis," as well as "mRNA analysis," Quesne and coworkers aimed to offer identification for a mixture of the multifarious undiagnosed phenotypes: "non-syndromic hearing loss" (NSHL), "aberrant skeletal phenotypes," and "considerable developmental delays," in four patients [70]. The WES detected a genetic variant (recessively inherited) in *PDZD7* which may elucidate the NSHL phenotype, proved by messenger RNA analysis to hinder gene expression in the affected persons since no *PDZD7* exons were amplified. In addition, microcephaly phenotype and developmental delays were defined by the chromosome microarray by identifying de novo unequal movement in chromosomes number 8 and 18. The skeletal phenotype was related to an autosomal dominant inheritance with a genetic variant in *COL1A1* leading to the identification of osteogenesis imperfecta. This work demonstrated phenotypic heterogeneity commonly found in rarely undetectable diseases and also the use of giving complete genomic analysis with supplementary validated analysis of mRNA to maximize the diagnostic yield.

Agrawal and coworkers [71] targeted use integration of whole-genome shotgun, protein, and messenger RNA analysis to assist in the identification of families with diverse neurogenic and myopathic phenotypes [71] to identify five possible pathogenic strains. In this case, a particular alteration in the *NEFL* gene was found in every affected member that had previously been related to "Charcot-Marie-Tooth" syndrome. This is an outstanding illustration of the influence of multiple omics analysis to give a cellular diagnosis of patients with undiagnosed rare phenotypes, while enhancing the formerly known medical phenotype. Abela et al. [72] used whole-exome sequencing with metabolomics to detect the indicative biomarkers of the mitochondrial aconitase deficiency.

6.2 *Pathogenic and Prognostic Biomarkers Can Be Detected by Integrated Multiple Omic Data Sets*

Favier and coworkers studied deficiency of mevalonate kinase, an auto-inflammatory recessively inherited disease with the involvement of multiple organs. A wide range of clinical presentations includes "hyperimmuno-globulinemia D syndrome," "periodic fever syndrome" and "mevalonic aciduria" [73]. The authors performed WES, RNA-Seq, as well as differential analysis of protein in a study of two sisters who presented polarized phenotypic heterogeneity in which both sisters had a homozygous driver variant in *MVK* but only one sibling had symptoms [74]. Their integrated analysis discovered an unusual transmutation in *STAT1* (the modifier gene) that led to the upregulation in mRNA as well as protein expression, which may account for a phenotype in the affected one. "Single omic" analysis only was not sufficient to find such mutations, so it is an excellent example of why such integrated multi-omics are important in detecting the basis of uncommon diseases and defining phenotypic heterogeneity that can make difficult patient care.

The discovery of prognostic biomarkers through analysis of multiple omic techniques was highlighted in numerous studies of unusual tumors including "adrenocortical carcinoma" (ACC), "sarcoma," "uveal melanoma," and "pseudomyxoma peritonei." Different predictive ACC groups discussed in three of the five included ACC studies [75–77], including three predictive molecular ACC subtypes clustered by the profile of methylation with an accuracy of 92.4% [76], two clusters through changes in methylation with recurrent genetic mutations (poor predictions) and micro RNA regulation (good predictions) [75]. In the research of uveal melanoma, four molecularly separate groups were found with the difference in the prognostic results: two related with better prognosis (disomy 3) and two with poor prognosis (monosomy 3) [78].

6.3 Assisting Early Diagnosis of Cancer

Early detection of cancer is important in treating it timely and also restricting cancer-related fatalities. "Liquid biopsy," the method based on non-invasive blood tests, increases the importance of detecting tumors prior to the appearance of symptoms [79]. The approach offers unparalleled benefits more than the surgical biopsy, as cancer tissue, if completely available, may be overly sensitive or low in cells. Non-invasive detection of mutations related to "circulating tumor DNA" (ctDNA) secreted from dying cancer cells in the blood shows positive promise. Conversely, the most important drawback is its low ratio among the entire "circulating cell-free DNA." The quantity of ctDNA available depends on the type of cancer and stage [80], the tumor load, and the treatment [81], among other factors. Thus, the methods based on a single biomarker linked with a tumor can produce an incompatible outcome with restricted sensitivity. Collaborative acquisition of numerous biomarkers or a combination of multiple approaches, e.g., integrating protein-DNA transmutations or mRNA expression and genome changes as biomarkers for early cancer stage, can improve the identification sensitivity of non-invasive liquid biopsy diagnosis significantly. Non-invasive blood tests included an investigation of KRAS mutations and the existence of four proteins in 221 patients with "pancreatic ductal adenocarcinomas." Such mutations were there in the plasma of only 30% of the patients. Conversely, the integrative study of these mutations with four protein biomarkers attained 99.5% specificity and 64% sensitivity [82]. Similarly, a multi-analyte blood test, "CancerSEEK" integrated the genetic modifications and protein expression in combination with artificial intelligence. On the basis of 61 amplicons inside 16 genes including 8 protein biomarkers, the trial was able to locate the tumor organ where it originated and detected the first five types of tumor (liver, ovary, pancreas, stomach plus esophagus cancer) with 69–98% sensitivity and 99% specificity. The level of AFP (alpha-fetoprotein) can be a biomarker in hepatocellular carcinoma, even though the low sensitivity of 39–65% along with specificity has made its use contentious [83]. However, the combined discovery of alpha-fetoprotein and RNA-profile of exosomes, with a strong focus on the expression of "miR-122" and "miR-148a," increased the discriminatory capability of the model to differentiate hepatocellular tumor from the liver cirrhosis by AUC of 0.931 [63]. Tumor-related RNA-derived from exosomes called "exoRNA" combined with circulating tumor DNA improved sensitivity to the detection of EGFR mutations in the plasma of "non-small cell lung cancer" (NSCLC) from 82 to 98% when compared with circulating tumor DNA alone [84]. These successful works prove that data integration carries significant potential for effective clinical use, and new strategies are expected to emerge from diagnostic practices.

6.4 Both Novel Treatment and Drug Re-Purposing Opportunities Can Be Identified Through Multi-omic Analysis

The care of patients with uncommon diseases usually depends on the management of symptoms, rather than causal cure, with limited treatment options available. For instance, Gara and coworkers [85] detected 156 differently methylated genes in adrenocortical carcinoma, involving hypermethylation of gene *CYP1B1*, which was revealed to have sensitivity to decitabine (a methylation inhibitor) in the adrenocortical carcinoma cell line. In addition, this work also observed that cell propagation occurs in altered genes *MEIS1, G0S2, GATA6, NCOA7, FAM1156A, KCTD12* following the treatment with oncostatin M [85]. However, even when the new curative targets are observed as outstanding candidates for clinical study, the cost of experiments frequently leads to pharmaceutical companies rejecting to check and produce the new drug. Of those new drugs that have been fortunate enough to be considered eligible for investment, the time frame from testing to clinical use is 12 years [86]. Therefore, drug re-purposing that has already been accepted for use in another disease has largely focused on finding treatments for rare diseases, especially for precise oncology medicine [87]. Identifying the potential for drug retaliation to overcome the lack of access to treatment was a strong recurring idea of multiple omic analyses of unusual tumor studies. For example, the drug "Ponatinib," commonly used to treat leukemia was discovered as a probable drug re-purposing chance for "small cell carcinoma" of the ovary hypercalcaemic type, via integrated analysis of proteome and transcriptome with functional cell-line and animal models [88].

7 Challenges and Future Perspectives in Multi-omics Data Integration

Integrating multi-omics data set to gain a complete understanding of biological processes and diseases comes with its own set of challenges. The basic diversity of individual omics data, the large size of the data sets leading to computational dynamic analysis, and the lack of studies that help prioritize a set of different tools make data integration and data analysis a challenging task. Most omics data is generated using a variety of platforms, which is why data storage and formats are very different. Most multi-omics integration analysis tools require data to be in certain formats (especially in the Matrix X Sample matrix), so each omics data needs to be processed. The step-by-step process includes data filtering, systematic sorting, batch results removal, and quality testing. It is necessary to carefully use these step-forward measures as they have a major impact on integration analysis. For example, the data filtering step plays an important role in sound filtering and reducing the number of features that go into integration models as many integration methods are more powerful on the computer which is why it is necessary to reduce the size of input data sets. However, determining the appropriate filtering methods is challenging due to the lack of universal standards. Perez-Riverol et al. [89] developed a workflow that could lead to feature selection from high-end omics data sets. In this regard, the development of new integration methods/tools should be considered to better manage large data sets.

The key to any analysis that includes the right choice of approach would address the biological question of interest. There are studies that make a compilation of compound tools, but they are not enough in terms of the selection tools in the context of the biological question that you are interested in. One such in-depth study is needed to guide the public in a better understanding of the various tools. Another factor that can add value to multi-omics data interpretation is clinical information. Currently, there is no solid way to combine omics data with non-omics data such as clinical metadata. Recent developments in the sector are underway in an effort to reduce challenges. Further advances in integrated multi-omics data analysis should aim to reduce the interoperability of multiple data sets and develop a framework that can assist in seamless multi-omics data analysis.

8 Conclusion

Cancer is a complex paradigmatic phenotype. Every single omic approach derived data type has its own warning and difficulty sets. There are, however, many ways to create an integrated multi-omic computational model. This chapter has thus been showing the present state of the data integration methods for a variety of cancer studies of complex phenotypes. The advancements in the field of this multi-omic analysis come from a variety of disciplines ranging from mathematical development to machine knowledge and artificial intelligence uses to the studies of single-cell sequencing and imaging. Nevertheless, the progress in data integration methods to combine several analytical methods into comprehensive and strong frameworks will offer the field unparalleled progress in the understanding of the complex biology of cancer and its impact on clinical settings. This field is rising rapidly and is presently in progress, with new algorithmic methods being released regularly.

References

1. Siegel, R. L., Miller, K. D., & Jemal, A. (2019). Cancer statistics, 2019. *CA: A Cancer Journal for Clinicians, 69*(1), 7–34.
2. Lawrence, M. S., Stojanov, P., Polak, P., Kryukov, G. V., Cibulskis, K., Sivachenko, A., Carter, S. L., Stewart, C., Mermel, C. H., Roberts, S. A., & Kiezun, A. (2013). Mutational heterogeneity in cancer and the search for new cancer-associated genes. *Nature, 499*(7457), 214–218.
3. Alyass, A., Turcotte, M., & Meyre, D. (2015). From big data analysis to personalized medicine for all: Challenges and opportunities. *BMC Medical Genomics, 8*(1), 1–2.
4. Yan, J., Risacher, S. L., Shen, L., & Saykin, A. J. (2018). Network approaches to systems biology analysis of complex disease: Integrative methods for multi-omics data. *Briefings in Bioinformatics, 19*(6), 1370–1381.
5. Hasin, Y., Seldin, M., & Lusis, A. (2017). Multi-omics approaches to disease. *Genome Biology, 18*(1), 1–5.
6. Chakraborty, S., Hosen, M., Ahmed, M., & Shekhar, H. U. (2018). Onco-multi-OMICS approach: A new frontier in cancer research. *BioMed Research International, 3*, 2018.
7. Fotouhi, S., Asadi, S., & Kattan, M. W. (2019). A comprehensive data level analysis for cancer diagnosis on imbalanced data. *Journal of Biomedical Informatics, 90*, 103089.
8. Khoshgoftaar, T. M., Fazelpour, A., Dittman, D. J., & Napolitano, A. (2015). Ensemble vs. data sampling: Which option is best suited to improve classification performance of imbalanced bioinformatics data? In 2015 IEEE 27th International Conference on Tools with Artificial Intelligence (ICTAI), 2015 Nov 9 (pp. 705–712). IEEE.
9. Zhang, B., Wang, J., Wang, X., Zhu, J., Liu, Q., Shi, Z., Chambers, M. C., Zimmerman, L. J., Shaddox, K. F., Kim, S., & Davies, S. R. (2014). Proteogenomic characterization of human colon and rectal cancer. *Nature, 513*(7518), 382–387.
10. Ren, S., Shao, Y., Zhao, X., Hong, C. S., Wang, F., Lu, X., Li, J., Ye, G., Yan, M., Zhuang, Z., & Xu, C. (2016). Integration of metabolomics and transcriptomics reveals major metabolic pathways and potential biomarker involved in prostate cancer. *Molecular & Cellular Proteomics, 15*(1), 154–163.
11. Tini, G., Marchetti, L., Priami, C., & Scott-Boyer, M. P. (2019). Multi-omics integration—A comparison of unsupervised clustering methodologies. *Briefings in Bioinformatics, 20*(4), 1269–1279.
12. Golubnitschaja, O., & Costigliola, V. (2012). General report & recommendations in predictive, preventive and personalised medicine 2012: White paper of the European association for predictive preventive and personalised medicine. *EPMA Journal, 3*(1), 1–53.
13. Wani, N., & Raza, K. (2019). Integrative approaches to reconstruct regulatory networks from multi-omics data: A review of state-of-the-art methods. *Computational Biology and Chemistry, 83*, 107–120.
14. Du, W., & Elemento, O. (2015). Cancer systems biology: Embracing complexity to develop better anticancer therapeutic strategies. *Oncogene, 34*(25), 3215–3225.

15. de Anda-Jáuregui, G., & Hernández-Lemus, E. (2020). Computational oncology in the multi-omics era: State of the art. *Frontiers in Oncology, 7*(10), 423.
16. Rohart, F., Gautier, B., Singh, A., Lê Cao, K. A. (2017). mixOmics: An R package for 'omics feature selection and multiple data integration. *PLoS Computational Biology, 13*(11), e1005752.
17. Zoppi, J., Guillaume, J. F., Neunlist, M., & Chaffron, S. (2021). MiBiOmics: An interactive web application for multi-omics data exploration and integration. *BMC Bioinformatics, 22*(1), 1–4.
18. Meng, C., Helm, D., Frejno, M., & Kuster, B. (2016). moCluster: Identifying joint patterns across multiple omics data sets. *Journal of Proteome Research, 15*(3), 755–765.
19. Kourou, K., Exarchos, T. P., Exarchos, K. P., Karamouzis, M. V., & Fotiadis, D. I. (2015). Machine learning applications in cancer prognosis and prediction. *Computational and Structural Biotechnology Journal, 1*(13), 8–17.
20. Streeter, O. E., Jr., Beron, P. J., & Iyer, P. N. (2017). Precision medicine: Genomic profiles to individualize therapy. *Otolaryngologic Clinics of North America., 50*(4), 765–773.
21. Wang, W., Baladandayuthapani, V., Morris, J. S., Broom, B. M., Manyam, G., & Do, K. A. (2013). iBAG: Integrative Bayesian analysis of high-dimensional multiplatform genomics data. *Bioinformatics, 29*(2), 149–159.
22. Reck, M., Rodríguez-Abreu, D., Robinson, A. G., Hui, R., Csőszi, T., Fülöp, A., Gottfried, M., Peled, N., Tafreshi, A., Cuffe, S., & O'Brien, M. (2016). Pembrolizumab versus chemotherapy for PD-L1–positive non–small-cell lung cancer. *New England Journal of Medicine, 10*(375), 1823–1833.
23. Luo, W. B. (1831). Pathview: AnR/Bioconductor package for pathway-based data integration and visualization. *Bioinformatics, 29*(14), 1830.
24. Sales, G., Calura, E., Cavalieri, D., & Romualdi, C. (2012). g raphite-a Bioconductor package to convert pathway topology to gene network. *BMC Bioinformatics, 13*(1), 1–2.
25. Koh, H. W., Fermin, D., Vogel, C., Choi, K. P., Ewing, R. M., & Choi, H. (2019). iOmic-sPASS: Network-based integration of multiomics data for predictive subnetwork discovery. *NPJ Systems Biology and Applications, 5*(1), 1.
26. Shi, Q., Zhang, C., Peng, M., Yu, X., Zeng, T., Liu, J., & Chen, L. (2017). Pattern fusion analysis by adaptive alignment of multiple heterogeneous omics data. *Bioinformatics, 33*(17), 2706–2714.
27. Wang, B., Mezlini, A. M., Demir, F., Fiume, M., Tu, Z., Brudno, M., Haibe-Kains, B., & Goldenberg, A. (2014). Similarity network fusion for aggregating data types on a genomic scale. *Nature Methods, 11*(3), 333–337.
28. Rappoport, N., & Shamir, R. (2019). NEMO: Cancer subtyping by integration of partial multi-omic data. *Bioinformatics, 35*(18), 3348–3356.
29. Lin, D., Zhang, J., Li, J., Calhoun, V. D., Deng, H. W., & Wang, Y. P. (2013). Group sparse canonical correlation analysis for genomic data integration. *BMC Bioinformatics, 14*(1), 1–6.
30. Zhou, Y., Liu, Y., Li, K., Zhang, R., Qiu, F., Zhao, N., & Xu, Y. (2015). ICan: an integrated co-alteration network to identify ovarian cancer-related genes. *PLoS One, 10*(3), e0116095.
31. El-Manzalawy, Y. (2018). CCA based multi-view feature selection for multi-omics data integration. In 2018 IEEE Conference on Computational Intelligence in Bioinformatics and Computational Biology (CIBCB), 2018 May 30 (pp. 1–8). IEEE.
32. Sadoughi, F., Afshar, H. L., Olfatbakhsh, A., Mehrdad, N. (2016). Application of canonical correlation analysis for detecting risk factors leading to recurrence of breast cancer. *Iranian Red Crescent Medical Journal, 18*(3).
33. Hulsen, T., Jamuar, S. S., Moody, A. R., Karnes, J. H., Varga, O., Hedensted, S., Spreafico, R., Hafler, D. A., & McKinney, E. F. (2019). From big data to precision medicine. *Frontiers in Medicine, 1*(6), 34.
34. Kelley, D. R., Reshef, Y. A., Bileschi, M., Belanger, D., McLean, C. Y., & Snoek, J. (2018). Sequential regulatory activity prediction across chromosomes with convolutional neural networks. *Genome Research, 28*(5), 739–750.

35. Alipanahi, B., Delong, A., Weirauch, M. T., & Frey, B. J. (2015). Predicting the sequence specificities of DNA-and RNA-binding proteins by deep learning. *Nature Biotechnology, 33*(8), 831–838.
36. Bernstein, B. E., Stamatoyannopoulos, J. A., Costello, J. F., Ren, B., Milosavljevic, A., Meissner, A., Kellis, M., Marra, M. A., Beaudet, A. L., Ecker, J. R., & Farnham, P. J. (2010). The NIH roadmap epigenomics mapping consortium. *Nature Biotechnology, 28*(10), 1045–1048.
37. Zhou, J., & Troyanskaya, O. G. (2015). Predicting effects of noncoding variants with deep learning–based sequence model. *Nature Methods, 12*(10), 931–934.
38. List, M., Hauschild, A.-C., Tan, Q., Kruse, T. A., Mollenhauer, J., & Baumbach, J. (2014). Classification of breast cancer subtypes by combining gene expression and DNA methylation data. *Journal of Integrative Bioinformatics, 11*, 236. https://doi.org/10.2390/biecoll-jib-2014-236
39. Kim, M., Oh, I., & Ahn, J. (2018). An improved method for prediction of cancer prognosis by network learning. *Genes, 9*(10), 478.
40. Drabovich, A. P., Saraon, P., Drabovich, M., Karakosta, T. D., Dimitromanolakis, A., Hyndman, M. E., Jarvi, K., & Diamandis, E. P. (2019). Multi-omics Biomarker Pipeline Reveals Elevated Levels of Protein-glutamine Gamma-glutamyltransferase 4 in Seminal Plasma of Prostate Cancer Patients*[S]. *Molecular & Cellular Proteomics, 18*(9), 1807–1823.
41. Pai, S., Hui, S., Isserlin, R., Shah, M. A., Kaka, H., & Bader, G. D. (2019). netDx: interpretable patient classification using integrated patient similarity networks. *Molecular Systems Biology, 15*(3), e8497.
42. Mostafavi, S., Ray, D., Warde-Farley, D., Grouios, C., & Morris, Q. (2008). GeneMANIA: A real-time multiple association network integration algorithm for predicting gene function. *Genome Biology, 9*(1), 1–5.
43. Huang, L., Brunell, D., Stephan, C., Mancuso, J., Yu, X., He, B., Thompson, T. C., Zinner, R., Kim, J., Davies, P., & Wong, S. T. (2019). Driver network as a biomarker: Systematic integration and network modeling of multi-omics data to derive driver signaling pathways for drug combination prediction. *Bioinformatics, 35*(19), 3709–3717.
44. Lehmann-Che, J., Poirot, B., Boyer, J. C., & Evrard, A. (2017). Cancer genomics guide clinical practice in personalized medicine. *Therapies, 72*(4), 439–451.
45. Rizvi, N. A., Hellmann, M. D., Snyder, A., Kvistborg, P., Makarov, V., Havel, J. J., Lee, W., Yuan, J., Wong, P., Ho, T. S., & Miller, M. L. (2015). Mutational landscape determines sensitivity to PD-1 blockade in non–small cell lung cancer. *Science, 348*(6230), 124–128.
46. Tsai, E. A., Shakbatyan, R., Evans, J., Rossetti, P., Graham, C., Sharma, H., Lin, C. F., & Lebo, M. S. (2016). Bioinformatics workflow for clinical whole genome sequencing at partners healthcare personalized medicine. *Journal of Personalized Medicine, 6*(1), 12.
47. Zhang, H., He, L., & Cai, L. (2018). Transcriptome sequencing: RNA-seq. In T. Huang (Ed.), *Computational systems biology* (pp. 15–27). Humana Press.
48. Aslam, B., Basit, M., Nisar, M. A., Khurshid, M., & Rasool, M. H. (2017). Proteomics: Technologies and their applications. *Journal of Chromatographic Science, 55*(2), 182–196.
49. Yakkioui, Y., Temel, Y., Chevet, E., & Negroni, L. (2017). Integrated and quantitative proteomics of human tumors. *Methods in Enzymology, 1*(586), 229–246.
50. Nesvizhskii, A. I. (2010). A survey of computational methods and error rate estimation procedures for peptide and protein identification in shotgun proteomics. *Journal of Proteomics, 73*(11), 2092–2123.
51. Mihăşan, M., Wormwood, K. L., Sokolowska, I., Roy, U., Woods, A. G., & Darie, C. C. (2019). Mass spectrometry-and computational structural biology-based investigation of proteins and peptides. In *Advancements of mass spectrometry in biomedical research* (pp. 265–287).
52. Gatto, L., & Christoforou, A. (2014). Using R and Bioconductor for proteomics data analysis. *Biochimica et Biophysica Acta (BBA)-Proteins and Proteomics,* 1844(1), 42–51.
53. Cox, J., & Mann, M. (2008). MaxQuant enables high peptide identification rates, individualized p.p.b.-range mass accuracies and proteome-wide protein quantification. *Nature Biotechnology, 26*, 1367–1372. https://doi.org/10.1038/nbt.1511

54. Armitage, E. G., & Ciborowski, M. (2017). Applications of metabolomics in cancer studies. In *Metabolomics: From fundamentals to clinical applications* (pp. 209–234).
55. Perrotti, F., Rosa, C., Cicalini, I., Sacchetta, P., Del Boccio, P., Genovesi, D., & Pieragostino, D. (2016). Advances in lipidomics for cancer biomarkers discovery. *International Journal of Molecular Sciences, 17*(12), 1992.
56. Petrosino, J. F. (2018). The microbiome in precision medicine: The way forward. *Genome Medicine, 10*(1), 1–4.
57. Routy, B., Le Chatelier, E., Derosa, L., Duong, C. P., Alou, M. T., Daillère, R., Fluckiger, A., Messaoudene, M., Rauber, C., Roberti, M. P., & Fidelle, M. (2018). Gut microbiome influences efficacy of PD-1–based immunotherapy against epithelial tumors. *Science, 359*(6371), 91–97.
58. Gopalakrishnan, V., Spencer, C. N., Nezi, L., Reuben, A., Andrews, M. C., Karpinets, T. V., Prieto, P. A., Vicente, D., Hoffman, K., Wei, S. C., & Cogdill, A. P. (2018). Gut microbiome modulates response to anti–PD-1 immunotherapy in melanoma patients. *Science, 359*(6371), 97–103.
59. Matson, V., Fessler, J., Bao, R., Chongsuwat, T., Zha, Y., Alegre, M. L., Luke, J. J., & Gajewski, T. F. (2018). The commensal microbiome is associated with anti–PD-1 efficacy in metastatic melanoma patients. *Science, 359*(6371), 104–108.
60. Hu, R., Wang, X., & Zhan, X. (2013). Multi-parameter systematic strategies for predictive, preventive and personalised medicine in cancer. *EPMA Journal, 4*(1), 1–2.
61. Cheng, T., & Zhan, X. (2017). Pattern recognition for predictive, preventive, and personalized medicine in cancer. *EPMA Journal, 8*(1), 51–60.
62. Zhan, X., Long, Y., & Lu, M. (2018). Exploration of variations in proteome and metabolome for predictive diagnostics and personalized treatment algorithms: Innovative approach and examples for potential clinical application. *Journal of Proteomics, 30*(188), 30–40.
63. Wang, Y., Zhang, C., Zhang, P., Guo, G., Jiang, T., Zhao, X., Jiang, J., Huang, X., Tong, H., & Tian, Y. (2018). Serum exosomal micro RNA s combined with alpha-fetoprotein as diagnostic markers of hepatocellular carcinoma. *Cancer Medicine, 7*(5), 1670–1679.
64. Curtis, C., Shah, S. P., Chin, S.-F., Turashvili, G., Rueda, O. M., & Dunning, M. J. (2012). The genomic and transcriptomic architecture of 2,000 breast tumours reveals novel subgroups. *Nature, 11*(486), 346–352.
65. Stemke-Hale, K., Gonzalez-Angulo, A. M., Lluch, A., Neve, R. M., Kuo, W. L., Davies, M., Carey, M., Hu, Z., Guan, Y., Sahin, A., & Symmans, W. F. (2008). An integrative genomic and proteomic analysis of PIK3CA, PTEN, and AKT mutations in breast cancer. *Cancer Research, 68*(15), 6084–6091.
66. Nam, H., Chung, B. C., Kim, Y., Lee, K., & Lee, D. (2009). Combining tissue transcriptomics and urine metabolomics for breast cancer biomarker identification. *Bioinformatics, 25*(23), 3151–3157.
67. Komurov, K., Tseng, J. T., Muller, M., Seviour, E. G., Moss, T. J., Yang, L., Nagrath, D., & Ram, P. T. (2012). The glucose-deprivation network counteracts lapatinib-induced toxicity in resistant ErbB2-positive breast cancer cells. *Molecular Systems Biology, 8*(1), 596.
68. Jayaram, S., Gupta, M. K., Raju, R., Gautam, P., Sirdeshmukh, R. (2016). Multi-omics data integration and mapping of altered kinases to pathways reveal gonadotropin hormone signaling in glioblastoma. *Omics: A Journal of Integrative Biology, 20*(12), 736–746.
69. Schrörs, B., Boegel, S., Albrecht, C., Bukur, T., Bukur, V., Holtsträter, C., Ritzel, C., Manninen, K., Tadmor, A. D., Vormehr, M., & Sahin, U. (2020). Multi-omics characterization of the 4T1 murine mammary gland tumor model. *Frontiers in Oncology, 23*(10), 1195.
70. Stabej, P. L., James, C., Ocaka, L., Tekman, M., Grunewald, S., Clement, E., Stanescu, H. C., Kleta, R., Morrogh, D., Calder, A., & Williams, H. J. (2017). An example of the utility of genomic analysis for fast and accurate clinical diagnosis of complex rare phenotypes. *Orphanet Journal of Rare Diseases, 12*(1), 1–8.
71. Agrawal, P. B., Joshi, M., Marinakis, N. S., Schmitz-Abe, K., Ciarlini, P. D., Sargent, J. C., Markianos, K., De Girolami, U., Chad, D. A., & Beggs, A. H. (2014). Expanding the phenotype associated with the NEFL mutation: Neuromuscular disease in a family with overlapping myopathic and neurogenic findings. *JAMA Neurology, 71*(11), 1413–1420.

72. Abela, L., Spiegel, R., Crowther, L. M., Klein, A., Steindl, K., Papuc, S. M., Joset, P., Zehavi, Y., Rauch, A., Plecko, B., & Simmons, T. L. (2017). Plasma metabolomics reveals a diagnostic metabolic fingerprint for mitochondrial aconitase (ACO2) deficiency. *PloS One, 12*(5), e0176363.
73. Favier, L. A., & Schulert, G. S. (2016). Mevalonate kinase deficiency: Current perspectives. *The Application of Clinical Genetics, 9*, 101.
74. Carapito, R., Carapito, C., Morlon, A., Paul, N., Jacome, A. S., Alsaleh, G., Rolli, V., Tahar, O., Aouadi, I., Rompais, M., & Delalande, F. (2018). Multi-OMICS analyses unveil STAT1 as a potential modifier gene in mevalonate kinase deficiency. *Annals of the Rheumatic Diseases, 77*(11), 1675–1687.
75. Assié, G., Letouzé, E., Fassnacht, M., Jouinot, A., Luscap, W., Barreau, O., Omeiri, H., Rodriguez, S., Perlemoine, K., René-Corail, F., & Elarouci, N. (2014). Integrated genomic characterization of adrenocortical carcinoma. *Nature Genetics, 46*(6), 607–612.
76. Zheng, S., Cherniack, A. D., Dewal, N., Moffitt, R. A., Danilova, L., Murray, B. A., Lerario, A. M., Else, T., Knijnenburg, T. A., Ciriello, G., & Kim, S. (2016). Comprehensive pan-genomic characterization of adrenocortical carcinoma. *Cancer Cell, 29*(5), 723–736.
77. Lippert, J., Appenzeller, S., Liang, R., Sbiera, S., Kircher, S., Altieri, B., Nanda, I., Weigand, I., Gehrig, A., Steinhauer, S., & Riemens, R. J. (2018). Targeted molecular analysis in adrenocortical carcinomas: A strategy toward improved personalized prognostication. *The Journal of Clinical Endocrinology & Metabolism, 103*(12), 4511–4523.
78. Hoadley, K. A., Yau, C., Hinoue, T., Wolf, D. M., Lazar, A. J., Drill, E., Shen, R., Taylor, A. M., Cherniack, A. D., Thorsson, V., & Akbani, R. (2018). Cell-of-origin patterns dominate the molecular classification of 10,000 tumors from 33 types of cancer. *Cell, 173*(2), 291–304.
79. Mattox, A. K., Bettegowda, C., Zhou, S., Papadopoulos, N., Kinzler, K. W., & Vogelstein, B. (2019). Applications of liquid biopsies for cancer. *Science Translational Medicine, 11*(507).
80. Bettegowda, C., Sausen, M., Leary, R. J., Kinde, I., Wang, Y., Agrawal, N., Bartlett, B. R., Wang, H., Luber, B., Alani, R. M., & Antonarakis, E. S. (2014). Detection of circulating tumor DNA in early-and late-stage human malignancies. *Science Translational Medicine, 6*(224), 224ra24.
81. Tie, J., Kinde, I., Wang, Y., Wong, H. L., Roebert, J., Christie, M., Tacey, M., Wong, R., Singh, M., Karapetis, C. S., & Desai, J. (2015). Circulating tumor DNA as an early marker of therapeutic response in patients with metastatic colorectal cancer. *Annals of Oncology, 26*(8), 1715–1722.
82. Cohen, J. D., Javed, A. A., Thoburn, C., Wong, F., Tie, J., Gibbs, P., Schmidt, C. M., Yip-Schneider, M. T., Allen, P. J., Schattner, M., & Brand, R. E. (2017). Combined circulating tumor DNA and protein biomarker-based liquid biopsy for the earlier detection of pancreatic cancers. *Proceedings of the National Academy of Sciences, 114*(38), 10202–10207.
83. Tian, M. M., Fan, Y. C., Zhao, J., Gao, S., Zhao, Z. H., Chen, L. Y., & Wang, K. (2017). Hepatocellular carcinoma suppressor 1 promoter hypermethylation in serum. A diagnostic and prognostic study in hepatitis B. *Clinics and Research in Hepatology and Gastroenterology, 41*(2), 171–80.
84. Krug, A. K., Enderle, D., Karlovich, C., Priewasser, T., Bentink, S., Spiel, A., Brinkmann, K., Emenegger, J., Grimm, D. G., Castellanos-Rizaldos, E., & Goldman, J. W. (2018). Improved EGFR mutation detection using combined exosomal RNA and circulating tumor DNA in NSCLC patient plasma. *Annals of Oncology, 29*(3), 700–706.
85. Gara, S. K., Wang, Y., Patel, D., Liu-Chittenden, Y., Jain, M., Boufraqech, M., Zhang, L., Meltzer, P. S., & Kebebew, E. (2015). Integrated genome-wide analysis of genomic changes and gene regulation in human adrenocortical tissue samples. *Nucleic Acids Research, 43*(19), 9327–9339.
86. Mohs, R. C., & Greig, N. H. (2017). Drug discovery and development: Role of basic biological research. *Alzheimer's & Dementia: Translational Research & Clinical Interventions, 3*(4), 651–657.
87. Pantziarka, P., & Meheus, L. (2018). Omics-driven drug repurposing as a source of innovative therapies in rare cancers. *Expert Opinion on Orphan Drugs, 6*(9), 513–517.

88. Lang, J. D., Hendricks, W. P., Orlando, K. A., Yin, H., Kiefer, J., Ramos, P., Sharma, R., Pirrotte, P., Raupach, E. A., Sereduk, C., & Tang, N. (2018). Ponatinib shows potent antitumor activity in small cell carcinoma of the ovary hypercalcemic type (SCCOHT) through multikinase inhibition. *Clinical Cancer Research, 24*(8), 1932–1943.
89. Perez-Riverol, Y., Kuhn, M., Vizcaíno, J. A., Hitz, M. P., & Audain, E. (2017). Accurate and fast feature selection workflow for high-dimensional omics data. *PloS One, 12*(12), e0189875.

Computational Intelligence Methods for Predicting Cancer Susceptibility from SNP Data

Saanya Yadav and Yasha Hasija

Abstract Cancer is a chronic disease where cells inside the body grow abnormally. It is a complicated disease with various molecular changes brought on by hereditary, environmental, and lifestyle factors. Human cancers for a long time avowed to be linked to genetic predisposition as well as causal environmental exposures. Cancers are most often recurring in many cases, implying that environmental factors are important in determining cancer risk. Multiple mutations in a lifetime, germline substitution in single nucleotide polymorphism, indel polymorphisms, and some constructional changes in chromosomes are all genomic causes of cancer. SNPs (Single nucleotide polymorphisms) act as biological markers and are evident in human DNA on gene promoter regions, coding DNA, non-coding DNA, and leader-trailer sequence making the 5′ and 3′ ends of untranslated regions. The different genomic elements in which any specific SNPs are situated determine the pathways for SNP-cancer interaction which is discussed in detail in this chapter. Moreover, it is being observed that external factors leading to changes in the genes owing to genetic code variations contribute to cancer risks concerning SNPs. Whole-genome SNP arrays are a helpful tool to uncover the association between SNPs and diseases like cancer, thanks to recent developments in high-throughput technologies. Computer intelligence-based machine learning approaches for handling classification problems can be used to predict cancer susceptibility models, gives reliable results for research and assessment. The approach studied in this chapter is to identify the mutations in genomic sequence that persists in the patients with cancer and forecast novel SNP-cancer interactions, to be used later for early detection with the help of computational intelligence. This discourse aims to give an all-inclusive overview of automated early diagnosis operations using SNP data and configure the future of cancer research.

Keywords Cancer · SNPs · SVM · Predictive models · Epigenetic · Classifier

---

S. Yadav · Y. Hasija (✉)
Department of Biotechnology, Delhi Technological University, New Delhi, Delhi, India
e-mail: yashahasija@dtu.ac.in

K. Raza (ed.), *Computational Intelligence in Oncology*, Studies in Computational Intelligence 1016, https://doi.org/10.1007/978-981-16-9221-5_24

1 Introduction

The latest revolution is combining medical-clinical knowledge with machine learning techniques. Machine learning and computer intelligence are inextricably linked. Machine Learning (ML) is an aforementioned category that is capable of learning to make predictions or judgments without being specifically taught to do so. The more data a machine learning model sees, the better it performs over time. Deep learning, a subcategory of ML which allows abstract representation of data via deep neural networks, have recently demonstrated their prospects in simulating human cognition and going beyond our intellectual limits in a variety of applications in a spectrum [1].

In the year 2020, a projected 19.3 million novel malignancies (over 18 million excluding non-melanoma skin carcinoma) were diagnosed across the globe, and over half of them succumbed to death because of cancer (9.9 million excluding non-melanoma skin cancer) [2]. Early cancer detection focuses on finding symptomatic individuals as soon as feasible so that they can receive the best therapy available. When treatment therapy for a deadly disease like cancer is delayed or ineffective, the survival's probability decreases, increasing treatment complications along with high expenditure. Early detection improves treatment outcomes by giving patients treatment at the earliest possible stage and is thus an essential public health approach [3]. Single nucleotide polymorphisms (SNPs) are thought to be the genetic foundation for and possible cancer indicators that cause individual variations in disease susceptibility. SNP-containing gene analysis is critical for cancer early detection and customized tailored treatment. Figure 1 shows the latest surge in research in these domains, as the situation demands more such methods.

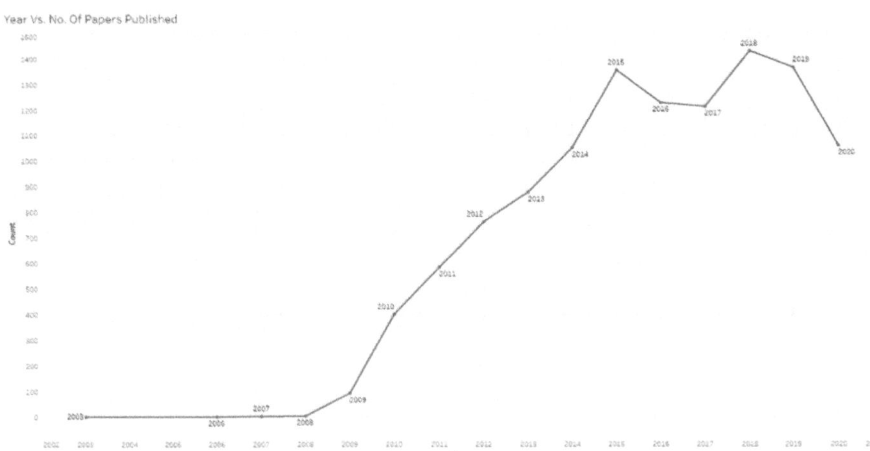

Fig. 1 Graph representing the number of papers published for computational intelligence in oncology taken from the MeSH tool of Pubmed. The trend tracebacks to two decades with a sudden increase from 2009 onwards

2 SNPs and Cancer Susceptibility

Single nucleotide polymorphism (SNP) is a mutation in DNA at a single point, which is passed on to generations and persists with time. Some of these SNPs are known to cause specific forms of cancer. Such links enable scientists to search for SNPs to assess someone's genetic susceptibility to being carcinogenic at an early stage [4].

Different SNPs are explained below on the basis of their location in DNA with their relation to oncology. In the genome, SNPs are found at the gene promoter region, exonal region of a gene, intronal region of a gene, and at untranslated regions of the gene.

2.1 Gene Promoter Region

The promoter region is located just upstream or close to a gene that will be transcribed. It is in this area that specific regulatory elements (cis-acting elements and specific transcriptional factors) will bind to aid in the transcription of RNA [5]. The promoter region consists of the TATA box, transcription binding sites, regulatory elements, CpG islands and many more [6]. Variations and polymorphisms in promoter regions influence susceptibility to cancer by interfering with epigenetic mechanisms (DNA methylation and modification in histone) [4].

Promoter activity is reduced with the occurrence of SNPs in the promoter region followed by a reduction in transcription of RNA [7]. Several transcription binding sites and factors are present in the promoter region. SNPs in promoter regions impede the binding of factors on transcription binding sites and decrease the speed of the process of transcription of the target gene. AT *CDH1* site, occupancy of SNPs promotes the production of tumors pertaining to the colon, breast, gastric, and prostate cancers [8]. In patients with breast carcinoma, SNPs enhance the promoter activity of the survivin gene by acting on GATA-1 transcription binding sites (cis-acting element) and increasing the chance of survival of oncogene [9]. The methylation of DNA is mainly due to the promoter gene CpG Island. SNPs present in this region are the source of many diseases. They exert on dinucleotides in CpG islands contributing to changes in DNA methylation, conversions in chromatin as well as silencing of target genes [10]. Polymorphism occurring in enzymes in promoters like DNA methyltransferase, methionine synthase have the ability to inhibit the overall synthesis of DNA in addition to promoting abnormal methylation of DNA in epigenetic mechanisms Cyclin A2's promoter region SNPs are seen to be linked with a higher chance of having colon, liver, and lung cancers SNP (rs672196) in the Nrf2 gene reduces the survival of patients with renal cancer if present [11].

2.2 Exonal SNPs

SNPs falling inside the coding region of DNA (exonal region) are termed as synonymous coding (cSNP) and non-synonymous based on the capacity to alter the protein sequence via replacing the amino acid in the codon sequence. Non-synonymous SNP can change the encoded codon sequence while synonymous SNP cannot replace any amino acid. Exonal SNPs influence genetic mechanisms linked to cancer susceptibility [4].

Amino acid mutation caused by non-synonymous cSNPs can alter the function of proteins. In the majority of variations, the mutation in the initial two bases of a codon leads to a new amino acid in the sequence. Changes in these sequences can impact the role of protein and its interactions by modifying the secondary structure of the protein through processes like phosphorylation and changing the number of bonding hydrogen. These mutations affect various cell signaling pathways and alleviate the oncogenic and tumor proteins. Exons of different genes contain over 13,000 known SNPs, with 58 percent of them being non-synonymous cSNPs [12]. Polymorphism in the tyrosine kinase domain (exonal region of DNA) is significant for malignancies. The Epidermal Growth Factor Receptor (EGFR), which functions as a receptor of this community, is been included in the advancements and progressions of different cancers as polymorphism in these areas leads to an increase in protein activity and sensitivity in Tyrosine kinase domains [13]. These polymorphisms also increase the property of tumorigenesis in cells by gaining the function of different proteins [14]. Mutations in synonymous cSNP generally do not cause amino acid substitution but possess the ability to alter the neighboring genes. Splicing of RNA, regulation of stability, and biomolecular structure of messenger RNA, as well as protein folding, are all affected by synonymous cSNPs. These alterations have a major impact on protein function, leading to variations in cellular responsiveness of stimuli to cell targets, which relates to unique patient reactions to medicines [15]. Based on in-silico analysis, synonymous SNPs can cause a variety of disorders by affecting gene regulation pertaining to microRNA and therefore modifying the expression of the gene [16]. Synonymous cSNPs can also change the pace at which the ribosomal binding to mRNA, altering the tendency of translation and the building framework and functionality of the resulting protein. Several mRNA secondary conformations and protein secondary foldings, such as helix folding, may also arise [17]. Furthermore, in the synonymous codon, codon use is not irregular, along with base structure formation is linked to the codon's second base location [18].

2.3 Intronal SNPs

Introns is that part of a DNA sequence that itself doesn't make any protein but assists in gene expressions in particular tissues, transcription as well as translation processes. Enhancers like cis-acting elements are present within introns to promote the procedure of initiation and elongation in transcription. We are aware that intron splicing manifolds the stability of the RNA is made. The SNPs functional in introns affect the splicing of mRNA of genes located in the vicinity and lncRNA binding. Thus, SNPs affect cancer susceptibility by epigenetic along with genetic pathways [19].

The cis-acting binding sites falling in intronal region positively affect gene expression which is a hive for harmful variants in genes [20]. Genome-based research found that the rs2981578 variant is the riskiest factor for breast cancer susceptibility in fibroblast growth sensory system factor 2. When cloned, this sequence showed extreme transcription factor FOXA1 in the binding region of the intronal region. The risk factor for breast cancer is related to FOXA1 and ESR1. SNP sequence in the TOX3 gene increases the affinity for complex DNA and has allele-specific proteins [21]. The C to T mutation in IRF4 enhances IRF4 translation through transcriptional repression, which is linked to a higher possibility of male acute lymphoblastic leukaemia [22]. Genomic imprinting is described as an epigenetic process responsible for genes to express in a way that is particular to their parent of origin. DNA methylation and histone modification (acetylation) is known to be the driving force behind this. Gene expression is influenced by SNPs in the areas that are imprinted. H19 gene decreases the cell material immediately after birth that is basically imprinted and codes for oncofetal RNA. H19 gene rs2839698 TC intronic SNP are protected from bladder cancer [23]. LncRNA (long non-coding RNA) found in the intronal region can rearrange and modify chromatin, alter histones, stimulate or suppress transcription along with tumor gene activity, alter the phenomena of splicing. SNP (rs2147578) genomic intronal variations in the intronal region at LAMC2-1:1 transcript affect microRNA-128-3p binding (occurs in the majority of tissues) and increase the chance of colorectal cancer. This polymorphism genotypes' cytosine-cytosine and guanine-guanine influence higher risk of contracting colorectal carcinoma [24]. Polymorphism in lnc region is known to increase the susceptibility of colorectal, gastric, and prostate cancers. The third intron lying in lncRNA is addressed as a short isoform for rs11672691 and possesses enhancing and promoting the ability for prostate cancer [25].

2.4 UTR Related SNPs

SNPs lying in 3′UTR and 5′UTR regions of mRNAs critically affect the process of translation. The 3′UTR regulates the stability of mRNA by polyadenylating RNA transcripts and the interactions with the regulatory proteins, messenger RNA, and miRNA [26]. These variations within UTRs are unruly as they change secondary folding and active binding sites of mRNA [27]. Signaling pathways of many cancer-related genes are altered due to these variations. mRNA folding, processing, and translation are affected by SNPs in the UTR region and have operational disruptive effects on mRNA survival [28].

SNPs in the 5′UTR have an impact on mRNA synthesis, transportation, longevity, and translation. Variation as SNPs in the 5′-UTR is found linked to numerous eukaryotic illnesses because they impact the accuracy of mRNA translation [29]. Ribosomes attach directly to the ribosome binding site of the 5′-UTR region of mammalian genes. A mutation of + 2756 Cytosine to Thymine in the 5′-UTR of the c-Myc gene increases the sensitivity and function of ribosome binding sites, increasing c-Myc production and carcinogenesis in multiple myeloma [30]. A -34 Guanine to Thymine mutation in the CDKN2A gene causes the creation of a novel upstream open reading frame that suppresses translation, leading to loss of allele function and an elevated chance of melanoma [31]. The 5′-UTR is involved in regulating transcription as well. The + 24 T/C mutation in the CR2 gene's 5′-UTR is linked to a greater susceptibility to nasopharyngeal cancer (NPC). Due to involvement in enhanced transcriptional function, those with the minor allele Cytosine have a higher chance of NPC than people with the Thymine allele [32].SNPs in the 3′-UTR and miRNAs can influence mRNA disintegration and the process of translation via changing miRNA binding sites [19]. Upon attaching to the 3′-UTR of the mRNA transcript, microRNAs impede translation and destabilize their desired complementary mRNAs. By breaking sequence complementarity, SNPs in the 3′-UTRs change how microRNAs recognize their targets [33]. Three SNPs in the 3′UTR of genes linked to cell interaction and mobility in the LPP gene were related with a substantially higher sensitivity to lung cancer among males in laminar tests by gender [34]. Nuclear receptors (NR1/2, PGR), genes involved in the primary doxorubicin metabolic route (SLC22A16), and the dox-progesterone-linked allele all influence the risk of mortality, tumor progression, or relapse of breast cancer. SNPs in the 3′UTR were shown to be substantially linked to a higher chance of recurrence-free survival and treatment responsiveness [35].

3 Commonly Used Computational Intelligence Methods

3.1 Support Vector Machine

Support vector machines (SVM) saw the light of the world by the works of Vapnik in 1963. These models maximize (support) separation margin (vector), which has become a powerful classification method that is also being used to categorize or subtype cancer genomics (Fig. 2) [36]. The concept of a support vector machine is popular because it provides high accuracy while using fewer computer services. SVMs are a type of machine that can be used for both categorization and retrogression. It is, however, frequently used for classification reasons.

SVM is an important yet effective technique for the categorization of arbitrary input data. After feeding the machine with metadata, the system performs in such a way that creates a hyperplane (also called decision boundary) separating the data into groups/classes. This categorization is then used for interpretation by identifying labels from vectors used in the analysis. SVM is a strong tool for the creation of a

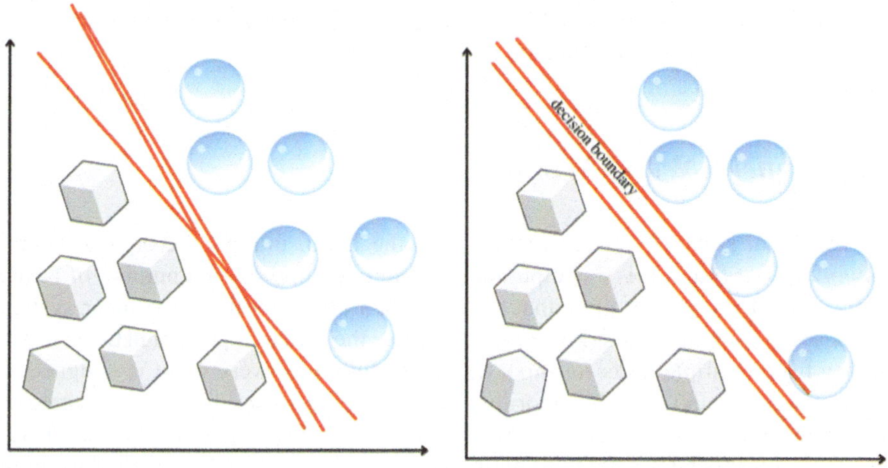

Fig. 2 We have two different datasets that need to be classified. Here we can have many dividing planes, but we will choose the plan which has the maximum margin for accurate results

classifier. It aims to create a hyperplane between a pair of classes that enables the prediction of markers from some feature vectors in space [37]. The hyperplane is aimed at the farthest data points that are far-flung from the nearest data values from all of the categories. Support vectors are the points in a plane that are the closest together and have an impact on the hyperplane or decision boundary's positioning and configuration. Take a look at the following dataset:

$$(x_1,\ y_1),\ (x_2,\ y_2),\ \ldots,\ (x_n,\ y_n),\quad x_i \in R^d \,\&\, y_i \in (-1,\ +1)$$

Here, x_i belongs to a dimensional vector used for representing our object of interest and y_i is the label for class for our compound i to be used in training.

The equation for hyperplane can be as below:

$$wx^N + m = 0$$

where w is the vector representing weight, input is represented as x and m is the bias. The w and m should follow the given equations for each component belonging to the input data training set because of the class label:

$$wx_i^N + m \geq +1 \text{ for } y_i = 1$$
$$wx_i^N + m \geq +1 \text{ for } y_i = -1$$

The goal of this model training lies in identifying w in addition to m such that the decision boundary partitions the input metadata as well as increases the bourn 1/ || w ||2. Support vectors will fall under x_i, where $y_i\ (wx_i^N + m) = 1$. SVM has been utilized in cancer classification since the early 2000s when increased microarray gene regulation information became accessible [36].

3.2 Artificial Neural Network

The Artificial Neural Network (ANN), like the brain, mimics the organic neural network of our brain. It is a computational system composed of a number of basic, highly linked processing units that interpret data based on their nonlinear system responses to external inputs (Fig. 3). They imitate the echelons present in the neurons as they have multiple ports for input, in this technology, every input is assigned to a value (weight) and then the algorithm decides to fire-focused on the aggregate of the inputs. This is the result of 3 levels of operational logical units, the first layer comprises the input dataset. Synthesizing this data using hidden layers and the output layer which generates the solution [38]. Its benefit over traditional programming is that it can handle issues for which there is no algorithmic answer or for which the approach is too complicated to find. ANNs are capable of performing statistical analyses such as linear, logistic, and nonlinear retrogression. It is difficult for artificial networks based on the neural pathways to comprehend the architecture of the method since they cannot seem to figure out how to use the classification system [39].

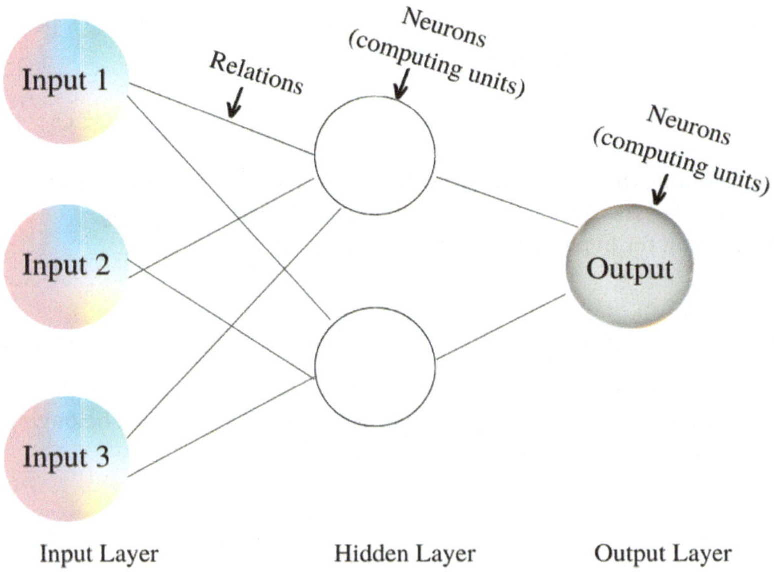

Fig. 3 A feed-forward Artificial Neural Network. These are extremely nonlinear, as here the transfer of data from the previous layer to the next layer is sigmoid and dependent on the linkage in the relations

The most commonly used ANNs are feed-forward networks. They send the weight input to the hidden layer (next layer) from the first layer. This network is used to identify a completely nonlinear correlation between certain input variables and one or more output variables. The network does this by connecting many layers of neurons as computing units and calculating outputs as synthesized functions of inputs [40]. Avoiding overfitting (having multiple neural layers) is the first conduct when utilizing ANNs. To get this outcome, one must be frugal and favor tiny networks, such as those included in a mono concealed layer. Observations have come about that one concealed layer is capable of estimating any non-linear combination accurately. Moreover, network size should be proportional to the quantity of metadata available for the teaching system. The parameters of ANNs, arbitrary inputs must fall in minimum a single grade lower than the number of target relations, at most times, preferably two [41]. The initial branches have an impact on the weights that are established at the end of the learning phase. Such events lead to irregularities in ANN algorithm results, which may be studied using ensemble runs with the objective, characterizing the most efficient model by reducing volatility and determining another more regress and mean of the various feed-forward neural networks algorithms [42]. Contrary to traditional statistical analysis, the ANNs can handle convolution even when the input size is very less and the variable-to-record ratio is imbalanced. In this way, the ANN model circumvents the dimensionality issue [38].

3.3 Decision Trees

A typical tree has a root system, offshoots, and leaves. In the Decision Tree, the same pattern is followed. It is made up of nodes in leaves and roots and has branches [43]. Decision trees, first presented in the 1960s, are among the most implicit data extraction devices. They have been extensively implemented in numerous fields because they are simple to use, subjective, and resilient even in the case of missing information [44].

The basic component of the decision tree is nodes. Three types of nodes can be put in use while working. A root node is a decision that divides all the input into a pair or more collective exclusive subsets. Internal nodes reflect one of the options accessible in the tree construction at that time. The end consequence of a series of decisions or occurrences is represented by leaf nodes. The other constituent of the decision tree branches. Branches are random events that emerge from the root and internal nodes. A grading of random events is deployed to create a DT model. A subtyping-based decision rule is shown by every way followed to leaf node from root node via internal one [45].

Splitting is a crucial step in this model. To segregate parent from child nodes of the desired entity, only input variables relevant to the desired variable are utilized. It is possible to engage both discrete and variables with a constant input (that are compressed in at least two or more types). This process of splitting persists until the halting conditions are fulfilled [46]. Stopping is another essential step for the model. When used to forecast succeeding reports, the more complicated a model is, the less trustworthy it becomes. When creating a decision tree, it is important to include halting rules to keep the model from getting too complicated. Stopping specifications must be chosen based on the analysis' aim as well as the dataset's features. And pruning, among all steps, is the one that can be a lifesaver. Stopping rules are ineffective in some instances. Growing a big tree initially and then pruning that to the ideal dimensions by deleting nodes having little extra details is another approach to create an efficient decision tree model. Pre and post are the two forms of pruning. To avoid the formation of unessential branches, pre-pruning employs Chi-square tests or numerous function optimization. After constructing a full decision tree, post-pruning is used to remove branches in a way that enhances the overall accuracy of a particular dataset [45].

3.4 Bayesian Networks

In comparison to many other ML approaches, Bayesian networks (BN) enable us to know about relations in effect and their causes using domain ideas in a more visually attractive and understandable manner, and they are employed to answer many alarming clinical issues. They do this in a natural way, encoding ambiguous domain knowledge [47]. They possess the capacity to naturally capture the cause and effect relationships between diagnostic or prognostic variables recorded in medicinal datasets [48]. BNs are highly employable because of their visual display nature that allows the information they comprise to be clearly recognized by a clinician and they can explicitly integrate foreknowledge while understanding the framework and variables of the system [49]. They make parameter estimation easier owing to their accurate recognition of the joint probability space; they also allow for cause-effect-based interventions in addition to observational inference. They can be used to interrogate any node in the network and are good at making predictions even when the data is insufficient [50]. BN is made up of a directed acyclic graph (DAG) with arbitrary values assigned at its nodes and the probability dispensation of a particular value of each parameter in the network given linked to its parents' values.

As we have seen, there are several algorithms for examining the data and giving new conclusions for different problems. These algorithms are based on a variety of approaches for changing feature weights and data constraints. ANNs have the unique feature to understand and model non-linear and complicated connections, it also offers no limitation on the dataset, while SVM is not suitable for large datasets [3] SVM is great with higher dimensions and low sample set and is memory efficient [51]. Output generated by decision trees is relatively easier to read and interpret and can work well even with less data cleaning. But like two sides of a coin, decision trees have their own flaws, when the main aim is to forecast the result of a continuous variable, they are less successful in making predictions [52]. The major drawback found while working with Bayesian Networks is the fact that there is no widely acknowledged way for creating a network from data. Bayesian Networks are also more extendable than other machine learning approaches. In order to add a new piece of evidence to a Bayesian Network, all that is required is the insertion of a few probabilities and a small number of graph edges [53]. Other than these models, some unsupervised approaches like Generative adversarial networks (GANs) are also being employed for scanning and interpreting medical imaging data, and are continuously enhancing their outputs by hybridizing with other models [54].

4 Predictive Models in Cancer Diagnosis

The above-mentioned knowledge when applied to real-world datasets results in creating predictions in prognosis and susceptibility of diseases, some of them are summarised below. Table 1 mentions some more studies that have been undertaken in the past.

4.1 Multiple Myeloma

Multiple myeloma (MM), a.k.a. Kahler's disease, is the cancer of plasmacytes, where some cells of plasma grow uncontrollably and crowd other essential cells. Multiple myeloma makes for about one percent of all cancers and thirteen percent of blood-related malignancies. The presence of carcinogenic plasmacytes in the bone's bone marrow region, anaemia, renal failure, a high calcium level, and changed or damaged bones are all signs of it [63]. Current diagnostics include bone marrow assessment, FISH, CT as well as MRI. Many alkylating drugs are used for its treatment [64]. Escalated tumor load, comorbidities, and organ dysfunction all have an impact on treatment outcomes and myeloma patients' ability to receive therapy. The patient will miss out on the best chance for therapy if the detection is delayed, and problems may arise that can only be reversed in rare cases [65].

Genome-wide association studies (GWAS) discovered some important SNP loci for multiple myeloma. SNP at 7p15.3 influences the gene expression for binding transformations for myeloma. *ATG5* SNP at 6q21, *JARID2,* and rs4888262 SNP affects the development of transcriptional repressor for MM. *ULK4* is involved in the autophagy of cells [66].

Gradient Boosting DT is observed to be a promising approach for early detection in multiple myeloma. SVM classifiers are a simplified machine learning approach to predict specific treatment options. The efficient approach for using these classifiers is building novel interpretations of gene-level regulations based on unsupervised and self-paced interpreting algorithms to discover underlying valuable insights, integrating clinical makers, SNPs, and therapies to build a more detailed patient description to find the target treatment [67]. Bone marrow streaks as digital images have

Table 1 Some recent models employed for predicting cancer susceptibility in various cancer

Type of cancer	Method employed	Year of study	Study population	Model performance	Reference
Breast cancer	Deep convolutional neural networks	2017	272 whole slide images	CI: 95%	[55]
	CDSS (Clinical Decision Support Systems)	2017	Database from WBCD, WDB, and WPBC	Specificity: 0.89 Sensitivity: 0.81	[56]
	Deep Convolutional Neural Networks	2016	Lung Image Database Consortium (LIDC)	Sensitivity: 78.7 ± 8.0 Specificity: 85.7 ± 6.8	[57]
Lung Cancer	Deep convolutional neural networks	2020	EMRs of 2 million patients from Taiwan	AUC of 0.90	[58]
	LCP-CNN	2019	1200 patients from some UK based hospitals	AUC of 0.89	[59]
	ANN	2018	NHIS survey datasets from 1997–2015	AUC of 0.86	[60]
Multiple Myeloma	Gradient Boosting Decision Tree	2021	4000 + routine blood & biochemical examination records from China	AUC of 0.97	[61]
	ANN	2021	500 patient dataset from USA	PPV: 0.97	[62]

Here, CI: Confidence Interval, Specificity: true negative rate, Sensitivity: True positive rate, AUC: Area under the ROC Curve, PPV: positive predictive value

been screened by SVM classifiers [68]. ANN can analyze non-linear data and multivariable datasets to diagnose the disease at early stages by recognizing input patterns, compiled with the interpretation from mass spectrometry [69].

4.2 *Breast Cancer*

Breast cancer is found as the most common form of cancer across the globe. It is identified in its advanced stages as a result of women's neglect in self-inspecting and low clinical assessment of breasts. Breast cancer is the result of improper immunological response and surveillance systems. A link between inherited and environmental variables has been declared as the underlying reasons for this cancer [70]. Clinicians check the breasts, the region around the neck and collarbone, and the armpits during a physical examination. Breasts are examined for any abnormalities, such as lumps or other breast cancer symptoms [71]. To minimize the percentage of diseased women, we need to raise the number of early-detected breast cancers, it is important to enhance the procedure for early detection of disease. Breast density is a simple mammographic indicator that has been related to an increased breast cancer risk [72]. According to the number of people carrying variants of a particular gene that increase the risk of breast cancer, SNPs contribute at least fourteen percent for the inheritance of breast malignant tumors [73].

A mammogram-based tumor detection method was performed by Thamari et al. The suggested approach is designed to address two issues. One problem is detecting tumors as suspicious areas with a low resolution to their backdrop, and the other is extracting characteristics that classify tumors. For contrast stretching of mammographic inputs, the filtered picture is employed. The image's backdrop is then removed using the top hat technique. For segmentation, the rebuilt image is utilized. For segmentation, the threshold approach is applied, and then the characteristics are retrieved from the segmented tumor region. The final step is to classify the data using the SVM classifier [74].

One of the studies [75] took 57,902 women in the model-based risk evaluating initiative for a cancer screening study, that gathered information on conventional risk factors and breast radiograph inputs (breast density). A subgroup of these people agreed to have 18 breast cancer predisposition SNPs genotyped in their saliva specimens (SNP18) [76]. They inferred the prediction power of SNP18 alone and when corrected for traditional risk variables in the paper. They found 100 percent compliance with the genotyping of all sampled SNPs.

Some more experiments have been conducted in this regard. SVM is used to assess whether the microcalcification is present in each pixel position in the mammography. Texture energy measurements by Laws are obtained in accordance with the region of interest to enhance the classification rate. Once the characteristics for every single ROI have been calculated, the SVM classifier may utilize them as input. 322 digital mammographic pictures from the MIAS database were used to test the technique [77]. SVM cocktails can also be used, as 12 different SVMs were hybridized to achieve higher accuracy in detection of the disease and outperformed the existing others [78].

4.3 Lung Cancer

Lung cancer is a kind of malignant tumor that initiates in the lung parenchyma and inside the bronchus. Long-term exposure to carcinogens, particularly cancer stick (cigarette) smoke, is considered to promote aberrant lung epithelial development. If the exposure is not halted, genetic changes will occur, as well as a change in protein regulation. The cell cycle is interrupted as a result, which promotes tumorigenesis [79]. A low-dose computed tomography scan is the most often used lung cancer screening tool, although it is only advised for certain age groups and has sparked many disputes over its benefits in lung cancer detection [80].

When physiological factors and inheritance-based variants (usually in the region of SNPs) are also included in the working model, ANN offers good prediction performance. For accurate remaining surviving time forecast along with sensitivity probe of the metadata, the statistics construction was a feedforward ANN. The rate of accuracy was used in the analysis of the data. Overfitting, which was primarily driven by a multi-dimensional (oversized) ANN working on the small input as metadata provided, posed a statistical risk of incorrect findings [81]. In another paper, lung cancer was distinguished from benign pulmonary disorders and healthy persons using the ANN model. To distinguish from pulmonary cancer patients and non-cancer people, or pulmonary carcinoma with types of ontologies, researchers used a feedforward ANN. This was based on overfitting hazards that were comparable [82].

Researchers have also used a lung-based database to look at characteristics other than the stage that can impact lung cancer 5-year durability. The researchers use a multifactorial retrogression model and an artificial neural network model with two concealed layers to predict abiding lifespan and investigate the impact age and BMI has on the body. Now, even if the dataset is relatively large, the danger of incorrect conclusions owing to overfitting still exists [83]. Another approach could be to use microRNAs negatively labeled for lung cancer to neutralize severe chronic stages of lung cancer. The model is trained using decision trees by TCGA and LUAD databases to learn to classify the status of cancer [84].

5 Challenges and Future Outlook

The disease of cancer is considered difficult to diagnose as compared to many other diseases. Hence, to be able to predict whether someone is a cancer patient or not, especially in the early stages of the illness, comes with added obstructions. The sampling of patient data must be done carefully with utmost care to avoid any inconsistencies in generalization since the models have to be as accurate as possible when deployed in production. Moreover, issues pertaining to security, integrity, and morality continue to exist in the domain of artificial intelligence.

However, in spite of the aforementioned issues, computational intelligence is the way to go. Once the deployed programs are trained and are approved to be used in production, these will not only save time but also reduce workload and expenditure. This will help healthcare institutions to save their finances which can be utilized to fulfill requirements in other domain(s).

6 Conclusion

With the increasing number of cancer patients, pathologists have been asked to continuously upgrade their diagnostic protocols, as they are time and energy-consuming. Machines, when programmed, can do these operations in seconds. The machine repeats the procedure after each iteration in order to improve it. In such instances, the ethical dilemma of many hands develops, since it is unclear to what extent physicians, programmers, hospitals, or suppliers bear moral or legal responsibility. As machine learning becomes more widely adopted, more attention will need to be paid to its future research for resolving the scope of errors and its feasible clinical integration. There are various strategies to choose from, each with its own set of advantages and disadvantages. Most of these machine learning approaches are available in open-source forms, making them simple to experiment with and apply to photos. There are several measures for measuring an algorithm's performance; nevertheless, one must be aware of the potential flaws that might lead to false metrics. Deep learning has been employed more recently, and it has the advantage of not requiring picture feature identification and calculation as a first step; instead, features are recognized as part of the learning process. Better statistical analysis of the disparate datasets employed would yield more accurate results and offer context for illness outcomes. New research is needed based on the creation of more public databases that would collect valid cancer datasets from all patients who have been diagnosed.

References

1. Deep Learning vs. Machine Learning: What's the difference? [Internet]. [cited 2021 Oct 8]. Available from: https://www.zendesk.com/blog/machine-learning-and-deep-learning/
2. Sung, H., Ferlay, J., Siegel, R. L., Laversanne, M., Soerjomataram, I., Jemal, A., et al. (2021). Global cancer statistics 2020: GLOBOCAN estimates of incidence and mortality worldwide for 36 cancers in 185 Countries. *CA: A Cancer Journal for Clinicians, 71*(3), 209–249.
3. ANN for Data Science | Basics Of Artificial Neural Network [Internet]. [cited 2021 Oct 7]. Available from: https://www.analyticsvidhya.com/blog/2021/07/understanding-the-basics-of-artificial-neural-network-ann/
4. Deng, N., Zhou, H., Fan, H., & Yuan, Y. (2017). Single nucleotide polymorphisms and cancer susceptibility (Vol. 8). Oncotarget. Impact Journals LLC, pp. 110635–110649.
5. Promoter [Internet]. [cited 2021 Jul 2]. Available from: https://www.genome.gov/genetics-glossary/Promoter
6. Addgene: Promoters [Internet]. [cited 2021 Jul 13]. Available from: https://www.addgene.org/mol-bio-reference/promoters/
7. Peltoketo, H., Piao, Y., Mannermaa, A., Ponder, B. A., Isomaa, V., & Poutanen, M., et al. (1994). A point mutation in the putative TATA box, detected in nondiseased individuals and patients with hereditary breast cancer, decreases promoter activity of the 17 beta-hydroxysteroid dehydrogenase type 1 gene 2 (EDH17B2) in vitro. *Genomics, 23*(1), 250–252.
8. Ben Nasr, H., Hamrita, B., Batbout, M., Gabbouj, S., Bouaouina, N., Chouchane, L., et al. (2010). A single nucleotide polymorphism in the E-cadherin gene promoter -160 C/A is associated with risk of nasopharyngeal cancer. *Clinica Chimica Acta, 411*(17–18), 1253–1257.

9. Boidot, R., Vegran, F., Jacob, D., Chevrier, S., Cadouot, M., Feron, O., et al. The transcription factor GATA-1 is overexpressed in breast carcinomas and contributes to survivin upregulation via a promoter polymorphism. *Oncogene, 29*(17):2577–2584.
10. Stirzaker, C., Song, J. Z., Davidson, B., & Clark, S. J. (2004). Transcriptional gene silencing promotes DNA hypermethylation through a sequential change in chromatin modifications in cancer cells. *Cancer Research, 64*(11), 3871–3877.
11. Yamaguchi, Y., Kamai, T., Higashi, S., Murakami, S., Arai, K., Shirataki, H., et al. (2019) Nrf2 gene mutation and single nucleotide polymorphism rs6721961 of the Nrf2 promoter region in renal cell cancer. *BMC Cancer, 19*(1), 1–9.
12. Tennessen, J. A., Bigham, A. W., O'Connor, T. D., Fu, W., Kenny, E. E., Gravel, S., et al. (2012). Evolution and functional impact of rare coding variation from deep sequencing of human exomes. *Science (New York, NY), 337*(6090), 64–69.
13. Raghav, D., Sharma, V., & Agarwal, S. M. (2013). Structural investigation of deleterious non-synonymous SNPs of EGFR gene. *Interdisciplinary Sciences, Computational Life Sciences, 5*(1), 60–68.
14. Honsa, E. S., Cooper, V. S., Mhaissen, M. N., Frank, M., Shaker, J., Iverson, A., et al. (2017). Rela mutant enterococcus faecium with multiantibiotic tolerance arising in an immunocompromised host. *mBio, 8*(1).
15. Hunt, R., Sauna, Z. E., Ambudkar, S. V., Gottesman, M. M., & Kimchi-Sarfaty, C. (2009). Silent (synonymous) SNPs: Should we care about them? *Methods in molecular biology (Clifton, NJ), 578*:23–39.
16. Wang, Y., Qiu, C., & Cui, Q. (2015). A large-scale analysis of the relationship of synonymous SNPs changing MicroRNA regulation with functionality and disease. *International Journal of Molecular Sciences, 16*(10), 23545–23555.
17. Lx, S., Jp, B., & Vp, S. (1999). Single-nucleotide polymorphisms can cause different structural folds of mRNA. *Proceedings of the National Academy of Sciences of the United States of America, 96*(14), 7871–7876.
18. Gupta, S. K., Majumdar, S., Bhattacharya, T. K., & Ghosh, T.C. (2000). Studies on the relationships between the synonymous codon usage and protein secondary structural units. *Biochemical and Biophysical Research Communications, 269*(3), 692–696.
19. Deng, N., Zhou, H., Fan, H., & Yuan, Y. (2017). Single nucleotide polymorphisms and cancer susceptibility. *Oncotarget, 8*(66), 110635.
20. Zhang, X., Bailey, S. D., & Lupien, M. (2014). Laying a solid foundation for Manhattan—'setting the functional basis for the post-GWAS era.' *Trends in Genetics, 30*(4), 140–149.
21. Robbez-Masson, L. J., Bödör, C., Jones, J. L., Hurst, H. C., Fitzgibbon, J., Hart, I. R., et al. (2013). Functional analysis of a breast cancer-associated FGFR2 single nucleotide polymorphism using zinc finger mediated genome editing. In M. Isalan (Ed.). *PLoS ONE, 8*(11), e78839.
22. Do, T. N., Ucisik-Akkaya, E., Davis, C. F., Morrison, B. A., & Dorak, M. T. (2010). An intronic polymorphism of IRF4 gene influences gene transcription in vitro and shows a risk association with childhood acute lymphoblastic leukemia in males. *Biochimica et Biophysica Acta (BBA)—Molecular Basis of Disease, 1802*(2), 292–300.
23. Verhaegh, G. W., Verkleij, L., Vermeulen, S. H. H. M., den Heijer, M., Witjes, J. A., & Kiemeney, L. A. (2008). Polymorphisms in the H19 gene and the risk of bladder cancer. *European Urology, 54*(5), 1118–1126.
24. Gong, J., Tian, J., Lou, J., Ke, J., Li, L., Li, J., et al. (2016). A functional polymorphism in lnc-LAMC2-1:1 confers risk of colorectal cancer by affecting miRNA binding. *Carcinogenesis, 37*(5), 443–451.
25. Hua, J. T., Ahmed, M., Guo, H., Zhang, Y., Chen, S., Soares, F., et al. (2018). Risk SNP-mediated promoter-enhancer switching drives prostate cancer through lncRNA PCAT19. *Cell, 174*(3), 564-575.e18.
26. Skeeles, L. E., Fleming, J. L., Mahler, K. L., & Toland, A. E. (2013). The impact of 3′UTR variants on differential expression of candidate cancer susceptibility genes. *PLOS ONE, 8*(3), e58609.

27. Sabarinathan, R., Wenzel, A., Novotny, P., Tang, X., Kalari, K. R., & Gorodkin, J. (2014). Transcriptome-wide analysis of UTRs in non-small cell lung cancer reveals cancer-related genes with SNV-induced changes on RNA secondary structure and miRNA target sites. *PloS one, 9*(1).
28. Aouacheria, A., Navratil, V., López-Pérez, R., Gutiérrez, N. C., Churkin, A., Barash, D., et al. (2007). In silico whole-genome screening for cancer-related single-nucleotide polymorphisms located in human mRNA untranslated regions. *BMC Genomics, 8*(1), 2.
29. Mendell, J. T., & Dietz, H. C. (2001). When the message goes awry. *Cell, 107*(4), 411–414.
30. Chappell, S. A., LeQuesne, J. P., Paulin, F. E., DeSchoolmeester, M. L., Stoneley, M., Soutar, R. L., et al. (2000). A mutation in the c-myc-IRES leads to enhanced internal ribosome entry in multiple myeloma: A novel mechanism of oncogene de-regulation. *Oncogene, 19*(38), 4437–4440.
31. Cazzola, M., & Skoda, R. C. (2000). Translational pathophysiology: A novel molecular mechanism of human disease. *Blood, 95*(11), 3280–3288.
32. Fan, Q., He, J.-F., Wang, Q.-R., Cai, H.-B., Sun, X.-G., Zhou, X.-X., et al. (2013). Functional polymorphism in the 5′-UTR of CR2 is associated with susceptibility to nasopharyngeal carcinoma. *Oncology Reports, 30*(1), 11–16.
33. Selbach, M., Schwanhäusser, B., Thierfelder, N., Fang, Z., Khanin, R., & Rajewsky, N. (2008). Widespread changes in protein synthesis induced by microRNAs. *Nature, 455*(7209), 58–63.
34. Yan, S., Sun, R., Wu, S., Jin, T., Zhang, S., Niu, F., et al. (2019). Single nucleotide polymorphism in the 3′ untranslated region of LPP is a risk factor for lung cancer: A case-control study. *BMC Cancer, 19*(1), 35.
35. Pamuła-Piłat, J., Tęcza, K., Kalinowska-Herok, M., & Grzybowska, E. (2020). Genetic 3′UTR variations and clinical factors significantly contribute to survival prediction and clinical response in breast cancer patients. *Scientific Reports, 10*(1), 5736.
36. Huang, S., Cai, N., Pacheco, P. P., Narrandes, S., Wang, Y., & Xu, W. (2018). Applications of support vector machine (SVM) learning in cancer genomics. *Cancer Genomics & Proteomics, 15*(1), 41–51.
37. Noble, W. S. (2006). What is a support vector machine? *Nature Biotechnology, 24*(12), 1565–1567.
38. Hy, S., Sl, H., Kt, L., & Cl, L. (2013). In-hospital mortality after traumatic brain injury surgery: A nationwide population-based comparison of mortality predictors used in artificial neural network and logistic regression models. *Journal of Neurosurgery, 118*(4), 746–752.
39. Yu, Z., Lu, H., Si, H., Liu, S., Li, X., Gao, C., et al. (2015). A highly efficient gene expression programming (GEP) model for auxiliary diagnosis of small cell lung cancer. *PloS One, 10*(5).
40. Bertolaccini, L., Solli, P., Pardolesi, A., & Pasini, A. (2017). An overview of the use of artificial neural networks in lung cancer research. *Journal of Thoracic Disease., 9*(4), 924–931.
41. Feng, F., Wu, Y., Wu, Y., Nie, G., & Ni, R. (2012). The effect of artificial neural network model combined with six tumor markers in auxiliary diagnosis of lung cancer. *Journal of Medical Systems, 36*(5), 2973–2980.
42. Santos-García, G., Varela, G., Novoa, N., & Jiménez, M. F. (2004). Prediction of postoperative morbidity after lung resection using an artificial neural network ensemble. *Artificial Intelligence in Medicine, 30*(1), 61–69.
43. Jadhav, S. D., & Channe, H. P. (2016). Efficient recommendation system using decision tree classifier and collaborative filtering. *International Research Journal of Engineering and Technology.*
44. Fallon, B., Ma, J., Allan, K., Pillhofer, M., Trocmé, N., & Jud, A. (2013). Opportunities for prevention and intervention with young children: lessons from the Canadian incidence study of reported child abuse and neglect. *Child and Adolescent Psychiatry and Mental Health, 7*(1).
45. Song, Y.-Y., & Lu, Y. (2015). Decision tree methods: Applications for classification and prediction. *Shanghai Archives of Psychiatry, 27*(2), 130–135.
46. Patel, N., Patel, S. P. B., & Prof, A. (2012). Study of various decision tree pruning methods with their empirical comparison in WEKA Saurabh Upadhyay. *International Journal of Computer Applications, 60*(12), 975–8887.

47. Sesen, M. B., Nicholson, A. E., Banares-Alcantara, R., Kadir, T., & Brady, M. (2013). Bayesian networks for clinical decision support in lung cancer care. In R. A. Calogero (Ed.) *PLoS ONE, 8*(12), e82349.
48. Daly, R., Shen, Q., & Aitken, S. (2011). Learning Bayesian networks: Approaches and issues. *The Knowledge Engineering Review, 26*(2), 99–157.
49. Julia Flores, M., Nicholson, A. E., Brunskill, A., Korb, K. B., & Mascaro, S. (2011). Incorporating expert knowledge when learning Bayesian network structure: A medical case study. *Artificial Intelligence in Medicine, 53*(3), 181–204.
50. Stojadinovic, A., Bilchik, A., Smith, D., Eberhardt, J. S., Ward, E. B., Nissan, A., et al. (2013). Clinical decision support and individualized prediction of survival in colon cancer: Bayesian belief network model. *Annals of Surgical Oncology, 20*(1), 161–74.
51. Top 4 advantages and disadvantages of Support Vector Machine or SVM | by Dhiraj K | Medium [Internet]. [cited 2021 Oct 7]. Available from: https://dhirajkumarblog.medium.com/top-4-advantages-and-disadvantages-of-support-vector-machine-or-svm-a3c06a2b107
52. Decision Tree—Overview, Decision Types, Applications [Internet]. [cited 2021 Oct 7]. Available from: https://corporatefinanceinstitute.com/resources/knowledge/other/decision-tree/
53. Scott McCloskey [Internet]. [cited 2021 Oct 7]. Available from: http://www.cim.mcgill.ca/~scott/RIT/researchPaper.html
54. Singh, N. K., & Raza, K. (2021). *Medical image generation using generative adversarial networks: A review* In Studies in Computational Intelligence, *932*, 77–96. https://doi.org/10.1007/978-981-15-9735-0_5
55. Ehteshami Bejnordi, B., Veta, M., Johannes van Diest, P., van Ginneken, B., Karssemeijer, N., Litjens, G., et al. (2017). Diagnostic assessment of deep learning algorithms for detection of lymph node metastases in women with breast cancer. *JAMA, 318*(22), 2199.
56. Oyelade, O. N., Obiniyi, A. A., Junaidu, S. B., & Kana, A. F. D. (2017). A modified select and test (ST) algorithm for medical diagnosis in an ad-hoc network environment. In *2017 IEEE 3rd International Conference on Electro-Technology for National Development (NIGERCON)* (pp. 19–23). IEEE.
57. Cheng, J.-Z., Ni, D., Chou, Y.-H., Qin, J., Tiu, C.-M., Chang, Y.-C., et al. (2016). Computer-aided diagnosis with deep learning architecture: Applications to breast lesions in US images and pulmonary nodules in CT scans. *Scientific Reports, 6*(1), 24454.
58. Yeh, M. C.-H., Wang, Y.-H., Yang, H.-C., Bai, K.-J., Wang, H.-H., & Li, Y.-C. (Jack). (2021). Artificial intelligence–based prediction of lung cancer risk using nonimaging electronic medical records: Deep learning approach. *Journal of Medical Internet Research, 23*(8), e26256.
59. Baldwin, D. R., Gustafson, J., Pickup, L., Arteta, C., Novotny, P., Declerck, J., et al. (2020). External validation of a convolutional neural network artificial intelligence tool to predict malignancy in pulmonary nodules. *Thorax, 75*(4), 306–312.
60. Hart, G. R., Roffman, D. A., Decker, R., & Deng, J. (2018). A multi-parameterized artificial neural network for lung cancer risk prediction. In Y. Qiu (Ed.). *PLOS ONE, 13*(10), e0205264.
61. Yan, W., Shi, H., He, T., Chen, J., Wang, C., Liao, A., et al. (2021). Employment of artificial intelligence based on routine laboratory results for the early diagnosis of multiple myeloma. *Frontiers in Oncology, 29*, 11.
62. Yenamandra, A., Hughes, C., & Maris, A. (2021). Artificial intelligence in plasma cell myeloma: Neural networks and support vector machines in the classification of plasma cell myeloma data at diagnosis. *Journal of Pathology Informatics, 12*(1), 35.
63. Morandi, F., Horenstein, A. L., Costa, F., Giuliani, N., Pistoia, V., & Malavasi, F. (2018). CD38: A target for immunotherapeutic approaches in multiple myeloma. *Frontiers in Immunology, 9*.
64. Rajkumar, S. V., & Kumar, S. (2020). Multiple myeloma current treatment algorithms. *Blood Cancer Journal, 10*(9), 1–10.
65. Pawlyn, C., Cairns, D., Kaiser, M., Striha, A., Jones, J., Shah, V., et al. (2020). The relative importance of factors predicting outcome for myeloma patients at different ages: results from 3894 patients in the Myeloma XI trial. *Leukemia, 34*(2), 604–612.
66. Mitchell, J. S., Li, N., Weinhold, N., Försti, A., Ali, M., van Duin, M., et al. (2016). Genome-wide association study identifies multiple susceptibility loci for multiple myeloma. *Nature Communications, 7*(1), 12050.

67. Povoa, L. V., Ribeiro, C. H. C., & da Silva, I. T. (2021). Machine learning predicts treatment sensitivity in multiple myeloma based on molecular and clinical information coupled with drug response. *PLOS ONE, 16*(7), e0254596.
68. Saeedizadeh, Z., Mehri Dehnavi, A., Talebi, A., Rabbani, H., Sarrafzadeh, O., & Vard, A. (2016). Automatic recognition of myeloma cells in microscopic images using bottleneck algorithm, modified watershed and SVM classifier. *Journal of Microscopy, 261*(1), 46–56.
69. Deulofeu, M., Kolářová, L., Salvadó, V., María Peña-Méndez, E., Almáši, M., Štork, M., et al. (2019). Rapid discrimination of multiple myeloma patients by artificial neural networks coupled with mass spectrometry of peripheral blood plasma. *Scientific Reports, 9*(1), 1–7.
70. Akram, M., Iqbal, M., Daniyal, M., & Khan, A. U. (2017). Awareness and current knowledge of breast cancer. *Biological Research, 50*(1), 33.
71. Kolb, T. M., Lichy, J., & Newhouse, J. H. (2002). Comparison of the performance of screening mammography, physical examination, and breast US and evaluation of factors that influence them: an analysis of 27,825 patient evaluations. *Radiology, 225*(1), 165–175.
72. McCormack, V. A., & Silva I dos, S. (2006). Breast density and parenchymal patterns as markers of breast cancer risk: A meta-analysis. *Cancer Epidemiology and Prevention Biomarkers, 15*(6), 1159–1169.
73. Eccles, S. A., Aboagye, E. O., Ali, S., Anderson, A. S., Armes, J., Berditchevski, F., et al. (2013). Critical research gaps and translational priorities for the successful prevention and treatment of breast cancer. *Breast Cancer Research, 15*(5), 1–37.
74. Ireaneus, Y., Rejani, A., & Selvi, S. T. (2009). Early detection of breast cancer using SVM classifier technique. *International Journal on Computer Science and Engineering, 1*(3), 127–130.
75. van Veen, E. M., Brentnall, A. R., Byers, H., Harkness, E. F., Astley, S. M., Sampson, S., et al. (2018). Use of single-nucleotide polymorphisms and mammographic density plus classic risk factors for breast cancer risk prediction. *JAMA Oncology, 4*(4), 476.
76. Turnbull, C., Ahmed, S., Morrison, J., Pernet, D., Renwick, A., Maranian, M., et al. (2010). Genome-wide association study identifies five new breast cancer susceptibility loci. *Nature Genetics, 42*(6), 504–507.
77. Dheeba, J., & Tamil Selvi, S. (2011). Classification of malignant and benign microcalcification using SVM classifier. In *2011 International Conference on Emerging Trends in Electrical and Computer Technology, ICETECT 2011* (pp. 686–690).
78. Wang, H., Zheng, B., Yoon, S. W., & Ko, H. S. (2018). A support vector machine-based ensemble algorithm for breast cancer diagnosis. *European Journal of Operational Research, 267*(2), 687–699.
79. Siddiqui, F., & Siddiqui, A. H. (2021). Lung cancer. In *Cambridge handbook of psychology, health and medicine* (2nd ed., pp. 605–606).
80. Cainap, C., Pop, L. A., Balacescu, O., & Cainap, S. S. (2020). Early diagnosis and screening in lung cancer. *American Journal of Cancer Research, 10*(7), 1993–2009.
81. Hsia, T., Chiang, H., Chiang, D., Hang, L., Tsai, F., & Chen, W. (2003). Prediction of survival in surgical unresectable lung cancer by artificial neural networks including genetic polymorphisms and clinical parameters. *Journal of Clinical Laboratory Analysis., 17*(6), 229.
82. Feng, F., Wu, Y., Wu, Y., Nie, G., & Ni, R. (2011). The effect of artificial neural network model combined with six tumor markers in auxiliary diagnosis of lung cancer. *Journal of Medical Systems, 36*(5), 2973–80.
83. Poullis, M., McShane, J., Shaw, M., Woolley, S., Shackcloth, M., Page, R., et al. (2012). Lung cancer staging: A physiological update. *Interactive CardioVascular and Thoracic Surgery, 14*(6), 743–749.
84. Sherafatian, M., & Arjmand, F. (2019). Decision tree-based classifiers for lung cancer diagnosis and subtyping using TCGA miRNA expression data. *Oncology Letters*

Realizing the Potential of Blockchain in Cancer Research

Shazmeen Shamsi and Sarah I. Rahman

Abstract One of the leading causes of preventable deaths across the globe with almost 10 million deaths in 2020. Scientists and researchers are working day in, day out to develop new methods for the earliest possible diagnosis of this disease and thus save millions of human lives. Today, the healthcare sector is miraculously backed by technologies like machine learning, the Internet of Things (IoT), and computational intelligence which aid in the early prediction of the disease with precision, thereby improving the chances of survival and also providing a better healthcare experience with lower treatment morbidity. Blockchain, the technology behind Bitcoin, is another revolutionary technology that can be combined with it. Blockchain is a kind of decentralized and distributed ledger which uses a peer-to-peer network to make a continuously growing chain of chronological records to form a digital ledger. The fact that it has no central authority offers numerous advantages like transparency, immutability, improved traceability, and enhanced security of the transactions being carried out. Blockchain has incredibly useful applications in cancer research ranging from secure data storage to full patient ownership of records. This chapter predominantly aims to highlight how its characteristics can be utilized to revolutionize cancer research and also discuss its future prospects.

Keywords Cancer · Artificial intelligence · Machine learning · Internet of Things · Blockchain

1 Introduction

William Mougayar, the author of the book 'The Business Blockchain', describes the blockchain as '*The blockchain cannot be described just as a revolution. It is a tsunami-like phenomenon, slowly advancing and gradually enveloping everything*

S. Shamsi
School of Computational and Integrative Sciences, Jawaharlal Nehru University, New Delhi, India
e-mail: shazmeen184002@st.jmi.ac.in

S. I. Rahman (✉)
School of Biotechnology, Jawaharlal Nehru University, New Delhi, India

K. Raza (ed.), *Computational Intelligence in Oncology*, Studies in Computational Intelligence 1016, https://doi.org/10.1007/978-981-16-9221-5_25

along its way by the force of its progression'. The preceding comment made by William Mougayar is something to ponder over. Blockchain technology is undoubtedly attracting a huge section of society due to its captivating potential. The vast amount of talk and anticipation generated by this technology is garnering the curiosity of an enormous number of people, both researchers and common mass, alike, potentially ushering in a new revolution. This chapter seeks to give its readers a quick but thorough grasp of the key components of this technology and its incredible applications in cancer research.

Man's ultimate motive is to completely modernize and automate his lifestyle so as to prosper and lead a lavish life. This seems accomplishable only through the expansion of science and technology. We are served with a multitude of really beneficial applications which aid in simplifying our tasks, not only with the rapid pace at which they work but also with the ease and efficiency of tasks performed. The technology revolution is gradually impacting every sector, communication, trade, research to the extent that it has slowly crept into and impacted the healthcare sector as well and is unquestionably posing to be a great asset for us. The world is making a gradual transition from conventional to contemporary technologies. This technological breakthrough has impacted almost every sphere of our lives. It must be mentioned that of all the sectors that have benefitted from this revolution, the healthcare sector is one of the most important ones and has definitely improved our quality of life. Apart from allowing us to store data with ease, it also helps in medical diagnosis, and today, real-time self-monitoring of our health condition is also possible, through virtual environments. This leads us to make one conclusion that mankind is slowly making a transition from real to virtual world, a glimpse of which could be seen during the COVID-19 pandemic, where each and every transaction, be it for financial, educational, or business purpose, was carried out on virtual platforms.

However, cybercriminals, with their nefarious skills, are always on the lookout for an opportunity to profit by compromising data related to the transactions in progress. Secure Internet transactions involving other parties aren't always reliable. The person making transactions is always at risk and has the fear of getting cheated. Blockchain successfully attempts to overcome all these hurdles and offers safe and secure transactions to be carried out.

Blockchain is a magical technology that can be used with nearly any other technology on the market today to enhance its benefits and make it safer and more secure to use. It is basically an online distributed ledger technology that preserves all the transactions in a time-stamped format, the copy of which is present on the ledger and maintained collectively by each and every 'peer' in the chain network. The best part is that the involvement of third parties is ruled out. Whenever a transaction is intended to be carried out, it is validated by at least 51% of the 'peers' in the network, and only then, block gets added to the chain. Blocks are analogous to the pages of a ledger, and the entire chain is analogous to the record book.

Blockchain is a breakthrough technology that came into being with the introduction of Bitcoin, a type of cryptocurrency. Everyone needs to understand the real potential of this new technology so that we may make the greatest use of it. When combined with the healthcare sector, it has the potential to redefine the power of this sector in a manner one could have never even imagined. It is predicted to change healthcare patterns, causing a shift away from paper based, insecure online transactions involving third parties toward secure, immutable online transactions.

This chapter provides the readers with an overview of blockchain technology. It is anticipated that the readers would have a thorough understanding not only of this remarkable technology but also its applications in the healthcare industry. The readers will also get an idea of how this technology works and its fundamental parts and features. We will also learn about the advantages of this technology over traditional practices and its limitations; following which, we will learn the practical applications in cancer research.

2 Need for Blockchain Technology

Satoshi Nakamoto's white paper 'Bitcoin: A Peer-to-Peer Electronic Cash System' was published on October 31, 2008, and it was the first time this idea was discussed. The article focuses on a 'peer-to-peer form of electronic currency', which enables Internet payments to be transmitted directly from one party to another without the involvement of a bank or other financial institution.

The demand for this technology developed as a result of the 2008 global banking crisis, which resulted in the collapse of investment. The Bitcoin cryptocurrency, which was the first practical use of this technology, offers several benefits, including efficiency, cost-effectiveness, dependability, and a secure mechanism for initiating and recording financial transactions while maintaining anonymity. With an ever-growing human population and urbanization, the number of transactions carried out is expected to expand exponentially, affecting the complexity, efficiency, and cost of present systems and, as a result, increasing their vulnerability [1].

To achieve their goals, contemporary digital transactions rely on trustworthy third parties. Whether these parties can truly be trusted or not is a huge question? Is it true that these third parties, who may be anybody from a government agency to a private owner, say that the transactions are conducted in a secure environment? According to studies, even while a few central authorities adhere to stringent standards to protect transaction privacy and security to the point of issuing certificates of assurance, these technologies are not infallible. In today's society, when everything is done with the click of a mouse, we also want technology that is efficient, quick, and inexpensive. The blockchain is the ideal solution to this problem. People do not need to pay money to a third party such as a bank or a government or private entity; instead, they keep their own records as digital ledgers that can be monitored with ease and precision because of the blockchain architecture's peer-to-peer, distributed, and decentralized nature. The world requires technology like blockchain, which provides a safe and secure platform for conducting transactions while also allowing total ownership and power over one's property and transparent transactions.

Because of its immutability, data saved on the network cannot be modified or erased, and this is a crucial characteristic that may be utilized to keep very sensitive and confidential data on the system. Another significant issue addressed by this technology is the problem of double spending. Because the records are kept exactly historically, it is simple to keep track of the money spent and prevent the issue and loss that double spending might cause [2]. Now that we've established its importance, let's go deeper into this technology.

3 Features of Blockchain

Some of the important features of blockchain are described as follows.

3.1 Decentralized

This refers to the fact that data and transactions are not managed by a governing authority or a third party. Because each entity in the chain has the same copy of the ledger, it is an open-ledger technology that assures full integrity among all members that are a part of the blockchain. Users are kept highly engaged, vigilant, and informed about all transactions that take place as a result of this feature [3]. To give you an idea of the benefits of these characteristics, consider the following:

- Eliminating the requirement for third parties speeds up the transaction process significantly.
- Data will never be destroyed since each user has a copy
- Transaction costs will be lower
- Scams are not a possibility.

Note: The two words described above may appear identical in context, but they are fundamentally distinct. Decentralization refers to the amount of control and authority that users share in decision-making, whereas dispersed network refers to the users' differing geographical locations. A decision is made in a decentralized network based on the votes of all nodes. As previously said, if at least 51% of the participants vote in favor of something, it is carried out; otherwise, it is rejected [4].

However, in a distributed system, the processing is shared among all players, but it may allow a central authority to make all decisions. Both of these characteristics are present in blockchain [5].

3.2 Distributed

This is a distributed technology that allows data and transactions to be synced and shared among all entities in the chain rather than being duplicated or transmitted. What has to be recognized is that the records/money can never be hacked or stolen because there is no central data storehouse and transactions are dispersed across all organizations. This also reduces the burden on a single server by spreading processing power among the network's many machines [6].

Advantages:

- Due to dispersed processing power, the output is better and more efficient.
- All members are assured of ownership since they actively engage in all transactions.
- Because each transaction is kept as an identical duplicate on all nodes, tampering with the data is impossible because any fraudulent behavior is readily recognized.

3.3 *Immutable*

Once data are put to the blocks, it cannot be altered since it is kept indefinitely on the blockchain network. This implies that data that were uploaded to the Bitcoin network when it was originally formed is still safe and secure and can be accessed with ease. In terms of this function, it differs from databases in that databases enable us to update and delete data stored on their network in addition to creating and adding data. In blockchain, however, this is not the case. While it allows us to create and add data, it does not allow us to update or delete it. It contributes to its security because all transaction records go back to day 1, and any attempt to tamper with the data is futile [7]. Both the sender and the recipient may be confident that their information will not be tampered with.

3.4 *Transparent*

When a single block or transaction between two people is added, it is mirrored in all the other blocks. As a result, nothing is concealed from anyone, and all modifications are visible to the public [8]. It is a beneficial trait. Let's have a look at how this works. Consider the case when a thief has acquired unauthorized access to the network and is impersonating someone else. He simply cannot make any transaction because, first and foremost, all transactions must be validated by all, and secondly and most importantly, the private key is a unique key that is nearly impossible to guess correctly, and if a person tries a few keys, all of his attempts are reflected on all blocks, allowing him to be easily traced.

3.5 Peer-To-Peer (P2P) Network

Peer-to-peer (P2P) networking: Blockchain enables safe transactions between two parties without the involvement of a third party. Each transaction is digitally signed through the use of cryptographic algorithms. Only, the actual receiver with knowledge of the sender's public key and his own private key may decode the code [9]. Hashing methods used for signature formation are critical because they function as a trapdoor, making it nearly hard for cybercriminals to get through.

4 How Blockchain Works?

We now know that all records in the digital ledger are kept in blocks that are protected by digital signatures. Digital signatures are kinds of electronic signatures that validate the authenticity of a transaction [10]. They are created using hashing algorithms that use public and private key encryptions. The sender signs the message using his/her private key and the receiver's public key, whereas the receiver is able to see the contents of the transaction using only his/her private key and the sender's public key. Blocks carrying the transactions are unchangeable and intangible. When new data are requested to be added to the blockchain on a public blockchain, the request is mirrored on all nodes in the network. If the transaction is accepted according to the consensus rules, it is timestamped and linked to the previous block to be added to the blockchain network. Because hackers may be ready and lucky enough to perform the 51 percent assault, the choice of which nodes would attach the block is crucial. As a result, the consensus algorithm technique that is employed becomes highly essential. The main steps in the approval and validation of a blockchain transaction are as follows (Fig. 1):

Step 1: A transaction request is made.
Step 2: All nodes in the network get the transaction request.
Step 3: Consensus protocols are used in order to validate/reject it.
Step 4: Approval and validation of the transaction.
Step 5: The block is added to the chain.
Step 6: Transaction occurs.

5 Convergence of Technology and Health Care

The convergence of modern technology with health care has the tendency to make the latter much more efficient and manageable. With the increasing availability of electronic health data (EHR), there is now more opportunity for both discovery and practical applications to improve health care. These include providing an accurate medical diagnosis, predicting diseases in the early stages, and disease analyses.

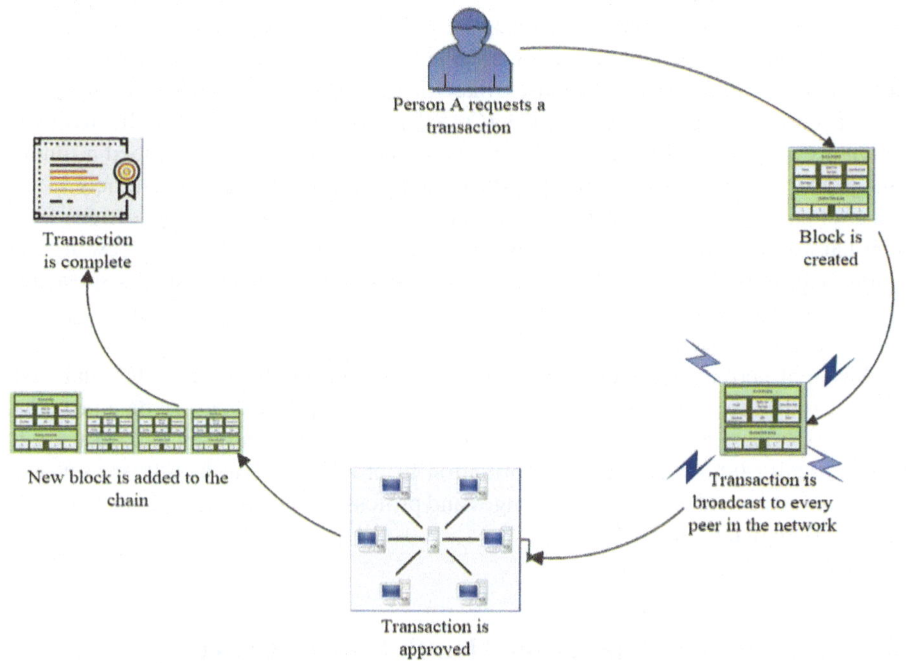

Fig. 1 Diagrammatic representation of how blockchain works

Smart health (s-health) is an explicit example of the integration of technology in health care. The industry of smartwatches, fitness trackers, and smart devices that constantly gather health data in abundance is growing rapidly. Unfortunately, the majority of this information is unstructured and cannot be used in predictive models. Deep learning and AI networks are known to effectively process large volumes of relatively messy data, including errors in labels and large numbers of input variables [11]. Also, they do not generally have to specify which variables are needed to be considered for prediction and in what combinations; instead, neural networks can learn representations of the key factors and interactions from the data itself. Due to these advantages, the use of ML in the realm of health care has become prevalent. The EHR data collected could be mined for several possible applications. The entire contents of the EHR like medications, admission details, and vital signs could be analyzed using ML algorithms to estimate the probability of a patient reacting adversely to antibiotics or to accurately measure the patient's risk of contracting a common hospital-acquired disease like clostridium difficile infection [12]. Forecasting tools to predict the event of a zoonotic disease outbreak are another area that has been explored using ML and is known to give fairly accurate results [13]. More number of variables gives and larger training datasets are known to make models better.

ML tools have been vastly applied to detect patterns in image data automatically to predict trends or for decision-making. The dataset varies according to the need of the user. Labeled radiology images, CT scans, PET scans, wound images, mammograms, X-rays are all examples of datasets that have been explored for potential therapeutic information. Many image databases like ImageNet, cancer imaging archive, and open access series of imaging studies (OASIS) have labeled datasets collected from hospitals or generated for research purposes. Guo et al. (2015) developed a fundus image analysis-based automatic classification and grading system for cataracts so that cataract patients can receive the preliminary classification and get suggestions from ophthalmologists timely, conveniently, and even remotely [14]. Many review articles doing a structural analysis of ML algorithms applied in s-health results show that the ML approach is used in many s-health applications such as glaucoma diagnosis, Alzheimer's disease [15].

Physical activity recognition is another important application of ML that will significantly save the cost and time of patients and hospitals. Sensory data provided by smartphones, fitness bands, and other wearable smart devices can be used to automatically infer meaningful information to provide several healthcare services like promoting healthy behavior changes and professional medical analysis like early heart failure detection [16].

6 Drawbacks of Traditional Health Care in Cancer Research

The past two decades have seen immense progress in the understanding of the cause and progression of cancer. The regulation and treatment have improved tenfold with the advancement of technology. Despite being widely studied, cancer still remains a major reason for morbidity and death. In 2018, there were 17 million new cancer cases in 2018 with 9.5 million deaths worldwide. By the next two decades, the numbers are expected to grow to a staggering 27.5 million new cancer cases and mortality reaching 16.3 million [17]. This is the figure for cases due to just population aging, while the burden may be even larger due to other risk factors such as smoking, unhealthy diet, and physical inactivity. This will lead to overwhelming pressure on oncologists and the healthcare system. With the aid of technology, the task of cancer diagnosis, making personalized treatment plans and patient care, can be speedup and made easier. Keeping health data readily available and letting patient track their own files can save a significant amount of time thus reducing the load on the medical management.

A patient diagnosed with cancer tends to be overcome with grief, confusion, and uncertainty. The dainty task of researching existing treatment methods and the possible side effects associated becomes a lot harder in those times. A user-friendly guide to give an easy-to-understand combined previous research on particular cancer would be a massive help. Moreover, the traditional paper records of the patient's medical reports become hard to manage. The electronic medical record system currently in use does not guarantee the privacy and security that is needed when it comes to storing sensitive health data collected from patients. The present cancer registry systems have the drawback of not having consistent information in both local and state databases. Local and state-level registry see regular changes with the ongoing patient treatment and quality control checks, respectively [18]. Thus, the researcher conducting a study using that dataset would have no way to know about the variations in the two databases and hence possibly leading to skewed results. Another downside to the current data storing process is the tedious, inefficient process of getting access to a patient's medical history records that eventually leads to a delay inpatient care. Miscommunication between the patient and doctors costs the healthcare industry millions every day that could have been avoided otherwise had there been an efficient system of quick data retrieval in place.

7 Applications of Blockchain Technology in Cancer Research

Blockchain, although a new technology, has several applications in cancer research and management, as described in the following section.

7.1 Medical Record Management

With the growing specialization of healthcare services and significant patient mobility, obtaining healthcare services across various hospitals for tests and treatment is quite frequent, especially for cancer patients, where care transition and coordination are very common [18]. Companies are coming up with open-access healthcare databases that house patient data under one roof while maintaining the integrity of health records. This will speed up the patient care process by providing easy speedup and up-to-date access to the medical history of patients which will be a boon, especially for high-stage cancer patients.

7.2 Palliative Care

Early sharing of electronic health records (EHR) between providers is critical for timely cancer patient care. Patients may look to consult a different doctor for a better understanding of their state before deciding on a treatment. Having access to an accurate history of patients' health data also goes a long way in optimizing post-treatment monitoring to give the best care. In practice, knowing the radiation dosage received during therapy, for example, may be critical in order to minimize potentially detrimental repercussions for the patient. The severity of the chronic disease, as well as patients' potential inability to manage their own medical history, as well as needed permission management processes, may make data exchange even more difficult, causing treatment delays.

7.3 Future Research

The prospect of adopting and developing blockchain technology (BCT) for healthcare data management has lately piqued industry and academic interest [19]. Blockchain is a peer-to-peer distributed technology that creates a shared, immutable, and transparent append-only record of all activities performed by all network members such as scientists, doctors, public health authorities, lab-tech. Easy sharing of genomic data provides a genetic perspective to cancer studies and leads to a better fundamental understanding of the disease. The use of encryption, digital signature, and hash function makes the data secure [20], and since the users have full control of their data, they can rest assured that their data are secure and will not be misused or tampered with.

7.4 Drugs and Equipment Regulation

The life-saving drugs used in cancer treatment often drill a hole in the pockets of many patients. Often duplicates of these costly drugs can be found. The need to ensure the legitimacy of drug suppliers and the quality of drugs is a high priority of the healthcare system. Blockchain can be applied to decentralize the pharmaceutical supply chain and provide transparency of the shipping process while also ensuring the waste treatment of waste generated. Product identification, tracing, and verification of clinical devices, medications, and other supplies can be easily done by implementing blockchain technology in the pharmaceutical supply chain. This can possibly reduce the breakdown supply chain in times of high demand like what occurred during COVID-19.

7.5 Insurance and Cost-Saving

Two factors are used to determine cost savings: the cost of patient-doctor contact and the cost of pharmacological research and development and it has been shown that incorporating blockchain will save money for hospitals, the pharmaceutical industry, and insurance companies [21, 22]. Data management solutions that blockchain-based intelligent contract technology can save money on managing multisite clinical trials at drug research facilities.

8 Future Directions

Though the banking industry was the first to use this technology, many other industries are anticipated to follow suit. The obstacles must be overcome, and new possibilities for scientists and researchers in this sector are likely to emerge as a result. The integration of this technology with other technologies such as the Internet of Things, computational intelligence, and machine learning is expected to result in massive changes throughout the world. There has been a surge in interest in blockchain technology for the delivery of safe and secure healthcare data management making it a more dependable way of diagnosis and treatment. In the future, blockchain might be a technology that helps with customized, genuine, and secure health care by combining all of a patient's real-time clinical data and presenting it in an up-to-date secure healthcare setting. Although as a new technology, blockchain too has its own limitations. Transparency and immutability, two highlighting features of blockchain may also prove to be a concern for large-scale execution. Data are being stored on nodes and thus visible to every ledger puts a high privacy risk on health data. Also, data protection rights of countries like the EU give owners the option of having their data erased, thus clashing with the 'append-only' ability of blockchain. Furthermore, duplicating voluminous data across every node will be inefficient and costly. As blockchain is still budding, much work is required to be done on the back end as well as making user interfaces for the technology to evolve and be implemented across a range of sectors [23].

9 Conclusion

This chapter enables us to understand that blockchain is a decentralized, distributed ledger that is transparent and immutable and maintains records as transactions in time-stamped blocks. It enables users to quickly make and verify transactions without relying on a central authority. It offers one-of-a-kind possibilities for reducing complexity, enabling trustless cooperation and generating safe and immutable data. We also learn about the limitations of traditional healthcare systems in cancer research and how blockchain comes to the rescue in solving major healthcare issues pertaining to cancer research. It has the potential to empower both patients and healthcare providers in real-time data exchange and also maintain the privacy of patients. It empowers patients with the ability to have full control of their data and never worry about misplacing any medical history record because everything that gets stored on blocks is immutable and intangible. Blockchain is finally gaining traction, with a slew of practical applications being deployed and investigated.

References

1. Xie, J., Tang, H., Huang, T., Yu, F. R., Xie, R., Liu, J., & Liu, Y. (2019). A survey of blockchain technology applied to smart cities: Research issues and challenges. *IEEE Communications Surveys & Tutorials., 21*(3), 2794–2830.
2. Maroufi, M., Abdolee, R., & Tazekand, B. M. (2019). *On the convergence of blockchain and internet of things (iot) technologies*. arXiv preprint arXiv:1904.01936.
3. Mettler, M. (2016). Blockchain technology in healthcare: The revolution starts here. In *2016 IEEE 18th International Conference on e-Health Networking, Applications and Services (Healthcom)* (pp. 1–3). IEEE.
4. Mamoshina, P., Ojomoko, L., Yanovich, Y., Ostrovski, A., Botezatu, A., Prikhodko, P., Izumchenko, E., Aliper, A., Romantsov, K., Zhebrak, A., & Ogu, I. O. (2018). Converging blockchain and next-generation artificial intelligence technologies to decentralize and accelerate biomedical research and healthcare. *Oncotarget, 9*(5), 5665.
5. Zhang, P., White, J., Schmidt, D. C., Lenz, G., & Rosenbloom, S. T. (2018). FHIRChain: Applying blockchain to securely and scalably share clinical data. *Computational and structural biotechnology journal., 1*(16), 267–278.
6. Hussein, A. F., ArunKumar, N., Ramirez-Gonzalez, G., Abdulhay, E., Tavares, J. M., & de Albuquerque, V. H. (2018). A medical records managing and securing blockchain based system supported by a genetic algorithm and discrete wavelet transform. *Cognitive Systems Research, 1*(52), 1–1.
7. Schöner, M. M., Kourouklis, D., Sandner, P., Gonzalez, E., & Förster, J. (2017). *Blockchain Technology in the Pharmaceutical Industry*. Frankfurt School Blockchain Center, Frankfurt, Germany.
8. Shae, Z., Tsai, J. (2018). Transform blockchain into distributed parallel computing architecture for precision medicine. In *2018 IEEE 38th International Conference on Distributed Computing Systems (ICDCS)* (pp. 1290–1299). IEEE.
9. Angeletti, F., Chatzigiannakis, I., & Vitaletti, A. (2017). The role of blockchain and IoT in recruiting participants for digital clinical trials. In *2017 25th International Conference on Software, Telecommunications and Computer Networks (SoftCOM)* (pp. 1–5). IEEE.
10. Fang, W., Chen, W., Zhang, W., Pei, J., Gao, W., & Wang, G. (2020). Digital signature scheme for information non-repudiation in blockchain: A state of the art review. *EURASIP Journal on Wireless Communications and Networking., 2020*(1), 1–5.
11. Bhardwaj, R., Nambiar, A. R., & Dutta, D. (2017). A study of machine learning in healthcare. In *2017 IEEE 41st Annual Computer Software and Applications Conference (COMPSAC)* (Vol. 2, pp. 236–241). IEEE.
12. Wiens, J., Campbell, W. N., Franklin, E. S., Guttag, J. V., & Horvitz, E. (2014). Learning data-driven patient risk str. jpegication models for Clostridium difficile. In *Open Forum Infectious Diseases* (Vol. 1, No. 2). Oxford University Press.
13. Han, B. A., Schmidt, J. P., Bowden, S. E., & Drake, J. M. (2015). Rodent reservoirs of future zoonotic diseases. *Proceedings of the National Academy of Sciences., 112*(22), 7039–7044.
14. Guo, L., Yang, J. J., Peng, L., Li, J., & Liang, Q. (2015). A computer-aided healthcare system for cataract classification and grading based on fundus image analysis. *Computers in Industry, 69*, 72–80.
15. Rayan, Z., Alfonse, M., & Salem, A. B. M. (2019). Machine learning and approaches in smart health. In *8th International Congress of Information and Communication Technology, ICICT 2019.*
16. Huynh-The, T., Hua, C. H., Tu, N. A., & Kim, D. S. (2020). Physical activity recognition with statistical-deep fusion model using multiple sensory data for smart health. *IEEE Internet of Things Journal., 8*(3), 1533–1543.
17. https://www.cancer.org/research/cancer-facts-statistics/global.html, n.d.
18. Kasten, J. E. (2020). Blockchain application to the cancer registry database. *International Journal of Healthcare Information Systems and Informatics (IJHISI), 15*(4), 70–87.

19. Peters, A. W., Till, B. M., Meara, J. G., & Afshar, S. (2017). Blockchain technology in health care: A primer for surgeons. *Bulletin of the American College of Surgeons, 12*, 1–5.
20. Haq, I., & Esuka, O. M. (2018). Blockchain technology in pharmaceutical industry to prevent counterfeit drugs. *International Journal of Computers and Applications, 975*, 8887.
21. Alam, M. T. & Raza, K. (2021). Blockchain technology in healthcare: making digital healthcare reliable, more accurate, and revolutionary. In *Translational Bioinformatics in Healthcare and Medicine* (pp. 81–96). Elsevier.https://doi.org/10.1016/B978-0-323-89824-9.00007-0
22. Radanović, I., & Likić, R. (2018). Opportunities for use of blockchain technology in medicine. *Applied Health Economics and Health Policy, 16*(5), 583–590.
23. Series, B. P. (2020). *Opportunities and challenges of blockchain technologies in health care* (pp. 1–12).

The manufacturer's authorised representative in the EU is Springer Nature Customer Service Centre GmbH, Europaplatz 3, 69115 Heidelberg, Germany. If you have any concerns regarding our products, please contact ProductSafety@springernature.com

Printed and bound by CPI Group (UK) Ltd, Croydon, CR0 4YY
30/09/2026
02225324-0019